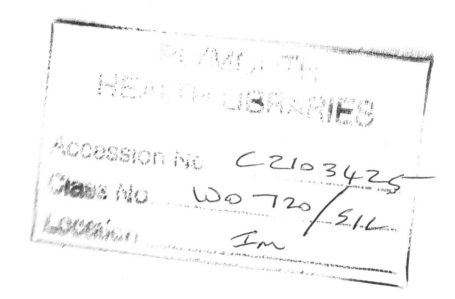

Geriatric Anesthesiology

Second Edition

Geriatric Anesthesiology

Second Edition

Jeffrey H. Silverstein
G. Alec Rooke
J.G. Reves
Charles H. McLeskey

Editors

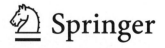 Springer

Jeffrey H. Silverstein, MD
Professor
Department of Anesthesiology, Surgery,
  and Geriatrics and Adult Development
Vice Chairman for Research
Associate Dean for Research
Mount Sinai School of Medicine
New York, NY, USA

G. Alec Rooke, MD, PhD
Professor
Department of Anesthesiology
University of Washington and the Veterans
  Affairs Puget Sound Health Care System
Seattle, WA
and
Visiting Professor of Anesthesia, Critical
  Care, and Pain Medicine
Harvard Medical School
Beth Israel Deaconess Medical Center
Boston, MA, USA

J.G. Reves, MD
Vice President for Medical Affairs
Dean, College of Medicine
Department of Anesthesiology/College
  of Medicine
Medical University of South Carolina
Charleston, SC, USA

Charles H. McLeskey, MD
Salt Lake City, UT, USA

Library of Congress Control Number: 2007926756

ISBN: 978-0-387-72526-0   e-ISBN: 978-0-387-72527-7

Printed on acid-free paper.

9 8 7 6 5 4 3 2 1

springer.com

To my Grandparents, Regina and David Silverstein and Blanche and Daniel Klein, MD. Their love and their sufferings provided endless opportunities and insights. I hope, and believe, they would have liked this result.

—JHS

To my Children, Douglas and Linnea.

—GAR

To Margaret Cathcart and her late Husband, Dr. John W. Cathcart.

—JGR

To my Parents, Marion and Hamilton McLeskey, who encouraged care and consideration for our elderly.

—CHM

Preface to the Second Edition

Do not go gentle into that good night,
Old age should burn and rave at close of day;
Rage, rage against the dying of the light.
Dylan Thomas

The goal of getting older is to age successfully. Unfortunately, the majority of our older patients will have acquired one or more chronic medical conditions as they age, and, even if a perfectly healthy older patient presents for surgery, that patient's ability to handle physiologic stress will be diminished, including the stress of surgery. Nearly half of all surgical procedures involve patients older than age 65, and that percentage is likely to increase as the U.S. population ages. Thus, the perioperative care of the older patient represents one of the primary future frontiers of anesthetic practice. Even though perioperative mortality has diminished for the elderly, as well as for the population in general, the growing number of cases spotlights perioperative morbidity and mortality as an important issue for patients and health care systems alike. The vision set forward by the first edition (i.e., to apply the growing body of knowledge in this subspecialty area to the everyday practice of anesthesiology) remains the mission and vision of this second edition. The editors believe that the updated contents of this edition represent an important opportunity to consolidate and organize the information that has been acquired since 1997 and to apply that knowledge to the current practice of anesthesiology.

Part I contains several new chapters on topics that may not always seem to be directly involved with anesthetic care, but are important to the future of medical and anesthesia care. An understanding of the aging process may lead to methods of slowing its progression, or at least of ameliorating some of its consequences, including the development of chronic disease. Most anesthesiology residency programs provide limited formal teaching of geriatric anesthesia. The editors believe the incorporation of relevant subspecialty material in the anesthesiology curriculum is needed to improve care for this patient population. The realities of reimbursement for services rendered to the older patient, either by Medicare or other payers, warrant the attention of all anesthesiologists who provide care for older patients. Ethics as applied to treatment of the older patient is also addressed. The medical management of this population is often complicated by issues such as patient goals that differ from physician expectations, physician "ageism," patient cognitive impairment, and the physician's failure to recognize the true risk of surgery and attendant recovery time. The last chapter of Part I reviews current knowledge and suggests research areas where the greatest impact on patient outcomes might be realized.

Parts II and III review the physiology of aging and the basic anesthetic management of the geriatric patient, and Part IV examines selected surgical procedures frequently performed in older patients. Not all of these chapters are specific to anesthetic management. Geriatric medicine is a broad field with many relevant topics. Wound healing is a perfect example. The reality is that anesthesiologists can likely have a positive impact on patient care by being better able to recognize conditions that may compromise skin when other medical professionals may fail to and, as a result, can improve protection of the skin, especially during long operating room cases. In contrast, polypharmacy and drug interactions, major topics in geriatric medicine, have direct relevance to anesthetic management. The cardiac surgery chapter is an example of how age affects outcomes after a specific type of surgical procedure. The unusual aspects of anesthetic management for cardiac surgery revolve mostly around the patient's underlying disease status rather than there being anything specific to cardiac anesthesia in the older patient beyond the principles delineated in Parts II and III.

For chapters similar to those in the first edition, an effort has been made to update content and incorporate studies that examine outcome. Such work helps us challenge conventional wisdom and sometimes test novel ideas that prove beneficial. Even the most casual reader of this textbook will recognize huge gaps in our present knowledge. It is not sufficient, for example, to take an understanding of the physiology of aging and draw conclusions regarding anesthetic management from that information. Oftentimes, however, we are forced to do just that when making anesthetic management decisions. The editors hope the future will provide better research and answers that advance the field of geriatric anesthesiology.

The editors thank the many authors of this text. In addition to their hard work, they responded to entreaties for revisions and updates with admirable patience and promptness. Their contributions expand our knowledge and will improve the care of elderly patients.

Lastly, the editors thank Stacy Hague and Elizabeth Corra from Springer. Without their vision and determination, this book would not exist.

Jeffrey H. Silverstein, MD
G. Alec Rooke, MD, PhD
J.G. Reves, MD
Charles H. McLeskey, MD

Preface to the First Edition

Approximately 14% of the current U.S. population is 65 years of age or older. By the year 2020, it is predicted that 20% or 60,000,000 Americans will reach this milestone. Further, if today's statistics continue unchanged, at least half of these individuals will undergo anesthesia and surgery, likely of increasing complexity, prior to their eventual demise. The geriatric patient population represents a huge and growing challenge for anesthesia providers the world over.

My interest in the anesthetic management of geriatric patients was kindled 15 years ago while on the faculty at Bowman Gray. One of our surgeons asked me to anesthetize his healthy 72-year-old father. All went well in the intraoperative and postoperative periods and he was discharged home in the customary time frame. However, my colleague later reported that he had observed subtle psychomotor changes in his father which persisted postoperatively for 7 weeks. It dawned on me that perhaps the geriatric patient is not simply an older adult, but rather, a truly different physiologic entity. What could explain the relatively commonly observed delayed postoperative return of normal mentation in the geriatric surgical patient? It is this and other unanswered questions regarding the anesthetic management of the elderly that stimulated the development of this text.

Geriatric Anesthesiology is designed to be a comprehensive text that methodically addresses the aging process while emphasizing important clinical anesthetic considerations. The first two sections of the text define the demographics of our aging population and describe age-related physiologic changes that occur in each major organ system. The third section addresses the multitude of factors that contribute to a safe and successful anesthetic with suggested adjustments in technique that may improve anesthetic management of the elderly. Topics range from preoperative evaluation and risk assessment to the altered effects of various classes of drugs with further discussion regarding positioning, thermoregulation, perioperative monitoring, and postoperative recovery. In addition, issues such as management of pain syndromes, outpatient anesthesia, medicolegal implications, and even special CPR techniques in this age group are considered. The fourth section identifies the ten most commonly performed surgical procedures in the elderly, and for each, offers recommended anesthetic techniques. The text ends with an intriguing exploration into future research opportunities in the field, including molecular mechanisms of aging.

Considerable energy has gone into the creation of this text. I am grateful for the significant efforts made by all the contributing authors and especially appreciate contributions made by the editors from Williams & Wilkins. The text would have been impossible to complete without the encouragement, dogged determination, and professionalism of Ms. Tanya Lazar and Mr. Carroll Cann. Tim Grayson was innovative and supportive during the original design and formulation of this project.

I am optimistic that this text will heighten the awareness of the very real clinical differences presented by the geriatric patient population. Perhaps by referring to appropriate sections in this text, anesthesia providers will be armed with a better understanding of the physiologic changes of aging and the recommended considerations and modifications of anesthetic technique, which we hope will contribute to an ever-improving outcome for the geriatric surgical patient population.

Charles H. McLeskey, MD

Contents

Contributors

James H. Abernathy, III, MD, MPH
Assistant Professor
Department of Anesthesia and
    Perioperative Medicine
Medical University of South Carolina
Charleston, SC, USA

Sheila R. Barnett, MD
Associate Professor
Department of Anesthesiology
Harvard Medical School
Beth Israel Deaconess Medical Center
Boston, MA, USA

Jack M. Berger, MD, PhD
Clinical Professor
Department of Anesthesiology
Keck School of Medicine
University of Southern California
Los Angeles, CA, USA

Shaul Beyth, MD, MSc
Department of Orthopedic Surgery
Hadassah Hebrew University Medical Center
Jerusalem, Israel

Harold Brem, MD
Associate Professor
Director, Wound Healing
Department of Surgery—Wound Healing Program
Columbia University Medical Center
New York, NY, USA

Charles Cain, MD, MBA
Clinical Professor
Department of Anesthesiology
Columbia University Medical Center
New York, NY, USA

Jeffrey L. Carson, MD
Richard C. Reynolds Professor of Medicine
Chief
Division of General Internal Medicine
Department of Medicine
UMDNJ—Robert Wood Johnson Medical School
New Brunswick, NJ, USA

Rodrigo Cartin-Ceba, MD
Critical Care Medicine Fellow
Department of Critical Care Service
Mayo Clinic
Rochester, MN, USA

David J. Cook, MD
Professor
Department of Anesthesiology
Mayo Clinic College of Medicine
Rochester, MN, USA

Gregory Crosby, MD
Associate Professor
Department of Anesthesiology
Brigham and Women's Hospital
Harvard Medical School
Boston, MA, USA

Deborah J. Culley, MD
Assistant Professor
Department of Anesthesiology
Brigham and Women's Hospital
Harvard Medical School
Boston, MA, USA

Melissa Doft, MD
Surgical Resident
Department of Surgery
Columbia University Medical Center
New York, NY, USA

Sylvia Y. Dolinski, MD, FCCP
Associate Professor
Department of Anesthesiology and Critical Care
Medical College of Wisconsin
Milwaukee, WI, USA

Thomas J. Ebert, MD, PhD
Professor and Vice-Chair for Education
Department of Anesthesiology
Medical College of Wisconsin
Milwaukee, WI, USA

James B. Eisenkraft, MD
Professor
Department of Anesthesiology
Mount Sinai School of Medicine
New York, NY, USA

Sheila J. Ellis, MD
Associate Professor
Department of Anesthesiology
University of Nebraska Medical Center
Omaha, NE, USA

Anna Flattau, MD
Assistant Professor
Department of Surgery and Family
   Medicine—Wound Healing Program
Columbia University Medical Center
New York, NY, USA

Lee A. Fleisher, MD
Robert D. Dripps Professor
Department of Anesthesiology and Critical Care
Chair of Anesthesiology and Critical Care
Hospital of the University of Pennsylvania
Philadelphia, PA, USA

Pamela Flood, MD
Associate Professor
Department of Anesthesiology
Columbia University
New York, NY, USA

Daniel M. Gainsburg, MD
Assistant Professor
Department of Anesthesiology
Mount Sinai School of Medicine
New York, NY, USA

Ognjen Gajic, MD, MSc, FCCP
Assistant Professor
Department of Internal Medicine
Mayo Clinic College of Medicine
Rochester, MN, USA

Maria F. Galati, MBA
Vice Chair, Administration
Department of Anesthesiology
Mount Sinai School of Medicine
New York, NY, USA

Michael S. Golinko, MD
Post-Doctoral Research Scientist
Department of Surgery—Wound Healing Program
Columbia University Medical Center
New York, NY, USA

Leanne Groban, MD
Associate Professor
Department of Anesthesiology
Wake Forest University School of Medicine
Winston-Salem, NC, USA

Andrew M. Hanflik, BS
Medical Student
Keck School of Medicine
University of Southern California
Los Angeles, CA, USA

Gary R. Haynes, MD, PhD
Professor
Department of Anesthesia and Perioperative Medicine
Medical University of South Carolina
Charleston, SC, USA

Paul J. Hoehner, MD, MA, FAHA
Director
Department of Cardiovascular and Thoracic
   Anesthesiology
Central Maine Heart Associates
Central Maine Heart and Vascular Institute
Lewiston, ME
Harvey Fellow in Theology
Ethics and Culture
Department of Religious Studies
University of Virginia Graduate School of Arts
   and Sciences
Charlottesville, VA, USA

Christopher J. Jankowski, MD
Assistant Professor and Consultant
Department of Anesthesiology
Mayo Clinic College of Medicine
Rochester, MN, USA

Jacqueline M. Leung, MD, MPH
Professor
Department of Anesthesia and Perioperative Care
University of California San Francisco
San Francisco, CA, USA

Michael C. Lewis, MD
Associate Professor
Department of Anesthesiology
Miller School of Medicine
University of Miami
Miami, FL, USA

Cynthia A. Lien, MD
Professor
Department of Anesthesiology
Weill Medical College of Cornell University
New York, NY, USA

Linda L. Liu, MD
Associate Professor
Department of Anesthesia and Perioperative Care
University of California San Francisco
San Francisco, CA, USA

Roger D. London, MD, MBA
Vice President and Medical Director
Flagship Patient Advocates
New York, NY, USA

Idit Matot, MD
Associate Professor
Department of Anesthesiology and Critical
    Care Medicine
Hadassah Hebrew University Medical Center
Jerusalem, Israel

Matthew D. McEvoy, MD
Assistant Professor
Department of Anesthesia and
    Perioperative Medicine
Medical University of South Carolina
Charleston, SC, USA

Kathryn E. McGoldrick, MD
Professor and Chair
Department of Anesthesiology
New York Medical College
Valhalla, NY, USA

Charles H. McLeskey, MD
Salt Lake City, UT, USA

Jessica Miller, MD
Fellow
Department of Pediatric Anesthesiology and
    Critical Care
Children's Hospital of Philadelphia
Philadelphia, PA, USA

Terri G. Monk, MD
Professor
Department of Anesthesiology
Duke University Health System
Durham, NC, USA

Stanley Muravchick, MD, PhD
Professor
Department of Anesthesiology and Critical Care
Hospital of the University of Pennsylvania
Philadelphia, PA, USA

Steven M. Neustein, MD
Associate Professor
Department of Anesthesiology
Mount Sinai School of Medicine
New York, NY, USA

J.G. Reves, MD
Vice President for Medical Affairs
Dean, College of Medicine
Department of Anesthesiology/College of Medicine
Medical University of South Carolina
Charleston, SC, USA

G. Alec Rooke, MD, PhD
Professor
Department of Anesthesiology
University of Washington and the Veterans Affairs
    Puget Sound Health Care System
Seattle, WA
Visiting Professor of Anesthesia, Critical Care, and
    Pain Medicine
Harvard Medical School
Beth Israel Deaconess Medical Center
Boston, MA, USA

Daniel I. Sessler, MD
Chair
Department of Outcomes Research
The Cleveland Clinic
Cleveland, OH, USA

Steven L. Shafer, MD
Professor
Department of Anesthesia
Stanford University
Palo Alto, CA
Professor
Department of Biopharmaceutical Sciences and
    Anesthesia
University of California San Francisco
San Francisco, CA, USA

Jeffrey H. Silverstein, MD
Professor
Department of Anesthesiology, Surgery,
  and Geriatrics and Adult Development
Vice Chairman for Research
Associate Dean for Research
Mount Sinai School of Medicine
New York, NY, USA

Juraj Sprung, MD, PhD
Professor
Department of Anesthesiology
Mayo Clinic College of Medicine
Rochester, MN, USA

Takahiro Suzuki, MD, PhD
Assistant Professor
Department of Anesthesiology
Nihon University Surugadai Hospital
Tokyo, Japan

Tamas A. Szabo, MD, PhD
Assistant Professor
Department of Anesthesiology
Ralph H. Johnson Veterans Administration
  Medical Center
Charleston, SC, USA

Bernadette Veering, MD, PhD
Associate Professor
Department of Anesthesiology
Leiden University Medical Center
Leiden, The Netherlands

David O. Warner, MD
Professor
Department of Anesthesiology
Mayo Clinic College of Medicine
Rochester, MN, USA

R. David Warters, MD
Professor
Department of Anesthesiology
Ralph H. Johnson Veterans Administration
  Medical Center
Charleston, SC, USA

Part I
Introduction to Clinical Geriatrics

Part I
Introduction to Climate Genomics

1
The Practice of Geriatric Anesthesia

Jeffrey H. Silverstein

The approach to and management of surgery and anesthesia in geriatric patients is different and frequently more complex than in younger patients. In caring for the elderly in the operating room, recovery room, and intensive care unit, the members of the perioperative medical team should be aware of the nature of aging physiology, the interaction of these alterations with pathologies, and the likelihood of multiple diagnoses and polypharmacy. The context of geriatric care encompasses multiple levels, stretching from primary care, through acute hospitalization, acute and subacute rehabilitation, nursing home care, and hopefully back to sufficient function to require additional primary care. By the nature of their practices, anesthesiologists and geriatricians have different approaches to patient care and the time frame over which such care occurs. In communicating with patients and geriatricians, one should understand that expectations for recovery are frequently different than in younger patients, marked by issues of maintenance of function and independence. There is an evolving understanding that specific approaches taken in the perioperative period have an impact that remains apparent months to years following surgery. Integrating care across this continuum can be difficult but invariably improves patient outcomes.

Geriatric medical care has evolved from an empiric specialty in the 1950s and 1960s to a largely evidence-based practice today. An excellent short reference guide called *Geriatrics at Your Fingertips* is available in a small pocket edition as well as on the Internet[1] (http://www.geriatricsatyourfingertips.org/). Perioperative geriatrics, however, is very much at the beginning of the process of developing sufficient primary data on which to base practice guidelines. There are few randomized controlled trials that provide class I evidence regarding perioperative care of the elderly, leaving the practitioner to extrapolate data from literature that has accumulated on geriatric care in other contexts, from retrospective reviews, and from the nonoperative geriatric literature.

This introductory chapter presents some of the common concepts of geriatrics and a general approach to caring for geriatric patients presenting for anesthesia and surgery. Virtually every chapter in this book elaborates on this foundation chapter. In approaching the elderly as patients, the anesthesiologist must understand that there is tremendous heterogeneity or variability in aging, both in the body as a whole as well as in individual systems. Thus, the alterations described in this and the following chapters are likely, on average, to be present in geriatric surgical patients. However, each individual patient will manifest these changes differently. The reader is encouraged to develop expertise and judgment and to identify those areas in need of improved approaches with the goal of developing an evidence-based practice for perioperative geriatrics.

Demography

As a result of nationwide improvements in health care, nutrition, education, and general living standards, the elderly account for an increasing percentage of the United States population (Figure 1-1). One in eight Americans were elderly (age 65 and older) in 1997. By 2030, according to the United States Bureau of the Census, one in five could be elderly. Between 2010 and 2030, as the baby boom generation reaches age 65, anesthesiologists will face a variety of challenges. The fastest-growing segment of the population is that aged 85 and older.

The average life expectancy in the United States is almost 72 years for men and 79 years for women. However, those who reach the age of 65 can expect to live 17.4 more years; a life expectancy of 82.4 years. There are racial disparities in longevity. In the United States, white men who reach age 65 can expect to live 15.7 more

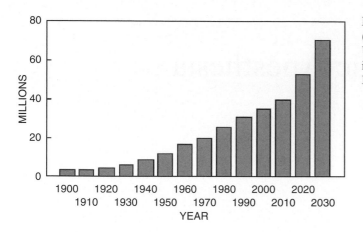

FIGURE 1-1. Growth of the Elderly Population, 1900–2030. (Reprinted from He W, Sengupta M, Velkoff VA, DeBarros KA. U.S. Census Bureau. Current Population Reports, P23-209, 65+ in the United States: 2005. Washington, DC: U.S. Government Printing Office; 2005.)

years whereas black men who reach 65 can expect to live 13.6 more years. Women are generally longer lived than men; however, the racial discrepancy is similar, with 19.4 and 17.6 additional years, respectively, of additional life expected for white and black women who reach age 65.

In 2004, 7.9 million patients over the age of 65 underwent a surgical procedure.[2] The number of patients over the age of 65 years who undergo noncardiac surgery has been projected to increase to 14 million over the next three decades[3] with similar increases expected for cardiac surgery. Seventy years ago, surgery was considered a desperate measure for patients older than 50 years of age, who were thought to be incapable of sustaining the rigors of even an inguinal hernia repair.[4] Advances in anesthesia during the past century have allowed surgeons to develop an extraordinary array of procedures with excellent outcomes in an increasingly aged population. Recent estimates confirm that the amount of surgical activity in the aging population is increasing.[5] Bolstered by the evolving demographics noted above, anesthesiologists can expect an ever-increasing portion of their overall workload to involve geriatric patients.

Definitions of Aging

Aging is a process of gradual and spontaneous change resulting first in maturation and subsequently decline through middle and late life. Senescence is the process by which the capacity for growth, function, and capacity for cell division are lost over time, ultimately leading to death. Aging comprises both a positive component of development (e.g., wisdom and experience) along with the negative component of physiologic and often cognitive decline.

Researchers and clinicians have found advantages in differentiating normal aging from age-related disease processes. Normal aging is those changes measured, on average, across the population. Some of these changes, for example, decrease in muscle mass, occur even in the well-conditioned, exercising elderly. In order to distinguish aging from disease, researchers have had to carefully screen patients for disease processes. This process has allowed gerontologists to determine that many long-held truisms concerning aging were not accurate. For example, it is now clear that aging per se does not involve neuronal loss in the brain, and cognitive decline is not an inevitable aspect of aging. Although it is evident to clinicians that diseases progressively accumulate in aging, many of these processes are no longer considered synonymous with increased age. That is not to suggest that aging is an innocent bystander, that is, that age-related disease accumulation could occur simply as a function of time. Lakatta and Levy,[6] in their studies of cardiac physiology, explained that age-related changes alter the substrate upon which disease processes evolve. In this conception, age affects the severity of disease manifestations for a given time at risk.

In contrast to normal aging, Rowe and Kahn[7] described the idea of successful aging. In successful aging, the deleterious effects of senescence are minimized such that the individuals suffer few of the unwanted features of aging. These individuals are vibrant and active into late age, with limited impairment. The combination of genetic and environmental status that leads to longevity is discussed in the chapter Theories of Aging (Chapter 3). The distinction between normal and successful aging highlights one of the principal phenomena in gerontology: that there is tremendous variability in aging between individuals of a given species. Although it is extremely convenient to categorize and even stereotype patients by age, chronological age is a poor predictor of physiologic aging.

Currently, morbidity, mortality, and recovery times for elderly patients undergoing surgery are substantially greater than those for younger patients.[8] (See also the section Surgical Outcomes and Functional Decline later in this chapter.) Age frequently alters the presentation of surgical illness. Symptoms of disease may be diminished, ignored, or inappropriately attributed to old age. Obtaining an accurate history can be challenging in the elderly. One of the results of the complexity of the patient population is an increased likelihood of preventable adverse events and consequences.[9] Thus, improving anesthetic care for geriatric patients represents the primary challenge of anesthesiology in the next few decades.

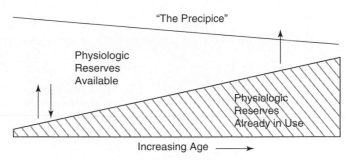

FIGURE 1-2. Schematic of homeostenosis. This diagram shows that maintaining homeostasis is a dynamic process. The older person uses or consumes physiologic reserves just to maintain homeostasis, and therefore there are fewer reserves available for meeting new challenges. (Reprinted with permission from Taffet GE. Physiology of aging. In: Cassel CK, Leipzig R, Cohen HJ, Larson EB, Meier DE, eds. Geriatric Medicine: An Evidence-Based Approach. 4th ed. New York: Springer; 2003.)

General Physiology of Aging

A homeostatic system is an open system that maintains its structure and functions by means of a multiplicity of dynamic equilibriums rigorously controlled by interdependent regulatory mechanisms.[10] Such a system reacts to change through a series of modifications of equal size and opposite direction to those that created the disturbance. The goal of these modifications is to maintain the internal balances. The term homeostenosis has been used to describe the progressive constriction of homeostatic reserve capacity. Another common means of expressing this idea is that aging results in a progressive decrease in reserve capacity. Diminishing reserve capacity can be identified at a cellular, organ, system, or whole-body level. As an example, glomerular filtration rate (GFR) progressively decreases with aging, limiting the capacity to deal with any stress on this excretory mechanism, be that a fluid load or excretion of medications or other toxic substances. Once again, the variability associated with aging is a key modifier of the decrease in physiologic function. So, although in general GFR decreases 1 mL/year, 30% of participants in a large study that defined this change had no change in GFR whereas others showed much greater decrements.[11] The concept of reserve has also been used in describing cognitive function.[12] Taffet has expanded the general interpretation of the decrease in physiologic reserve to emphasize that the reserve capacity is not an otherwise invisible organ capacity but the available organ function that will be used to maximal capacity by the elderly to maintain homeostasis (Figure 1-2). When the demands exceed the capacity of the organ or organism to respond, pathology ensues. This is ever more likely as aging decreases the capacity of any system to respond. The concept of organ reserve will be invoked in many chapters of this textbook.

Frailty

A term frequently applied to elderly patients is "frail." One would expect the frail elderly to be at higher risk for functional decline following surgery. Unfortunately, much like Justice Potter Stewart's 1964 definition of obscenity, most physicians can identify frailty when they see it, but a clinically relevant scientific definition has been elusive. Linda Fried and colleagues[13] have defined frailty, focusing primarily on muscle loss, or sarcopenia, as a clinical syndrome in which three or more of the following criteria are present: unintentional weight loss (10 lbs. in past year), self-reported exhaustion, weakness (grip strength), slow walking speed, and low physical activity. In the initial evaluation of the participants from the Cardiovascular Health Study (5317 men and women 65 years and older), the overall prevalence of frailty was 6.9%.[13] Frailty is perceived, in this context, as a cyclical decline that perpetuates itself (Figure 1-3). Frailty has been described as a form of predisability, which is distinct from functional impairment.[14] However, in the setting of sarcopenia, further muscle loss associated with surgical illness could be functionally disastrous. Indeed, Wolfe[15,16] has recently shown that the catabolic response to the stress of surgery and the subsequent loss of muscle mass is of even greater concern in the elderly. Frailty as a specific measure has not been prospectively characterized as a preoperative risk factor. The American Society of Anesthesiologists physical status score does not easily capture frailty, although clinicians may factor significant frailty into their assessment of a patient's physical status. Current research efforts should help define the relevance of frailty in the assessment and management of elderly patients.

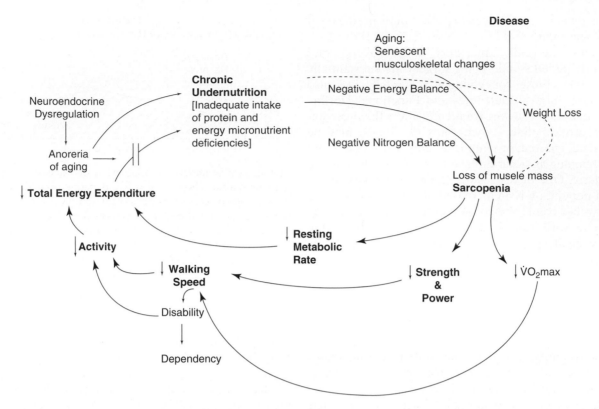

FIGURE 1-3. Cycle of frailty hypothesized as consistent with demonstrated pairwise associations and clinical signs and symptoms of frailty. (Reprinted with permission from Fried LP, Tangen CM, Walston J, Newman AB, Hirsch C, Gottdiener J, Seeman T, Tracy R, Kop WJ, Burke G, McBurnie MA; Cardiovascular Health Study Collaborative Research Group. Frailty in older adults: evidence for a phenotype. J Gerontol A Biol Sci Med Sci. 2001 Mar; 56(3):M146–56.)

Surgical Outcomes and Functional Decline

Traditional surgical outcomes include morbidity and mortality within a defined period following a procedure, frequently 30 days. Data from the Veterans Administrations National Surgical Quality Improvement Program (NSQIP) provides the most current insight into surgical outcomes for elderly patients. Hamel et al.[17] reported on 26,648 patients aged ≥80 (median age 82) and 568,263 patients <80 (median age 62) from the NSQIP database. Thirty-day mortality varied by procedure but was always higher for patients >80 (Table 1-1). Mortality was low (<2%) for many common procedures (transurethral prostatectomy, hernia repair, knee replacement, carotid endarterectomy, vertebral disc surgery, laryngectomy, and radical prostatectomy). The incidence of complications increased, but probably more important was that the impact of complications on mortality and functional recovery increased with age. Twenty percent of patients >80 had one or more complications, and the presence of a complication increased mortality from 4% to 26%. Respiratory and urinary tract complications were the most common.

For the mid- to late-life patient, symptoms and disability are the principal outcomes of most disease processes. They may become the focus of protracted care. In order to conceptualize disability in a format that supports medical and survey research, Verbrugge and Jette[18] elucidated The Disablement Process. The pathway to disability (Figure 1-4) begins with a disease or pathology. Impairments occur at the organ-system level and are dysfunctional and structural abnormalities in specific body systems, such as cardiovascular or neurologic. Functional limitations subsequently occur at the organism, or entire

TABLE 1-1. Thirty-day mortality for operations.

	<80 years	>80 years
General surgery	4.3	11.4
Vascular surgery	4.1	9.4
Thoracic surgery	6.3	13.5
Urologic surgery	0.7	1.9
Neurosurgery	2.4	8.6
Otolaryngological surgery	2.5	8.8
Orthopedic surgery	1.2	8.3

Source: Hamel et al.[17]

Note: Median age for the <80 group = 62 years, median age for >80 = 82 years.

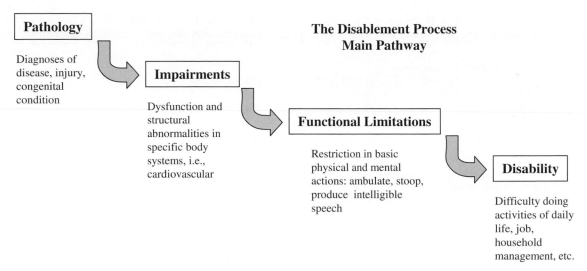

FIGURE 1-4. The disablement process: main pathway. (Adapted with permission from Verbrugge and Jette.[18])

being, level and comprise restrictions in basic physical and mental abilities such as ambulation, reaching, bending, and communicating intelligibly. Disability occurs when there is an insurmountable gap between an individual and environmental demands such that their expected social role is compromised. Intra-individual (e.g., age, socioeconomic status) and extra-individual (e.g., acute medical events, preventive interventions) factors can influence the Disablement Process in either direction. These factors may be preexisting or new occurrences.

The goals of therapy for a geriatric patient are frequently motivated by a desire to avoid disability and preserve or perhaps improve functional status. The most common measures of functional status are called activities of daily living (ADL) and instrumental activities of daily living (IADL)[19] (Tables 1-2 and 1-3). ADLs are those basic activities fundamental to self-care whereas IADLs are those functions necessary to live independently. ADLs and IADLs are subjective reported measures. In a research context, it is common to include objective measures of function to assess strength, time to perform specific activities, or distance covered in a fixed period of time. Measurement of cognitive function by neuropsychologic tests is analogous to measures of physical function. In general medical patients, there has been extensive research regarding both the basis for functional decline as well as approaches to improving outcomes in elderly patients hospitalized for acute illness. Many of the published clinical trials studied variations of the comprehensive geriatric assessment, described below.

The disablement process model is the theoretical basis for a model of elements that influence functional recovery after elective major surgery (Figure 1-5). There are two types of preexisting factors or determinants: 1) variable elements of function that may be modifiable or amenable to interventions; 2) relatively fixed elements in the context of daily living, which shape function and the roles of the variable elements, but may not be feasible targets for improving recovery. Variable elements are a comprehensive array of psychosocial, behavioral, and preoperative biomedical factors that can influence the evolution of function directly or indirectly through their influences on, and/or interaction with, other determinants. These elements are potentially amendable to intervention prior to an elective surgical procedure. Fixed elements are a separate constellation of contextual factors of daily living in which determinants and functional evolution interact and unfold. Anesthesia incorporates pharmacologic techniques to eliminate pain and the stress response attendant to surgical procedures. Within the acute event, there are surgical options (e.g., laparoscopic procedures) that may decrease the stress of the surgical procedure as well as the potential for anesthetic choices that may impact the trajectory of recovery. The model is qualitatively similar to a model for acute medical illness developed by Palmer et al.[20] and provides a framework for the identification of potential interventions to enhance postoperative recovery, prevent disability, and prolong independence in elders undergoing surgery.

The impact of surgery on functional outcomes in elderly patients has been most clearly described by Lawrence et al.[21] in their report on a prospective cohort of 372 patients, 60 years or older, undergoing abdominal surgery by surgeons in private practice and two university-affiliated hospitals in the San Antonio area. The participants were assessed preoperatively and postoperatively at 1, 3, and 6 weeks, 3 and 6 months, using self-report and performance-based measures ADL, IADL, the Medical Outcomes Study Short Form-36 (SF-36) Physical Component and Mental

TABLE 1-2. Activities of daily living. In each category, circle the item that most closely describes the person's highest level of functioning and record the score assigned to that level (either 1 or 0) in the blank at the beginning of the category.

A. Toilet   _____
1. Care for self at toilet completely; no incontinence   1
2. Needs to be reminded, or needs help in cleaning self, or has rare (weekly at most) accidents   0
3. Soiling or wetting while asleep more than once a week   0
4. Soiling or wetting while awake more than once a week   0
5. No control of bowels or bladder   0

B. Feeding   _____
1. Eats without assistance   1
2. Eats with minor assistance at meal times and/or helps with special preparation of food, or in cleaning up after meals   0
3. Feeds self with moderate assistance and is untidy   0
4. Requires extensive assistance for all meals   0
5. Does not feed self at all and resists efforts of others to feed him or her   0

C. Dressing   _____
1. Dresses, undresses, and selects clothes from own wardrobe   1
2. Dresses and undresses self with minor assistance   0
3. Needs moderate assistance in dressing and selection of clothes   0
4. Needs major assistance in dressing but cooperates with efforts of others to help   0
5. Completely unable to dress self and resists efforts of others to help   0

D. Grooming (neatness, hair, nails, hands, face, clothing)   _____
1. Always neatly dressed and well-groomed without assistance   1
2. Grooms self adequately with occasional minor assistance, e.g., with shaving   0
3. Needs moderate and regular assistance or supervision with grooming   0
4. Needs total grooming care but can remain well-groomed after help from others   0
5. Actively negates all efforts of others to maintain grooming   0

E. Physical ambulation   _____
1. Goes about grounds or city   1
2. Ambulates within residence or about one-block distance   0
3. Ambulates with assistance of (check one) a ( ) another person, b ( ) railing, c ( ) cane, d ( ) walker, e ( ) wheelchair   0
    1. _____ Gets in and out without help.
    2. _____ Needs help getting in and out
4. Sits unsupported in chair or wheelchair but cannot propel self without help   0
5. Bedridden more than half the time   0

F. Bathing   _____
1. Bathes self (tub, shower, sponge bath) without help   1
2. Bathes self with help getting in and out of tub   0
3. Washes face and hands only but cannot bathe rest of body   0
4. Does not wash self but is cooperative with those who bathe him or her   0
5. Does not try to wash self and resists efforts to keep him or her clean   0

Source: Lawton and Brody.[19]
Scoring interpretation: For ADLs, the total score ranges from 0 to 6. In some categories, only the highest level of function receives a 1; in others, two or more levels have scores of 1 because each describes competence at some minimal level of function. These screens are useful for indicating specifically how a person is performing at the present time. When they are also used over time, they serve as documentation of a person's functional improvement or deterioration.

Component Scales (PCS, MCS), Geriatric Depression Scale (GDS), Folstein Mini-Mental State Exam (MMSE), timed walk, functional reach, and hand-grip strength. The mean recovery times were: MMSE, 3 weeks; timed walk, 6 weeks; ADL, SF-36 PCS, and functional reach, 3 months; and IADL, 6 months (Figure 1-6). Mean grip strength did not return to preoperative status by 6 months. This result, that most functional recovery takes 3 to 6 months or longer, provides an indication of the impact that surgery makes on an elderly population. It should be noted that this cohort was accumulated before the popularity of laparoscopic procedures, so the stress of surgery and the recovery period may now be, on average, shorter.

In preparing a patient for surgery, informing him or her regarding the prolonged time that it will take to recover to preoperative status or better can be extremely important. Patients who understand that recovery is a prolonged process are less likely to become discouraged and more likely to continue prolonged efforts to regain strength and endurance.

Approach to the Patient

Although a variety of investigations in elderly patients have explored specific issues in geriatric care, a comprehensive evidence-based approach to the perioperative care of the elderly is not available in 2007. Therefore, the current approach is based on the few studies that have addressed these issues directly, extrapolation from studies

TABLE 1-3. Instrument (independent) activities of daily living. In each category, circle the item that most closely describes the person's highest level of functioning and record the score assigned to that level (either 1 or 0) in the blank at the beginning of the category.

A. Ability to use telephone	_____
1. Operates telephone on own initiative; looks up and dials numbers	1
2. Dials a few well-known numbers	1
3. Answers telephone but does not dial	1
4. Does not use telephone at all	0
B. Shopping	_____
1. Takes care of all shopping needs independently	1
2. Shops independently for small purchases	0
3. Needs to be accompanied on any shopping trip	0
4. Completely unable to shop	0
C. Food preparation	_____
1. Plans, prepares, and serves adequate meals independently	1
2. Prepares adequate meals if supplied with ingredients	0
3. Heats and serves prepared meals or prepares meals but does not maintain adequate diet	0
4. Needs to have meals prepared and served	0
D. Housekeeping	_____
1. Maintains house alone or with occasional assistance (e.g., domestic help for heavy work)	1
2. Performs light daily tasks such as dishwashing, bedmaking	1
3. Performs light daily tasks but cannot maintain acceptable level of cleanliness	1
4. Needs help with all home maintenance tasks	1
5. Does not participate in any housekeeping tasks	0
E. Laundry	_____
1. Does personal laundry completely	1
2. Launders small items; rinses socks, stockings, etc.	1
3. All laundry must be done by others	0
F. Mode of transportation	_____
1. Travels independently on public transportation or drives own car	1
2. Arranges own travel via taxi but does not otherwise use public transportation	1
3. Travels on public transportation when assisted or accompanied by another	1
4. Travel limited to taxi or automobile with assistance of another	0
5. Does not travel at all	0
G. Responsibility for own medications	_____
1. Is responsible for taking medication in correct dosages at correct time	1
2. Takes responsibility if medication is prepared in advance in separate dosages	0
3. Is not capable of dispensing own medication	0
H. Ability to handle finances	_____
1. Manages financial matters independently (budgets, writes checks, pays rent and bills, goes to bank); collects and keeps track of income	1
2. Manages day-to-day purchases but needs help with banking, major purchases, etc.	1
3. Incapable of handling money	0

Source: Lawton and Brody.[19] Copyright by the Gerontological Society of America.
Scoring interpretation: For IADLs, from 0 to 8. In some categories, only the highest level of function receives a 1; in others, two or more levels have scores of 1 because each describes competence at some minimal level of function. These screens are useful for indicating specifically how a person is performing at the present time. When they are also used over time, they serve as documentation of a person's functional improvement or deterioration.

that provide some insight into the broader care of elderly surgical patients, and some general suggestions derived from the experience of the author and his colleagues.

Stanley Muravchik nicely delineated the approach to the preanesthetic assessment of the elderly by specifying an organ-based vertical approach, as opposed to the horizontal approach of traditional diagnostic medicine (Figure 1-7). The specific age-related changes to major organ systems as well as the interaction between aging and disease processes are each covered in individual chapters in this book. For each organ system, the anesthesiologists should determine the functional status and attempt to assess the reserve capacity. In some cases, reserve capacity can be directly tested, as in a cardiac stress test. Many systems, particularly many of the homeostatic mechanisms of concern in the elderly, e.g., the autonomic nervous system, immune system, or even thermoregulatory control, remain difficult to assess. Neither baseline function nor reserve capacity have easily administered tests with reliable results for these systems. Maintenance of intraoperative normothermia can be a challenging goal in some elderly patients, although it is difficult to predict which will be particularly resistant.[22] (See Chapter 8.) The clinician should be attempting to distinguish age-related changes from disease, acknowledging that there are important interactions between the two, and that it can

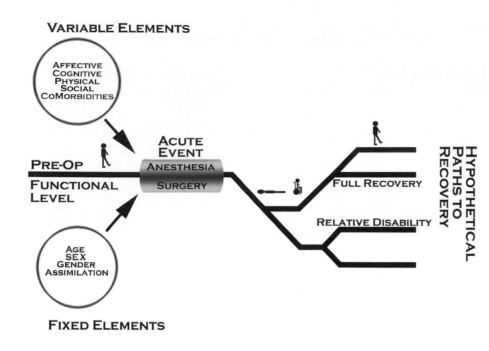

VARIABLE ELEMENTS

AFFECTIVE
COGNITIVE
PHYSICAL
SOCIAL
COMORBIDITIES

PRE-OP

FUNCTIONAL
LEVEL

ACUTE
EVENT
ANESTHESIA
SURGERY

FULL RECOVERY

RELATIVE DISABILITY

HYPOTHETICAL
PATHS TO
RECOVERY

AGE
SEX
GENDER
ASSIMILATION

FIXED ELEMENTS

FIGURE 1-5. This model, developed by Valerie Lawrence, MD, from the University of Texas Medical Center at San Antonio, Texas, and Jeffrey H. Silverstein, MD, from the Mount Sinai School of Medicine in New York, divides preoperative elements into those that are potentially variable and those that are not amenable to preoperative alteration. An important aspect is the management of the acute event. The combination of these factors determines the functional outcomes of patients undergoing surgery.

be difficult to determine what is aging and what is actual disease.

In addition to a focus on senescent physiology of standard organ systems, proper evaluation in elderly patients requires attention to areas that are not frequently evaluated in younger patients (Table 1-4). Sometimes it is difficult to imagine an anesthesiologist evaluating a patient's pressure points for early skin breakdown or specifically asking a patient about incontinence. The thrust of this chapter is that *someone* on the perioperative team must be cognizant of these issues. The team taking care of the patient has to have both the acute event and the recovery period as their focus of cooperation.

The skin and musculoskeletal system can undergo tremendous alterations. Up to 10% of elderly patients develop serious skin breakdown during prolonged operations in which pressure is exerted over debilitated areas.[23] Patients with severe arthritis, other limitations of range of motion, or prosthetic joints should, to the extent possible, be positioned on an operating room table in a position they find comfortable before the induction of anesthesia. This avoids severe strain on ligaments and joints that can be severely painful in the postoperative period.

The elderly take a large percentage of the medications prescribed in the United States. Patients frequently consume multiple medications. The management of these medications is frequently chaotic. The patient may present a bag full of prescription bottles and is not totally sure which one they take, or, somewhat more likely, convey a few of the many medications that they have been prescribed. Many of these medications have interactions

with drugs used by anesthesiologists in the perioperative period. These issues are presented in some detail in Chapter 14.

Acquiring information can be challenging and may involve discussion with not only the patient, but also their immediate caregiver as well as reference to previous medical records. A comprehensive approach to caring for the geriatric surgical patient may assign some of the assessment goals to the geriatrician, anesthesiologist, or surgeon. Additional time should be scheduled to accomplish an appropriate preoperative assessment. The area in which the preoperative assessment is conducted should be relatively quiet and well lit.

Hearing loss is a common complaint and should be generally understood by the anesthesiologist. Presbyacusia generally involves impaired sensitivity, particularly to higher pitched sounds, a derangement in loudness perception, impaired sound localization, and a decrease in time-related processing tasks. The summary behavior is frequently expressed as "I can hear you, but I can't understand you." The examiner can maximize the potential for communicating effectively with the patient by placing themselves 3–6 feet away, directly facing the patient. Use deliberate, clear speech at a somewhat slower (not comically or sarcastically) rate. The general tendency to speak louder needs to be tempered by the realization that shouted speech is often perceived as distorted by the elderly who are hard of hearing. Hearing aid technology has expanded dramatically and includes a variety of both external and surgically implantable technologies.[24] In general, patients should always be interviewed with their hearing aids in

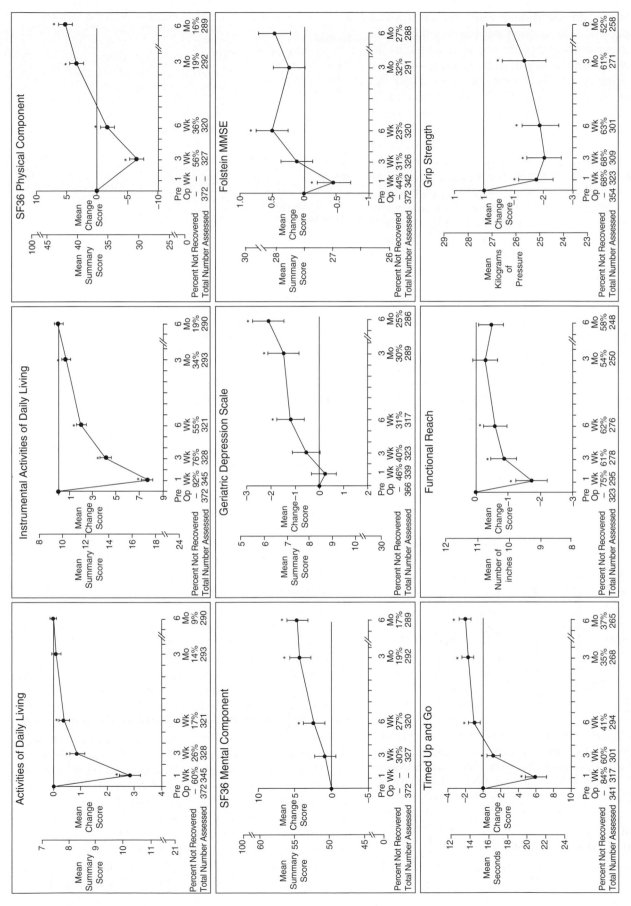

FIGURE 1-6. Functional recovery after major abdominal operation. Recovery is shown as mean individual change from preoperative baseline and 95% confidence intervals, with worsened function below a zero line representing preoperative status; a score of −1 indicates a one-point worsening relative to the preoperative baseline. An additional "shadow" y-axis is shown for orientation to mean summary or total scores. Asterisks indicate statistically significant differences from preoperative baseline, adjusted for multiple comparisons. MMSE, Mini-Mental State Exam; SF36, Medical Outcomes Study Short Form-36. (Reprinted with permission from Lawrence et al.[21])

place, and, barring an operation in which the ear is within the sterile operative field, hearing aids can be left in during surgery. Modern hearing aids do not pose a risk to the patient associated with the use of electrocautery and, if not within the primary electrical path, are not at risk for damage from electrocautery units. Having the hearing aid in place assists communication during emergence and in the postanesthesia care unit.

Loss of visual acuity is also common in the elderly. Visual acuity is included in a number of geriatric-care paradigms, including those that approach the prevention of perioperative delirium by means of making visual orientation easier. Cataracts can be particularly problematic. Before major surgery that is truly elective and schedulable, such as a total hip replacement, serious thought should be given to correcting the patient's vision if they have bilateral dense cataracts. Although less likely to have major impact, given the opportunity, a visit to an eye doctor to maximize visual acuity, perhaps through a change in correction, may be beneficial to the patient. The patient may be better able to read and utilize rehabilitation aids.

A particularly important issue in perioperative geriatrics is the role of the geriatrician. In the 1980s, geriatricians began evaluating a concept generally referred to as comprehensive geriatric assessment (CGA). CGA is a multidimensional, interdisciplinary, diagnostic process to identify care needs, plan care, and improve outcomes of frail older people.[25] The benefits of CGA are to improve diagnostic accuracy, optimize medical treatment, and improve medical outcomes (including functional status and quality of life).

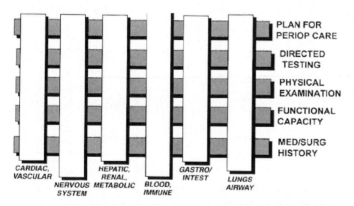

FIGURE 1-7. Organ system–based vertical approach to preoperative assessment of the elderly patient by an anesthesiologist differs from the traditional diagnostic approach because it applies the various techniques of inquiry (shaded bars) sequentially to each major organ system (open bars) in order to assess organ function and functional reserve. The primary objective of preoperative assessment should be evaluation of physical status rather than the identification of specific underlying disorders. (Reprinted with permission from Muravchick S. Preoperative assessment of the elderly patient. Anesthesiol Clin North Am 2000;18(1):71–89, vi.)

TABLE 1-4. Focus areas for assessment of geriatric patients.

Medical
Organ function and reserve
Medical illnesses
Medications
Nutrition
Dentition
Hearing
Vision
Pain
Urinary incontinence

Mental
Cognitive status
Emotional status
Spiritual status

Physical
Functional status
Balance and gait
Falls

Environmental
Social, financial status
Environmental hazards

In the perioperative arena, cooperative programs that feature some version of CGA have been evaluated. The most common perioperative environment for these programs has been hip fracture services. In a review of orthogeriatric care, Heyburn and colleagues[26] described four models that have been applied to hip fracture patients: the traditional model in which care is directed by the orthopedic surgeon and medical queries are directed to a consultant; the second is a variation in which multidisciplinary rounds with geriatricians and surgeons increase awareness of cross-specialty issues; the third involves early postoperative transfer to a geriatric rehabilitation unit; and the fourth is combined orthogeriatric care in which the patient is admitted to a specialized ward where care is coordinated by geriatricians and orthopedic surgeons. Delirium is a common complication following hip fracture and has been the primary outcome of interest for some of these studies. (See also Chapters 9 and 24.) Edward Marcantonio conducted a randomized trial of proactive geriatric consultation based on a structured protocol for patients with hip fractures (Table 1-5). The intervention reduced delirium by more than one-third.

In his review for the Freeman lecture, Rubenstein succinctly summed up the general state of affairs when he remarked that, despite the relatively consistent body of evidence supporting the utility of CGA and other geriatric follow-up programs, they have failed to be instituted on a wide scale. Soon after the initial successful reports, the institution of prospective payment diagnostic related groups (DRG) as part of the Medicare program made any additional stay in the hospital unprofitable. In fact, although CGA is effective at preventing rehospitaliza-

TABLE 1-5. Module with recommendations from Marcantonio's Active Geriatric Consultation.

1. Adequate central nervous system oxygen delivery:
   a) Supplemental oxygen to keep saturation >90%, preferably >95%
   b) Treatment to increase systolic blood pressure >2/3 baseline or >90 mm Hg
   c) Transfusion to keep hematocrit >30%
2. Fluid/electrolyte balance:
   a) Treatment to restore serum sodium, potassium, glucose to normal limits (glucose <300 mg/dL, <16.5 mmol/L for diabetics)
   b) Treat fluid overload or dehydration detected by examination or blood tests
3. Treatment of severe pain:
   a) Around-the-clock acetaminophen (1 g four times daily)
   b) Early-stage breakthrough pain: low-dose subcutaneous morphine, avoid meperidine
   c) Late-stage breakthrough pain: oxycodone as needed
4. Elimination of unnecessary medications:
   a) Discontinue/minimize benzodiazepines, anticholinergics, antihistamines
   b) Eliminate drug interactions, adverse effects, modify drugs accordingly
   c) Eliminate medication redundancies
5. Regulation of bowel/bladder function:
   a) Bowel movement by postoperative day 2 and every 48 hours
   b) D/c urinary catheter by postoperative day 2, screen for retention or incontinence
   c) Skin-care program for patients with established incontinence
6. Adequate nutritional intake:
   a) Dentures used properly, proper positioning for meals, assist as needed
   b) Supplements: 1 can Ensure, 3 cans Ensure for poor oral intake
   c) If unable to take food orally, feed via temporary nasogastric tube
7. Early mobilization and rehabilitation:
   a) Out of bed on postoperative day 1 and several hours daily
   b) Mobilize/ambulate by nursing staff as tolerated, such as to bathroom
   c) Daily physical therapy; occupational therapy if needed
8. Prevention, early detection, and treatment of major postoperative complications:
   a) Myocardial infarction/ischemia—electrocardiogram, cardiac enzymes if needed
   b) Supraventricular arrhythmias/atrial fibrillation—appropriate rate control, electrolyte adjustments, anticoagulation
   c) Pneumonia/chronic obstructive pulmonary disease—screening, treatment, including chest therapy
   d) Pulmonary embolus—appropriate anticoagulation
   e) Screening for and treatment of urinary tract infection
9. Appropriate environmental stimuli:
   a) Appropriate use of glasses and hearing aids
   b) Provision of clock and calendar
   c) If available, use of radio, tape recorder, and soft lighting
10. Treatment of agitated delirium:
   a) Appropriate diagnostic workup/management
   b) For agitation, calm reassurance, family presence, and/or sitter
   c) For agitation, if absolutely necessary, low-dose haloperidol 0.25–0.5 mg every 4 hours as needed; if contraindicated, use lorazepam at same dose

Source: Marcantonio ER, Flacker JM, Wright RJ, Resnick NM. Reducing delirium after hip fracture: a randomized trial. J Am Geriatr Soc 2001;49(5):516–522.

tion, the financial incentives of the DRG system (see Chapter 2) favor multiple hospitalizations for multiple medical problems. However, some perioperative CGA programs have cut down on length of stay.[27] When a CGA program is instituted, it is essential that there is a mechanism for operationalizing the recommendations generated by the assessment. Programs with only consultation are less effective than programs in which there is a clear mechanism to institute and follow up on recommendations. Current methods for covering the costs of perioperative care have not favored the development of these programs. In the presence of evidence that such programs work, clinicians caring for elderly surgical patients are challenged to organize a care plan that facilitates rapid recovery and prevents complications. The team caring for the patient should understand the current functional status of the patient and be able to enter into reasonable discussion with the patient and/or their immediate family concerning realistic goals of surgical care.

Organizations and Resources in Geriatric Anesthesia

Perioperative care of the elderly is an important issue. For many years, the American Society of Anesthesiologists has maintained a Committee on Geriatrics. Among other educational and research efforts, the Committee maintains the Syllabus on Geriatric Anesthesiology which can be found on the ASA's Web site, www.asahq.org/clinical/geriatrics/geron.htm. The Society for the Advancement of Geriatric Anesthesia (SAGA) was formed in 1999 with the mission of improving the care of older patients having surgery. SAGA sponsors an annual meeting and provides organizational guidance for individuals interested in the perioperative care of the elderly (www.sagahq.org). A longer-standing effort in the United Kingdom is the Age Anaesthesia Association (www.aaa-online.org.uk/). The American Geriatrics Society has developed a Section on Surgical and Related Specialties that organizes educational efforts as well as supports a number of research funding opportunities to support investigation into perioperative geriatrics (www.americangeriatrics.org/specialists/). The Section supports the Geriatric Syllabus for Specialists as well as the Research Agenda Setting Process.[28]

Conclusion

This introductory chapter outlines the broad scope of perioperative geriatric care and provides a perspective with which to utilize the information in the remainder of this text. Geriatric care is, by nature complex, multidisciplinary, and evolving. There is much yet to be learned in the area of perioperative geriatrics, but still many practices and procedures are known and can be used to improve the quality of perioperative care today.

References

1. Reuben DB, Herr KA, Pacala JT, Pollock BG, Potter JF, Semla TP. Geriatrics at Your Fingertips. 8th ed. New York: American Geriatrics Society; 2006.
2. DeFrances CJ, Podgornik MN. 2004 National Discharge Survey. 371. 5-4-2006. Hyattsville, MD: National Center for Health Statistics. Advance Data from Vital and Health Statistics.
3. Mangano DT. Preoperative risk assessment: many studies, few solutions. Is a cardiac risk assessment paradigm possible? Anesthesiology 1995;83:897–901.
4. Ochsner A. Is risk of operation too great in the elderly? Geriatrics 1927;22:121.
5. Klopfenstein CE, Herrmann FR, Michel JP, Clergue F, Forster A. The influence of an aging surgical population on the anesthesia workload: a ten-year survey. Anesth Analg 1998;86:1165–1170.
6. Lakatta EG, Levy D. Arterial and cardiac aging: major shareholders in cardiovascular disease enterprises. Part I. Aging arteries: a "setup" for vascular disease. Circulation 2003;107:139–146.
7. Rowe JW, Kahn RL. Human aging: usual and successful. Science 1987;237:143–149.
8. Tiret L, Desmonts JM, Hatton F, Vourch G. Complications associated with anaesthesia: a prospective survey in France. Can Anaesth Soc J 1986;33:336–344.
9. Rothschild JM, Bates DW, Leape LL. Preventable medical injuries in older patients. Arch Intern Med 2000;160:2717–2728.
10. de Rosnay J. Homeostasis: resistance to change. Heylighen F, Joslyn C, Turchin V, eds. Brussels: Pincipia Cybernetica; 1997. Available at: http://cleamc11.vub.ac.be/homeosta.html.
11. Lindeman RD. Renal physiology and pathophysiology of aging. Contrib Nephrol 1993;105:1–12.
12. Whalley LJ, Deary IJ, Appleton CL, Starr JM. Cognitive reserve and the neurobiology of cognitive aging. Ageing Res Rev 2004;3:369–382.
13. Fried LP, Tangen CM, Walston J, et al. Frailty in older adults: evidence for a phenotype. J Gerontol A Biol Sci Med Sci 2001;56:M146–M156.
14. Morley JE, Haren MT, Rolland Y, Kim MJ. Frailty. Med Clin North Am 2006;90:837–847.
15. Wolfe RR. The underappreciated role of muscle in health and disease. Am J Clin Nutr 2006;84:475–482.
16. Wolfe RR. Optimal nutrition, exercise, and hormonal therapy promote muscle anabolism in the elderly. J Am Coll Surg 2006;202:176–180.
17. Hamel MB, Henderson WG, Khuri SF, Daley J. Surgical outcomes for patients aged 80 and older: morbidity and mortality from major noncardiac surgery. J Am Geriatr Soc 2005;53:424–429.
18. Verbrugge LM, Jette AM. The disablement process. Soc Sci Med 1994;38:1–14.
19. Lawton MP, Brody EM. Assessment of older people: self-maintaining and instrumental activities of daily living. Gerontologist 1969;9:179–186.
20. Palmer RM, Counsell S, Landefeld CS. Clinical intervention trials: the ACE unit. Clin Geriatr Med 1998;14:831–849.
21. Lawrence VA, Hazuda HP, Cornell JE, et al. Functional independence after major abdominal surgery in the elderly. J Am Coll Surg 2004;199:762–772.
22. Sessler DI. Perianesthetic thermoregulation and heat balance in humans. FASEB J 1993;7:638–644.
23. Aronovitch SA. Intraoperatively acquired pressure ulcer prevalence: a national study. J Wound Ostomy Continence Nurs 1999;26:130–136.
24. Kim HH, Barrs DM. Hearing aids: a review of what's new. Otolaryngol Head Neck Surg 2006;134:1043–1050.
25. Rubenstein LZ, Joseph T. Freeman award lecture: comprehensive geriatric assessment—from miracle to reality. J Gerontol A Biol Sci Med Sci 2004;59:473–477.
26. Heyburn G, Beringer T, Elliott J, Marsh D. Orthogeriatric care in patients with fractures of the proximal femur. Clin Orthop Relat Res 2004;(425):35–43.
27. Vidan M, Serra JA, Moreno C, Riquelme G, Ortiz J. Efficacy of a comprehensive geriatric intervention in older patients hospitalized for hip fracture: a randomized, controlled trial. J Am Geriatr Soc 2005;53:1476–1482.
28. Solomon DH, LoCicero J, Rosenthal RA, eds. New Frontiers in Geriatrics Research. An Agenda for the Surgical and Related Medical Specialties. New York: American Geriatrics Society; 2004.

2
Demographics and Economics of Geriatric Patient Care

Maria F. Galati and Roger D. London

Anesthesiologists in geriatric practice care primarily for patients who are insured via Medicare, the federal health insurance program for citizens over the age of 65. The Medicare program has grown steadily in complexity and cost since its inception in 1965. It is expected to come under significant financial pressure as the population of the United States ages and the costs of providing health care continue to grow at ever-increasing rates.

This chapter is intended to provide those anesthesiologists who care for the geriatric patient population with an introduction to key health policy issues related to the Medicare program and to facilitate understanding of the demographics and economics of geriatric care with special emphasis on Medicare. The first part of the chapter is a general introduction and overview of the demographic and financial issues facing Medicare in the near future. The second part of the chapter raises some of the major policy issues that are specific to the practice of anesthesiology under the Medicare program.

Medicare Demographics and Financing Issues

The Enactment of the Medicare Program

Medicare is the federal program that provides health care insurance to all citizens who are at least 65 years old and to some disabled Americans. The program was enacted in 1965 with passage of one of the most important pieces of domestic legislation of the post-World War II period, but the legislative process that preceded it was marked by years of debate and controversy.

From the Eisenhower administration forward, the United States government struggled with how best to meet the high cost of health care for the elderly. Results of the 1950 census revealed that since 1900 the aged population had grown from 4% to 8% of the total population. Two-thirds of the elderly had annual incomes of less than $1000, and only 1 in 8 had health insurance.[1] In response to the crisis, bills proposing hospital insurance for the aged were introduced in every Congress from 1952 through 1965.[2]

Legislators recognized and feared the power of organized medicine to thwart passage of legislation that involved government-sponsored health insurance. Therefore, when the Johnson Administration made its proposal, it included only a mandatory plan for covering hospital expenses for the elderly. This plan is what eventually became known as "Medicare Part A."

It was the Chairman of the House Ways and Means Committee in 1965, Congressman Wilbur Mills, who fashioned a compromise that led to the creation of "Medicare Part B," a voluntary plan for coverage of physician expenses for the elderly that was acceptable to the American Medical Association (AMA). In the compromise proposal for Medicare Part B, physician expenses were to be reimbursed on "usual and customary" charges as long as they were "reasonable."[3] Physicians also retained the right to bill patients directly and in excess of the amount reimbursed by the government.

On July 30, 1965, President Lyndon Johnson enacted the Medicare and Medicaid programs by signing the Social Security Act of 1965 with these words:

There are men and women in pain who will find ease. There are those alone and suffering who will now hear the sound of approaching help. There are those fearing the terrible darkness of despair and poverty—despite long years of labor and expectation—who will now see the light of hope and realization.[4]

The Organization and Funding of Medicare

The Social Security Administration administered the Medicare program from 1965 until 1977, when Medicare was reorganized under the Health Care Financing Administration (HCFA) within the Department of Health, Education and Welfare. In July 2001, HCFA was renamed the Centers for Medicare and Medicaid Services (CMS).[5] In 1966, the

Medicare program covered more than 19 million citizens over the age of 65. Coverage for the disabled began in 1973 and, as of 2003, the program served more than 40 million Americans: 35 million elderly and 6 million disabled.[6]

The Medicare program provides coverage to the aged, the permanently disabled, and people with end-stage renal disease under two parts: Hospital Insurance (HI) or Medicare Part A, and Supplementary Medical Insurance (SMI) or Medicare Part B. The Medicare + Choice managed-care plan, also known as the "Medicare Advantage" program or Medicare Part C, was added by the Balanced Budget Act of 1997 and allows beneficiaries to opt for enrollment in private-sector–managed Medicare insurance plans. The Medicare Prescription Drug Improvement and Modernization Act of 2003 became effective in 2006, and extended a new prescription drug benefit to Medicare beneficiaries known as Medicare Part D.

The CMS contracts with private-sector agents to administer Medicare program services, including provider enrollment and claims administration processes. Contractors that process Part A claims are known as fiscal intermediaries and those that administer Part B claims are known as carriers. These contractors are usually insurance companies, many of which are Blue Cross-Blue Shield plans around the United States that can act as both fiscal intermediaries and contractors. Contractors are barred by law from making a profit on services provided to the Medicare program.

Enrollment in Medicare Part A is automatic for eligible beneficiaries and covers inpatient hospital care, after-hospital care in skilled nursing facilities, hospice care, and some home health services. Beneficiary enrollment in Medicare Part B is voluntary and covers physician services, outpatient hospital services, diagnostic tests, some home health services, and medical equipment and supplies. By law, 25% of Part B program costs must come from beneficiary premiums.

Employers and employees who make mandatory contributions to the Part A Hospital Insurance Trust Fund finance the majority of the Medicare program costs. Other funding sources include general tax revenues, and the premiums, deductibles, and copayments paid by the beneficiaries. Of the Medicare program's annual expenses ($214.6 billion in 1997), 89% are funded by people under the age of 65 in the form of payroll and income taxes and interest from the trust fund. Only 11% comes from monthly premiums paid by the beneficiaries.[7]

Twenty-First Century Realities and the Future of the Medicare Program

Baby Boomer Demographics

The so-called "baby boomer generation," the post-World War II Americans born between 1946 and 1964, will have a significant impact on the demographics of our society and on the Medicare program. It is predicted that as the boomers age, the number of people in the United States aged 65 years and older is expected to roughly double to 77 million by the year 2030.[8]

Given the existing Medicare funding system, it is clear that the aging of the American population will bring fiscal pressures to bear on the Medicare program in two ways. There will be more retired beneficiaries, as boomers age and live longer than their parents, and there will be fewer workers to pay for the retiree expenses.[9]

It is predicted that the over-65 age group will grow from approximately 13% of the total population in 2000 to 20% in 2030 and will remain above 20% for at least several decades thereafter.[10] In addition, life expectancies are continuing to increase, and typical boomers are projected to live approximately 2 years longer than their parents did, spending more years in retirement (Figure 2-1). At the same time, the labor force is expected to grow much more slowly than the population of retirees, resulting in many fewer workers per retiree. In 2000, there were 4.8 people ages 20 to 64 for each person age 65 or older. This ratio is expected to decrease to approximately 2.9 people ages 20 to 64 for each person age 65 or older by 2030 (Figure 2-2).

Although baby boomers report an intention to work longer than their parents did, it remains to be seen whether employers will accommodate this expectation and what effect this may have on the projected decrease in the worker–retiree ratio. Thus, retirement of the baby boomer generation will strain the already vulnerable Medicare program. The Social Security and Medicare

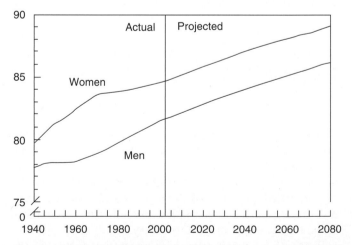

FIGURE 2-1. Life expectancy of 65-year-olds. (From Congressional Budget Office based on Social Security Administration. The 2003 annual report of the Board of Trustees of the Federal Old-Age and Survivors Insurance and Disability Insurance Trust Funds. March 17, 2003. p. 86. Available at: www.ssa.gov/OACT/TR/TR03/tr03.pdf.)

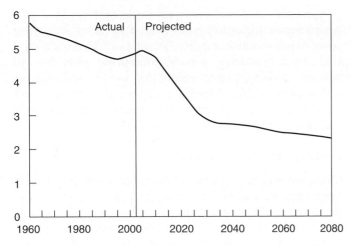

FIGURE 2-2. Ratio of population ages 20 to 64 to population ages 65 and older. (From Congressional Budget Office based on Social Security Administration. The 2003 annual report of the Board of Trustees of the Federal Old-Age and Survivors Insurance and Disability Insurance Trust Funds. March 17, 2003. p. 82. Available at: www.ssa.gov/OACT/TR/TR03/tr03.pdf.)

Boards of Trustees are predicting that starting in 2010, when the baby boom generation begins to retire, the Hospital Insurance Trust Funds will experience rapidly growing annual deficits leading to fund exhaustion by 2019.[11] The report also predicts that the Supplemental Medical Insurance Trust Fund, which pays for physician services and the new prescription drug benefit, will have to be funded by large increases in premiums and increased transfers from general revenues.

Baby Boomer Expectations

The baby boomer generation will bring millions of people into the Medicare program and these new beneficiaries will also bring with them a new set of expectations. Baby boomers constitute the first generation born to the Medicare program and the first with significant experience with managed medical insurance plans. Baby boomers also include a significant number of women with working experience and, in general, are more affluent than their forebears. They expect to enter retirement with more assets and with high expectations of the retirement experience.

A survey conducted by Roper Starch Worldwide for the American Association of Retired Persons (AARP) and entitled, "Baby-Boomers Envision Their Retirement: An AARP Segmentation Analysis," examined the expectations, attitudes, and concerns of the baby boomers as they approach retirement. There were several key attitudinal findings from the survey. Most baby boomers believe that they will still be working during their retirement years. This is unlike previous generations and has

important implications for employers as well as the Medicare program.

Only one in five boomers expects to move to a new geographic area when they retire and almost one in four expects to receive an inheritance that will affect their retirement planning. Only approximately 35% expect that they will have to scale back their lifestyle during retirement and only 16% believe that they will have serious health problems when they are retired (AARP op. cit.). These are very optimistic views of the extent to which baby boomers' retirement years will be disrupted by particular life events.[12]

Less optimistic conclusions emerged when the survey examined attitudes toward Social Security and Medicare: 55% had a very or somewhat favorable view of Social Security and 60% had a favorable view of Medicare. However, only 46% said that they were very or somewhat knowledgeable about Medicare and only 40% were confident that Medicare would be available to them during retirement. Indeed, baby boomers were much less confident in their abilities under Medicare to access care, choose their own doctors, or to consult specialists at the same level as under their current health plan (AARP op. cit.).

Medicare Coverage Gaps

These less optimistic baby boomer attitudes may reflect an astute appreciation of the limitations of the Medicare program. Benefits under the Medicare program are significantly limited. One study has found that 80% of employer-sponsored fee-for-service plans cover a larger proportion of medical expenses than Medicare does.[13]

Medicare has not traditionally covered services such as long-term nursing care, outpatient prescription drugs, or routine vision, dental, hearing, and foot care. The Balanced Budget Act of 1997 extended coverage to include annual mammograms, Pap smears, prostate and colorectal screenings, diabetes management, and osteoporosis diagnosis. In December 2003, when the new prescription drug benefit was signed into law, it was projected that average out-of-pocket prescription drug spending for Medicare beneficiaries would be lower; however, it was also expected that 25% of beneficiaries would actually pay more as a result of the new coverage.[14] Furthermore, it is estimated that 3.1 million low-income subsidy-eligible beneficiaries are not receiving this assistance and therefore still face financial barriers in accessing necessary prescription drugs.[15] It will take years to fully assess the impact of this latest change in Medicare benefits on beneficiaries, providers, and the program itself.

Medicare beneficiaries rely on privately purchased or government-sponsored supplemental insurance plans to "tie in" and complement the array of services covered by the Medicare program. Supplemental insurance coverage

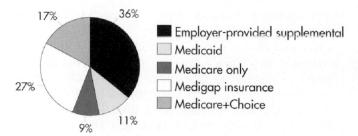

FIGURE 2-3. Supplemental insurance status of Medicare beneficiaries, 1999. (From Rice and Bernstein.[16])

for these services has been historically provided by Medicaid plans (for the poor) and by so-called "Medigap" policies for those able to afford additional coverage.

In 1999, approximately 91% of Medicare beneficiaries relied on supplemental insurance plans. Of those with supplemental insurance, 27% purchased Medigap insurance and 36% received supplemental insurance related to employment. An additional 17% were enrolled in Medicare + Choice plans and 11% qualified for coverage through Medicaid. The remaining 9% had no supplemental coverage (Figure 2-3).[16] In 1996, Medigap premiums across the nation ranged from $233 annually for the least-expensive basic coverage, to $2205 annually for the most comprehensive plan.[17]

Some employers, mostly large companies, also sponsor plans that cover retired workers and their spouses. In 2006, 35% of firms with more than 200 employees offered retiree health benefits, with 77% of firms in this category covering Medicare-eligible retirees. In 1988, before implementation of the Part D drug benefit, 66% of large firms offered retiree coverage.[18]

The poorest Medicare recipients have their medical costs paid in part by the Medicaid program. Of these "dual eligibles," those with incomes and resources substantially below the federal poverty line are entitled to full Medicaid coverage. Specifically, eligibility for full Medicaid coverage is determined by whether an individual qualifies for Supplemental Security Income, an income maintenance program designed for very poor aged, disabled, and blind Americans. Thus, Medicaid provides complementary coverage for a portion of Medicare beneficiaries.

Unlike Medicare, Medicaid coverage includes benefits such as prescription drugs, hearing aids, and payment for nursing home services. The Medicaid program also makes premium payments and pays a portion of Medicare deductibles and other copayments required of beneficiaries. Because this assistance must be claimed by beneficiaries through an application process, a substantial portion of potentially eligible low-income individuals, perhaps as many as 3.9 million, do not receive this aid.[19]

As a result of these various coverage options, Medicare beneficiaries are either not covered at all or are partly covered in a somewhat unpredictable way. This variability challenges practicing geriatric medicine providers to become knowledgeable about the specific situation in which each of their Medicare-eligible patients can find themselves, especially as it may relate to the patient's ability to comply with treatment plans.

Prescription Drug Benefit

Medicare was late in providing prescription drug coverage compared with most private insurance plans, and the universal public health plans in other developed nations, that have traditionally provided this benefit as an important part of comprehensive health coverage. Drug therapies can reduce the need for hospitalization by effectively managing chronic health problems of the elderly such as heart disease, diabetes, and depression. Chronically ill patients have been found to underuse essential medications because of cost considerations and to suffer serious health consequences, including an increased number of emergency room visits and inpatient admissions, as a result.[20]

In 1998, 73% of noninstitutionalized Medicare beneficiaries had drug coverage of some kind for at least a portion of the year through supplemental insurance, such as managed Medicare plans, employer-sponsored plans, and Medigap plans.[21] However, the out-of-pocket spending by older Americans for prescription drugs amounts on average to 50% of total costs, compared with just 34% of costs for those under age 65.[22] The prices of the prescription drugs used most often by the elderly have been increasing in recent years. Expensive new brand-name drugs, some of which are more effective than the older drugs that they are superseding, are being brought to market at an increasingly rapid rate.[23]

In a recent nationwide survey of chronically ill older adults, it was reported that 33% underuse prescription drugs because of concerns about out-of-pocket drug costs. Furthermore, 66% of these patients failed to discuss their intention to underuse medications with a clinician citing that no one asked about their ability to pay and that they did not believe that providers could offer any assistance.[20]

Impact on the Near-Poor

It is the near-poor, those with annual incomes between $10,000 and $20,000, who are most often caught in the prescription drug cost quandary. In 1999, only 55% of the near-poor had coverage for the entire year and more than 20% of those with prescription drug coverage received it via a Medicare Advantage plan. Access to prescription drugs and levels of reimbursement for prescription drugs has decreased significantly under these managed-

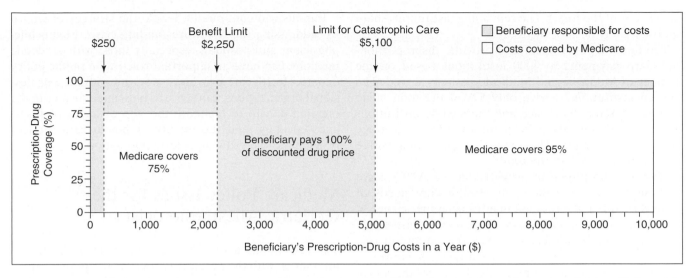

FIGURE 2-4. Prescription drug coverage under Medicare effective 2006. (Reproduced with permission from Iglehart.[25] Copyright © 2004 Massachusetts Medical Society. All Rights Reserved.)

Medicare plans since the Balanced Budget Act of 1997. As a result, the near-poor had higher out-of-pocket costs for prescription drugs in 1999 than other Medicare beneficiaries who were poorer (and therefore, Medicaid-eligible), and those with higher incomes.[24] Unfortunately, the new prescription drug benefit may not lead to a significant reduction in out-of-pocket prescription drug costs for these near-poor beneficiaries who will incur costs that fall through gaps in the coverage (Figure 2-4).

In the intervening years before implementation of the new prescription drug benefit, there were some opportunities for the more than 33% of beneficiaries with no prescription drug benefits at all. Between 2004 and 2006, Medicare beneficiaries were eligible for drug-discount cards that were expected to save them up to 10%–15% on their total drug costs. In addition, beneficiaries with incomes below 135% of the federal poverty level were eligible for a $600 per year subsidy.[25] These opportunities expired when the new drug benefit took effect in 2006.

Medicare and the Academic Health Center

The Medicare program has many shortcomings and, over the next two decades, significant reform will be required to maintain even the current level of protection that it offers to America's elderly. This looming crisis in health care insurance for the elderly as well as the more than 40 million uninsured is of great concern to lawmakers and the public but should also be of great concern to health care providers, hospitals, and physicians, who rely on Medicare as a significant source of their revenues. In 2000, payments made by the Medicare program accounted for 31% of total national spending on hospital

care and 21% of total national spending on physician and clinical services.[26]

Physicians in academic practice have even greater reason to be interested in the plight of the Medicare program. In addition to the significant flow of funds received by Academic Health Centers (AHCs) in the form of clinical revenues, AHCs are dependent on the Medicare program for support of graduate medical education (GME) and care provided to indigent patients. All undergraduate medical students and almost 50% of all residents are trained in AHCs, which also provide most of the charity care and medical specialty services such as neonatal, burn and trauma intensive care, and organ transplant services.[27]

Graduate Medical Education Payments

Since the initiation of the Medicare Prospective Hospital Payment System in the mid-1980s, GME payments have been made to AHCs to reimburse them for Medicare's share of the costs of resident physician education. AHCs are eligible for two types of reimbursements: direct GME, covering direct costs such as resident and faculty salaries and benefits; and indirect GME, recognizing the relatively larger inpatient costs at hospitals with teaching programs.

The Federal government has provided more than $100 billion in GME support to AHCs since the mid-1980s. These funds are distributed to approximately 1000 institutions based on the number of residents trained, their costs in the reference year 1985, and their share of Medicare beneficiaries served. The top ten AHCs receive an average of $60 million each (12% of the total), and the next 40 institutions receive approximately $30 million each (24% of the total). The remaining institutions share approximately 64% of the total.[27]

The Federal government also provides disproportionate share payments to 4000 institutions based on the number of Medicare and Medicaid patients served. The top ten institutions receive only 5% of the total or an average of $20 million each and the next 40 institutions receive approximately 11% of the total for an average of $10 million each. The remaining institutions share approximately 85% of the total.[27]

Hospital and physician providers at the AHCs serve important roles in meeting the health care needs of underserved populations and in advancing the science of health care through education and research. These providers are paid by Medicare to play this important role in shaping the future of the health care system. However, the same federal system continually challenges these providers to maintain a commitment to education, research, and charity care despite declining reimbursement for these important activities.

"Pay for Performance" Initiatives

The CMS has recognized the need to provide incentives to hospital and physician providers who can innovate to create improved patient outcomes at lower costs. Several demonstration projects are in place to provide hospitals with reimbursement bonuses if they meet quality standards and report their results to CMS.

Physicians got their first opportunity to apply to Medicare's physician Pay for Performance (P4P) initiative effective in April 2005. The CMS selected 10 physician group practices, with 200 or more physicians, which were eligible to earn performance payments in addition to usual fee-for-service payments. The payments were based on how well the groups managed the care of patients to prevent complications and avoidable hospitalizations thereby enhancing quality and reducing costs under both Part A and Part B of the Medicare program.[28] These programs do not reward academic activities such as teaching, research, and grant work. Therefore, success of P4P programs in the academic setting will depend on how much of physician compensation is based on clinical activity.[29]

Summary

Many solutions to the looming Medicare crisis have been proposed. Common reform measures include changes to the age of eligibility, linking premiums to beneficiary incomes, increasing revenues via higher payroll taxes or counting Medicare benefits as taxable income, and altering the concept of Medicare as a defined benefit program.

Pundits will continue to debate the strategy of choice for addressing the Medicare funding crisis. Meanwhile, physicians and hospitals, especially those with academic missions, can have an important role in the public policy debate. Health care providers, working with their professional organizations, can serve as patient advocates in the ongoing debate to facilitate the improvement of insurance coverage and the quality of health care services provided to the growing elderly population.

Medicare Policy Issues for the Geriatric Anesthesiologist

The regulations and processes governing a physician's interaction with the Medicare program are quite complex and a full description is well beyond the scope of this chapter. However, it is the authors' intention to provide the practicing geriatric anesthesiologist with an introduction to policy issues specific to the practice of Anesthesiology under the Medicare program. These key issues include:

1) Participation status in the Medicare program
2) Medicare's Resource Based Relative Value System (RBRVS) for physician reimbursement
3) Medicare's rules for the anesthesia care team
4) Compliance-related issues for anesthesiologists

The CMS provides a specialty-specific page on its Web site that is dedicated to Medicare regulations and information specific to the practice of Anesthesiology. Physicians interested in further study of Medicare claims processing, fees and policies for the reimbursement of anesthesia services should consult CMS's anesthesiologist Web page at: http://www.cms.hhs.gov/center/anesth.asp.

Anesthesiologist Participation in the Medicare Program

The decision to enroll as a participating provider in the Medicare program is one of the first decisions that an anesthesiologist faces when starting a clinical practice. Anesthesiologists employed in geriatric practice can expect that the Medicare program will be the primary insurer for most of their patients. Anesthesiologists, who typically encounter their patients in an operating room setting where they are not the patient's primary provider, need to be aware of the political, patient satisfaction, and reimbursement issues related to their participation status in the Medicare program.

In 1990, only 30.8% of anesthesiologists participated in the Medicare program; this was the lowest rate of participation as a percentage of physicians by medical specialty. By 2003, participation by anesthesiologists had increased to 95.5%. This rate of participation closely matches that of physicians in related practices such as surgery, cardiovascular disease, ophthalmology, orthopedic surgery, pathology, radiology, urology, and nephrology.[30]

It is likely that the anesthesiologist's obligation to care for all surgical patients and new Medicare rules limiting charges from nonparticipating providers, influenced anesthesiologist enrollment decisions in the 1990s. Unfortunately, as anesthesiologist Medicare participation rates increased dramatically in the period from 1990 to 2003, the Medicare anesthesia conversion factor in the same period was decreased by almost 20%.[31] One might speculate that, during a decade of significant growth in managed care and public outcry concerning increasing health care costs, the pressures from patients, colleagues, local government, affiliated institutions, and the Medicare charge limitations combined to favor participation by anesthesiology providers.

In general, participation in the Medicare program by anesthesiologists is a voluntary decision. [Medicare participation by Certified Registered Nurse Anesthetists (CRNAs) and Anesthesiologist Assistants (AAs) is mandatory.[32]] However, some states encourage physician participation through legislative actions and regulatory requirements, such as in The Commonwealth of Massachusetts, where Medicare participation is a condition of medical licensure. Physicians can consult with their local Medicare carrier or their regional CMS office for local Medicare participation requirements.[33]

Physicians who enroll as participating providers enter into a 1-year, automatically renewable agreement to accept assignment for all covered services provided to Medicare beneficiaries. When a physician accepts assignment, they agree to accept the Medicare allowable charge as payment in full for the covered services rendered. After patients satisfy an annual deductible, Medicare pays 80% of the approved allowable charge. The remaining 20% is termed the "coinsurance" and it is the responsibility of the patient to pay this and any remaining portion of the annual deductible. Participating providers must bill the patient, or the patient's Medigap insurance plan, for coinsurance, deductible, and charges not covered by the Medicare Part B program.

In addition to the likely political and patient satisfaction advantages to Medicare participation, there are also financial and administrative opportunities. The most significant are that Medicare fee schedule allowances are 5% higher for participating physicians, and assigned Medicare claims filed with Medigap insurance information are automatically forwarded by Medicare to supplemental insurance carriers for processing of coinsurance and deductible charges.[34] A copy of the Medicare Participating Physician or Supplier Agreement (Form CMS-460) is available at http://www.cms.hhs.gov/cmsforms/downloads/cms460.pdf.

Medicare Payment Methodologies for Anesthesia Services

Medicare's Resource Based Relative Value System

In 1992, Medicare implemented the Resource Based Relative Value System (RBRVS) that established a Medicare Fee Schedule (MFS) of national values for each clinical procedure code. The value comprises three relative value units that represent the physician's work effort in rendering the service, the practice's overhead expenses for items such as rent, office staff salaries and supplies, and malpractice insurance premiums. Under RBRVS, Medicare also implemented a new definition of allowed charges that paid physicians based on the lesser of the submitted charge or the new relative value scale fee-schedule–based amount.[35]

At the time of the introduction of the MFS in 1992, Anesthesiology had already had a relative value scale for anesthesia payment in place for 30 years.[36] The American Society of Anesthesiologists (ASA) Relative Value Guide, adopted almost in its entirety by the HCFA in 1989, uses values that represent components of anesthesia services: the base unit value related to the complexity of the service performed; and the time units based on the actual time the anesthesiologist spends with a patient.

Note the CMS definition of anesthesia time:

Anesthesia time means the time during which an anesthesia practitioner is present with the patient. It starts when the anesthesia practitioner begins to prepare the patient for anesthesia services in the operating room or an equivalent area and ends when the anesthesia practitioner is no longer furnishing anesthesia services to the patient, that is, when the patient may be placed safely under postoperative care. . . .[37]

Medicare does not reimburse for modifier units, such as those designated by the ASA recognizing physical status, extremes of age, or unusual risk.[38]

Medicare reimburses anesthesia services via a separate methodology under RBRVS that uses the sum of procedure-specific relative value units and the variable time units. The sum of these units is then multiplied by an anesthesia-specific conversion factor that is corrected for geographic cost differences. It was the retention of the time unit factor in the anesthesia payment methodology that drove HCFA to create a separate anesthesia conversion factor under RBRVS.

The Medicare Fee Schedule for Anesthesia Services

The distinction in the MFS for anesthesiologists has disadvantaged the specialty. A good illustration of the problem is the differential between Medicare and private insurance fees for anesthesiologists versus the differential for other medical and surgical specialists. The AMA reports that Medicare's conversion factor for physician services represents approximately 83% of the conversion factor paid by private insurers. For anesthesiologists, the Medicare conversion factor represents less than 40% of a private insurer's rate. Therefore, Medicare payments for anesthesia services are less than half of Medicare payments for other medical and surgical services.[39]

The ASA has raised this issue of disparity in Medicare fees many times with the AMA/Specialty Society Relative Value Update Committee (RUC). The RUC is the body charged with reviewing and advising CMS on updates to work-related relative value units that are required, by law, at least every 5 years. In the first 5-year review, HCFA acknowledged the undervaluation and approved a nearly 23% increase in work values for anesthesia procedures, effective January 1, 1997.[40] In the fee schedule effective after the second 5-year review, CMS again received endorsements for reconsideration of the anesthesia work relative value units but responded with an insignificant adjustment.[41]

The MFS is often referenced by private insurers as a standard in setting physician reimbursement rates. It is also common for physicians from other specialties, who enjoy a more favorable Medicare-to-private insurer fee ratio, to suggest the MFS as a proxy for valuing physician services. This often occurs during joint negotiations such as those used in dividing fees for contracts paid on a global basis to physician groups. Anesthesiologists are disadvantaged when the MFS is used in this manner. It is, therefore, important for anesthesiologists to remain active in the discussion of these physician payment disparities and to work to educate others and thereby mitigate the effect of these disparities in the Medicare system and beyond.

Proposed Changes to the Anesthesia Payment Methodology

Anesthesiologists are involved in these important public policy debates via the activities of their professional society, the ASA, and the ASA Political Action Committee. In late 2003, the ASA charged the "Task Force to Study Payment Methodology" with studying the relationship of the anesthesiology payment methodology to Medicare's relative value payment system. The Task Force projected the threat of decreasing revenues from the ongoing undervaluation of anesthesia services under Medicare, the adoption of the MFS and payment policies by private insurers, and the projected increase in numbers of Medicare beneficiaries in the United States.

The Task Force estimated that, with Medicare beneficiaries representing approximately 30% of anesthesia services nationwide, a blended conversion factor of Medicare and private insurers is $40.25. When Medicare accounts for 50% of services, the blended conversion factor will decrease to $33.75. Furthermore, if the MFS becomes the model for a single-payer system, they predict that the blended conversion factor will decrease to $17.50 (personal communication, Karin Bierstein, Esq., American Society of Anesthesiologists, November 30, 2004).

The Task Force has been exploring a flat fee payment methodology that would capture elements both of the time and the complexity of care for a continuous period of anesthesia for each operative period, involving one or more surgical procedures. This methodology would rely on a greatly expanded anesthesia code set that would incorporate an average anesthesia time representative of procedures performed in both the private practice and academic settings.

The Task Force recommendations for a new Medicare anesthesia payment methodology will be presented to the RUC and, if approved, will be reflected in future fee schedule revisions. The principles of the new methodology were announced in the following Task Force resolution passed by the ASA House of Delegates in October 2004:

RESOLVED, That the Executive Committee in consultation with the Administrative Council is authorized to propose a restructuring of Medicare payments for anesthesia services based on the following principles:

That any new coding system must accurately reflect both the complexity and duration of the associated surgical procedures to compensate for the elimination of separately reported anesthesia time;

That the inevitable influence of a uniform Medicare conversion factor on payment rates in the private sector be thoroughly considered; and

That any transition to a uniform Medicare conversion factor must be based on a value sufficient to protect the specialty, as a whole and in aggregate, from economic damage.

These resolutions were referred for further study, and the ASA does not expect that a modification in the anesthesia payment methodology will occur in the near term.[42]

The Sustainable Growth Rate Formula

The CMS uses a Sustainable Growth Rate (SGR) system to determine annual changes in the physician fee schedule. This system compares physician spending based on the volume and intensity of services provided against spending targets tied to inflation and the gross domestic product, and adjusts physician fee schedules accordingly to meet the targets. In 2002, this process resulted in a 5.4% reduction in physician fees, and the need for ongoing reductions was predicted up through 2016. This triggered congressional interventions that overrode the SGR system in the years 2003, 2004, and 2005 and mandated a Government Accounting Office (GAO) review of the problem.[43]

Anesthesiologists have a large stake in securing the success of these efforts, and other efforts to reform the

Medicare payment methodology specific to anesthesia services. However, it is important to note that unless there is modification of the SGR statute, any updates to the MFS must meet spending targets and, therefore, where one physician group gains, others must lose.

In a period when the Medicare program faces many economic challenges, it is unlikely that the interests of any one group of physicians will prevail without a strong, well-targeted political effort. A focus of this political effort in the future will be the discussion of the looming problem of access to anesthesia care by the ever-growing numbers of Medicare beneficiaries.

The Anesthesia Care Team

There are a variety of ways for anesthesiologists to provide services for reimbursement under Part B of the Medicare program. Medicare reimburses the services of an anesthesiologist when the physician personally provides them or if an anesthesia care team provides them under medical direction or supervision. Anesthesia claims modifiers are used to denote whether services were provided personally, "medically directed," or "medically supervised." Medicare reduces reimbursement based on the series of claims modifiers that denote how the services were delivered (Table 2-1).

The anesthesia care team is defined as an anesthesiologist working with any of the following professionals:

CRNAs
AAs
Residents or interns
Student Nurse Anesthetists (SNAs)[44]

In most cases, when an anesthesiologist and a CRNA are providing a single anesthesia service, Medicare recognizes the service as if personally performed by the anesthesiologist.

Medical Direction Versus Supervision of Concurrent Procedures

When an anesthesiologist is involved in directing up to four concurrent procedures, Medicare recognizes the services as concurrent medical direction and sets out specific guidelines for documentation and reimbursement of these services. (See Compliance section for documentation requirements.)

Anesthesiologists are allowed to furnish additional services to other patients under an exception to the four concurrent case limits. This exception, which varies by state, generally applies to the following services, if they do not "substantially diminish the scope of control exercised by the physician" providing the medical direction:

Addressing an emergency of short duration in the immediate area;
Administering an epidural or caudal anesthetic to ease labor pain;
Providing periodic, rather than continuous monitoring, of an obstetric patient;
Receiving patients entering the operating suite for the next surgery;
Discharging patients in the recovery room; or
Handling scheduling matters.[44]

When services are provided in excess of four concurrent cases and the allowed exceptions, the services will fail to meet the medical direction requirements. These services are provided under what Medicare terms medical "supervision" and are reimbursed to the physician at a fraction of the MFS allowable through limits in billing for base and time units. Under the supervision requirements,

TABLE 2-1. CMS Anesthesia Care Team Claims Modifiers Matrix.

Modifier	CMS definition	Payment % of allowable to provider
AA	Anesthesia services performed personally by anesthesiologist	100% to anesthesiologist
AA/GC	Anesthesia services performed personally by anesthesiologist with resident involvement	100% to anesthesiologist
QK	Medical direction of up to 4 concurrent anesthesia procedures involving qualified individuals	50% to anesthesiologist 50% to qualified provider*
QK/GC	Medical direction of up to 4 concurrent anesthesia procedures involving 2–4 residents	50% to anesthesiologist
QX	CRNA service with anesthesiologist medical direction (reported by CRNA)	50% to CRNA
QY	Medical direction of CRNA by anesthesiologist for 1 case (reported by anesthesiologist)	50% to anesthesiologist
AD	Medical supervision by a physician; more than 4 concurrent anesthesia procedures	3 base units, no time units. 1 unit if anesthesiologist documented presence at induction

Source: Author's compilation from Medicare Carriers Manual, Part 3: Claims Process. Transmittal 1690, Section 4830, Claims for Anesthesia Services Performed on and after January 1, 1992. Department of Health and Human Services, The Health Care Financing Administration. Published January 5, 2001.
*Residents are not qualified for reimbursement.

the physician must still ensure that a qualified individual performs any procedure in which they do not personally participate.[45]

Requirements of the Attending Physician Relationship

Physicians in academic practice fall under additional Medicare requirements that govern the "attending physician" relationship. This relationship exists when an attending anesthesiologist provides care to a patient in a teaching hospital involving anesthesia residents.

In 1992, when RBRVS was introduced, a new rule was announced that was to eliminate the practice of full reimbursement for an anesthesiologist medically directing two concurrent cases with anesthesia residents. The ASA was able to persuade Medicare to postpone implementation of the new rules until 1994; however, the impact of this change has been significant. The ASA estimates that the cost to academic anesthesiology programs of this change alone exceeds $50 million annually.[46] The ASA has been working to encourage CMS to restore full payment for two concurrent teaching cases.

In January 2004, CMS took an interim step toward changes in the reimbursement guidelines for medical direction of residents. The new rule expands billing options for teaching anesthesiologists who are involved in providing care with residents for two concurrent anesthesia cases. In the new ruling, anesthesiologists can choose to bill the usual base units and anesthesia time only for the period they are actually present with the resident if they are present throughout pre- and postanesthesia care and if this is documented.

In the rule, CMS has also included language that allows the attending anesthesiologist to determine if a request for payment of the full time payment for both cases is warranted. This request must be provided with written documentation that he/she spent "sufficient time" with each patient considering factors such as patient condition, residents' experience, proximity of the operating rooms, and the actual time the attending anesthesiologist spent in each operating room in making the determination.[47] Anesthesiologists choosing to use the interim rule as a revenue opportunity must weigh potential benefits against the compliance risks and the investments in faculty education and system modifications needed to support a new documentation and billing process.

Compliance Issues

All physicians who interact with the Medicare program are obligated to assure that their business practices conform to the requirements of the program. This can be a daunting task because although a busy participating physician can delegate Medicare transaction authority to others, he/she retains all of the responsibility and risks related to the actions of his/her agents. Furthermore, the stakes for providers are high. Physicians who are found to be in violation of Medicare regulations can suffer both civil and criminal penalties as well as exclusion from the program. Physician practices can minimize the risks by adopting comprehensive compliance plans and assuring thorough internal controls, and training for all physicians and staff.

The Office of the Inspector General (OIG) does not mandate the adoption of compliance programs, but they have formulated seven fundamental elements of an effective compliance program. These elements are:

- Implement written policies, procedures, and standards of conduct
- Designate a compliance officer and compliance committee (e.g., a billing clerk and physician in a small practice)
- Conduct effective training and education
- Develop effective lines of communication
- Enforce standards through well-publicized disciplinary guidelines
- Conduct internal monitoring and auditing
- Respond promptly to detected offenses and develop corrective action plans[48]

Anesthesiologists should consult with their compliance officers to gain what should be an in-depth understanding of their obligations as providers in the Medicare program. An introduction to some of the key compliance issues affecting anesthesia practice, including reassignment of benefits, Medicare fraud and abuse initiatives, and medical record documentation follows.

For further information on compliance programs, one should consult the OIG postings in the Federal Register and on the OIG Web site at http://oig.hhs.gov/fraud/complianceguidance.html.

Reassignment of Medicare Benefits

Anesthesiologists who provide care to Medicare beneficiaries undertake responsibility for compliance with myriad complex and sometimes conflicting regulations. Anesthesiologists who practice in a group or academic setting, where administrative duties for billing and collections are delegated and Medicare payments are frequently reassigned to another entity, should be best informed of these responsibilities.

When a physician reassigns benefits under the Medicare program, they legally authorize another person or entity to bill Medicare on their behalf and to receive payments that would otherwise be sent directly to them. However, despite this written delegation of authority, the physician retains all responsibility for ensuring that the claims made on their behalf are in full compliance with Medicare regulations. In addition, the physician retains responsibility for assuring that their agent meets all confidentiality obligations and other state and federal regulations.

Even the best-intentioned physician may encounter difficulties in determining how to meet his/her obligations for compliance with Medicare regulations. The GAO tested the accuracy of carriers' responses to inquiries in a telephone audit. The GAO asked staff at the Medicare carriers to respond to "frequently asked questions" concerning physician billing procedures that were taken from the carriers' own Web sites. The GAO survey report concluded that physicians who do call their carriers with questions would "more often than not receive wrong or inaccurate answers." These problems were attributed to limits on resources for information system modernization and oversight activities, and limits on CMS's authority imposed by the Congress and Executive branches.[49]

Medicare Fraud and Abuse

Although the federal government has chosen to limit CMS resources for facilitating its administrative mission, it has significantly increased resources for the investigation of fraud and abuse. Public administration experts have noted that these resources could be better spent on preventive measures such as improved management of the program and effective measures to monitor and deter inappropriate payments, thereby minimizing the need for enforcement. However, this has not occurred and, as of 2000, CMS spent more than 25% of its total administrative expenses in its campaign against fraud and abuse.[49]

Many federal agencies are involved in protecting the Medicare program and ensuring provider compliance with all regulations. The OIG in the Department of Health and Human Services investigates suspected Medicare fraud or abuse and develops cases against providers. It has the authority to audit and inspect CMS programs and to act against individual providers with civil money penalties and/or exclusion from participation in all federal health care programs. The OIG also has authority to refer cases to the United States Department of Justice for criminal or civil action.[50] In its 2006 semiannual report, the OIG evidenced an active role in combating waste, fraud, and abuse, citing savings of more than $38.2 billion, 3425 exclusions, 472 criminal actions against individuals and entities, and 272 civil actions.[51]

Medicare defines fraud as "the intentional deception or misrepresentation that an individual knows to be false or does not believe to be true and makes, knowing that the deception could result in some unauthorized benefit to himself/herself or some other person." Abuse relates to practices that directly or indirectly result in unneces-

sary costs to the Medicare program. It is similar to fraud but is found when there is no evidence that the acts were committed knowingly, willfully, and intentionally.[52]

Some examples of fraud that should be immediately apparent to providers include activities such as the falsification of records, billing for services that were not furnished, or misrepresenting the type of service provided by using inappropriate codes. However, other actions that also constitute fraud and abuse may not be as apparent to providers. These include providing incentives to Medicare patients not provided to other patients such as the routine waiving or discounting of patient coinsurance and deductible payments. Other actions include billing Medicare on a higher fee schedule than other patients, breaching the agreements to accept assignment or participate in the Medicare program, or failing to provide timely refund of overpayments made by Medicare and beneficiaries.[52]

Physicians at Teaching Hospitals: Office of the Inspector General Initiative

Physicians in academic practice have been made most keenly aware of government efforts to enforce compliance with Medicare rules. Over the past decade, the government recovered $149 million from 15 universities that failed to document compliance with Medicare payment policies related to attending physician supervision of services provided with resident involvement.[49]

The Physicians at Teaching Hospitals (P.A.T.H.) initiative of the OIG has had long-lasting and costly effects on academic practices. Physician groups that paid settlements or were subject to civil or criminal prosecution were required to enter into multi-year Institutional Compliance Agreements with the federal government. These agreements impose requirements that closely follow the structure of a compliance program but can be more stringent.[53] They obligate practices to develop and adhere to a rigorous set of compliance standards involving audits of physician billing practices and annual physician and staff education, under threat of additional penalties. AHCs have reported that annual compliance program costs, after P.A.T.H. settlement, are absorbing millions of dollars.[54]

Documentation Requirements

Medical record documentation is the primary source used for judging compliance with Medicare regulations. Documentation should be timely and must support the medical necessity of the service as well as the level and scope of service provided. As with all medical record documentation, it must be legible and signed by the provider. Bills should not be submitted unless adequate documentation exists for the services.

Documentation of Anesthesia Time

The prominence of time in the Medicare reimbursement methodology for anesthesiologist services drives documentation requirements. Since January 1, 1994, Medicare has reimbursed anesthesia time based on the actual number of minutes of anesthesia provided calculated in fractions of 15-minute units, rounded to one decimal place.[37] This standard for the precise documentation and reporting of anesthesia time presents challenges, especially in practices without automated anesthesia record-keeping systems.

Unsynchronized timepieces within the operating room suite can create disparities in timekeeping documentation as recorded by the anesthesiologist and other members of the surgical team such as nurses, perfusionists, and surgeons. Unsynchronized timepieces between anesthetizing locations and a lack of diligence can also cause an anesthesiologist to create the appearance of overlap of anesthesia services (i.e., concurrency) when indeed the services were provided consecutively. These discrepancies frequently become apparent upon subsequent audit of the documentation when it is more difficult to initiate corrections.

Documentation of Medical Direction

When an anesthesiologist is involved in directing up to four concurrent procedures, Medicare recognizes the services as concurrent medical direction.

Documentation of concurrent medical direction must support the physician's completion of "7 steps." This documentation evidences that the physician:

Performs a preanesthesia examination and evaluation;
Prescribes the anesthesia plan;
Personally participates in the most demanding procedures in the anesthesia plan, including, if applicable, induction and emergence;
Ensures that a qualified individual performs any procedures in the anesthesia plan that he or she does not perform;
Monitors the course of anesthesia administration at frequent intervals;
Remains physically present and available for immediate diagnosis and treatment of emergencies; and
Provides indicated postanesthesia care.[44]

In May 2004, CMS issued new interpretive guidelines for surveyors regarding the documentation of the inpatient postanesthesia assessment as required in the Hospital Conditions of Participation for the Medicare Program. The revision allows the postanesthesia follow-up to be performed and documented by the individual who administered the anesthesia, or by a delegated practitioner who is qualified to administer anesthesia.[55]

Documentation by Teaching Physicians

In January 1997, Medicare imposed a requirement for use of the "GC" claim modifier to denote the involvement of residents in the delivery of anesthesia services and to certify that the teaching anesthesiologist was present during key portions of the service and immediately available during other parts of the service. In 1999, CMS extended the requirement to include a written attestation from the attending physician that these requirements were met.[56]

In November 2002, CMS implemented revised guidelines governing the documentation requirements for teaching physicians who care for patients with the involvement of resident physicians. These requirements restrict payment for teaching physician services to those that support the presence of the teaching physician during key portions of an anesthesia procedure and during the entire time for separately reimbursable procedures such as line and catheter insertions.

The most complex of these guidelines govern the documentation of teaching physician involvement with residents in the provision of evaluation and management services. Interested physicians should consult the Medicare Carriers Manual, Section 15016 for specifics of these guidelines. However, there are important general principles that the anesthesiologist should follow in all cases whether or not the resident and teaching physician services are provided contemporaneously:

- Teaching physicians cannot evidence their presence and participation via documentation of these activities by the resident or by "countersigning" a resident's note. They may reference the resident's note in their own note, but must independently document presence and participation in the critical portions of the service.
- The composite of the teaching physician's note and the resident's note may be used to support the medical necessity and level of service billed.[57]

Physician providers must be proactive in assuring compliance with the complex and dynamic requirements of participation in the Medicare program. Development of a compliance program, review of physician billing and documentation, and ongoing education and training of providers and staff will help physicians minimize compliance risk.

Summary

Medicare is the primary health plan serving our nation's elderly, an important source of revenue for physician and hospital providers, and a major underwriter of medical education and charity care in the United States. The program will experience growing, annual deficits starting in 2010 when Medicare costs are first predicted to exceed financing sources as the baby boomers begin to retire. In the interim, strategies for dealing with the impending crisis in Medicare will be a continual source of debate and providers should be represented in the discussions.

A large majority of anesthesiologists in the United States are enrolled as participating providers in the Medicare program. Many of the rules and regulations governing their interactions with the program are unique to the practice of anesthesiology and have significant implications for how clinical and business operations are conducted and whether, indeed, participation remains a viable strategy for anesthesiologists in the future. Geriatric anesthesiologists, by virtue of their subspecialty focus, should be best informed of Medicare policy issues and should participate in ongoing discussions to reshape Medicare as it enters an uncertain future.

References

1. Corning PA. The evolution of Medicare . . . from idea to law. Available at: http://www.ssa.gov/history/. Accessed September 28, 2004.
2. Gluck MG, Reno V, eds. Reflections on Implementing Medicare. Washington, DC: National Academy of Social Insurance; 2001:43.
3. Marmor TR. The Politics of Medicare. Chicago: Aldine Publishing; 1973.
4. Gluck MG, Reno V, eds. Reflections on Implementing Medicare. Washington, DC: National Academy of Social Insurance; January 2001:iii.
5. U.S. Social Security Administration. http://www.ssa.gov/history/. Accessed September 28, 2004.
6. The Centers for Medicare and Medicaid Services. http://ww.cms.hhs.gov/MedicareEnRpts. Accessed October 17, 2004.
7. Iglehart JK. The American health care system: Medicare. Health Policy Rep 1999;340:327–332.
8. Moon M. Health policy 2001: Medicare. N Engl J Med 2001; 344:928–931.
9. Lubitz J, Beebe J, Baker C. Longevity and Medicare expenditures. N Engl J Med 1995;332:999–1003.
10. U.S. Census Bureau. www.census.gov/population/www/projections/natdet-D1A.html. Accessed October 18, 2004.
11. The Centers for Medicare and Medicaid Services. http://ww.cms.hhs.gov/publications/trusteesreport. Accessed October 18, 2004.
12. http://www.AARP.org/econ/boomer. Accessed October 9, 2004.
13. Center for Medicare Education. http://www.medicareed.org/resources. Accessed October 18, 2004.
14. Estimates of medicare beneficiaries' out-of pocket drug spending in 2006. Available at: http://www.kff.org. Accessed November 24, 2004.
15. The Medicare prescription drug benefit. Available at: http://www.kff.org/medicare. Accessed December 8, 2006.
16. Rice T, Bernstein J. Supplemental Health Insurance for Medicare Beneficiaries. Medicare Brief No. 6.

    Available at: http://www.nasi.org/Medicare/Briefs/medbr6.htm. Washington, DC: National Academy of Social Insurance; November 1999.
17. Rowland D, Feder J, Seliger Keenan P. Managed care for low-income elderly people. Generations: Q J Am Soc Aging 1998(Summer);22:45.
18. Kaiser Family Foundation and Health Research and Educational Trust. Employer health benefits: 2006 summary of findings. Available at http://www.kff.org/insurance/7527/upload/7528.pdf. Washington, DC. Accessed December 8, 2006.
19. Families USA Foundation. Shortchanged: Billions Withheld from Medicare Beneficiaries. Publication No. 98-103. Washington, DC. July 1998. p. 1.
20. Piette JD, Heisler M, Wagner TH. Cost-related medication underuse. Arch Intern Med 2004;164:1749–1755.
21. Poisal JA, Murray L. Growing differences between Medicare beneficiaries with and without drug coverage. Health Aff 2001;20:74–85.
22. Davis M, Poisal J, Chulis G, et al. Prescription drug coverage, utilization, and spending among Medicare beneficiaries. Health Aff 1999;18:231–243.
23. National Institute for Health Care Management Research and Education Foundation. Factors affecting the growth of prescription drug expenditures. Available at http://www.hihcm.org. Accessed July 9, 1999.
24. The Commonwealth Fund. Caught in Between: Prescription Drug Coverage of Medicare Beneficiaries Near Poverty. Issue Brief No. 669. New York; August 2003.
25. Iglehart J. The new Medicare prescription-drug benefit—a pure power play. N Engl J Med 2004;350:826–833.
26. The Centers for Medicare and Medicaid Services. http://www.cms.hhs.gov/charts/series/sec3-C.pdf. Accessed December 3, 2004.
27. National Academy of Science. The Roles of Academic Health Centers in the 21st Century: A Workshop Summary. Washington, DC; 2002.
28. The Centers for Medicare and Medicaid Services. http://www.cms.hhs.gov/media. January 31, 2005, release accessed February 7, 2005.
29. Vuletich M. Pay for performance: is it right for an academic practice? MGMA Connex 2005;69.
30. The Centers for Medicare and Medicaid Services. http://www.cms.hhs.gov/researchers/pubs/datacompendium/2003. Accessed October 18, 2004.
31. The Centers for Medicare and Medicaid Services. http://www.cms.hhs.gov/faca/ppac/oral_asa.pdf. Accessed November 29, 2004.
32. The Centers for Medicare and Medicaid Services. http://www.cms.hs.gov/manuals/14_car/3btoc.asp. Chapter 17. Accessed December 6, 2004.
33. The Centers for Medicare and Medicaid Services http://www.cms.hhs.gov/about/regions/professionals.asp. Accessed December 6, 2004.
34. Centers for Medicare and Medicaid Services. Medicare Resident and New Physician Guide: Helping Health Care Professionals Navigate Medicare. 7th ed. Baltimore: Centers for Medicare and Medicaid Services; August 2003:16.
35. The Centers for Medicare and Medicaid Services www.cms.hhs.gov/publications/overview. Accessed November 29, 2004.

36. Ogunnaike BO, Giesecke AH. ASA Relative Value Guide (RVG): a defining moment in fair pricing of medical services. ASA Newslett 2004;68:15–17.

37. Medicare carriers' manual. Part 3. Chapter 15, Section G. Rev. 1690 p. 15. Available at: http://www.cms.hhs.gov/manuals. Accessed November 1, 2004.

38. The Centers for Medicare and Medicaid Services. http://www.cms.hhs.gov/physicians/pfs/wrvu-ch1.asp. Accessed November 29, 2004.

39. Bierstein K. Medicare is still the wrong benchmark. ASA Newslett 2002;66:25–27.

40. Scott M. The American Society of Anesthesiologists. http://www.asahq.org/newsletters/1997/-1_97/washington_0197.html. Accessed October 12, 2004.

41. The Centers for Medicare and Medicaid Services. http://www.cms.hhs.gov/faca/ppac/oral_asa.pdf. Accessed November 29, 2004.

42. Novak LC, Cohen NA. The American Society of Anesthesiologists. http://www.asahq.org/Newsletters/2005/09-05/whatsNew09_05.html. Accessed December 8, 2006.

43. U.S. Government Accountability Office. http://www.gao.gov/docsearch/abstract.php?rptno=GAO-05-85. Accessed October 20, 2004.

44. Carrier's manual. Part 3. Chapter 8. Available at: http://www.cms.hhs.gov/manuals/14_car/3b8000.asp. Accessed November 1, 2004.

45. Carrier's manual. Part 3. Chapter 8. Revision 1690, Section 15018. Fee schedule for physicians' services. Available at: http://www.cms.hhs.gov/manuals/pm_trans/R1690B3.pdf. Accessed December 6, 2004.

46. Hannenberg A, Scott M. The American Society of Anesthesiologists. http://www.asahq.org/Newsletters/2002/12_02/hannenberg.html. Accessed October 12, 2004.

47. The Centers for Medicare and Medicaid Services. http:/// www.cms.hhs.gov/manuals/ CMS transmittal 34, December 24, 2003. Accessed December 7, 2004, and 8310 conditions for payment of charges—anesthesiology services, rev. 1287/pp. 8–53. Accessed November 1, 2004.

48. The Centers for Medicare and Medicaid Services. http://www.cms.hhs.gov/medlearn/mrnp-guide.pdf. p. 121. Accessed October 17, 2004.

49. Iglehart J. The Centers for Medicare and Medicaid Services. N Engl J Med 2001;345:1920–1924.

50. The Centers for Medicare and Medicaid Services. http://www.cms.hhs.gov/medlearn/mrnp-guide.pdf. p. 9. Accessed October 17, 2004.

51. Office of Inspector General. http://www.oig.hhs.gov/publications/docs/semiannual/2006. Accessed December 8, 2006.

52. The Centers for Medicare and Medicaid Services. http://www.cms.hhs.gov/medlearn/mrnp-guide.pdf. pp. 124–126. Accessed October 17, 2004.

53. The Centers for Medicare and Medicaid Services. http://www.cms.hhs.gov/medlearn/mrnp-guide.pdf. pp. 131–132. Accessed October 17, 2004.

54. Swann M. Fast-tracking compliance training in academic practices. Am Coll Med Pract Exec Coll Rev 1999;16:61–88.

55. The Centers for Medicare and Medicaid Services. Interpretive guidelines §482.52(b)(4). Available at: http://www.cms.hhs.gov/manuals/107_som/som107_appendixtoc.asp. Accessed January 31, 2005.

56. The Centers for Medicare and Medicaid Services. http://www.cms.hhs.gov/manuals/. CMS transmittals 1690 and 1723, January 5, 2001 and September 26, 2001. Accessed November 1, 2004.

57. The Centers for Medicare and Medicaid Services. http://www.cms.hhs.gov/medlearn/mrnp-guide.pdf. pp. 134–135. Accessed October 17, 2004.

3
Theories of Aging

Stanley Muravchick

"Gerontology" refers to the application of the various scientific disciplines to the study of aging. Aging manifests itself in most organisms as a gradual decline in the capacity to maintain anabolic processes or to respond to environmental change. Degenerative changes in both the physical structure and the functional capacity of organs and tissues are the clinical characteristics of human aging. In all species, regardless of how aging makes itself apparent, the implied consequence of aging is an increased probability of death as a function of time.

Longevity can be expressed either in terms of lifespan or life expectancy (Figure 3-1). Lifespan is an idealized, species-unique parameter that quantifies maximum attainable age under optimal environmental conditions. Life expectancy represents an empirical estimate of typical longevity under prevailing or predicted circumstances. Increased life expectancy is therefore a socioeconomic, not a biologic, phenomenon. Consequently, biogerontologists usually limit the scope of their investigations to the physiologic and biochemical mechanisms of aging and to those biologic factors that determine lifespan.

Concepts of Aging

It is clear that genetics are intrinsically and fundamentally involved in aging and therefore in longevity, but exactly how this occurs is only now being established. Almost a century ago, a controversial and apparently flawed study of chick fibroblasts cells grown in vitro suggested that immortality might be achievable in the absence of all noxious or detrimental environmental influences.[1] However, it now seems that freedom from senescence may be possible only for cancer cells, not for fully differentiated cells or functional tissues.[2] Therefore, at least for the foreseeable future, human aging and death are inevitable realities.

The precise mechanisms that underlie the aging process and ultimately determine lifespan in biologic systems remain unknown. To date, no single theory of aging has explained satisfactorily all the observed patterns of human senescence or accounted for the differences between human aging and the aging of other species.[3] In general, however, theories of aging fall into two major categories. One category encompasses nonrandom, predictable, and centrally determined or preprogrammed processes. The other grouping includes several theories that describe random or "stochastic" mechanisms.

Programmed Aging

Theories of programmed or predetermined aging are similar in that they invoke a common theme of a "biologic clock" or "life pacemaker" that confers the unique longevity of each species. For example, there is good correlation between species lifespan and the number of cell doublings that can be expected when cells of a single type such as an embryonic fibroblast are taken from a wide variety of animals and grown in culture.[4] This suggests that there may be an intracellular mechanism that limits reproductive capacity, or perhaps there is a section of the nuclear genome that provides a species-specific phenotype dedicated to lifespan. Similarly, the "codon restriction theory" suggests that there are programmed changes in the capacity of cells that vary the kinds of proteins that will be generated during different stages of life.[5]

If either of these theories are valid, experimental manipulation of the "pacemaker" or "clock" sections of the genome should produce dramatic changes in lifespan. Every genomic segment is, however, also subject to the processes of natural selection that affect the entire genome.[6] There is little selective evolutionary advantage for a species to survive past the age of sexual maturity and rearing of offspring. For humans, for example, this would require a lifespan of only 30–40 years.[7] Because reproductive capacity seems to be the major determinant of species survival, phenotypic changes that favor longevity without altering fecundity should be unaffected by

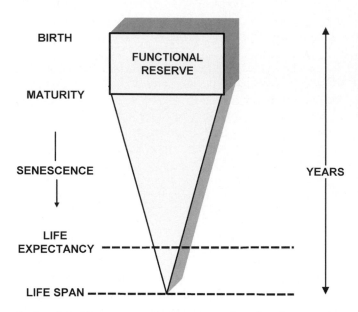

FIGURE 3-1. The concept of organ system functional reserve has been described as a "wedge" broadest at birth that then declines progressively after maturity. Applying this concept to human aging, genetically determined organ system functional reserve may determine lifespan but life expectancy reflects "real world" estimates of human longevity given extrinsic environmental factors. (Data from Jazwinski SM. Longevity, genes, and aging. Science 1996;273:54–59.)

evolutionary processes. Consequently, evolutionary theories of aging and longevity are unable to support the concept that there are specific genes that cause aging or control lifespan.[8] A "programmed aging" locus would have no species survival value and therefore would not be expected to persist intact in the genome throughout the long time course of evolution, although some evidence suggests that human cellular senescence could be a manifestation of evolutionary pressures to prevent malignant transformation.[9]

In fact, favorable changes in the genome segments that control reproduction and enhance species survival could have deleterious effects on postmaturation viability and lifespan. Senescence characterized by decreasing viability may be the price to be paid to sustain immortality of the species-specific germline at the expense of individual survival.[10] A genomic locus that determines lifespan is rarely found in nature unless the reproduction of that species requires the death of the mature adult as the final step of the reproductive process. This phenomenon is seen in plants, insects, and some fishes where the linkage between reproduction and death is mediated by programmed neuroendocrine mechanisms.[11]

Mammals express a well-defined aging phenotype with great similarities between mammalian species, yet many amphibians, reptiles, and sharks and other primitive fishes fail to show obvious physical signs of aging. Mammalian

aging could therefore have evolved along with other unique phenotypic mammalian characteristics, and it may not be the same process as the age-related biologic phenomena seen in some nonmammals.[12] Examination of the properties of genetic variation in Drosophila also supports the concept that aberrancies and mutations may not be nearly as important in determining longevity as is the underlying species phenotype.[13]

An external pacemaker tissue or organ must also be present to coordinate the aging-related interactions between tissues and multiple organ systems that characterize normal senescence, especially in humans. Therefore, this type of theory usually requires that neuroendocrine or immune mechanisms have a central role in processes of aging. Despite considerable investigation and some early data suggesting the importance of changes in hypothalamic activity in aging,[14] however, there has been little objective evidence that a neuroendocrine or other hormonal "pacemaker" tissue as envisioned actually exists. It is therefore highly unlikely that aging or longevity are precisely programmed genetic events.[15]

Stochastic Aging

Stochastic aging theories include a thermodynamic perspective that looks at increases or decreases in specific entropy production (SEP). In effect, viability is seen as a struggle against breakdown of intracellular order and structure. Growth and development represent an increase in order but aging is characterized as a breakdown in biologic order and an increase in randomness.[16] The higher and more complex the organism, the greater the maximum SEP. Biologic stress and aging have similar thermodynamic properties and their underlying principles have been described using common parameters.[17] Cells and tissues are conceptualized as "open systems" that are subject to energy and material flux and therefore require active energy expenditure to maintain physical order. They are in a nonequilibrium or "far-from-equilibrium" steady state. From this perspective, "normal" aging is an evolving, slowly changing state characterized by increased cell damage (less order) and decreased bioenergetic capacity. SEP therefore declines during aging as the ability to extract energy from the environment decreases.

In simplest terms, stochastic theories propose that physical and biochemical signs of aging may be a simple function of time and probability. The now-classic "genetic wear and tear" or "error-catastrophe" theory of aging is an example of this group. Originally, it suggested that degradation of the integrity of nuclear DNA (nDNA) over time generated random errors of genomic reproduction and transcription that accumulate. Eventually, the essential molecules needed for cell viability are no longer synthesized.[18] Progressive compromise of cellular and tissue function over time, therefore, produces the physical and clinical signs of aging. This theory predicts that there is an age-related increase in the fraction of proteins that are functionally defective, and that the error rate eventually rises exponentially as the key components of protein synthesis are themselves subject to defects or shortages.

Overall, however, the evidence that mammalian aging is a random breakdown in biologic order because of life-long accumulation of genomic errors caused by genetic mutations, remains very weak.[19] At least in human cells, faulty protein accumulates slowly throughout adulthood and the geriatric years and damage to the cells and micro-architecture seems to reflect secondary, not primary, errors in amino acid sequence. Nor does biologic order deteriorate at an accelerating or exponential rate.

It is true, however, that many of the enzymes that accumulate in the tissues of older subjects are less active and more susceptible to heat inactivation and proteolysis,[20] but these seem to be oxidized proteins that appear gradually, usually with methionine moieties or as various "glycated" molecules. Biologic amines can react non-enzymatically with glucose and other reducing sugars to form yellow-brown or fluorescent crosslinked complexes. They are precursors to irreversibly bound crosslinking agents called advanced glycation end products (AGEs). Advanced glycation, originally seen in vitro, now is known to occur in living tissues. AGEs randomly interconnect lipoproteins and proteins and disrupt uniform molecular alignment, reducing elasticity and increasing "stiffness" in tissues containing structural collagen.[21]

AGEs in the vascular tree may accumulate even more rapidly with chronic exposure to high levels of reducing sugars, as occurs in poorly controlled diabetics, and may predispose to intravascular plaque formation and produce loss of cardiovascular elasticity.[22] Ethanol is metabolized in vivo to acetaldehyde which then produces a chemically stabilized complex that resists rearrangement in the presence of reducing sugars and therefore does not progress to AGE formation. This may explain the so-called "French paradox," by which moderate chronic ethanol ingestion, for example, daily wine consumption, seems to confer a significant degree of protection from coronary artery disease.[23] Work in laboratory animals confirms that drugs or chemicals that block glycation or act as "crosslink breakers"[24] may reverse at least some of the clinical stigmata of the senescent cardiovascular system. However, confirmation of this concept in human studies has yet to be reported.

Aging is also associated with a progressive decline in the ability of cells and organelles to scavenge and degrade these and other types of defective proteins.[25] Normally, oxidized proteins undergo preferential degradation within the cell by the proteasomal system. There is a multicatalytic protease complex—the proteasome—as well as numerous other regulatory factors involved in the degradation of oxidized proteins.[26] The proteasome is present in the cytosol, nucleus, and endoplasmic reticulum of mammalian cells, but is itself subject to oxidative deterioration during aging and therefore may become progressively less effective in older individuals.[27]

Telomere shortening is another form of stochastic nDNA damage that has been invoked as a possible source of age-related decline. Located at the ends of eukaryotic chromosomes and synthesized by telomerase, telomeres are the genomic units that maintain the length of chromosomes. Human cancer cells demonstrate high telomerase activity. However, although there is a general association between cellular senescence and telomere shortening in vitro,[28] there is little evidence that telomere shortening is intrinsically associated with, or causally related to, normal human aging. Similarly, there is general correlation between species longevity and nDNA repair capacity but no firm evidence that the ability to recover from random nDNA damage is, in fact, progressively or universally compromised in older human subjects.

Other potential stochastic mechanisms include random nDNA methylation, a process that correlates with transcriptional silence of many genes. When nDNA mutations occur, enzyme systems that repair DNA are a second line of defense designed to return nDNA to its original genetic integrity. Another potential genomic mechanism for aging, therefore, is compromised expression of the enhancer and repressor/suppressor elements that, in turn, activate or inhibit gene expression, particularly of the components of DNA repair mechanisms. This may become important in cancer biology because tumor genes are not expressed until the environmental stimuli that maintain the suppression are removed. A similar process could be important in aging. A third possible mechanism of aging at the cellular level relates to messenger RNA (mRNA) production. Many proteins and enzymes decrease in concentration with aging. This seems in some cases to be a direct result of decreases in the mRNA levels which encode the protein. Hence, age-related limitation of the rate or accuracy of the transcription of mRNA from nDNA may be involved.

Altered Receptor Systems

Recent research in the discipline of molecular pharmacology has generated huge amounts of data with regard to biologic receptor systems, especially within the nervous system. With aging, there are decreases in acetylcholine synthesis and release as well as reduction of muscarinic receptor plasticity. This suggests a causal connection between impairment of central cholinergic function and aging. A "cholinergic" theory of aging[29] is even more attractive given the clear role of cholinergic deficiencies in Alzheimer-type dementia[30] and perhaps other age-related neurodegenerative disorders. Gamma-aminobutyric acid (GABA), a major inhibitory neurotransmitter, is an important site of drug action for anesthetic agents and another possible locus for aging within the nervous system. GABA receptors and other ligand-gated ion channels have been shown to have decreased specificity to their agonist molecules in older adults.[31] Although the demonstration of consistently decreased anesthetic requirement in older adults[32] is another intriguing clue supporting the concept of a link between aging and altered neurotransmitter dynamics, these observations have yet to be formulated into a coherent theory of aging that proposes a fundamental role for central nervous system receptors.

Oxidative Stress

Not all stochastic theories of aging focus on the state of DNA within the cell nucleus. Reactive oxygen species (ROS) or "free radicals" are routinely produced in the mitochondria as a byproduct of aerobic metabolism and oxidative phosphorylation.[33] If allowed to accumulate to high levels, ROS such as superoxide, impose a state of "oxidative stress" within the cell that can damage or destroy organelle and even molecular microarchitecture.[34] These toxic effects may be direct or they may be the consequences of a cascade of biochemical events. Investigations of oxidative phosphorylation in aging mitochondria confirm that aging is associated with both progressive decreases in mitochondrial energy generation[35] and increased levels of defective mitochondrial DNA (mtDNA),[36] presumably because of excessive ROS. Older mitochondria also demonstrate a loss of membrane potential and a decrease of both fusion and fission activity.[37] It is less clear whether increased ROS levels in the cytosol of a cell can damage nDNA, which is centrally located in the nucleus and relatively shielded from oxidation.

According to this general concept, sustained and life-long oxidative stress compromises the enzymatic machinery required for full bioenergetic capacity and also damages the mtDNA needed for synthesis of enzymes such as glutathione peroxidase and superoxide dismutase. These enzymes protect cells from metabolic byproducts by scavenging ROS as they are produced in the mitochondria. Two centuries ago, the renowned scientist Joseph Priestly, discoverer of oxygen's life-sustaining properties, speculated quite presciently that too much oxygen might lead to premature failure of oxidative processes. Therefore, from this perspective at least, aging at a cellular level can be considered a form of chronic oxygen toxicity. ROS, the byproducts of aerobic metabolism that is essential for life in all higher organisms, may generate a "vicious cycle" of progressive bioenergetic

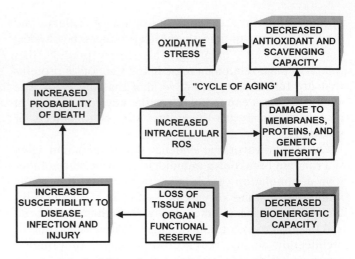

FIGURE 3-2. Insidious increases in concentrations of reactive oxygen species (ROS) throughout the adult years generate a "cycle of aging" that may explain both the decreased bioenergetic capacity that characterizes senescent tissues and the increased morbidity and mortality exhibited by a geriatric patient population. (Data from Ozawa.[66])

failure and functional compromise in the mitochondria (Figure 3-2).

Reconciling the Theories

Nevertheless, purely stochastic theories such as those invoking oxidative stress fail to explain the dramatically different patterns of aging that are seen in various animals despite the fact that virtually all species share a common ecosystem, have similar metabolic processes and byproducts, and are exposed to similar catabolic environmental forces. In fact, aging may reflect the degenerative consequences of a lifetime of exposure to the byproducts of aerobic metabolism that have not been successfully detoxified by the genetically determined processes available to protect the integrity of the cell genome, maintain normal neurotransmitter dynamics, and preserve full bioenergetic capacity (Figure 3-3). Viewed as progressive failure of a species-specific, genetically predetermined capacity to avoid or repair random damage to proteins, lipids, nDNA, and mtDNA by ROS, a concept that identifies accumulated oxidative stress as the underlying driving force of aging is compatible with most aging theories, both stochastic and nonstochastic.[38] Nor does the consistency of observed lifespan for a given species necessarily imply a discrete "biologic clock" or a "lifespan" gene for each species. Rather, it may reflect the net effect of many genes in the phenotype of each species whose expression influences the aging and longevity of that life form. These genetic factors have been described as "gerontogenes."[39]

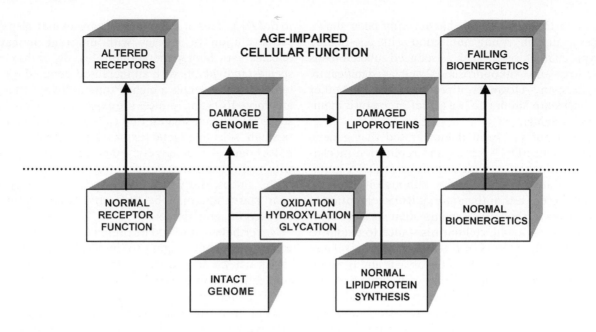

FIGURE 3-3. Proposed molecular mechanisms of aging include damage to the cellular and mitochondrial genome and disruption of cellular microarchitecture, including membrane-bound receptor complexes.

It is becoming plausible, therefore, that lifespan may reflect a stochastic interaction between the genetically determined biochemical and physiologic attributes of each species and the internal and external destructive factors that disorder biologic systems.[40] Consequently, exploring how each species is equipped genetically to deal with metabolic and environmental stress, therefore, has become a fundamental and crucial step in understanding the molecular biology of aging. The "theory of disposable soma" postulates that some species have increased their reproductive capacity in exchange for decreased lifespan.[41] However, other evolution theory suggests that the longer-lived species have evolved because of their greater degree of genetic investment in a more durable soma, including mechanisms, many perhaps complex and requiring considerable cell resources, that enhance cellular resistance to stress. "Hormesis," the low-level state of chronic oxidative stress that induces expression of genes that can increase the effectiveness of stress responses in mammals (also described as ischemic, hypoxic, or anesthetic "preconditioning"), may be more easily initiated in some species than in others. In fact, stress-induced expression of genes that facilitate cell repair is well established: cold stress has been shown to prolong lifespan in the nematode *Caenorhabditis elegans*[42] and heat stress significantly increases longevity of the fruit fly, *Drosophila melanogaster*.

Birds, and perhaps other nonmammalian species, also possess a mitochondrial lipid structure that is more resistant to oxidative damage than that of mammals.[43] This may confer a special adaptation that prevents the age-related tissue damage seen in mammals that is caused by ROS or AGEs. Avian lifespan is markedly prolonged relative to that of most mammals with comparable metabolic rates. Bird mitochondria also produce significantly less ROS than those of mammals, but it is not clear whether their specific bioenergetic capacity is significantly different.[44] In the nematode *C. elegans*, a genetic mutation with increased activities of antioxidative enzymes also has lifespan significantly greater than the wild-type strain.

Point mutations and deletions of mtDNA accumulate in adult humans, monkeys, and some laboratory rodents. Although these mutations are only a small proportion of total mtDNA and are randomly or clonally distributed in different tissues, the amount of defective mtDNA found in the heart and brain of mammalian species ranging in maximum lifespan from 3.5 to 46 years has been shown to be inversely correlated with lifespan. In addition, genetically altered mice that express a proofreading-deficient version of mtDNA polymerase develop into a young adult mouse phenotype with a three- to fivefold increase in mtDNA point mutations and increased mtDNA deletions. In these mice, the increased number of somatic mtDNA mutations has recently been shown to be associated in young adulthood with age-related phenotypic characteristics such as reduced subcutaneous fat, hair loss, and osteoporosis as well as significantly reduced lifespan.[45] However, it remains unclear whether these changes are similar to, or actual premature manifestations, of aging.

It has also not yet been demonstrated that genetic manipulation of mtDNA repair and replication mechanisms can produce mice with decreased mtDNA mutation rates and increased longevity, although it has been shown that there is less mitochondrial ROS generation in long-lived than in short-lived mammalian species. Most relevant to human aging, cellular resistance to oxidative stress has recently been shown to be closely correlated with mammalian longevity. Skin fibroblasts and lymphocytes from eight mammalian species with a range of lifespans show a direct correlation between cellular resistance to chemical, alkaline, and oxidative stress and the maximum lifespan of the species.[46] These results agree with the concept that ROS in mitochondria produce accumulating oxidative damage to mtDNA[47,48] (Figure 3-4) and perhaps to other key cellular components that in some way is related to the aging rate of each mammalian species.[49]

The theory that aging is a direct consequence of the accumulation of oxidative damage caused by ROS is consistent with the observed effectiveness of caloric restriction as a therapy that prolongs the life expectancy of laboratory rodents.[50] Caloric restriction may lower mitochondrial ROS levels and may reduce oxidative damage

to mtDNA. This or a similar mechanism may also explain the evolution of species with different longevities.[51] Species with higher metabolic rates, or, within a given species, individuals with an increased demand for oxidative energy may have a higher "rate of living" that generates more ROS and reduces life expectancy. Alternatively, some recent data suggest that caloric restriction, perhaps through selective gene expression, actually increases mitochondrial bioenergetic efficiency and is associated with suppression of metabolic stress responses.[52] Changes in the glucose–fatty acid cycle that occur in response to near starvation may be protective when calories are reduced in aging tissues.[53]

Nevertheless, it would be premature to attribute aging, in particular human aging, to simple bioenergetic deterioration caused by oxidative stress.[54] There is a general correlation between species longevity and the capacity to repair damaged DNA but evidence that the ability to recover from random oxidative DNA damage is progressively or universally compromised in older human subjects remains elusive.[55] In addition, although several investigations have confirmed that defective mtDNA increases in the cells of older subjects, it is not established that this produces a critical reduction of the macromolecules needed for normal bioenergetics.[56] In addition, the interaction between ROS and the bioenergetic apparatus is now known to be far more complex than was once believed. Peroxiredoxins represent a group of at least six isoforms of a multifunctional peroxidase.[57] They have recently been identified in many species and are believed to provide protection against the low-level oxidative stress associated with peroxide accumulation yet they do not appear to influence longevity.[58] Similarly, the overexpression of superoxide dismutase and catalase enhances resistance to experimental oxidative stress but decreases, rather than increases, lifespan of transgenic *Drosophila melanogaster*.[59] Taken together, these observations suggest that normal lifespan reflects a subtle and complex equilibrium between the byproducts of oxidative metabolism and endogenous mechanisms that respond to oxidative stress.

Human Aging and Geriatrics

The term "geriatrics" was coined at the start of the twentieth century[60] to describe the clinical subspecialty area of medicine that focuses on care of the elderly patient. But, as yet, there is still no consensus as to when the "geriatric" era begins in human subjects or whether any single physiologic marker can unequivocally identify a patient as "elderly." Therefore, establishing rigid or finite chronologic definitions of the term "geriatric" has little value other than for administrative, actuarial, or epidemiologic applications. Nevertheless, although it may have

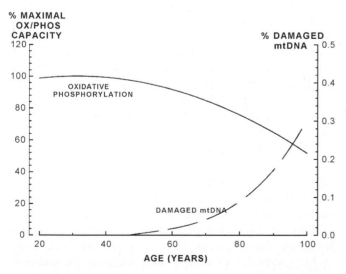

FIGURE 3-4. Recent studies of human tissues support the evolving concept that accumulation of damaged mitochondrial DNA (mtDNA) in the early geriatric era leads to a progressive decline in bioenergetic capacity and oxidative phosphorylation. (Data from Mandavilli et al.[47])

increased rapidly from the onset of human evolution until about 100,000 years ago, when the brain weight/body ratio of our hominid ancestors stabilized at the current value for modern humans,[61] empirical evidence and historical anecdote suggest that human lifespan has remained constant at about 120 years for at least the past 20 centuries.

In contrast, the past century has seen dramatic advances in medical science and health care that have greatly increased life expectancy in industrialized societies, especially in Japan and the United States, increasing the relative "agedness" of those societies.[62] However, the increased life expectancy so often invoked in discussions of "the graying of America" is a socioeconomic, rather than a biologic, phenomenon that steadily enlarges that fraction of the general human population considered "elderly." If, in fact, maximum human lifespan is fixed but life expectancy increases in response to elimination of disease and other external threats to longevity, the human survival curve may continue to undergo the "rectangularization"[63] that results in the compression of age-related morbidity and mortality into the later years of the geriatric era.[64] Yet, there is some evidence that human lifespan may not yet have reached its ultimate maximum value. The time perspective of metrics used in modern biology is so limited relative to the many millennia of human existence that subtle increases in lifespan may actually be occurring undetected.

Clinical Studies of Aging

All geriatricians accept increased interindividual variability as a hallmark of their patient populations. As they age, adults continually exhibit a progressively more varied array of physical responses to concurrent disease states which, in turn, reflect their lifelong exposure to environmental and socioeconomic conditions and to the accumulated stigmata of prior traumatic injuries and medical therapies. Prolonged longevity also enables complete expression of intrinsic genetic qualities in all their subtle physiologic manifestations. In effect, people are never more alike than they are at birth, nor more different or unique than when they enter the geriatric era.

Therefore, interpretation of clinical studies of human aging remains difficult and progress in understanding mechanisms of aging has been correspondingly slow. Yet, much has been learned about the relative strengths and weaknesses of the various forms of epidemiologic investigation used by gerontologists and geriatricians. Cross-sectional studies measure physiologic parameters simultaneously in young and in elderly subjects. Changes caused by undiagnosed age-related disease may be erroneously attributed to aging, and this experimental design cannot be controlled for cohort-specific factors such as nutritional and environmental history, genetic back-

ground, or prior exposure to infectious agents. Cross-sectional designs do not provide sufficient evidence for the interdependence of aging-related changes and therefore they probably should not serve as the final basis for theories and hypotheses of aging.[65]

Longitudinal designs provide a much stronger basis for inference regarding rates and characteristics of human aging. They require that the investigator obtain repeated measurements in each individual subject over several decades. Each subject therefore generates his own "young adult" control value for comparison with subsequent measurements. If any of the subjects in a longitudinal study eventually manifest signs of age-related disease, their data points can be excluded from the study, thereby leaving behind a smaller but more homogeneous group of healthy elderly subjects. Survival to and through adulthood and beyond also permits the full expression of even the subtlest genetic differences between individuals that might not be fully apparent over shorter lifespan intervals. In longitudinal studies, the signs and symptoms of aging become progressively more apparent or severe with increasing chronologic age. Any changes in structure or function that are not found in all members of a geriatric population, or those changes that do not seem to have a direct relationship between severity and chronologic age, can be attributed to age-related disease rather than to aging itself.

Although difficult and expensive to organize and maintain, long-term longitudinal studies have therefore produced substantial amounts of extremely valuable data related to human aging. Nevertheless, this methodology has some pitfalls. It requires establishing a chronologic "starting point" for the geriatric era, an arbitrary value that may change significantly during the study because of increases in life expectancy. In addition, the validity and utility of the data may be compromised by the inevitable evolution or revision of physiologic concepts and the refinement of measurement techniques that invariably occur over the time periods required to study human aging. Last, it is difficult to attract new physician scientists to a form of clinical investigation in which the answers to the scientific questions that are being asked may not be known during the lifetime of the investigator himself.

Summary

There is currently great scientific interest and experimental activity under way to fully define the role of long-term oxidative stress as a cause of increasing damage to mtDNA and intracellular protein.[66] As awareness of the roles of mitochondrial genetics and oxidative stress in mechanisms of senescence and death has increased among biogerontologists, the various theories of aging have begun to coalesce and unify. Genetically determined ability to scavenge ROS and to repair accumulated or randomly acquired damage to intracellular enzymes and organelles does, in general, correlate with longevity, both in humans and in other species that show phenotypic change with age. Declining bioenergetics and a reduction in capacity for oxidative phosphorylation also seems to explain the age-related clinical deterioration of maximal organ function that inevitably occurs throughout human adulthood, even in the most fit older subjects. In fact, many researchers already believe that it is progressive failure of mitochondrial bioenergetics that produces normal human aging as well as many aspects of age-related degenerative disease.[67]

References

1. Carel A. On the permanent life of tissues outside of the organism. J Exp Med 1912;15:516–528.
2. Hayflick L. The limited in vitro lifetime of human diploid cell strains. Exp Cell Res 1965;57:614–636.
3. Hayflick L. Biologic and theoretical perspectives of human aging. In: Katlic MR, ed. Geriatric Surgery: Comprehensive Care of the Elderly Patient. Baltimore: Urban and Schwarzenberg; 1990:3–21.
4. Hayflick L. The biology of human aging. Am J Med Sci 1973; 265:433–445.
5. Strehler BL. Aging: concepts and theories. In: Viidik A, ed. Lectures on Gerontology. New York: Academic Press; 1982: 1–57.
6. Gershon H, Gershon D. Paradigms in aging research: a critical review and assessment. Mech Ageing Dev 2000;117: 21–28.
7. Bidder GP. Senescence. Br Med J 1932;15:5831.
8. Ameisen JC. On the origin, evolution, and nature of programmed cell death: a timeline of four billion years. Cell Death Diff 2002;9:367–393.
9. Troen BR. The biology of aging. Mt Sinai J Med 2003;70: 3–22.
10. Kirkwood TB. Sex and ageing. Exp Gerontol 2001;36:413–418.
11. Sacher GA. Molecular versus systemic theories on the genesis of aging. Exp Gerontol 1968;3:265–271.
12. de Magalhaes JP, Toussaint O. The evolution of mammalian aging. Exp Gerontol 2002;37:769–775.
13. Partridge L. Evolutionary theories of ageing applied to long-lived organisms. Exp Gerontol 2001;36:641–650.
14. Finch CE. Neuroendocrine mechanisms and aging. Fed Proc 1979;38:178–183.
15. Harman D. Aging: overview. Ann NY Acad Sci 2001;928: 1–21.
16. Strehler BL. Genetic instability as the primary cause of human aging. Exp Gerontol 1986;21:283–319.
17. Toussaint O, Schneider ED. The thermodynamics and evolution of complexity in biological systems. Comp Biochem Physiol A Molec Integr Physiol 1998;120:3–9.
18. Orgel LE. The maintenance of the accuracy of protein synthesis and its relevance to ageing. Proc Natl Acad Sci USA 1963;49:517–521.
19. Orgel LE. The maintenance of the accuracy of protein synthesis and its relevance to ageing; a correction. Proc Natl Acad Sci USA 1970;67:1476.
20. Stadtman ER. Protein oxidation in aging and age-related diseases. Ann NY Acad Sci 2001;928:22–38.
21. Lee AT, Cerami A. Role of glycation in aging. Ann NY Acad Sci 1992;663:63–70.
22. Ulrich P, Cerami A. Protein glycation, diabetes, and aging. Recent Prog Horm Res 2001;56:1–21.
23. Al Abed Y, Mitsuhashi T, Li H, et al. Inhibition of advanced glycation end product formation by acetaldehyde: role in the cardioprotective effect of ethanol. Proc Natl Acad Sci USA 1999;96:2385–2390.
24. Vaitkevicius PV, Lane M, Spurgeon H, et al. A cross-link breaker has sustained effects on arterial and ventricular properties in older rhesus monkeys. Proc Natl Acad Sci USA 2001;98:1171–1175.
25. Reznick AZ, Lavie L, Gershon HE, et al. Age-associated accumulation of altered FDP aldolase B in mice: conditions of detection and determination of aldolase half life in young and old animals. FEBS Lett 1981;128:221–224.
26. Stolzing A, Grune T. The proteasome and its function in the ageing process. Clin Exp Dermatol 2001;26:566–572.
27. Gray DA, Tsirigotis M, Woulfe J. Ubiquitin, proteasomes, and the aging brain. Sci Aging Knowledge Environ 2003: 2003(34):RE6.
28. Ahmed A, Tollefsbol T. Telomeres and telomerase: basic science implications for aging. J Am Geriatr Soc 2001;49: 1105–1109.
29. Gallagher M, Colombo PJ. Ageing: the cholinergic hypothesis of cognitive decline. Curr Opin Neurobiol 1995;5: 161–168.
30. Yew DT, Li WP, Webb SE, et al. Neurotransmitters, peptides, and neural cell adhesion molecules in the cortices of normal elderly humans and Alzheimer patients: a comparison. Exp Gerontol 1999;34:117–133.
31. McGeer EG, McGeer PL. Age changes in the human for some enzymes associated with metabolism of catecholamines, GABA, and acetylcholine. Adv Behav Biol 1975;16: 287–305.
32. Munson ES, Hoffman JC, Eger EI II. Use of cyclopropane to test generality of anesthetic requirement in the elderly. Anesth Analg 1984;63:998–1000.
33. Nagy IZ. On the true role of oxygen free radicals in the living state, aging, and degenerative disorders. Ann NY Acad Sci 2001;928:187–199.
34. Sohal RS, Weindruch R. Oxidative stress, caloric restriction, and aging. Science 1996;273:59–63.
35. Knight JA. The biochemistry of aging. Adv Clin Chem 2000; 35:1–62.
36. Wei YH, Lee HC. Oxidative stress, mitochondrial DNA mutation, and impairment of antioxidant enzymes in aging. Exp Biol Med 2002;227:671–682.
37. Jendrach M, Pohl S, Voth M, Kowald A, Hammerstein P, Bereiter-Hahn J. Morpho-dynamic changes of mitochondria during ageing of human endothelial cells. Mech Ageing Dev 2005;126:813–821.
38. Golden TR, Melov S. Mitochondrial DNA mutations, oxidative stress, and aging. Mech Ageing Dev 2001;122: 1577–1589.

39. Rattan SI. Ageing, gerontogenes, and hormesis. Indian J Exp Biol 2000;38:1–5.
40. Skulachev VP. Programmed death phenomena: from organelle to organism. Ann NY Acad Sci 2002;959:214–237.
41. Mangel M. Complex adaptive systems, aging and longevity. J Theor Biol 2001;213:559–571.
42. Lithgow GJ, Walker GA. Stress resistance as a determinate of *C. elegans* lifespan. Mech Ageing Dev 2002;123:765–771.
43. Herrero A, Barja G. H_2O_2 production of heart mitochondria and aging rate are slower in canaries and parakeets than in mice: sites of free radical generation and mechanisms involved. Mech Ageing Dev 1998;103:133–146.
44. Holmes DJ, Fluckiger R, Austad SN. Comparative biology of aging in birds: an update. Exp Gerontol 2001; 36:869–883.
45. Trifunovic A, Wredenberg A, Falkenberg M, et al. Premature ageing in mice expressing defective mitochondrial DNA polymerase. Nature 2004;429:417–423.
46. Kapahi P, Boulton ME, Kirkwood TB. Positive correlation between mammalian life span and cellular resistance to stress. Free Radic Biol Med 1999;26:495–500.
47. Mandavilli BS, Santos JH, Van Houten B. Mitochondrial DNA repair and aging. Mutat Res 2002;509:127–151.
48. Sugiyama S, Hattori K, Hayakawa M, et al. Quantitative analysis of age-associated accumulation of mitochondrial DNA with deletion in human hearts. Biochem Biophys Res 1991;180:894–899.
49. Barja G, Herrero A. Oxidative damage to mitochondrial DNA is inversely related to maximum life span in the heart and brain of mammals. FASEB J 2000;14:312–318.
50. Masoro EJ, Bertrand H, Liepa G, et al. Analysis and exploration of age-related changes in mammalian structure and function. Fed Proc 1979;38:1956–1961.
51. Barja G. Endogenous oxidative stress: relationship to aging, longevity and caloric restriction. Ageing Res Rev 2002;1: 397–411.
52. Lee C-K, Klopp RG, Weindruch R, et al. Gene expression profile of aging and its retardation by caloric restriction. Science 1999;285:1390–1392.
53. Heininger K. Aging is a deprivation syndrome driven by a germ-soma conflict. Ageing Res Rev 2002;1:481–536.
54. Huang H, Manton KG. The role of oxidative damage in mitochondria during aging: a review. Front Biosci 2004;9: 1100–1117.
55. Lieber MR, Karanjawala ZE. Ageing, repetitive genomes and DNA damage. Nat Rev Mol Cell Biol 2004;5:69–75.
56. Maklashina E, Ackrell BA. Is defective electron transport at the hub of aging? Aging Cell 2004;3:21–27.
57. Rhee SG, Chae HZ, Kim K. Peroxiredoxins: a historical overview and speculative preview of novel mechanisms and emerging concepts in cell signaling. Free Radic Biol Med 2005;38:1543–1552.
58. Immenschuh S, Baumgart-Vogt E. Peroxiredoxins, oxidative stress, and cell proliferation. Antioxid Redox Signal 2005;7:768–777.
59. Bayne AC, Mockett RJ, Orr WC, Sohal RS. Enhanced catabolism of mitochondrial superoxide/hydrogen peroxide and aging in transgenic Drosophila. Biochem J 2005;391(Pt 2): 277–284.
60. Nascher IL. Geriatrics. NY Med J 1909;90:358–359.
61. Hofman MA. Energy metabolism, brain size and longevity in mammals. Q Rev Biol 1983;58:495–512.
62. Schneider EL, Reed JD Jr. Life extension. N Engl J Med 1985;312:1159–1168.
63. Comfort A. The Biology of Senescence. 3rd ed. New York: Elsevier; 1979:414 pp.
64. Fries JF. Aging, natural death, and the compression of morbidity. N Engl J Med 1980;303:130–135.
65. Hofer SM, Sliwinski MJ. Understanding ageing: an evaluation of research designs for assessing the interdependence of ageing-related changes. Gerontology 2001;47:341–352.
66. Ozawa T. Genetic and functional changes in mitochondria associated with aging. Physiol Rev 1997;77:425–464.
67. Calabrese V, Scapagnini G, Giuffrida Stella AM, et al. Mitochondrial involvement in brain function and dysfunction: relevance to aging, neurodegenerative disorders and longevity. Neurochem Res 2001;26:739–764.

4
Ethical Management of the Elderly Patient

Paul J. Hoehner

Because of the increasing growth of the elderly population, geriatric care is rapidly emerging as a unique medical specialty in its own right. Advancements in medical science and changes in the health care delivery system that impact the care of the elderly are accompanied by myriad ethical dilemmas that confront not only the physician and patient, but social workers, nursing home staff, and relatives. Settings involving the extremes of age and illness are the most complex in ethical deliberation. Although anesthesiologists may confront a variety of ethical issues, such as patient confidentiality, care of Jehovah's Witnesses, substance abuse, and so forth, this chapter will focus on those issues unique to and more likely to be encountered in the elderly patient.

Social Views of Aging

Social views of aging are inherently present and basically informative within any application of ethical principles to ethical problems involving the elderly. Therefore, it is important to recognize that one's view of aging can and will influence both clinical decision making as well as the application of ethical principles to individual concrete situations. Although contemporary views of aging are complex and varied, Gadow[1] helpfully outlines a spectrum of views, each of which contribute to the apparent social and moral value of the elderly patient and the resolution of ethical problems. First, aging can be viewed as the antithesis of health and vigor. This negative interpretation of the aging process is expressed in deceptively "objective" descriptions of the clinical changes in aging as "deterioration," "disorganization," and "disintegration," from the level of psyche to the level of cellular physiology. Gadow points out, however, that there is nothing a priori degenerative about changes in aging unless one "uncritically accepts as the only ideal of health the condition that younger individuals manifest."[1,2] Furthermore, it is a mistake to think of the elderly as gener-

ally sick and impaired. Patricia Jung notes that, "Clearly, to expose as false those myths that portray the old as inescapably and increasingly physically decrepit, mentally incompetent, desexualized persons best kept isolated in nursing homes is an important first step toward discerning what it means to age."[3] For many, old age is not a time of disability or disease; instead it is a time of remarkably good health. According to one government study, 72.3% of noninstitutionalized elderly persons described their health as "excellent," "very good," or "good," and only 27.6% described their health as "fair" or "poor."[4] Nevertheless, this same study showed that in 1990 persons over the age of 65 experienced more than two and a half times the number of days of activity restriction because of acute and chronic conditions as persons between the ages of 25 and 44, with 37.5% of people over the age of 65 experiencing some activity limitation caused by chronic conditions. Health care workers, whose contact with the elderly is naturally skewed toward those who are acute or chronically ill, and/or institutionalized, are especially prone to this unambiguously negative account found in the "decline model" that so powerfully dominates our cultural interpretation of aging.

Second, aging can be viewed as an unwelcome reminder of our mortality. Medicine, at least a little like Shelley's modern Prometheus,[5] tends to seek for and attain progress within the human condition in ways that defy its own ability to know what to do next. Shaped by the pervasive story of our therapeutic culture,[6] health care workers and their patients are driven by an interest in longevity that reaches far beyond the merely academic, emanating as it does from a desire to avoid suffering and certainly from a fear of death. Growing old in our therapeutic culture encourages us to desire perpetual youthfulness and gives us the power to strive for it (to some degree successfully, or, at least, cosmetically), but also forces us to ask just how old we really want to live to be. And as we age, for how long and in what ways do we care for ourselves? Advances in medicine bring new psychologic and ethical challenges, both for those who are older and for those who are living with and caring for them. For instance, the more natural and acceptable mortality is thought to be for the elderly, the more unthinkable it is for the non-elderly. This view can lead to the avoidance of the elderly as symbols of the unthinkable.

Medical and social views of aging can reflect the full diversity of a spectrum ranging from the philosophy that the elderly have *less* social and moral value than other individuals, to the other extreme of having *greater* value than others. The most positive of all attitudes is that of the elderly as a cultural treasure, a repository of wisdom, and an embodiment of history. Gadow[1] also observes another emerging perspective that treats the elderly as underprivileged citizens. This view bypasses the question of the intrinsic value of the elderly for society and brings them "out of the closet" to become recipients of our benevolence toward them as an "oppressed" group. The potential danger with this view is that by designating the elderly as "handicapped" individuals, and thereby as a special group needing services, the beneficiaries remain subordinate to the benefactor and may even become victim to the extremes of unwarranted paternalistic care.

A development inherent to the rise of geriatric medicine as a specialty is the view of aging as a clinical entity in its own right. Positively, aging is viewed as a unique human phenomenon worthy of specialized attention. The elderly are not health deviants but present special problems as well as special strengths not found in other populations. Surely this is a welcome view that will, and has already, greatly contributed to the understanding and care of many issues unique to this growing population (the focus of this textbook being one example). Negatively, the subspecialty approach to geriatric medicine may become a model for a broader social approach to the elderly whereby aging would be of interest as a "highly specific class of unusual phenomena, bearing little relation to the more general features of experience shared by persons of all ages."[1] Aging may be viewed not as a normal life process, with little or no purpose, but as a disease in itself. Yet much of what has been assumed mistakenly to be the "plight" of the elderly is in fact the consequence of specific pathologies not properly associated with aging. Chronic illnesses and degenerative diseases often associated with aging are frequently a result of lifestyle choices. Although aging may be associated with some rote memory loss, recent studies repeatedly indicate that the basic cognitive competence of the elderly does not deteriorate with age. There is some evidence of positive growth in certain more complex, integrative mental abilities. Peter Mayer notes in his essay "Biological Theories about Aging" that even physical changes such as osteoporosis among postmenopausal women and immune system decline which were once presumed to be

an inevitable result of growing old are now understood to be the consequence of specific medical conditions or other factors such as malnutrition.[7]

Ethical Principles

In our modern society, categories of right and wrong or decisions regarding the "good" are frequently characterized by competing rational philosophical theories (such as deontology, utilitarianism, natural law), as cultural and tradition-dependent artifacts, or as arising from individualistic or relativistic (e)motives. The classic paradigm of modern medical ethics, often referred to as "principlism," originated in a pragmatic attempt to overcome the impasse of these competing ethical theories in order to derive common and self-evident "principles" that would serve to guide a common language/paradigm of biomedical ethical decision making. This almost universally accepted paradigm of modern medical ethics revolves around the principles of respect for personal autonomy, beneficence, nonmaleficence, and justice. This paradigm, which has been extensively discussed in many basic medical ethics texts, will be assumed for the remainder of this chapter.

Recent work in medical ethics has focused on alternative frameworks based on such concepts as "virtue ethics," the "narrative life," and "personhood." These concepts may overcome some of the philosophical limitations of the traditional approach and provide a more firm theoretical grounding that can thereby proceed to the level of principles more appropriate for use in the elderly population. One exemplary approach is that of Spielman[8] who appropriates the moral anthropology of Hauerwas to build a more adequate principled approach to geriatric ethics. Hauerwas emphasizes an ethic of virtue that grows out of his conviction that "what one does or does not do is dependent on possessing a 'self' sufficient to take responsibility for one's actions."[9] Three aspects of the self, which are relevant to applying Hauerwas' work, are its temporal dimension, its social dimension, and its tragic or limited dimension.

Unlike the standard account of post-Kantian ethics in which the moral life is seen in terms of obedience to a set of rational, timeless principles, Hauerwas presents character, developed within the context of a particular story or narrative, as the key to the moral life. According to this temporal dimension, life is not seen as a series of discontinuous decisions but rather as a challenge to be faithful to a true story or history. Contemporary ethical theory tends to view the ideal human as a self-sufficient, independent moral agent, without social ties. Hauerwas' social dimension emphasizes the fact that we are all historical beings and cannot avoid being part of larger communities. Our ability to think and our ability to act are embedded in a social structure in which even the descriptions of our actions depend on language, which is a public possession. Human existence also has a necessarily tragic or limited dimension. Medicine cannot eradicate suffering and death in our lives. By using MacIntyre's characterization of medicine as a tragic profession, Hauerwas suggests that medical ethics cannot be limited to casuistic analyses of particular sets of problems and issues. He notes the continuity between the kind, of issues raised by medicine and the rest of our lives and raises important issues involved in the practice of medicine relative to the elderly, such as limited resource allocation. Hauerwas shows that not only are the history and the relationships of the self significant, but that the limitations inherent in medical treatment of the elderly cannot be ignored.[10]

Figure 4-1 illustrates how the temporal, social, and tragic or limited dimensions of human existence can be used to develop principles more appropriate to developing a geriatric ethic according to Spielman. The dimensions of temporality and sociality can be recognized in the increasing dependence on others as one ages. A more useful principle than autonomy is one of continuity. This principle may be stated as: "Act so that you avoid disrupting the continuity of past, present, and future values, commitments, and relationships in older people's lives." The purpose of the principle is to prevent the loss, as one ages, of a sense of the unity of one's life. Balancing the aspects of limitation and sociality helps to recognize and not ignore the elderly patient's social needs and desire to maintain some degree of independence. This avoids the temptation of caregivers to rely on institutional care when independence cannot be maintained. Silverstone[11] notes that the tendency for the physician to view chronically impaired patients with a biomedical disease-oriented framework contributes to a hospital-like solution to the patient's problems. This principle can be stated: "seek out the appropriate level of support and care for older patient," a level of care that maximizes independence and maintains the highest level of functioning. Because complete independence is usually neither possible nor desirable, "interdependence" with friends, relatives, and service providers more aptly describes this principle. Finally, the aspects of limitation and temporality suggest the principle of normality. Aging does not have to be seen as a disease or as a form of deviance. This principle would argue against treating every age-related change as a disease or problem to be solved. Rather, the aging process is valued, given the limitations it imposes, as a normal part of the human life narrative.

Informed Consent in the Elderly

Respect for Personal Autonomy

Many ethical conundrums in medical ethics are the result of specific principles coming into conflict in specific cases. The principle of respect for personal autonomy is sometimes taken to be *the* overriding principle in modern ethical deliberation. However, respect for personal autonomy does not, and should not, exhaust moral deliberation. Other principles are important and not only when autonomy reaches its limits. Childress notes that focusing on the principle of respect for personal autonomy can foster indifference and that the principles of care and beneficence are important even in discussions of informed consent. The role played by the principle of respect for personal autonomy is one of setting limits, such that, "without the limits set by the principle of respect for autonomy, these principles (beneficence, nonmaleficence, and justice) may support arrogant enforcement of "the good" for others."[12] Yet, the principle of respect for autonomy is not absolutely binding and does not outweigh all other principles at all times. Two different approaches have been used by ethicists to resolve conflicts or apparent contradictions between competing principles. First is to construct an a priori serial ranking of the principles, such that some take absolute priority over others. Second, principles can be viewed as prima facie binding, competing equally with other prima facie principles in particular circumstances. This view requires one to view more closely the complexities and particularities of individual cases and is more situational in context. The prima facie principle of respect for autonomy can be overridden or justifiably infringed when the following conditions are satisfied: (1) when there are stronger competing principles (proportionality); (2) when infringing on the principle of respect for personal autonomy would *probably protect* the competing principles (effectiveness); (3) when infringing the principle of respect for personal autonomy is *necessary* to protect the competing principle(s) (last resort); and (4) when the infringement of the principle of respect for personal autonomy is the *least intrusive or restrictive* in the circumstances, consistent with protecting the competing principle(s) (least infringement).[12]

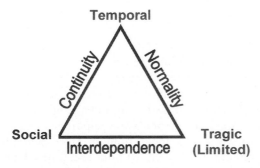

FIGURE 4-1. Principles of a geriatric ethic derived from Hauerwas' dimensions of human nature. (Adapted with permission from Spielman.[8])

Shared Decision Making

Aside from the legal requirements and the specter of malpractice, recent discussions of "informed consent" have focused on the concept of "shared decision making" and the clinical-therapeutic role of the informed consent process in improving patient care. These discussions recognize that there should be a collaborative effort between physicians and patients to arrive at appropriate treatment decisions. The physician brings knowledge and trained judgment to the process, whereas the patient brings individual and unique priorities, needs, concerns, beliefs, and fears. Focusing on the process of informed consent, as opposed to bare legal requirements, increases a patient's participation in his or her own care, which may result in increased patient compliance and self-monitoring. Informed consent as "teaching" (indeed, the origin of the word "doctor" is from "teacher") further diminishes patients' misconceptions or inaccurate fears about their situation and prospects and may improve patient recovery or comfort with a better understanding of the care that is being provided. No good data are available regarding these "therapeutic" effects of informed consent, and further studies seem warranted. Despite these theoretical positive aspects, issues surrounding informed consent remain vexing for physicians in a number of clinical situations from both legal and ethical perspectives. Even the ideal model of "shared decision making" does not address many of the realities of medical practice, including emergency situations, conflicts of interest, and questions of futility.

By emphasizing informed consent as a temporal "process," one can avoid the pitfalls of viewing informed consent as a single event. Informed consent can never be reduced to a signature on a consent form. "Perhaps the most fundamental and pervasive myth about informed consent is that informed consent has been obtained when a patient signs a consent form. Nothing could be further from the truth, as many courts have pointed out to physicians who were only too willing to believe this myth."[13] Although a matter of routine in many institutions because they are seen as providing protection against liability, informed consent forms actually provide very little. The informed consent form does have value in that it provides an opportunity for the patient to read the information on the form and to create a *locus* for the appropriate patient–physician discussion that is the key element. An informed consent form merely documents that the "process" of informed consent has taken place.

Traditionally, consent to anesthesia in the past was subsumed under the consent to the surgical procedure and included within the surgery consent form. The anesthesiologist was one step removed from the formal consent process. Today, separate specific consent for anesthesia is required in most states. It is imperative that the

TABLE 4-1. Elements of the process of informed consent.

Threshold elements (preconditions)
  Decision-making capacity or competency
  Freedom or voluntariness and absence of overriding state or legal
    interests

Informational elements
  Adequate disclosure of material information
  Recommendation
  Understanding

Consent elements
  Decision
  Authorization

anesthesiologist make a concerted effort to adequately complete this process with the patient and, when appropriate, the patient's family regarding the anesthetic procedure and adequately document in a note the patient's consent on the chart or anesthetic record (above and beyond any signature on a standard form issued by a ward clerk).

Beauchamp and Childress[14] have broken down the process of informed consent into seven elements (Table 4-1). These include threshold elements or preconditions, which include (1) decision-making capacity or competency of the patient, (2) freedom or voluntariness in decision making, including absence of overriding legal or state interests; informational elements including (3) adequate disclosure of material information, (4) recommendations, and (5) an understanding of the above; consent elements, which include (6) decision by the patient in favor of a plan and (7) authorization of that plan. Several of these elements can pose particular challenges in the elderly population.

Threshold Elements

Decision-Making Capacity

Physicians are frequently faced with the problem of making treatment decisions for elderly patients who no longer have decision-making capacity. Many diseases and conditions that can make continued life contingent on life-prolonging therapies can also destroy or substantially impair a person's decision-making capacity and are more likely to do so in older people. In addition, Alzheimer's disease and other forms of dementia are more likely to be present in older persons. One estimate is that 5% to 7% of persons over 65, and 25% of those over 84, suffer from severe dementia.[15] Assessment of decision-making capacity even in cases of mild dementia can be particularly difficult.[16] Decision-making capacity requires: (1) a capacity to understand and communicate, (2) a capacity to reason and deliberate, and (3) possession of a set of values and goals.[17–19] Although there is general agreement regarding these three requirements, there is no single, universally accepted standard of decision-making capacity. This is because decision-making capacity is not an all-or-nothing concept. Decision making is also a task-related concept and the requisite skills and abilities vary according to the specific decision or task. The relevant criteria should also vary according to the risk to a patient. Basically, one must ask the following questions: Does the patient understand his or her medical condition? Does the patient understand the options and the consequences of his or her decision? Is the patient capable of reasonable deliberation? Is the patient able to communicate his or her decision? Does the patient possess a coherent set of values and/or goals? Several reviews provide helpful discussions of the clinical assessment of elderly patients' decision-making capacity within these contexts.[20–22] Instruments such as the MacArthur Competence Assessment Tool-Treatment (MacCAT-T) may provide a flexible yet structured method with which physicians and other caregivers can assess, rate, and report patients' abilities relevant for evaluating capacity to make treatment decisions.[23]

Informed consent in the elderly patient presents other unique aspects.[24] Sugarman et al.[25] conducted a structured literature review in the published empiric research on informed consent with older adults (aged 60 years and older). Diminished understanding of informed consent information was associated with older age and with fewer years of education. Although showing some impairment in their quality of reasoning, the elderly are able to reach reasonable risk-taking decisions to the same degree as young adults.[26,27]

To what extent must a patient "understand" his or her condition, treatment options, and risks?[28] If fully "informed" is meant to mean fully "educated"[29] then "informed" consent may be seen as an impossible standard. However, the primary object of information is to facilitate the patients' care rather than providing a litany of possible complications in order to avoid a lawsuit. Factual knowledge is used, not as an end in itself, but as a means to extend the patients' own understanding in such a way as to meet their own unique priorities, needs, concerns, beliefs, and fears so that they may decide about their care in the manner in which they normally make similar choices. This will vary from patient to patient and with the risks of the procedure involved. It is a mistake to assume that a patient must understand information to the same extent and in the same manner as a physician, or even as a well-educated layman. This may indeed be seen as just as paternalistic as not permitting patients to participate in decision making at all.[13]

Visual and hearing impairments and diminished memory and comprehension in the elderly patient require the clinician to exercise particular caution when obtaining informed consent.[30] One must also be careful to avoid the mistake of equating recall, a standard endpoint in many studies on the adequacy of informed consent and which may be problematic in the elderly, with understanding and comprehension. Meisel and Kuczewski[13] note that, "While it may be true that someone who cannot retain information for a few seconds might not be said to understand it, people often make reasonable decisions but cannot later recall the premises that supported the reasoning or the process that led to the conclusion." Distant recall of the informed consent process may be an indicator of the adequacy of a patient's understanding, but its absence says little about the patient's understanding at the time of consent. Physicians also tend to underestimate patients' desire for information and discussion and, at the same time, overestimate patients' desire to make decisions.[31–33] Elderly patients and their physicians often differ on patient quality-of-life assessments that may be associated with clinical decisions.[34] These studies and others underscore the need for clear communication, individualization, and compassion in obtaining adequate informed consent in the elderly. New strategies to maximize comprehension of informed consent information (e.g., storybooks, videos, and so forth) also may be useful.[25]

Assessment of patient capacity to enter into the process of informed consent or competency to make rational medical decisions is a complicated issue. Much has been written on the criteria for determining individual capacity and the legally defined characteristic of "competency."[19,35–38] Competency, unlike the decision-making capacity, is a legal term and an all-or-nothing concept specific to a given task. In the absence of a clear medical diagnosis such as delirium or unconsciousness, decisions regarding competency must be made with assistance from psychiatric services, ethics consult services, and/or legal counsel. In general, decisions must be made in these situations on the patient's behalf, either by "substituted judgment" (a decision based on what the patient would have wanted, assuming some knowledge of what the patient's wishes would have been) with or without the help of proxy consent or by a decision made according to the "best interests" of the patient on the basis of a balancing of a "benefit versus burdens" ratio. An appropriate hierarchy for surrogate decision makers is delineated, for example, in a provision of the Virginia Health Care Decisions Act (Code of Virginia §54.1–2981) as follows: 1. A legally appointed guardian or committee. 2. The patient's spouse if no divorce action has been filed. 3. An adult son or daughter of the patient. 4. The patient's parent. 5. An adult brother or sister of the patient. 6. Any other relative of the patient in descending order of relationship. It must be remembered that the caregiver has an ethical obligation to evaluate the competency of the surrogate's decisions with regard to (1) lack of conflict of interest,

(2) reliability of the evidence of the patient's desires on which the surrogate is relying, (3) the surrogate's knowledge of the patient's own value system, and (4) the surrogate's responsible commitment to the decision-making process.[39] All these situations involve complex issues and, again, may require the assistance of hospital ethics committees or consult services.

Voluntariness

A second threshold element is one of freedom or voluntariness. Here one asks the question of whether the patient's decision is free from external constraints. These constraints can consist of myriad social, familial, and even financial factors that can be difficult, if not impossible, to sort out. However, it is not true that the principle of respect for autonomy is at odds with *all* forms of heteronomy, authority, tradition, etc. Competent individuals may autonomously choose to yield first-order decisions (i.e., their decisions about the rightness and wrongness of particular modes of conduct) to a professional, family, spouse, or to a religious institution. In these instances, the person is exercising second-order autonomy in selecting the professional, person, or institution to which they choose to be subordinate. In these cases, second-order autonomy becomes central.[40] The distinguishing feature becomes whether the second-order decision was free and voluntary. Frequently, elderly patients decide on specific treatment options with respect for the opinions of family members, or a concern for their psychologic, physical, and/or financial well-being. As Waymack and Taler observe, "It is often the case that health care professionals find themselves in the care of elderly patients where, because of the nature of chronic care, families often ask or are asked to play a significant role."[41] It is perfectly appropriate for elderly patients to consider the preferences of loved ones, and they should not automatically be encouraged to make decisions concerning treatment options, particularly life-extending treatments, for exclusively self-regarding or purely selfish reasons. Moreover, although undue pressure and influence are clearly improper, it is a mistake to assume that any advice and counsel from family members constitutes undue pressure or influence. However, when elderly patients possess decision-making capacity, generally they and only they have the moral authority to decide how much weight to give the preferences and interests of family members. While it is true that elderly patients can have ethical obligations toward family members that have a bearing on treatment decisions and the interests of family members can be "ethically relevant whether or not the patient is inclined to consider them,"[42] they should generally retain decision-making authority even if physicians believe that they are failing to give due consideration to the interests of family members.[43]

Informational Elements

Adequate Disclosure

The first of the informational elements of informed consent is adequate disclosure. This is the process of properly informing the patient of his or her diagnosis, prognosis, treatment options, risks, and possible outcomes. The anesthesiologist should reveal the specific risks and benefits of each anesthetic option, the complications of instrumentation of the airway, the risks and benefits of invasive monitoring, the presence and use of a fallback plan, and basis for the anesthesiologist's recommendations.[44] "Transparency" is a useful term describing the openness by which the anesthesiologist discusses the treatment plans with a patient. By "thinking out loud" regarding the options and plans, the anesthesiologist communicates the thought processes that he is making that is going into his or her recommendation, thus allowing the patient to understand and participate in this process. Most patients and parents of patients want assurance and explanation regarding anesthesia, not necessarily detailed and exhaustive information.

The discussion of risks and hazards of the diagnostic or therapeutic options, as well as information about anticipated pain or suffering, are, in theory and practice, the most troublesome aspects of informed consent. According to the President's Commission for the Study of Ethical Problems in Medicine and Biomedical and Behavioral Research, "Adequate informed consent requires effort on the part of the physician to ensure comprehension; it involves far more than just a signature on the bottom of a list of possible complications. Such complications can be so overwhelming that patients are unable to appreciate the truly significant information and to make sound decisions."[19] The law does not require one to give a list of every possible complication of a planned procedure (which may inflict an undue amount of emotional distress), but only a "reasonable" amount of information. Negligence is not failure to achieve a good outcome, nor failure to disclose all remote risks.[45]

But just how does one define "reasonable"? The courts have had difficulty as well assessing what a "reasonable" standard of disclosure may be. The most cited standard is the professional practice standard.[46] This standard defines reasonable disclosure as what a capable and reasonable medical practitioner in the same field would reveal to a patient under the same or similar circumstances. Some courts have ignored this prevailing standard of disclosure and shifted the focus from the professional community as forming the standard to the patients themselves. It focuses on the "new consumerism" in health care, an extension of the patient's right of self-determination, where the patient is viewed as consumer of health care and the physician as provider.[47] The "reasonable patient standard" asks what a reasonable patient would consider *reasonable* and *material* to the decision of whether to consent to a procedure offered. The burden, however, is still on the physician to ascertain just what is reasonable and material for a hypothetical "reasonable patient." This recognizes a significant shift in consent law. As legal standards continue to evolve, the reasonable patient standard may become more commonly accepted and eventually displace the professional practice standard as the majority opinion in American informed consent law. A further extension of this line of thinking is the "subjective person standard." This standard recognizes that all patients are different, there is no hypothetical "reasonable person," and hence the standard of disclosure must recognize not only the local standard of care but individual patient needs and idiosyncrasies as well. One important factor in all the above is the notion of "causality," i.e., would additional information have affected this particular patient's decision? What specific, individual concerns did the patient have that would have most affected his or her decision whether or not they are part of the local standard of care for disclosure? The risk of vocal cord damage from a routine intubation may be so small as to not require mentioning in the normal situation (although this is debatable). It may, however, be very important for a professional singer in opting between regional or general anesthesia.

Recommendation and Understanding

Providing a recommendation and patient understanding are the other two informational elements in the informed consent process. The principle of patient autonomy does not require the physician to present the information in a totally neutral manner, if this were even possible. Indeed, part of the informed consent process is to present information to the patient in a way that buttresses a physician's recommendations. Persuasion is a justifiable way for educating patients. This is different from manipulation, which is defined as inappropriately causing a certain behavior, and coercion, which is actually threatening a patient with a plausible punishment so the patient will act in a certain way.

Assessing patient understanding of the information presented can be a difficult issue, especially if "standard" consent forms are relied upon. In one study, 27% of postoperative surgical patients signing consent forms did not know which organ had been operated upon, and 44% did not know the nature of the procedure.[48] Cassileth et al.[49] showed that 55% of cancer patients could list only one of the major complications for chemotherapy within 1 day of signing consent forms. Other studies have shown that risk-specific consent forms do not aid retention[50] and that decision makers often sign consent forms that they do not understand.[51] Attempts must be made to educate patients according to their individual needs and, as has been stated

previously, not to assume a patient must have complete understanding, but only that necessary given their own particular situation to come to a reasonable decision. This will vary from patient to patient and from situation to situation, and consent forms cannot be relied upon to provide this information, no matter how detailed.

Consent Elements: Decision and Autonomous Authorization

Finally, there are the two consent elements: decision and autonomous authorization. The patient must be able to reach a decision and authorize the physician to provide the care decided upon. The physician must document the consented-to technique as well as the invasive monitoring to be used. The patient may consent either verbally or in writing, both are ethically and legally just as valid. It may be more difficult to provide evidence of verbal consent after the fact, however, making it all the more important to document adequately the patient's response in the chart. Although lack of an objection is not equivalent to an authorization, cooperation of patients during performance of a procedure in the absence of overt verbal authorization has usually been deemed equivalent to implied consent and sufficient in cases specifically addressing these issues.[52]

Advance Directives

Advance directives are statements that a patient makes, while still retaining decision-making capacity, about how treatment decisions should be made when they no longer have the capacity to make those decisions. California was the first state to legalize the "living will" in 1976; by 1985, 35 states and the District of Columbia had enacted similar laws. In 1991, the Patient Self-Determination Act (PSDA) became federal law involving all Medicare and Medicaid providers. The PSDA provides that all health care providers must give all patients written information at the time of their admission advising them of their rights to refuse any treatments and to have an advance directive. The presence of an advance directive must be documented in the patient's record, and discrimination against a person because they do or do not have an advance directive is prohibited.

There are two general forms of advance directives. Living wills are documents stating the desires of the patient for treatment alternatives, usually to die a "natural" death and not to be kept alive by advanced life-support measures. In many states, the patient may also stipulate wishes regarding fluid and nutrition discontinuation in the event of persistent vegetative state. Living wills become effective on the determination of "terminal illness" or when death is imminent (within 6 months) or

TABLE 4-2. Living will.

Strengths
1. Allows the physician to understand the patient's wishes and motivations.
2. Extends the patient's autonomy, self-control, and self-determination.
3. Relieves the patient's anxiety about unwanted treatment.
4. Relieves physician's anxiety about legal liability.
5. Reduces family strife and sense of guilt.
6. Improves communication and trust between patient and physician.

Weaknesses
1. Applicable only to those in persistent vegetative state or the terminally ill (patients who have a disease that is incurable and who will die regardless of treatment).
2. Death must be imminent (likely to occur within 6 months).
3. Ambiguous terms may be difficult to later interpret.
4. There is no proxy decision maker, so:
   • It requires prediction of final illness scenario and available treatment.
   • It requires physician to make decisions on the basis of an interpretation of a document.

Source: Junkerman C, Schiedermayer D. Practical Ethics for Students, Interns, and Residents. 2nd ed. Hagerstown, MD: University Publishing Group; 1998. Copyright © 1998 by University Publishing Group. Used with permission. All rights reserved.

when two physicians make the diagnosis of persistent vegetative state. The strengths and weaknesses of the living will are outlined in Table 4-2. Living wills have several weaknesses, including the frequent lack of specific instructions and the impossibility of any person foreseeing all the contingencies of a future illness.[53] Therefore, many advocate an alternative form of advance directive known as a Power of Attorney for Healthcare (PAHC). A PAHC provides for the appointment of a person to act as a health care agent, proxy, or surrogate to make treatment decisions when the patient is no longer able. The PAHC allows a person to add specific directives and often will give the designated agent authority to have feeding tubes withheld or withdrawn. Most PAHCs become effective when two physicians, or one physician and a psychologist, determine that the patient no longer has decision-making capacity. However, this requirement is not universal, and individual state statutes may vary. Table 4-3 lists the advantages of the PAHC that may make it a better option than a living will. Individual state statutes may differ regarding certain components such as witnesses and need for notarization. Whichever form of advance directive a patient chooses to use, both serve a valuable role in preventing ethical dilemmas if designed properly and implemented.

In many instances, elderly patients who lack decision-making capacity have neither executed an advance directive nor previously discussed their preferences regarding treatment options. Even when surrogates are available, disagreements among parties (particularly family members with vested interests), legal or regulatory obstacles, or other problems may hinder a clear decision-making process. The American Geriatric Society Ethics Committee has published a position statement that outlines a strategy for dealing with these situations.[54] They recommend that health care providers and institutions develop methods to make decisions for incapacitated persons without surrogates and to establish mechanisms for intra-institutional conflict resolution, such as an ethics committee, to mediate conflicting situations. They also recommend that surrogate decision-making laws and policies should not hinder the patient's ability to die naturally and comfortably. Evidence from competent patients in similar circumstances should shape the plan of care for an individual patient in the absence of evidence that the patient's wishes would be otherwise.[54] Other strategies include the "prior competent choice" standard, which stresses the values the patient held while competent. The "best interest standard" moves the focus to the patient's subjective experience at the time the treatment is considered.[21]

TABLE 4-3. Power of Attorney for Healthcare (PAHC).

Activation of PAHC
Lack of decision-making capacity must be certified by two physicians or one physician and a psychologist who have examined the patient. Until then, the patient makes all the decisions.

Advantages
1. Physician has someone to talk with—a proxy, a knowledgeable surrogate—who can provide a substituted judgment of how the patient would have chosen. If the agent is unable to provide a substituted judgment, the agent and physician together can use the best-interest standard (how a reasonable person might choose in consideration of the benefit–burden concept of proportionality).
2. Provides flexibility; this decreases ambiguity and uncertainty because there is no way to predict all possible scenarios.
3. Authority of agent can be limited as person desires.
4. Avoids family conflict about rightful agent.
5. Provides legal immunity for physicians who follow dictates.
6. Allows appointment of a nonrelative (especially valuable for persons who may be alienated from their families).
7. Most forms can be completed without an attorney.
8. Principal may add specific instructions to the agent, such as the following: "I value a full life more than a long life. If my suffering is intense and irreversible, or if I have lost the ability to interact with others and have no reasonable hope of regaining this ability even though I have no terminal illness, I do not want to have my life prolonged. I would then ask not to be subjected to surgery or to resuscitation procedures, or to intensive care services or to other life-prolonging measures, including the administration of antibiotics or blood products or artificial nutrition and hydration." (Adapted with permission from Bok S. Personal directions from care at the end of life. N Engl J Med 1976;295:362–369.)

Source: Junkerman C, Schiedermayer D. Practical Ethics for Students, Interns, and Residents. 2nd ed. Hagerstown, MD: University Publishing Group; 1998. Copyright © 1998 by University Publishing Group. Used with permission. All rights reserved.

There remains an urgent role for physicians to educate their patients, their institutions, and their legislatures regarding the important role of advance directives in clinical decision making and the need to remove legislative and institutional hindrances to providing excellent care to dying patients and their families. Although playing an important role in unique circumstances, advance directives are not a substitute for adequate communication among physicians, patients, and family about end-of-life decision making and, in themselves, do not substantially enhance physician–patient communication or decision making.[55]

Do-Not-Attempt-Resuscitation Orders in the Operating Room

The anesthesiologist is most likely to come into contact with ethical issues involving advance directives when a patient is scheduled for surgery with a "do-not-resuscitate" (DNR, or the preferred and more realistic terminology "do-not-attempt-resuscitation," DNAR[56]) order on the chart. As many as 15% of patients with DNAR orders will undergo a surgical procedure.[57] Wenger et al.[58] studied a subgroup of the SUPPORT (Study to Understand Prognoses and Preferences for Outcomes and Risks of Treatment) database and found that of 745 patients presenting to the operating room (OR), 57 had a DNAR order. Operative procedures ranged in complexity and risk from tracheostomy and vascular access to liver transplantation and coronary artery bypass grafting. Twenty of the 57 patients had their DNAR order reversed preoperatively. Two of these patients suffered an intraoperative cardiac arrest and were resuscitated. Both patients subsequently died postoperatively. Only one patient without DNAR order reversal arrested during surgery and died without attempted resuscitation.

Anesthesiologists and surgeons are generally reluctant to proceed with surgical intervention if they are not allowed to intervene in the dying process. They feel that consent for anesthesia and surgery implies consent for resuscitation and is inconsistent with a DNAR order.[59,60] Anesthesiologists tend to claim that the induction and maintenance of anesthesia can often involve creating conditions in which resuscitation is required.[59] Indeed, anesthesia itself has at times been referred to as a "controlled resuscitation." Because anesthetic agents or procedures may create conditions requiring resuscitation, the anesthesiologist ought to have the right to correct those conditions when possible. Surgeons and physicians doing other procedures use similar arguments to claim that if cardiac or pulmonary arrest is a consequence of their actions they should be allowed to prevent or reverse those conditions. In a 1993 survey of anesthesiologists by Clemency and Thompson,[60] almost two thirds of the respondents *assumed* DNAR suspension in the perioperative period and only half discussed this assumption with the patient/guardian.

This dilemma represents a classic problem in the principled approach to medical ethics: the conflict of two or more prima facie ethical principles. If the physician chooses to act paternalistically to provide what is believed to be the best treatment at the time, he is giving precedence to the concept of beneficence over the patient's autonomy. If, however, the physician acts to preserve patient autonomy, he may feel that the duty to do good, as directed by the principle of beneficence, has been compromised. Further complicating the issue is that "DNAR" has multiple definitions and interpretations and involves a spectrum of procedures that the general public is not aware of.[61]

Although automatic suspension of DNAR orders during a surgical procedure and for an arbitrary period postoperatively is the most unambiguous and straightforward policy, it is now argued that this is inappropriate.[62,63] Statements from both the American Society of Anesthesiologists and the American College of Surgeons recognize that this policy effectively removes patients from the decision-making process, even if they are willing to accept the risk of operative mortality. They recommend instead a policy of "required reconsideration" of the DNAR order, as the patient who undergoes a surgical procedure faces a different risk/benefit ratio. Both statements are, however, ambiguous about just how resuscitation is to be handled in the OR. Two alternatives are presented: (1) to suspend the DNAR order in the perioperative period, and (2) to limit resuscitation to certain procedures and techniques. Because of the complexities surrounding the nature of resuscitation, public misconceptions and lack of awareness of these complexities, and the desire to honor the goals reflected in a patient's decision to forgo CPR, a third alternative has been proposed involving a values-centered[61] or goal-directed[64] approach. By ascertaining the patient's goals, values, and preferences rather than individual procedures, the anesthesiologist is given greater flexibility in honoring the objectives of the DNAR order within the clinical context of the arrest. Although seeking to honor both the autonomy of the patient and the physician's duty to beneficence within the spirit of the original DNAR order, this alternative is not without its problems.[65] The establishment of a physician–patient relationship that will facilitate a full understanding of a patient's values and goals is a daunting, if not impossible, task for the anesthesiologist confronted with the demands of a limited preoperative encounter. These concerns may be even more profound in the elderly population.[66] Physicians have not been good at predicting the wishes of their patients regarding resuscitation in other situations, even after discussion has taken place.[67–69] It does, however, provide a third alternative and recognizes that, despite its practical limitations and high regard for patient autonomy in our society, there must always exist a degree of physician–patient trust in any clinical encounter.

Anesthesiologists need to be actively involved in their own institutions to develop policies for DNAR orders in the OR. Open communication among the anesthesiologist, surgeon, and patient or family must exist to reach an agreement about DNAR status. Appropriate exceptions to suspension of a DNAR order in the OR should be honored. Timing of reinstitution of DNAR status should also be addressed and agreed upon before the procedure. Actual experience shows that very few times will a patient insist on a DNAR status during the procedure.

Treatment Futility

With respect to informed consent, what if the patient's decision is counter to the recommendations of the anesthesiologist or amounts to something the anesthesiologist regards as dangerous? Must the physician necessarily do whatever a patient wants? In short, no. In nonemergent circumstances, physicians are not obligated to provide care that they feel is not in their patients' best interest. "First, do no harm" is the operative principle in these situations. It is important again to distinguish in these cases the negative and positive rights based on or related to the principle of respect for personal autonomy and to recognize that the limits on positive rights may be greater than the limits on negative rights. For example, the positive right to request a particular treatment may be severely limited by appropriate clinical standards of care, physician judgment, or just allocation schemes. Clinicians should, however, be very cautious when making this claim and should only do so if absolutely convinced that no other options are available.

Occasionally, physicians have found it necessary to justify unilaterally deciding that certain medical interventions (such as CPR) are "futile" and withhold these interventions even when a patient or a patient's family wants them. The notion of medical futility is particularly confusing and open to different interpretations and abuses. "Futility" can be defined in several senses. "Strict sense futility" or "medical" futility is defined when a medical intervention has no demonstrable physiologic benefit, e.g., when there have been no survivors after CPR under the given circumstances in well-designed studies, or in cases of progressive septic or cardiogenic shock despite maximal treatment. There are no obligations for physicians to provide medically futile treatment, even when families want "everything done." Unilateral decisions to withhold treatment (such as DNAR orders) are appropriate under these circumstances. Usually a DNAR order

may be written on the basis of "futility" when two or more staff physicians concur in writing and give justification for their decision. The patient or surrogate need not agree with the decision but must be notified. If there is disagreement, an ethics consultation may be appropriate and helpful.

It is rare that a given medical intervention is unlikely to have any physiologic effect whatsoever and hence futility may also be defined in a "less strict sense." In this instance, there may be a low survival rate but the rate is not zero. In this case, although the physician may have the particular expertise to determine whether a particular intervention is reasonable according to a particular standard of reasonableness, setting a particular standard involves a value judgment that goes beyond that expertise. For example, a 79-year-old cancer patient wants CPR in the event that he suffers cardiopulmonary arrest because he believes that *any* chance that CPR will restore cardiopulmonary function is worthwhile and that *any* prolongation of his life is also valuable and worthwhile (for instance, by allowing for a family member to return from overseas). Whereas the physician may assess that the chance of CPR restoring function is $x\%$, x is greater than zero and whether the chance of restoring function is reasonable, valuable, or worthwhile only if it is greater than $x\%$ depends primarily on the patient's own values. Unilateral decisions may not be appropriate in this instance, and discussions with the patient and family should be initiated to provide information and advice.

Whereas a physician may have the expertise to assess whether a particular intervention is likely to achieve a specified outcome, determining whether an outcome is an appropriate or valuable objective for a patient is dependent on the patient's own value judgments. A medical intervention can be futile in a third sense when it will have no reasonable chance to achieve the patient's goals and objectives. For example, CPR is futile in this sense if there is no reasonable chance that it will achieve the patient's goal of leaving the hospital and living an independent life. Because medical interventions are futile in relation to the patient's goals, this sense of futility provides a very limited basis for unilateral decisions to withhold medication interventions that patients want. The American Medical Association Council of Judicial and Ethical Affairs has commented that resuscitative efforts "would be considered futile if they could not be expected to achieve the goals expressed by the informed patient. This definition of futility not only respects the autonomy and value judgments of individual patients but also allows for the professional judgment and guidance of physicians who render care to patients."[70]

Because the term "futility" tends to communicate a false sense of scientific objectivity and finality and to obscure the inherent evaluative nature of the judgments, it is recommended that physicians avoid using the term to justify unilateral decisions to withhold life-sustaining treatment. Rather, physicians should explain the specific grounds for concluding that interventions generally, or particular life-sustaining measures, are inappropriate in the given circumstances. Whereas the statement that a given intervention is futile tends to discourage discussion, explaining the grounds for a given judgment in light of the circumstances and with an understanding of the patient's own values and goals tends to invite discussion and point it in the right direction.

Treatment Redirection and Palliative Care

Jean Paul Sartre said that "the meaning of life is found in death," and how we deal with the aging process determines how we deal with death and our philosophy of life. This is most important for the physician and patient when faced with end-of-life decision making involving treatment redirection and palliative care options.

Treatment redirection refers to that point in the patient's care plan when the patient or surrogate, along with the health care team, recognizes the need to move from aggressive curative treatment to supportive palliative care. The 1995 SUPPORT study found that as many as 50% of patients were subjected to burdensome, curative treatment because the patient, family, and physician had not recognized or discussed the realities of the patient's condition.[71] Potter suggests three barriers to meeting the need for treatment redirection.[72] First, clinicians and patients often are narrowly focused on curative or ameliorative intervention. Lack of communication between the physician, who assumes that "they want everything done," and the patients and families, who have different expectations, contributes to this problem. Furthermore, patients and their families often assume that physicians have reliable knowledge about what therapies are effective and which are not because of their intense focus on curative treatment. A study by Feinstein and Horwitz,[73] however, shows that evidence-based medical decisions can only be claimed for less than 20% of clinical situations.

Second, physicians and patients are often reluctant or unable to discuss palliation as a treatment option.[74] Although evidence suggests that physicians are more willing to withhold or withdraw treatment from seriously ill patients,[57] patients and families continue to report that there is a lack of physician communication in the area of shifting treatment to palliative care.[75] Disparity of beliefs and preferences causes much of this communication problem.

Finally, there is a lack of knowledge of and confidence in palliative care by both physicians[76] and society.[77] Part of the problem is that patients are referred to palliative care and hospice programs far too late in their hospital course to do any good. Furthermore, Potter notes that, "although there is a growing trend toward patients wanting to be in control of their own death, cultural diversity factors, belief in the power of medical technology, and a strong tendency to deny death prevent a working consensus about how to approach the experience of dying."[72] Patients and their families may also be suspicious that palliative care is a way to save money, a form of rationing, although there is no empirical evidence that palliative care is more cost effective.[78]

Effective treatment-redirection involves three sequential steps.[72] First, there must be a system to recognize clues, both patient signals and physiologic signs, to indicate that the current form of treatment may not be wanted or may not be warranted.[79] Second, there must be deliberation as part of the informed consent process that focuses on the appropriateness of the current treatment options. Potter reminds one that "because the patient is embedded in a social context of family and friends, there must be an inclusive attitude that searches out the wider origin of beliefs and preferences in the patient's moral community."[72] Furthermore, the health care providers themselves must analyze their own personal beliefs and preferences that can create biases and distort clinical judgment. An open dialog is a necessary part of the deliberation process. Third and finally, there must be an implementation plan that activates excellent palliative care.[80] The aim is for both the patient and the health care team to make a smooth transition from the ultimate goal of curing to that of caring.

End-of-Life Care

End-of-life palliative care options and decision making have become increasingly complicated as new forms of therapy and pain control become available. Pain control in the terminal stages of many illnesses is one of the primary goals of effective palliative care and is an area in which anesthesiologists have a great deal to offer. One of the most pervasive causes of anxiety among patients, their families, and the public is the perception that physicians' efforts toward the relief of pain are sadly deficient. Studies indicate that their fears may be justified. In a study of 1227 elderly patients, approximately 20% experienced moderate or severe pain during the last month of life and the final 6 hours before death.[81] In another study of a random sample of 200 elderly community residents in the last month before death, 66% had pain all or most of the time.[82] Pain influenced behavioral competence, perceived quality of life, psychologic well-being, depression, and diminished happiness. A recent editorial raises concern that medical, radiation, and surgical oncologists are not effectively treating the pain of patients with cancer.[83]

Fear of inadequate pain relief during the terminal stages of illness may be responsible for the increasing interest in euthanasia and physician-assisted suicide (PAS). It is now commonly accepted that the administration of large quantities of narcotic analgesics is not euthanasia when the purpose is to alleviate pain and suffering, not to shorten the life of the patient. Wanzer et al.[84] note that:

In the patient whose dying process is irreversible, the balance between minimizing pain and suffering and potentially hastening death should be struck clearly in favor of pain relief. Narcotics and other pain medications should be given in whatever dose and by whatever route is necessary for relief. It is morally correct to increase the dose of narcotics to whatever dose is needed, even though the medication may contribute to the depression of respiration or blood pressure, the dulling of consciousness or even death, providing the primary goal of the physician is to relieve suffering. The proper dose of pain medication is the dose that is sufficient to relieve pain and suffering, even to the point of unconsciousness.

In this regard, there is clearly a strong need for increased physician and patient education as well as careful ethical analysis.

The terminal stages of the dying process can be accompanied by a number of other disturbing symptoms, both for the family and the patient. Symptoms recorded in the last 48 hours of life include noisy and moist breathing (death rattle), restlessness and agitation, incontinence of urine, dyspnea, retention of urine, nausea and vomiting, sweating, jerking, twitching, plucking, confusion, and delirium.[85–87] Appropriate palliative care must take into account the comfort and care of the patient with regard to these symptoms as well.[88,89]

Despite even the highest quality of palliative care, many patients still report significant pain 1 week before death,[90] some of whom request help in hastening death. Furthermore, patients request a hastened death not simply because of unrelieved pain, but because of the wide variety of other unrelieved physical symptoms in combination with loss of meaning, dignity, and independence.[91]

Confusion may exist about the physician's moral responsibility for contributing to the patient's death. The principle of double effect has an important role in ethical decision making in these instances. Double effect acknowledges that the intent and desired effect of treatment is mitigation of symptoms rather than cessation of life, even though life may be shortened. As frequently formulated, the principle stipulates that one may rightfully cause evil (shortening of life) through an act of choice (treatment of pain) if four conditions are verified: (1) the act itself, apart from the evil caused, is good or at least indifferent; (2) the good effect of the act is what the

agent intends directly, only permitting the evil effect; (3) the good effect must not come about by means of the evil effect; and (4) there must be some proportionately grave reason for permitting the evil effect to occur.[92]

Public and professional debate and confusion over PAS continues even after its legalization in Oregon, the trials of Jack Kevorkian in Michigan, and the experience in the Netherlands. Anesthesiologists should be particularly concerned with the debate for two reasons: (1) because of their unique skills, anesthesiologists may have a very active role as practitioners of euthanasia,[93] and (2) the fear of uncontrolled pain relief, an area that anesthesiologists can provide particular expertise, is a primary motivation for euthanasia and PAS.[94]

PAS differs from euthanasia in that the physician is not the direct agent in PAS whereby in euthanasia the physician is the direct agent. However, not all ethicists agree that PAS and euthanasia differ significantly because of agency. The 1994 edition of the American Medical Association Code of Medical Ethics states that PAS and euthanasia are, "fundamentally incompatible with the physician's role as healer, would be difficult or impossible to control, and would pose serious societal risks."[95] The Second Edition (1989) of the American College of Physicians Ethics Manual reads, "Although a patient may refuse a medical intervention and the physician may comply with this refusal, the physician must never intentionally and directly cause death or assist a patient to commit suicide."[96] The position statement of the American Geriatrics Society Ethics Committee recommends that, "For patients whose quality of life has become so poor as to make continued existence less preferable than death, the professional standard of care should be that of aggressive palliation, not that of intentional termination of life. . . . Laws prohibiting VAE [voluntary active euthanasia] and PAS should not be changed."[97] A study by Koenig et al.[98] showed that the majority of elderly patients attending a geriatrics clinic did not favor legalization of PAS. Furthermore, relatives of these patients could not consistently predict the patients' attitudes or agree among themselves. Recently, public and professional attitudes toward PAS and euthanasia have shifted. The Third Edition (1993) of the American College of Physicians Ethics Manual, although maintaining that physicians should make relief of suffering in the terminally ill patient their highest priority, does not include the strict prohibition included in the previous edition and is much more ambiguous regarding PAS and euthanasia.[99]

The politics of euthanasia and PAS remain controversial. Physicians should be concerned that renewed interest in euthanasia and PAS will not divert attention from the pressing concerns of adequate pain control, treatment of depression, and symptom management in the terminally ill and should actively seek alternate ways to address patient worries regarding loss of control, indignity, and dependence during the final stages of an illness. The elderly, particularly the severely demented, are at the cutting edge of the debate over PAS and VAE. "Senicide" is a very real entity in cultural anthropology. It is not unthinkable that in our aging society, pressure will mount to take moral guidance from anthropologic data, with economic concerns replacing the nomadic.[100] Physicians need to resolve not to let public policy matters interfere with their duty to the health and welfare of their individual patients, regardless of age, and to maintain a commitment to both healing and caring. Anesthesiologists can provide a unique service to their physician colleagues, patients, and general population through education and consultation regarding chronic pain and symptom control in the terminally ill. Measures must go beyond education and become an established part of quality assurance.[101] Anesthesiologists can contribute by assisting their hospitals with means to monitor the treatment of patients in pain. Despite the growing acceptance among the general population and the medical community regarding physician involvement in euthanasia, it is not compatible with the healer's mission and art. At its core, killing patients should never be the means by which symptoms or sufferings, psychologic or physical, are relieved.

Resource Allocation and the Elderly

Concerned over the increasing cost of health care in the United States, many health care policy makers claim that health care rationing is unavoidable. Rationing by age seems to offer a means of reducing spending on health care.[102] Many patient-selection decisions in the United States, such as for heart transplantation, intensive care, and kidney dialysis and transplantation, have long been based on age criteria.[103–106] A recent study by Hamel et al.[107] concludes that older age was associated with higher rates of decisions to withhold ventilator support, surgery, and dialysis even after adjustments for differences in patients' prognoses and preferences. Older patients with coronary artery disease were less likely to undergo invasive and noninvasive testing,[108–110] although studies in octogenarians show that coronary artery bypass surgery is highly cost effective and improves their quality of life in a manner equal to that of a younger population.[111–113] "Age-rationing" implies that elderly patients are denied access to potentially beneficial health care services to which younger patients are not denied access. This is to be distinguished from cost-containment measures that merely result in withholding medical services that are not expected to benefit these patients.[114]

There are several arguments advanced to defend the denial of access to scarce and/or costly medical care to the elderly. One argument is to suggest that elderly patients are not medically suitable candidates for certain

life-sustaining measures. Even if these measures were to succeed, the quality of elderly patients' lives, because of continued ill health and chronically poor functioning, will remain poor. Extending life under such circumstances is not deemed to provide a substantial benefit. This argument is "ageist" at its core because it is based on false universal generalizations regarding all elderly patients. Although the chances of experiencing ill health and impaired functioning increase with age, many elderly people are medically suitable candidates for a wide range of treatment options, and many enjoy good health and unimpaired functioning. A patient's overall health status is generally a more reliable indicator of medical suitability than age alone.

Another defense of age-rationing holds that greater benefits are obtained when life-extending treatments are received by younger patients. These benefits include overall social welfare (because younger persons are more productive than the elderly) and cost effectiveness (because younger patients can be expected to benefit more and at a lower cost).[115] There are three major difficulties with this line of argument. First, it again is ageist in its underlying generalizations. It assumes that elderly persons are unproductive and fails to take into account other standards of productivity (general health status, employment history, and current employment status, etc.). Second, elderly persons who would fail to receive treatments and who would die because of age rationing would bear the burdens, but they would not enjoy any of the benefits derived from the increased productivity that is said to result from this argument. The shift in the benefit–burden ratio to a particular class on the basis of age reveals its injustice and inherent age bias. Finally, even if it can be claimed that it is more cost effective to deny certain classes of people access to beneficial health care, this fails to provide a reason for it being fair or just. Justice can require greater expenditures.

The economic, social, and public policy issues are enormously complicated and beyond the scope of this chapter. Rationing scarce medical resources purely on the basis of a certain age cut-off, however, does not seem to be ethically justifiable.[114,116–118] The growing support in the United States for age criteria in health care does not have a sound medical basis. Support more likely reflects certain social, economic, or even philosophical attitudes and values not universally shared by society or by other cultures. This is different from saying that age cannot be taken into account as a predictor of medical benefit or prognosis. Kilner[119] endorses the use of age as a "symptom" or "rule of thumb" in relation to medical assessments of patients. He states that age "may serve as a tool the physician uses in applying a medical criterion, not as a criterion in its own right." Both the acute physiology and chronic health evaluation (APACHE) III and the SUPPORT model include age as one prognostic element, along with other physiologic variables. In neither study does age seem to have a major role, compared with other variables.[120,121] Physicians must utilize the best available data on treatment outcomes and costs and assume responsibility for developing criteria for appropriateness and medical necessity across the spectrum of patient age and economic status. Physicians should practice appropriateness-based, not cost-based medicine.[122] The rapid changes occurring in the health care system and the recurring emphases on "bottom-line" management require physicians to be involved in allocation decisions at both the professional and public policy level. Rationing policies and managed care plans must be accompanied by full disclosure to patients regarding the limits to their care resulting from these policies and plans, along with a process of patient advocacy and appeal. Gag rules that restrict such disclosures are inherently unethical.[123]

Clinical Research and the Elderly Patient

The elderly patient with severe dementia or depression, or incapacitated in the critical care or emergency setting, represents an extremely vulnerable population, not unlike that of young children or infants, and presents unique dilemmas in the area of clinical research ethics. The ethical issues raised can be summarized as one of balancing: (1) protecting potentially vulnerable research participants, and (2) advancing knowledge and providing potentially beneficial new therapies for a special group of patients. These issues become most manifest when dealing with psychiatric patients, children, and the adult or elderly incapacitated patient, usually in a critical care or emergency setting.[124–130]

In terms of the elderly population in particular, there is no doubt or argument against the proposition that including the elderly, even those incapacitated or suffering from severe dementia or depression, in clinical research designed to benefit this particular population is both important and necessary. Simply to exclude such patients from clinical research trials because they lack the capability for providing informed consent subjects the entire population of such patients to a trial-and-error, anecdotally driven practice of medicine that may, ultimately, end up doing more harm to these patients and result in increased and unnecessary morbidity and mortality in the long term. Balanced against this noble task of advancing our knowledge base for the benefit of future patients, is the necessity of maintaining high ethical standards in the process and protecting those participants in current research trials who may or may not directly benefit from being subject to the nontherapeutic particularities and randomization of a research program design. The focus on the prior concern is on the many, i.e., the

entire population of patients who will potentially benefit from such studies. The focus on the latter is the one, i.e., the individual patient who, by voluntary informed consent, has forfeited the right to individualized and purely therapeutic concern for participation in the artificial environment of the research protocol, whereby the focus of concern will be primarily on the efficient and statistically valid accumulation of specific information for the sake of future benefits. For this reason, patients who elect to participate in clinical research studies are protected from study designs that impose more than minimal risk, that are not designed with expectations to maintain or improve the condition of the patient, or that are flawed in their design such that a valid answer to an appropriate question cannot be obtained. The bar for protection needs to be raised to a higher level for those patients who are incapacitated and cannot understand the nature of the research proposal and/or cannot provide appropriate consent to participate. These patients represent a particularly vulnerable population that can easily be exploited.

Proxy or surrogate consent has a longstanding history in the realm of the purely therapeutic clinical situation. But to what extent does the ethical reasoning inherent in proxy or surrogate consent still apply in the clinical research situation and can the ethical conclusions drawn from the purely therapeutic physician/patient situation be univocally transferred to the physician-researcher/patient-subject research situation? It is common for clinical researchers to presuppose that there is no problem with transferring the standards of proxy consent that exist in the therapeutic relationship into the domain of clinical research.

There are two major difficulties with this view. These difficulties stem from a close examination of the two theoretical foundations upon which proxy or surrogate consent to treatment rests. The first relies on the ability of close family members, friends, or appointed surrogates to provide evidence of the patient's own wishes as to what they would want in a particular foreseeable circumstance (substituted judgment). This can either be through personal knowledge or through available written documents executed by the patient beforehand. Few patients, however, actually end up discussing relative issues in any direct way with friends, family, or their physicians regarding their future medical care.[14,131] Even fewer are likely to discuss involvement in clinical research trials in the event they are incapacitated by an injury or illness. Even when these discussions have been conducted, studies show that surrogates and physicians do not accurately predict patient wishes, in both therapeutic and research situations.[128,132–134] Many ethicists have raised the question as to whether anyone can speak with authority for "what the patient would have wanted" and question whether this "mythological foundation" for proxy consent should, in fact, be abandoned. Yet even if a case could be made that sickness, illness, and death are universal concerns that can provide at least a point of "sympathy" for a close friend or relative and thereby provide a modest grounding for substituted judgment, this is categorically different from choices that involve participating in medical research. Choosing to forgo the "therapeutic" for the "experimental" is, with few extenuating circumstances, a uniquely personal decision, a decision that is grounded on the individual particularities of any given research protocol. If this foundation for substituted judgment (speaking for what the patient would have wanted) in the therapeutic situation is in any sense called into question, it certainly must be even more so in the experimental situation. Richard McCormick[135] states, "Whether a person *ought* to do such things [enroll in a research study] is a highly individual affair and cannot be generalized in the way the good of self-preservation can be. And if we cannot say of an individual that he *ought* to do these things, proxy consent has no reasonable presumptive basis."

The second foundation for proxy or surrogate consent is that of speaking for the "best interest" of the patient. Therapeutic decisions are often made, in the absence of any compelling evidence of what the patient specifically would have wanted, on the basis of what would be in the best interest of the patient (in emergency situations, treatment is often assumed to be in the "best interest" of any patient until proven otherwise). Yet it is difficult to apply this to the research situation, for in this situation the "best interest" of the patient is always relegated to the needs of the study design (e.g., randomization to a particular treatment group). To think otherwise is to fall victim to the so-called "therapeutic misconception."[136–138] Even physician-investigators are prone to blur clinical trial and patient care such that their attention is diverted from the inherent conflicts between the pursuit of science and the protection of research participants.[139] The ethical challenge is to define the limits on the kinds of research risks that the proxy can accept on behalf of a noncompetent patient/subject. Most ethicists and institutional review boards (IRBs) would agree that if the research is potentially beneficial or presents minimal risks and that the knowledge that may be gained would be important to the class of subjects under study, it would be appropriate for a surrogate or proxy to grant consent on behalf of the patient/subject. But how does one define what "minimal risk" and reasonable benefit is within the context of any given research proposal? Similarly, how does one balance the risks against the potential benefits for the subjects or against the knowledge the research may produce?

In a recent commentary, Karlawish[130] proposes that a distinction should be made between risks that are justified by potential benefits for the subjects and risks that are not justified by those benefits. Proxy consent is permissible if the risks posed by the components of the research that do not offer potential benefits for the subjects are no more than minimal and are justified by the importance of the knowledge to be gained. The risks posed by components with potential benefits are justified by the state of equipoise: the expert consensus is that the interventions being compared are within the standard of care so that equilibrium exists in the balance between risks and benefits in the intervention and control groups.

Federal regulations for the protection of research participants, known as the "common rule," require that research involving "vulnerable" subjects include "additional safeguards" and that the investigator obtains informed consent from a "legally authorized representative."[140] Although the rule does not describe safeguards in detail, and most states have not addressed the question of who is legally authorized to provide consent, it does underscore the necessity of protecting vulnerable patients *and their families* from exploitation. One possible consideration (variously proposed by others) is to provide for two patient surrogates, one of which would be the normal surrogate that would be provided for in the strict therapeutic context, and the other a court-designated or IRB-approved representative that would be able to look after the particular interests of the patient and family within the research context. Consent would be required from both, and either would be able to withdraw the patient from the clinical trial at any time. Truog et al.[141] have noted, "The most effective protection against exploitation comes not from the process of informed consent, but, rather, from the careful oversight and scrutiny of conscientious institutional review boards." If this is the case, then review and control boards, particularly those of organizations responsible for the publication and dissemination of the results of research studies, need to take their role very seriously. The identification and discussion of ethical flaws in current research studies need to be more openly discussed in the mainstream medical literature in the hope that these discussions would elevate the level of ethical practices in human research conducted by physician-scientists.[142]

Summary

1. A clinician's own view of aging can and will influence both clinical decision making as well as the application of ethical principles to individual concrete situations. Aging does not have to be seen as a disease or as a form of deviance but rather, the aging process can be valued given the limitations it imposes as a normal part of the human life narrative. Furthermore, the geriatric patient can present with a number of unique perioperative ethical dilemmas that can challenge accepted medical ethics paradigms.

2. Informed consent is a temporal "process" and can never be reduced to a signature on a consent form. Proper informed consent is centered on the notions of open communication and shared decision making. Compassion, understanding, and creativity are necessary to overcome many of the challenges geriatric patients present to the formal elements of the informed consent process.

3. Advance directives are statements that a patient makes, while still retaining decision-making capacity, about how treatment decisions should be made when they no longer have the capacity to make those decisions. There are two general forms of advance directives: living wills and PAHC. PAHCs have several advantages over living wills. Although playing an important role in unique circumstances, advance directives are not a substitute for adequate communication among physicians, patients, and family about end-of-life decision making.

4. Anesthesiologists need to be actively involved in their own institutions to develop policies for DNAR orders in the OR. Open communication among the anesthesiologist, surgeon, and patient or family must exist to reach an agreement about DNAR status. Clinicians should not automatically assume DNAR status to be suspended in the OR and appropriate exceptions to suspension of a DNAR order in the OR should be honored. Timing of reinstitution of DNAR status should also be addressed and agreed upon before the procedure and carefully documented.

5. "Futility" is a value-laden term and tends to communicate a false sense of scientific objectivity and finality. It is recommended that clinicians avoid the use of the term and focus on explaining the specific grounds for concluding that particular interventions are inappropriate in the given circumstances. Whereas the statement that a given intervention is futile tends to discourage discussion, explaining the grounds for a given judgment in light of the circumstances and with an understanding of the patient's own values and goals tends to invite discussion and point it in the right direction.

6. There are times when clinicians, patients, and their families need to redirect care from aggressive curative treatment to supportive palliative care without a sense of "abandoning" the patient. Anesthesiologists have an active role in end-of-life palliative care, both in terms of pain and symptom management. Inadequate pain relief in the terminal stages of most diseases is a continuing problem. Anesthesiologists can contribute by assisting their hospitals with means to monitor the treatment of patients in pain. Despite the growing acceptance among the general population and the medical community regarding physician involvement in euthanasia, it is not compatible with the healer's mission and art. Whereas there are times the dying process should not be prolonged, it should not be intentionally hastened either. At its core, killing patients should never be the means by which symptoms or sufferings, psychologic or physical, are "relieved."

7. "Age rationing" implies that elderly patients are denied access to potentially beneficial health care services to which younger patients are not denied access. This is to be distinguished from cost-containment measures that merely result in withholding medical services that are not expected to benefit these patients.

8. Some elderly patients in particular settings (such as with severe dementia or depression, or incapacitated in a critical care or emergency setting) are extremely vulnerable, similar to young children or infants, and may present unique dilemmas in the area of clinical research ethics. Whereas including the elderly in clinical research designed to benefit this particular population is both important and necessary, there is the equal and sometimes competing necessity of maintaining high ethical standards in the process and protecting those patients in research trials who may or may not directly benefit from being subject to the nontherapeutic particularities and randomization of a research program design.

References

1. Gadow S. Medicine, ethics, and the elderly. Gerontologist 1980;20(6):680–685.
2. Leach E. Society's expectations of health. J Med Ethics 1977;1(85):89.
3. Jung PB. Differences among the elderly: who is on the road to Bremen? In: Hauerwas S, Stoneking CB, Meador KG, Cloutier D, eds. Growing Old in Christ. Grand Rapids: William B. Eerdmans; 2003:115.
4. US Department of Health and Human Services. Vital and Health Statistics: Current Estimates from the National Health Survey, 1990, Series 10: Data from the National Health Survey, No. 181. Hyattsville, MD: DHHS, Publication No. [PHS] 92-1509; 1991.
5. Shelley M. Frankenstein: Or, The Modern Prometheus. London: Penguin Books; 1994.
6. Rieff P. The Triumph of the Therapeutic: Uses of Faith after Freud. New York: Harper & Row; 1966.
7. Mayer PJ. Biological theories about aging. In: Silverman P, ed. The Elderly as Modern Pioneers. Bloomington, IN: Indiana University Press; 1987:21.
8. Spielman BJ. On developing a geriatric ethic: personhood in the thought of Stanley Hauerwas. J Relig Aging 1989; 5(1/2):23–33.
9. Hauerwas S. A Community of Character: Toward a Constructive Christian Social Ethic. Notre Dame: University of Notre Dame Press; 1981.
10. Hauerwas S, Bondi R, Burrell DB. Truthfulness and Tragedy. Notre Dame: University of Notre Dame Press; 1977.
11. Silverstone B. Preface. In: Haug MR, ed. Elderly Patients and Their Doctors. New York: Springer; 1981:xii.
12. Childress JF. The place of autonomy in bioethics. Hastings Cent Rep 1990;20:12–17.

13. Meisel A, Kuczewski M. Legal and ethical myths about informed consent. Arch Intern Med 1996;156:2521–2526.
14. Beauchamp TL, Childress JF. Principles of Biomedical Ethics. Oxford: Oxford University Press; 1994.
15. US Congress Office of Technology Assessment. Losing a Million Minds: Confronting the Tragedy of Alzheimer's Disease and Other Dementias. Washington, DC: US Government Printing Office; 1987.
16. Marson DC, McInturff B, Hawkins L, Bartolucci A, Harrell LE. Consistency of physician judgments of capacity to consent in mild Alzheimer's disease. J Am Geriatr Soc 1998;45(4):453–457.
17. Buchanan AE, Brock DW. Deciding for Others: The Ethics of Surrogate Decision Making. Cambridge: Cambridge University Press; 1989.
18. President's Commission for the Study of Ethical Problems in Medicine and Biomedical Research. Deciding to Forgo Life-Sustaining Treatment. Washington, DC: US Government Printing Office; 1982.
19. President's Commission for the Study of Ethical Problems in Medicine and Biomedical Research. Making Health Care Decisions, Volume One: Report. Washington, DC: US Government Printing Office; 1992.
20. Appelbaum PS, Grisso T. Assessing patients' capacities to consent to treatment. N Engl J Med 1988;319(25):1635–1638.
21. Fellows LK. Competency and consent in dementia. J Am Geriatr Soc 1998;46(7):922–926.
22. Fitten LJ, Lusky R, Hamann C. Assessing treatment decision-making capacity in elderly nursing home residents. J Am Geriatr Soc 1990;38(10):1097–1104.
23. Grisso T, Appelbaum PS, Hill-Fotouhi C. The MacCAT-T: a clinical tool to assess patients' capacities to make treatment decisions. Psychiatr Serv 1997;48(11):1415–1419.
24. Ratzan RM. Informed consent in clinical geriatrics. J Am Geriatr Soc 1984;32(3):176.
25. Sugarman J, McCrory DC, Hubal RC. Getting meaningful informed consent from older adults: a structured literature review of empirical research. J Am Geriatr Soc 1998;46(4):517–524.
26. Dror IE, Katona M, Mungur K. Age differences in decision making: to take a risk or not? Gerontology 1998;44(2):67–71.
27. Stanley B, Guido J, Stanley M, Shortell D. The elderly patient and informed consent: empirical findings. JAMA 1984;252(10):1302–1306.
28. Lieberman M. The physician's duty to disclose risks of treatment. Bull NY Acad Med 1974;50:943–948.
29. Ingelfinger FJ. Informed (but uneducated) consent. N Engl J Med 1971;287:465–466.
30. Taub HA. Informed consent, memory, and age. Gerontologist 1980;20(6):686–690.
31. Johnston SC, Pfeifer MP. Patient and physician roles in end-of-life decision making. End-of-Life Study Group. J Gen Intern Med 1998;13(1):43–45.
32. Stiggelbout AM, Kiebert GM. A role for the sick role. Patient preferences regarding information and participation in clinical decision-making. Can Med Assoc J 1997;157(4):383–389.
33. Strull WM, Lo B, Charles G. Do patients want to participate in medical decision making? JAMA 1984;252(21):2990–2994.
34. Starr TJ, Pearlman RA, Uhlmann RF. Quality of life and resuscitation decisions in elderly patients. J Gen Intern Med 1986;1:373–379.
35. Midwest Bioethics Center Ethics Committee Consortium. Guidelines for the determination of decisional incapacity. Midwest Bioethics Cent Bull 1996:1–13.
36. Weinstock R, Copelan R, Bagheri A. Competence to give informed consent for medical procedures. Bull Am Acad Psychiatry Law 1984;12(2):117–125.
37. Roth LH, Meisel A, Lidz CW. Tests of competency to consent to treatment. Am J Psychiatry 1977;134:279–284.
38. Grisso T, Appelbaum PS. Assessing Competence to Consent to Treatment: A Guide for Physicians and Other Health Professionals. Oxford: Oxford University Press; 1998.
39. Pinkerton JV, Finnerty JJ. Resolving the clinical and ethical dilemma involved in fetal-maternal conflicts. Am J Obstet Gynecol 1996;175(2):289–295.
40. Dworkin G. Autonomy and behavior control. Hastings Cent Rep 1976;6(1):23–28.
41. Waymack MH, Taler GA. Medical Ethics and the Elderly: A Case Book. Chicago: Pluribus; 1988.
42. Hardwig J. What about the family? Hastings Cent Rep 1990;20(2):8.
43. Nelson JL. Taking families seriously. Hastings Cent Rep 1992;22(4):6–12.
44. Waisel DB, Truog RD. Informed consent. Anesthesiology 1997;87(4):968–978.
45. Crooke D. Ethical issues and consent in obstetric anesthesia. In: Birnbach DJ, Sanjay S, Gatt SP, eds. Textbook of Obstetric Anesthesia. New York: WB Saunders; 2000:744–753.
46. Waltz JR, Scheunemann T. Informed consent and therapy. Northwestern Univ Law Rev 1970;64:628.
47. Gild WM. Informed consent: a review. Anesth Analg 1989;68:649–653.
48. Byrne J, Napier A. How informed is signed consent? Br Med J 1988;296:839–840.
49. Cassileth BR, Zupkis RV, Sutton-Smith K, March V. Informed consent—why are its goals imperfectly realized? N Engl J Med 1980;302:896–900.
50. Clark SK, Leighton BL, Seltzer JL. A risk-specific anesthesia consent form may hinder the informed consent process. J Clin Anesth 1991;3:11–13.
51. Waisel DB, Truog RD. The benefits of the explanation of the risks of anesthesia in the day surgery patient. J Clin Anesth 1995;7:200–204.
52. Knapp RM. Legal view of informed consent for anesthesia during labor. Anesthesiology 1990;72(1):211.
53. Teno JM, Licks S, Lynn J, et al. Do advance directives provide instructions that direct care? SUPPORT Investigators. Study to Understand Prognoses and Preferences for Outcomes and Risks of Treatment. J Am Geriatr Soc 1997;45(4):508–512.
54. American Geriatrics Society Ethics Committee. Making treatment decisions for incapacitated older adults without advance directives. J Am Geriatr Soc 1996;44(8):986–987.

55. Teno JM, Lynn J, Wenger N, et al. Advance directives for seriously ill hospitalized patients: effectiveness with the patient self-determination act and the SUPPORT intervention. SUPPORT Investigators. Study to Understand Prognoses and Preferences for Outcomes and Risks of Treatment. J Am Geriatr Soc 1997;45(4):500–507.

56. Jonsen AR, Siegler M, Winslade WJ. Clinical Ethics. 4th ed. New York: McGraw-Hill; 1998.

57. La Puma J, Silverstein MD, Stocking CB, Roland D, Siegler M. Life-sustaining treatment: a prospective study of patients with DNR orders in a teaching hospital. Arch Intern Med 1988;148(2193):2198.

58. Wenger NS, Greengold NL, Oye RK, Kussin P, Phillips RS. Patients with DNR orders in the operating room: surgery, resuscitation, and outcomes. J Clin Ethics 1997;8:250–257.

59. Truog RD. "Do-not-resuscitate" orders during anesthesia and surgery. Anesthesiology 1991;74(3):606–608.

60. Clemency MV, Thompson NJ. "Do not resuscitate" (DNR) orders and the anesthesiologist: a survey. Anesth Analg 1993;76:394–401.

61. Thurber CF. Public awareness of the nature of CPR: a case for values-centered advance directives. J Clin Ethics 1996;7(1):55–59.

62. Committee on Ethics, American College of Surgeons. Statement on advance directives by patients: do not resuscitate in the operating room. Am Coll Surg Bull 1994; 79:29.

63. Committee on Ethics, American Society of Anesthesiologists. Ethical guidelines for the anesthesia care of patients with do not resuscitate orders or other directives that limit treatment (1993). 1997:12–13. ASA Standards, Guidelines and Statements.

64. Truog RD, Waisel DB, Burns JP. DNR in the OR: a goal-directed approach. Anesthesiology 1999;90(1):289–295.

65. Jackson SH, Van Norman GA. Goals- and values-directed approach to informed consent in the 'DNR' patient presenting for surgery: more demanding of the anesthesiologist? Anesthesiology 1999;90(1):3–6.

66. Sayers GM, Schofield R, Aziz M. An analysis of CPR decision-making by elderly patients. J Med Ethics 1997; 23:207–212.

67. Krumholz HM, Phillips RS, Hamel MB, et al. Resuscitation preferences among patients with severe congestive heart failure: results from the SUPPORT Project. Circulation 1998;98(648):655.

68. Rosin AJ, Sonnenblick M. Autonomy and paternalism in geriatric medicine. The Jewish ethical approach to issues of feeding terminally ill patients, and to cardiopulmonary resuscitation. J Med Ethics 1998;24:44–48.

69. Uhlmann R, Pearlman R, Cain K. Physicians' and spouses' predictions of elderly patients' resuscitation preferences. J Gerontol 1988;43:M115–M121.

70. American Medical Association Council on Ethical and Judicial Affairs. Guidelines for the appropriate use of do-not-resuscitate orders. JAMA 1981;265(14):1868–1871.

71. SUPPORT Investigators. A controlled trial to improve care for seriously ill hospitalized patients. The study to understand prognoses and preferences for outcomes and risks of treatments (SUPPORT). JAMA 1995;274(20): 1591–1598.

72. Potter RL. Treatment redirection: moving from curative to palliative care. Bioethics Forum 1998;14(2):3–9.

73. Feinstein AR, Horwitz RI. Problems in the 'evidence' of 'evidence-based medicine.' Am J Med 1997;103:529–535.

74. Weeks JC, Cook EF, O'Day SJ, et al. Relationship between cancer patients' predictions of prognosis and their treatment preferences. JAMA 1998;279(1709):1714.

75. Hanson LC, Danis M, Tulsky JA. What is wrong with end-of-life care? Opinions of bereaved family members. J Am Geriatr Soc 1997;45:1339–1344.

76. Bulger RJ. The quest for mercy: the forgotten ingredient in health care reform. West J Med 1997;167:362–373.

77. Lynn J, Teno JM, Phillips RS, et al. Perceptions by family members of the dying experience of older and seriously ill patients. Ann Intern Med 1997;126(2):97–106.

78. Emanuel E. Cost savings at the end of life. Crit Care Med 1996;25:1907–1914.

79. Randolph AG, Guyatt GH, Richardson WS. Prognosis in the intensive care unit: finding accurate and useful estimates for counseling patients. Crit Care Med 1998;26(4): 767–772.

80. Rudberg MA, Teno JM, Lynn J. Developing and implementing measures of quality of care at the end of life: a call for action. J Am Geriatr Soc 1997;45(4):528–530.

81. Kaiser HE, Brock DB. Comparative aspects of the quality of life in cancer patients. In Vivo 1992;6(4):333–337.

82. Moss MS, Lawton MP, Glicksman A. The role of pain in the last year of life of older persons. J Gerontol 1991;56: P51–P57.

83. Cherny NI, Catane R. Professional negligence in the management of cancer pain. Cancer 1995;76(2181):2185.

84. Wanzer SH, Federman DD, Adelstein SJ, et al. The physician's responsibility toward hopelessly ill patients: a second look. N Engl J Med 1989;320(13):844–849.

85. Lichter I, Hunt E. The last 48 hours of life. J Palliat Care 1990;6(4):7–115.

86. Martin EW. Confusion in the terminally ill: recognition and management. Am J Hosp Palliat Care 1990;73:20–24.

87. Massie MJ, Holland J, Glass E. Delirium in terminally ill cancer patients. Am J Psychiatry 1983;140(8):1048–1050.

88. Voltz R, Borasio GD. Palliative therapy in the terminal stage of neurological disease. J Neurol 1997;244(Suppl 4): S2–S10.

89. Power D, Kearney M. Management of the final 24 hours. Ir Med J 1992;85(3):93–95.

90. Coyle N, Adelhardt J, Foley KM, Portenoy RK. Character of terminal illness in the advanced cancer patient. J Pain Symptom Manage 1990;5:83–93.

91. Back AL, Wallace JI, Starks HE, Pearlman RA. Physician-assisted suicide and euthanasia in Washington State. JAMA 1996;275:919–925.

92. May WE. Double effect. In: Reich WT, ed. Encyclopedia of Bioethics. New York: The Free Press; 1978:316–320.

93. Benrubi GI. Euthanasia—the need for procedural safeguards. N Engl J Med 1992;326(3):197–199.

94. Jonsen AR. To help the dying die: a new duty for anesthesiologists? Anesthesiology 1993;78(2):225–228.

95. American Medical Association Council on Ethical and Judicial Affairs. Code of Medical Ethics: Current Opinions

with Annotations. Chicago: American Medical Association; 1994.

96. American College of Physicians Ethics Committee. Ethics Manual. 2nd ed. Ann Intern Med 1989;111(245):335.

97. American Geriatrics Society Ethics Committee. Physician-assisted suicide and voluntary active euthanasia. J Am Geriatr Soc 1995;43(5):579–580.

98. Koenig HG, Wildman-Hanlon D, Schmader K. Attitudes of elderly patients and their families toward physician-assisted suicide. Arch Intern Med 1996;156(19):2240–2248.

99. American College of Physicians Ethics Committee. Ethics Manual. 3rd ed. Ann Intern Med 1992;117:947–960.

100. Post SG. Euthanasia, senicide, and the aging society. J Religious Gerontol 1991;8(1):57–65.

101. Hill CS. When will adequate pain treatment be the norm? JAMA 1995;274:1880–1881.

102. Hamel MB, Phillips RS, Teno JM, Lynn J, Galanos AN, Davis RB. Seriously ill hospitalized adults: do we spend less on older patients? SUPPORT Investigators. Study to Understand Prognoses and Preference for Outcomes and Risks of Treatment. J Am Geriatr Soc 1996;44:1043–1048.

103. Evans RW, Yagi J. Social and medical considerations affecting selection of transplant recipients: the case of heart transplantation. In: Cowan DH, ed. Human Organ Transplantation. Ann Arbor: Health Administration Press; 1987:27–41.

104. Kjellstrand CM. Age, sex, and race inequality in renal transplantation. Arch Intern Med 1988;148:1305–1309.

105. Kjellstrand CM, Logan GM. Racial, sexual and age inequalities in chronic dialysis. Nephron 1987;45:257–263.

106. McClish DK, Powell SH, Montenegro H, Nochomovitz M. The impact of age on utilization of intensive care resources. J Am Geriatr Soc 1987;35(11):983–988.

107. Hamel MB, Teno JM, Goldman L, et al. Patient age and decisions to withhold life-sustaining treatments from seriously ill, hospitalized adults. Ann Intern Med 1999;130:116–125.

108. Gurwitz JH, Osganian V, Goldberg RJ, Chen ZY, Gore JM, Alpert JS. Diagnostic testing in acute myocardial infarction: does patient age influence utilization patterns? The Worcester Heart Attack Study. Am J Epidemiol 1991;134:948–957.

109. Bearden DM, Allman RM, Sundarum SV, Burst NM, Bartolucci AA. Age-related variability in the use of cardiovascular imaging procedures. J Am Geriatr Soc 1993;41:1075–1082.

110. Naylor CD, Levinton CM, Baigrie RS, Goldman BS. Placing patients in the queue for coronary surgery: do age and work status alter Canadian specialists' decisions? J Gen Intern Med 1992;7:492–498.

111. Sollano JA, Roe EA, Williams DL, et al. Cost-effectiveness of coronary artery bypass surgery in octogenarians. Ann Surg 1998;228(3):297–306.

112. Ott RA, Gutfinger DE, Miller M, et al. Rapid recovery of octogenarians following coronary artery bypass grafting. J Card Surg 1997;12(5):309–313.

113. Kirsch M, Guesnier L, LeBesnerais P, et al. Cardiac operations in octogenarians: perioperative risk factors for death and impaired autonomy. Ann Thorac Surg 1998;66(1):60–67.

114. Jecker NS, Pearlman RA. Ethical constraints on rationing medical care by age. J Am Geriatr Soc 1989;37:1067–1075.

115. Avorn J. Benefit and cost analysis in geriatric care: turning age discrimination into health policy. N Engl J Med 1984;310(20):1294–1301.

116. Cassel CK, Neugarten B. The goals of medicine in an aging society. In: Binstock RH, Post SG, eds. Too Old for Health Care? Controversies in Medicine, Law, Economics, and Ethics. Baltimore: Johns Hopkins University Press; 1991.

117. Dougherty CJ. Ethical problems in healthcare rationing. Testimony to the Senate Special Committee on Aging. Health Prog 1991;72:32–39.

118. Evans JG. Aging and rationing [editorial]. Br Med J 1991;303:869–870.

119. Kilner JF. Age as a basis for allocating lifesaving medical resources: an ethical analysis. J Health Polit Policy Law 1988;13(3):405–423.

120. Knaus WA, Harrell FE, Lynn J, et al. The SUPPORT prognostic model. Objective estimates of survival for seriously ill hospitalized adults. Study to understand prognoses and preferences for outcomes and risks of treatments. Ann Intern Med 1995;122(3):191–203.

121. Knaus WA, Wagner DP, Draper EA, et al. The APACHE III prognostic system. Risk prediction of hospital mortality for critically ill hospitalized adults. Chest 1992;102(6):1919–1920.

122. Rosenfeld KE, Pearlman RA. Allocating medical resources: recommendations for a professional response. J Am Geriatr Soc 1997;45(7):886–888.

123. Biblo JD, Christopher MJ, Johnson L, Potter RL. Ethical issues in managed care: guidelines for clinicians and recommendations to accrediting organizations. Bioethics Forum 1996;12(1):MC/1–MC/24.

124. Karlawish JHT, Sachs GA. Research on the cognitively impaired: lessons and warnings from the emergency research debate. J Am Geriatr Soc 1997;45(4):474–481.

125. Capron AM. Incapacitated research. Hastings Cent Rep 1997;27(2):25–27.

126. Prabhu VC, Kelso TK, Sears TD. An update on the PEG-SOD study involving incompetent subjects: FDA permits an exception to informed consent. IRB 1994;16(1–2):16–18.

127. Haimowitz S, Delano SJ, Oldham JM. Uninformed decision making: the case of surrogate research consent. Hastings Cent Rep 1997;27(6):9–16.

128. Warren JW, Sobal J, Tenney JH, et al. Informed consent by proxy: an issue in research with elderly patients. N Engl J Med 1986;315(18):1124–1128.

129. American College of Physicians. Cognitively impaired subjects. Ann Intern Med 1989;111(10):843–848.

130. Karlawish JHT. Research involving cognitively impaired adults. N Engl J Med 2003;348(14):1389–1392.

131. Baskin SA, Morris J, Ahronheim JC, Meier DE, Morrison RS. Barriers to obtaining consent in dementia research: implications for surrogate decision-making. J Am Geriatr Soc 1998;46(3):287–290.

132. Coppolino M, Ackerson L. Do surrogate decision makers provide accurate consent for intensive care research? Chest 2001;119(2):603–612.

133. Emanuel EJ, Emanuel LL. Proxy decision making for incompetent patients. JAMA 1992;267:2067–2071.

134. Secker AB, Meier DE, Mulvihill M, Paris BE. Substituted judgment: how accurate are proxy predictions? Ann Intern Med 1991;115:92–98.

135. McCormick R. Proxy consent in the experimentation situation. Perspect Biol Med 1974;18(1):2–20.

136. Appelbaum PS, Roth LH, Lidz CW, Benson P, Winslade W. False hopes and best data: consent to research and the therapeutic misconception. Hastings Cent Rep 1987; April(17):2–20.

137. Hochhauser M. "Therapeutic misconception" and "recruiting doublespeak" in the informed consent process. IRB 2002;24(1):11–12.

138. Miller FG, Rosenstein DL. The therapeutic orientation to clinical trials. N Engl J Med 2003;348(14):1383–1386.

139. Miller FG, Rosenstein DL, DeRenzo EG. Professional integrity in clinical research. JAMA 1998;280:1449–1454.

140. Department of Health and Human Services. Common rule, 45 CFR 46. Federal policy for the protection of human subjects; notices and rules. Federal Register 1991;56: 28003–28032.

141. Truog RD, Robinson W, Randolph A, Morris A. Is informed consent always necessary for randomized, controlled trials? N Engl J Med 1999;340(10):804–807.

142. Sade RM. Publication of unethical research studies: the importance of informed consent. Ann Thorac Surg 2003; 75(2):325–328.

5
Teaching Geriatric Anesthesiology to Practitioners, Residents, and Medical Students

Sheila J. Ellis

Care of the geriatric patient will continue to grow in importance as the geriatric proportion of the population continues to grow. The increasing life expectancy in the United States and improvements in medical care allow expansion of surgical procedures into populations once considered too unstable or frail to recover from the stress of surgery. Geriatric patients undergo the same range of surgical procedures as younger patients. Some procedures, such as cataract surgery or prostate resection, may be performed more frequently in the geriatric patient. Virtually every medical provider will need to have a thorough understanding of the needs, complications, and changes in the elderly. Thus, education in geriatric anesthesia is essential.

Geriatrics in Educational Programs

Medical School

Ideally, the introduction to geriatrics begins in medical school. The geriatric curriculum in medical schools has grown a great deal in the past several decades. The Longitudinal Study of Training and Practice in Geriatric Medicine by the Association of Directors of Geriatric Academic Programs found that in the academic year 2000 to 2001, 116 of 125 (93%) responding medical schools included geriatric topics as part of an existing required course, and 10 of 125 (8%) had a separate required course. Electives with geriatric topics were offered as separate courses in 68 schools (54%) and as part of an elective course in 35 institutions (28%).[1]

Anesthesiology Residency

The formal course of geriatric education usually concludes with the end of medical school. However, it is now recognized that structured geriatric education should be included in anesthesiology training. The Accreditation Council for Graduate Medical Education (ACGME) requires "appropriate didactic instruction and sufficient clinical experience in managing problems of the geriatric population" in accredited anesthesiology residency programs.[2] The type and amount of clinical experience that qualifies as sufficient and the amount of appropriate didactic instruction remains undefined.

The joint American Board of Anesthesiology (ABA)/American Society of Anesthesiologists (ASA) content outline for in-training examinations also includes a section titled "Geriatric Anesthesia/Aging: The Pharmacological Implications, MAC Changes and the Physiological Implications on CNS, Circulatory, Respiratory, Renal, and Hepatic Organ Systems." This is a very incomplete list, obviously.

Geriatrics as Part of Core Competencies

Residency education in geriatrics can be used to establish a curriculum to meet the updated required ACGME competencies. ACGME requires evidence of training and proficiency in six core areas, including patient care, medical knowledge, practice-based learning and improvement, interpersonal and communication skills, professionalism, and systems-based practice (Table 5-1).[3]

Communication Skills

Incorporating these competencies into a geriatric curriculum may provide a method to evaluate these principles while advancing geriatric education. A preoperative assessment of a confused patient can be an opportunity to teach and assess residents on communication skills. Interacting with the patient's caregiver provides an opportunity for development of interpersonal skills.[4] This preoperative assessment may be complicated because the

TABLE 5-1. Core competencies of accreditation council for graduate medical education.

Patient care
Medical knowledge
Practice-based learning and improvement
Interpersonal and communication skills
Professionalism
Systems-based practice

confused patient may have difficulty transmitting a complete medical history. Sensory changes such as hearing loss may challenge the anesthesia trainee to utilize additional modalities for clear communication, such as hearing amplification devices or written communication. Transmitting information to the elderly patient regarding preoperative medication usage and oral intake requires the ability to assess patient understanding. All of these communication skills can be directly observed or can be videotaped for discussion and additional feedback.

Teaching residents the skills needed for completing such a challenging preoperative assessment can be accomplished in a similar manner by direct observation or through a media presentation. A taped interview can be used to show students and residents methods for eliciting information and increasing the information obtained by improved interpersonal communication. Providing written instructions for patients can demonstrate improvement in communication skills.

Communication with other health care providers is also an important component of care of the elderly patient. Multiple providers may be involved such as primary care physicians, specialist physicians, home health attendants, and caregivers. Maintaining appropriate and adequate communication with all of these sources should be encouraged and evaluated.

Systems-Based Practice

A discussion of end-of-life issues and do-not-resuscitate orders in the perioperative period may be a way to teach systems-based practice. Systems-based practice requires an awareness of the larger context and system of health care. It is essential to understand what a do-not-resuscitate order means in the perioperative period. The institutional requirements regarding such notations can be reviewed while assessing or reconsidering such an order with the patient or surrogate. Clarification and, if necessary, modification of a do-not-resuscitate order should be documented in the medical record. This discussion can be integrated into the larger experience of health care beyond the immediate anesthetic needs. Such a discussion can also be useful to educate the resident and student in the core competency of professionalism and adherence to ethical principles in care of the patient.

Practice-Based Learning and Improvement

Practice-based learning and improvement requires the ability to determine an area that needs improvement, identify and apply an intervention, and measure impact of the intervention.[5] Patient-based learning and improvement seeks to improve patient care through appraisal of scientific evidence. Perioperative beta blockade can be a rich source of material for practice-based learning. The ability to recognize the current practice regarding perioperative use of beta blockade and the appropriate application of this therapy can be an important part of geriatric education. Incorporating these competencies into a geriatric curriculum can be a very effective method both for teaching the student and resident geriatric anesthesia, and providing a place for evaluation and assessment for the educational program.

Importance of Geriatric Training

For completion of anesthesiology residency, specific criteria must be fulfilled for pediatrics, including experience with a set number of anesthetics on a child younger than 1 year of age. In adult patients, the emphasis is on physiologic changes and specialized procedures, not on the age of the patient. By requiring a set number of cardiac procedures, for example, the trainee in anesthesiology will most likely include a number of elderly patients, but this is not guaranteed. It is possible that a resident could have an adequate number of cardiovascular procedures without performing the majority of these cases on geriatric patients. Does this matter? Is there a difference in cardiovascular disease in patients 45 versus 85 years of age? The disease processes may have widely varying causes, and the patients may have very different intraoperative and postoperative courses. Elderly patients may present with atypical presentations of common problems such as angina that may delay or alter treatment.

The older patient has the potential for many adverse perioperative events. The hazards of hospitalization and surgery in the elderly include adverse drug events, delirium, functional decline, infection, malnutrition, thromboembolism, and untreated or undertreated pain.[6] Hospitalization is often followed by an irreversible decline in functional status and a change in quality and style of life. Only 20% of patients in a large group returned to their preoperative functional level after repair of a hip fracture.[7] In a study of community-dwelling, noninstitutionalized patients aged 70 years or older hospitalized for acute medical illness, 31% of the patients declined in activities of daily living (ADL) at discharge compared with baseline after a mean length of admission of 8.6 days. At a 3-month follow-up, 40% reported disabilities related to ADL or instrumental ADL such as meal preparation or shopping for groceries compared with preadmission baseline.[8]

Therefore, it is important to have exposure to and experience with elderly patients, not just to diseases frequently seen in elderly patients. As a practical matter, a sampling of cases on a typical day at a hospital, ambulatory setting, or pain clinic servicing a general population will provide a number of elderly patients. The key should be to look at the patients in these settings as valuable educational opportunities. We believe that a resident diary of the number of patients cared for over the age of 75 would be important to determine if residents were exposed to an adequate number of geriatric patients.

Growth of Geriatric Anesthesia

The subspecialty fellowship in gerontology continues to grow with 338 fellows in training programs during 2001–2001.[9] However, the number of trainees in fellowship programs still falls short of the number needed to serve the expanding geriatric population.

The field of geriatric anesthesiology is relatively new. The Society for the Advancement of Geriatric Anesthesiology (SAGA) was established in the United States in 2000. There is also the Age Anaesthesia Association that functions in the United Kingdom. As of 2004, there is not a fellowship or subspecialty track in geriatrics for anesthesiology trainees. There is a dearth of specific citations in the medical literature related to the teaching of geriatric anesthesiology. It is expected that the recognition of geriatric anesthesia as a separate entity and the need for further expertise will fuel this branch of anesthesia.

Teaching Geriatrics

Education in geriatric anesthesia is a process that can be defined separately from teaching. Teaching implies an activity by an individual or a group causing another person to know new facts or how to accomplish a new task. The focus is on the teacher, not the learner.[10]

However, education is a broader process that results in a change in behavior on the part of the student. The focus of education is the learner, not the teacher.[10] The desired end result is not a specific ability to perform a task, or retention of a set of data. The goal is a change in behavior based on experiences. These experiences may be from direct interaction, indirect observations, or a more remote learning from lectures, but the desired end result is the same. If the instruction produces a change in behavior (and, most likely, attitude), education has been achieved.

Who is the target audience for education in geriatric anesthesia? Certainly residents in anesthesiology, student nurse anesthetists, student anesthesiology assistants, and medical students are focus groups for this training, and fully trained anesthesiologists through continuing medical education. Other individuals who will participate in anesthesia and the other aspects of patient care are also important and should be included when considering the establishment or expansion of an education program for geriatric anesthesia. Preoperative and postoperative recovery nurses, emergency room personnel, anesthesia technicians and anesthesia aides, and respiratory therapists can be included in geriatric education. Primary care physicians and surgeons certainly should be exposed to geriatric issues regarding perioperative medicine.

All of these groups are adult learners who should be independent and self-directed.[11] There may be many different reasons for seeking further education but the usual common factor is a desire for improvement as a clinician. Whereas formal training programs serve a large number of adult learners, there are many who utilize other educational avenues. This may take the form of self-study continuing medical education courses, lectures at medical meetings, Internet-based learning, and other opportunities. The desire for professional improvement and the active search for educational sources make adult learners very involved in their own education. The self-direction and independence of adult learners is a key trait in producing changes in their behavior.

Adult learners also use their own experiences as a resource for learning. They may view the current experience differently based on their background from others without a similar amount of experience. This can enhance education but must be acknowledged and accepted, not rejected by educators.[12] For example, an anesthesiology resident with a prior career in nephrology may treat acid-base management in the operating room differently from a resident without this experience. A faculty member who can acknowledge the experience of the student in this situation will not only provide better clinical care but also enhance the education of the student. This approach validates the adult learner and makes the learner more receptive to education in other areas. The previous learning may color the education of the adult learner so the educator must work to integrate and build on this, not reject the learning and, in doing so, reject the learner.

Principles to guiding adult teaching include having the learner be an active contributor and utilize as much as possible the current knowledge and experience in the learner.[11] Learning should closely relate to understanding and solving real problems that the learner will encounter. There should be opportunities for practice, with assessment and constructive feedback from the educator.

Developing a Geriatric Curriculum

Faculty Development

In developing a program for teaching geriatric anesthesia, the prime consideration is to identify an individual who will develop geriatric expertise and an interest in geriatric education. A leader who will take responsibility is vital. This key person, it is hoped, will provide a core of other people who can be viewed as mentors to facilitate and maintain a geriatric curriculum. In other faculty members with specific areas of interest or expertise, increased knowledge and emphasis on geriatrics can be used to supplement the geriatric anesthesia experts. For example, a cardiovascular anesthesiologist may provide education in the changes in cardiac function in the elderly whereas an anesthesia provider with advanced skills in regional anesthesia may provide insight into peripheral nerve blocks in this population.

An impediment to faculty development in geriatric anesthesiology can be the attitude that geriatric anesthesiology is not sufficiently interesting or academically rigorous enough to justify the effort toward further development. Because general anesthesiologists already care for older patients, many do not feel the need to develop skills or devote additional clinical or academic time that is already in short supply. This attitude can be countered by the requirements for geriatric anesthesia education from ACGME and the ASA/ABA content outline, the growth in this area in number of patients and understanding of aging, and the likelihood for career advancement.

The designation of a geriatric anesthesia faculty member can be an opportunity for personal career growth. The emergence of geriatric anesthesia as a distinct subspecialty can allow anesthesiologists to interact with gerontologists, pharmacists, ethicists, and other specialists. As an expanding field, there will be multiple possibilities for research, publication, and leadership. The recognition of a host of common perioperative problems in the elderly such as postoperative cognitive dysfunction and postoperative delirium that have important long-term consequences can be an area of research and academic interest.

Assessment of Resources

After identifying the person (or persons) who has an interest in geriatric anesthesia and educating others in this field, there should be an assessment of the resources available for increasing expertise. Is there a Department of Geriatrics at the educational institution that will partner with the anesthesiology department? If not, one could seek local experts in geriatrics in other fields who would be willing to provide mentoring and advice. Creat-

TABLE 5-2. Resources for teaching geriatric anesthesia.

Faculty development programs
Society for Advancement of Geriatric Anesthesia (SAGA)
Age Anaesthesia Association (United Kingdom)
American Society of Anesthesiologists Syllabus for Geriatrics
Portal of Geriatrics Online Education (POGOe)
American Geriatrics Society
   Geriatrics Syllabus for Specialists
   Geriatrics at Your Fingertips
Stanford University Geriatrics Education Resource Center
The John A. Hartford Foundation Consortium for Geriatrics in
   Residency Training

ing a network with others interested in geriatric anesthesia can provide support, information, and guidance. This can be aided by joining societies and organizations that promote and specialize in geriatrics and geriatric anesthesiology.

Membership in geriatric-oriented organizations can provide resources such as didactic lectures, speakers, journals, and meetings. For anesthesia providers, there is the SAGA in the United States and Age Anaesthesia Association in the United Kingdom (vide supra). Membership in the American Geriatric Society (AGS) promotes interaction with geriatric-oriented individuals in surgical and related subspecialties, national educational meetings, and monthly journals. The ASA has a geriatric syllabus available at no cost on their Web site.[13] Organizations such as these can provide lists of current, peer-reviewed geriatric articles in the medical literature, available educational grants, geriatric-related meetings, and speakers (Table 5-2).

Specific institutions may choose to develop multidisciplinary or specialty-specific seminars for faculty development in geriatrics.[14] Grants may provide funds for providing speakers and resources for these seminars or internal faculty with current geriatric expertise may be utilized to lead this expansion of geriatric expertise.

Determining a Program's Needs

Once the geriatric anesthesia specialists have been identified and outfitted with resources, there should be an assessment of departmental needs. One method to determine the needs and desires of the learners is to survey the students and residents. This can be done to discover areas of interest or areas that are inadequately covered by the current curriculum. Determining the aspects of caring for the elderly patient that are troubling or rewarding may be helpful. Do the residents and students think the geriatric curriculum, teaching, and experience are adequate? If not, what would they change? Assessing the confidence in teaching geriatric skills to fellow residents or students may determine areas for improvement.

The faculty can also be surveyed to find areas of expertise and interest that may be utilized for teaching geriatric anesthesia. The surveys may be repeated to assess the efficacy of the geriatric curriculum, and evaluation and feedback from the learners may help to guide needed changes.

A survey used at the University of Nebraska Medical Center sought information regarding the anesthesiology residents' confidence in performing specific tasks with the elderly patient such as functional assessment, discussion of advance directives and end-of-life issues, assessment of nutritional status, evaluation of sensory changes, risk and benefit discussion of proposed surgery, management of postoperative pain, evaluation for depression, and determination of the patient's social support (personal communication, Dr. Edward Vandenberg, Omaha, NE, May 5, 2004). The survey also included the residents' self-assessment of ability to distinguish between delirium and dementia and provide appropriate care for each, utilize information on aging physiology and age-related pharmacologic changes, and discuss relevant regulations regarding Medicare. The survey assessed the residents' desire to learn more about the above topics. This information was gathered on an annual basis to determine the areas of change desired in the curriculum as well as an assessment of the efficacy of the current curriculum.

TABLE 5-3. Sample geriatric curriculum for an anesthesiology residency.

A. Physiology of aging
  1. Gerontology
  2. Cardiovascular
  3. Respiratory
  4. Central and autonomic nervous system
  5. Renal and hepatic
B. Pharmacology of aging
  1. Induction agents
  2. Opioids
  3. Neuromuscular blockade
  4. Sedatives and hypnotics
  5. Cardiovascular medications
C. Preanesthetic evaluation
  1. Anesthetic risk and the elderly
  2. Guidelines for cardiac evaluation for noncardiac surgery
  3. Age-related disease
  4. Managing medical illness in the surgical patient
  5. Atypical presentations of common diseases in the elderly
D. Pain control in the elderly patient
  1. Acute pain control
  2. Chronic pain management
E. Regional anesthesia
F. Ethics and palliative care in geriatrics
G. Postoperative delirium and postoperative cognitive dysfunction
H. Special concerns in caring for the elderly
  1. The elderly ambulatory surgery patient
  2. Critical care
  3. Sedation and procedures in remote locations
  4. The elderly trauma patient

Producing a Geriatric Curriculum

After an assessment of the department's resources and needs is completed, a curriculum for geriatric education can be developed. Multiple teaching modalities should be incorporated into the development of this curriculum. There may be considerable overlap between the curriculum for residents and medical students although it may be necessary to condense the curriculum and didactics for medical students. Medical students' exposure to geriatrics will likely be covered in primary care rotations or separate geriatric clerkships. In many schools of medicine, it is part of a longitudinal educational continuum over at least 2 years. Geriatric anesthesia can be included in these or in the anesthesiology rotation.

Sample Curriculum

Table 5-3 shows an example of a geriatric curriculum for an anesthesiology residency.

Didactics

The geriatric curriculum can be integrated into the educational program of the residency program as a specific dedicated geriatric unit or integrated into the educational cycle of each subspecialty rotation. At the University of Nebraska Medical Center, the residency curriculum is 18

months in length so that residents are exposed to the entire didactic schedule twice during residency. The geriatric curriculum is inserted into the appropriate block. For example, during the time frame for preanesthesia evaluation and anesthetic risk, a lecture is given focusing on the preanesthetic evaluation of the geriatric patient and perioperative beta blockade is emphasized.

For didactic lectures, speakers may be utilized from complementary departments including gerontology, pharmacology, surgery, and internal medicine. Visiting professors can also be invited to provide information.

Discussion Groups

Journal clubs may be used to provide a more informal setting for a geriatric discussion group. This can be led and organized by the faculty member responsible for geriatric education or residents, and can provide interaction outside of the operating room. Case conferences and problem-based learning discussions allow specific examples and small group discussions that may provide for a more personal level of interaction and feedback. Such discussions with more relevant, reality-based learning in a smaller group may be more interesting to the adult learner than limiting geriatric education to lectures. Problem-based learning discussions can be based on actual cases or can be altered to incorporate a variety of teaching points in a concise manner.

Journal clubs, problem-based learning discussions, and case conferences are excellent opportunities to discuss current controversies in medical care, examine the medical literature, and reinforce topics covered in didactic lectures.

Reference Books

A library of geriatric anesthesiology references is helpful for consolidating information in an easily accessible location. There are multiple textbooks in geriatric medicine, gerontology, geriatric anesthesia, and geriatric surgery that should be available for consultation. These books should be available to the department members. The "Geriatric Syllabus for Specialists" and "Geriatrics at Your Fingertips," produced by the AGS, are valuable, pocket-sized resources that can be maintained in a reference library or acquired for each resident.

Computer-Based Materials

Internet-based resources are growing both in number and accessibility. The Portal of Geriatrics Online Education (POGOe) is an online clearinghouse that provides a single source of peer-reviewed educational products for those interested in geriatric education. Their site, www. pogoe.org, is funded by a grant from the Donald W. Reynolds Foundation to the Association of Geriatric Academic Programs. Physicians in training and practicing physicians may use the programs available.

Other educational materials that may be utilized are computer-based self-instruction modules in geriatrics. These may be available via the Internet or on CD or DVD formats. The Stanford University Geriatrics Education Resource Center and other locations have teaching resources available. An initiative funded by the John A. Hartford Foundation has developed the Consortium for Geriatrics in Residency Training. Institutions or individual faculty members may also choose to develop their own educational materials tailored to their specific requirements. Web-based computer modules can be created or utilized from sites such as POGOe or the Stanford University Geriatrics Education Resource Center to be used for education of medical students or residents. These offerings may also be available to practitioners who are not in a formal training program. Such computer modules can be case-oriented and allow the learner to progress at his or her own pace. This can expose the student or resident to topics that may not be covered in a clinical situation and allow for immediate feedback and evaluation. Pre- and postmodule examinations can be used to determine information retention. If further discussion and evaluation is desired, a faculty-led discussion session can emphasize learning points and provide another avenue for those using the modules to provide feedback and evaluation. The Web-based modules can either be tailored to medical student or resident educational needs, or both groups can use the same module.

Simulation

The use of simulators for education is increasing as a greater number of institutions acquire the equipment and gain experience with the advantages of simulation education. The simulators can be used for multiple types of cases and provide a wide range of experience for the student and trainee. Simulation should include patients with coexisting morbidities and intraoperative and postoperative changes in organ systems, as well as providing experience with life-threatening processes or rare conditions that may not be experienced by the trainee in a clinical situation. Simulation can be primarily software based or may have intricate mannequins, creating the feel and responsiveness of an actual geriatric patient. There are many types available, from whole-body simulators to specific airway or regional anesthesia modes. Receiving feedback and constructive criticism with objective data can be a very valuable part of the experience. The encounters may be videotaped, and the computer will maintain information on each action. An advantage of simulators is the ability to teach all levels of learners and a wide variety of careers such as anesthesia practitioners, critical care nurses, allied health professionals, and medical students.

Evaluation of Curriculum

The effectiveness of a geriatric anesthesia curriculum must be evaluated; this can be accomplished in a number of ways. If the geriatric curriculum is covered in a core unit, a posttest can be used to determine informational retention and attainment of basic facts and knowledge. A pretest before introduction of the geriatric curriculum could be useful to gauge the change in basic knowledge that will be demonstrated in the posttest. An evaluation of attitude change and self-perception of knowledge may be garnered from a survey of the participants.

Behavioral change is the ultimate desire of education. The ability to measure a change in behavior is difficult but may be reflected in the learner's professionalism and practice patterns. In a residency program, the use of 360-degree evaluations may be a useful tool for assessment. Faculty members, nurses, and other health care and support personnel can evaluate the resident attitudes and actions. The use of patient and family comments can be utilized in a constructive manner to note positive aspects of performance as well as areas for improvement. Feedback with suggestions for improvement can be given to the residents and students.

Summary

The number of geriatric patients is certain to increase. It is recognized that the academic programs in anesthesiology need to address the topic of geriatric anesthesia and prepare students to care for elderly patients. The expected growth in the older population and the increase in the number of operations for patients defined as elderly demand a well-trained profession able to meet the needs of this group. There are many avenues of medical knowledge such as postoperative cognitive dysfunction that are just beginning to be explored, along with further insight into the physiologic changes of aging and the effects of coexisting medical conditions.

The medical school curriculum has changed in the past several decades to reflect an increased emphasis on geriatrics in the primary care fields. Beyond the primary care fields, the establishment of geriatric specialists has been lagging. The education of students and residents in geriatric anesthesiology will require an increased emphasis in these training programs.

Establishing a geriatric anesthesiology curriculum requires an understanding of the needs of the adult learner who is self-directed, independent, and driven by internal motivation and the need for self-improvement. The adult student brings a set of experiences that can serve as a resource for further education but must be acknowledged and validated by the teacher. The desire for education that is practical and useful in everyday situations places an emphasis on teaching methods that utilize this, such as problem-based learning or case-oriented discussions with less desire for traditional lectures.

Identifying a single individual to be responsible for geriatric anesthesiology education is imperative. Identifying and encouraging other faculty interested in geriatric anesthesia is a key component in establishing and maintaining a geriatric curriculum. This interest can be enhanced by the realization that a great opportunity exists to have an impact on a field that is rapidly growing and gaining in recognition. Even one individual can have an effect on an institution and, by networking with other similarly interested people locally and at a distance, on the profession as a whole.

The involvement in geriatric anesthesia and geriatric societies provides a source of information and benefits such as scholarly journals, meetings, and educational opportunities.

Development of a geriatric anesthesia program requires an inventory of a department's resources and needs. Surveys and evaluations can be used to determine areas of strength or inadequate coverage in the current or proposed curriculum. Many modalities may be incorporated in the educational program including faculty lectures, visiting speakers, computer-based modules, journal clubs, case conferences and problem-based learning groups, simulations, discussion groups, and Internet-based resources. Educational materials may be tailored to a specific anesthesia program or adapted from available sources such as the POGOe.

Increasing geriatric anesthesiology education in a residency program may allow incorporation of core competencies required for graduate medical education. Education and evaluation in practice-based learning and improvement, professionalism, and systems-based practice can be used in conjunction with geriatric anesthesiology. Proficiency in medical knowledge, patient care, and communication are all essential attributes for geriatric anesthesiology.

Geriatric anesthesiology and geriatric anesthesia education will continue to grow and improve. By focusing time and resources on training anesthesia providers in the care of the elderly patient, the results will be better trained practitioners who can meet the needs of this growing population. The field of anesthesiology must incorporate geriatric anesthesiology education in all levels of its teaching.

References

1. The Association of Directors of Geriatric Academic Programs. Longitudinal study of training and practice in geriatric medicine. Available at: www.adgapstudy.uc.edu. Accessed August 13, 2004.
2. Accreditation Council for Graduate Medical Education. Program requirements for anesthesiology. Available at: www.acgme.org/downloads/RRC_progReq.040pr703_u804.pdf. Accessed January 15, 2007.
3. Accreditation Council for Graduate Medical Education. Outcome project, general competencies. Available at: www.acgme.org/outcome/comp/compMin.asp. Accessed January 15, 2007.
4. Barnett SR. Geriatric education: "Start low, go slow." ASA Newslett 2004;68(5):9–10.
5. Lynch DC, Swing SR, Horowitz DS, et al. Assessing practice-based learning and improvement. Teach Learn Med 2004;16(1):85–92.
6. Interdisciplinary Leadership Group of the American Geriatrics Society. A statement of principles: toward improved care of older patients in surgical and medical specialties. J Am Geriatr Soc 2000;48:699–701.
7. Creditor MC. Hazards of hospitalization in the elderly. Ann Intern Med 1993;118(3):219–223.
8. Sager MA, Franke T, Inouye SK, et al. Functional outcomes of acute medical illness and hospitalization in older persons. Arch Intern Med 1996;156(6):645–652.
9. Warshaw GA, Bragg EJ, Shaull RW, et al. Geriatric medicine fellowship programs: a national study from the Association of Directors of Geriatric Academic Programs' Longitudinal Study of training and practice in geriatric medicine. J Am Geriatr Soc 2003;51(7):1023–1030.
10. Schwartz AJ. Teaching anesthesia. In: Miller RD, ed. Anesthesia. 6th ed. New York: Churchill Livingstone; 2005: 3105–3117.

11. Kaufman DM. Applying educational theory in practice. BMJ 2003;326:213–216.
12. Newman P, Peile E. Valuing learners' experience and supporting further growth: educational models to help experienced adult learners in medicine. BMJ 2002;325: 200–202.
13. American Society of Anesthesiologists. Syllabus on geriatric anesthesiology. Available at: www.asahq.org/clinical/geriatrics/syllabus.htm. Accessed August 15, 2004.
14. Williams BC. Building geriatrics curricula in medical and surgical house officer programs through faculty development. Acad Med 2002;77(5):458.

6
Research Priorities in Geriatric Anesthesiology*

Christopher J. Jankowski and David J. Cook

The implications of an aging population on the practice of anesthesiology are profound. Normal aging results in diminished functional reserve across organ systems. These normal physiologic changes and age-related disease combine to limit the ability of the elderly to tolerate the stress of the perioperative period. Thus, geriatric issues affect every aspect of the care provided by the anesthesiologist.

For example, age-related physiologic changes and disease make the preoperative evaluation of geriatric patients more complex than that of younger patients. Baseline functional reserve is often difficult to assess because of limits in physical ability, either from deconditioning, age-related disease, cognitive impairment, or a combination of the three. The same issues make the maintenance of intraoperative homeostasis more challenging in this population. Finally, geriatric issues such as postoperative respiratory complications and cognitive changes, as well as acute and chronic pain management can make postoperative care challenging.

Despite these issues, surprisingly little research has been done to address the perioperative care of the aged, per se. This chapter will review some of the literature pertaining to this population in order to identify potentially fruitful areas of research.

First, some of the normal physiologic changes that occur with aging will be reviewed. This is essential to frame any discussion of preoperative assessment or intra- and postoperative management. Second, the preoperative evaluation of the older surgical patient will be discussed. Third, research related to the intraoperative management of geriatric patients will be described. Last,

the chapter will address geriatric issues in postoperative management, emphasizing postoperative respiratory and cognitive complications, as well as acute and chronic pain management. Each section will conclude with a list of potential research agenda items. The end of the chapter identifies research agenda items of the highest priority.

Physiologic Changes Relevant to Perioperative Care

The physiology of aging bears on preoperative assessment, intraoperative and postoperative management, and the types and likelihood of major adverse events. Age-related changes in cardiac, respiratory, neurologic, renal, and pharmacokinetics have been well defined. The most important generalization from physiologic studies of aging is that the basal function of the various organ systems is relatively uncompromised by the aging process. However, functional reserve, specifically the ability to compensate for physiologic stress, is reduced (Figure 6-1). This has profound implications for the preoperative assessment and the perioperative care of geriatric patients.

Cardiovascular Changes

Numerous changes in cardiovascular function with aging have implications for anesthetic care. With aging, a progressive decrease in the elasticity of the arterial vasculature leads to an increase in systolic blood pressure. Diastolic blood pressure increases through middle age and typically decreases after age 60.[1] There is also a decrease in the cross-sectional area of the peripheral vascular bed, resulting in higher peripheral vascular resistance.[2] A decrease in the peripheral vasodilatory response to β-adrenergic stimulation may also contribute to the hypertension of aging.[3]

*This chapter is based on work performed for "New Frontiers in Geriatrics Research: An Agenda for Surgical and Related Medical Specialties," a component of the American Geriatrics Society's Geriatrics-for-Specialists Initiative (GSI), funded by the John A. Hartford Foundation of New York. With permission of the American Geriatrics Society.

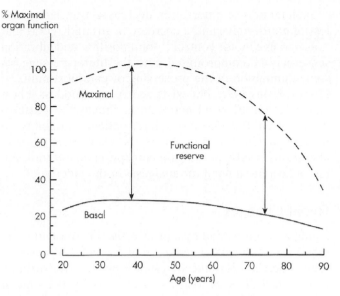

% Maximal
organ function

FIGURE 6-1. Functional reserve is the difference between maximal (broken line) and basal (solid line) function. Aging inevitably reduces functional reserve even in individuals who are physiologically "young." The configuration of the curve for "basal" function is adapted from longitudinal measurements of total (not weight-specific) basal metabolic rate. (Reprinted with permission from Muravchick S. Geroanesthesia: Principles for Management of the Elderly Patient. St. Louis: Mosby-Year Book; 1997.)

Progressive ventricular hypertrophy develops in response to increased afterload and leads to cellular hypertrophy and deposition of fibrotic tissue. Ventricular hypertrophy increases wall stress and myocardial O_2 demand, making the ventricle more prone to ischemia.

Although intrinsic contractility and resting cardiac output are unaltered with aging, ventricular hypertrophy and stiffening limit the ability of the heart to adjust stroke volume.[4] Ventricular hypertrophy impairs the passive filling phase of diastole. Thus, ventricular preload is more dependent on the contribution of atrial contraction. At the same time, fatty infiltration and fibrosis of the heart increases the incidence of sinus, atrioventricular, and ventricular conduction defects.[5,6] In addition, there are decreases in myocardial responsiveness to catecholamines; maximal heart rate response is correspondingly decreased.[4,7,8] The reduction in ventricular compliance and the attenuated response to catecholamines compromise the heart's ability to buffer decreases in circulatory volume resulting in a disposition to hypotension. Similarly, even modest increases in circulatory volume lead to congestive heart failure.

From the standpoint of perioperative hemodynamic stability, age-related changes in the autonomic control of heart rate, cardiac output, peripheral vascular resistance, and the baroreceptor response[9–13] are as important as the chronic changes in the myocardium and vasculature.

It is evident that age-related changes in the cardiovascular system involve alterations in both mechanics and control mechanisms; the same can be said of the pulmonary system.

Pulmonary Changes

The pulmonary system also undergoes age-related changes independent of comorbid disease processes. Functionally, there are remarkable parallels with changes in the heart. With aging, the thorax becomes stiffer.[14,15] This may not be evident in the sedentary patient, but reduced chest wall compliance increases the work of breathing and reduces maximal minute ventilation.[14,16] Loss of thoracic skeletal muscle mass further aggravates this process.[17] Because of a decrease in elastic lung recoil, the closing volume increases such that it exceeds functional residual capacity by age 65.[18] Inspiratory and expiratory functional reserve decrease with aging, and the normal matching of ventilation and perfusion becomes impaired.[19,20] The latter process increases the alveolar-arterial O_2 gradient and decreases the resting PaO_2.[18,21] The respiratory response to hypoxia diminishes in the aged[22] (Figure 6-2). In addition, ciliary function and cough are reduced.[15] Finally, pharyngeal sensation and the motor function required for swallowing are diminished in the elderly.[23,24]

These changes have important implications in the perioperative period. First, it is difficult to predict from a preoperative interview how an inactive, elderly patient will respond to the perioperative respiratory challenges.

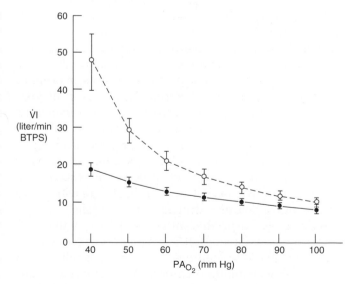

$\dot{V}I$
(liter/min
BTPS)

PA_{O_2} (mm Hg)

FIGURE 6-2. Ventilatory response (V_I) to isocapnic progressive hypoxia in eight young normal men (broken line) and eight normal men aged 64–73 (solid line). Values are means ± SEM. (Reprinted with permission from Kronenberg and Drage.[22])

Anesthetics, postoperative pain, the supine position, narcotics, as well as thoracic and upper abdominal operations impair pulmonary function and further depress respiratory drive.[14,25,26] Although blood gas analysis or spirometric tests may offer some value before thoracic operations, the alterations in pulmonary function after surgery are complex and typically not predictable from preoperative pulmonary function testing.[14,20,27] Age-related changes in pulmonary mechanics and respiratory control increase the risk of postoperative hypoxia[28,29] and perioperative aspiration in the elderly.[23,30]

Neurologic Changes

Pulmonary and cardiac complications account for much of the morbidity and mortality in older surgical patients. However, neurologic morbidity affects many patients as well. Also, age-related degenerative changes in the central and peripheral nervous systems contribute to a variety of other morbidities. In themselves, neurologic complications have a dramatic impact on length of stay, discharge disposition, functional status, and quality of life.

Independent of any comorbid process, both the central and peripheral nervous systems are affected by aging.[31] There is a loss of cortical gray matter through middle age, resulting in cerebral atrophy,[32] although how much of this is attributable to aging itself versus degenerative diseases is a subject of ongoing investigation.[33] At the level of the neuron, there is a reduction in the complexity of neuronal connections, a decrease in the synthesis of neurotransmitters, and an increase in the enzymes responsible for their postsynaptic degradation.[33–35] Although cerebral metabolism, blood flow, and autoregulation generally remain intact,[32] neuronal loss and the deficiency of neurotransmitters limit the ability of the older brain to integrate multiple neural inputs. This has been described as a loss of "fluid" intelligence. Neuronal loss and demyelinization also occur in the spinal cord.[36] Functionally, there are changes in spinal cord reflexes and reductions in proprioception. There are also important decreases in hypoxic and hypercarbic respiratory drive.[22,37] Decreases in visual and auditory function further complicate the ability of the nervous system to acquire and process information. This combination of changes limits the ability of the older patient to understand and process information in the perioperative period and probably contributes to postoperative delirium, drug toxicity, and falls.

Aging is also associated with neuronal loss in the autonomic nervous system. Both sympathetic and parasympathetic ganglia lose neurons, and there is fibrosis of peripheral sympathetic neurons. Peripheral autonomic neuronal loss is associated with impairment of cardiovascular reflexes. At the same time, decreases in adrenoceptor responsiveness result in increased adrenomedullary output and plasma catecholamine concentrations.[11,13,36]

Skeletal muscle innervation decreases, translating into loss of motor units, and a decrease in strength, coordination, and fine motor control.[38] Joint position and vibration sense may be compromised, and the literature suggests some diminution in the processing of painful stimuli.[39–42] However, this effect, if it exists, seems to be modest at best and does not affect all nerve types equally.[42–45] Furthermore, given the enormous inter-patient variability in nervous system function and in the experience of pain, alterations in subtypes of pain perception do not translate into a decreased need for analgesia in the elderly.[44–48]

Renal Changes

Aging is accompanied by a progressive decrease in renal blood flow and loss of renal parenchyma.[49,50] By age 80, renal blood flow is reduced by half. Renal cortical atrophy results in a 30% decrease in nephrons by the end of middle age.[49,51] Furthermore, aging is associated with sclerosis of nephrons so that some of those remaining are dysfunctional.[50,52] Together, these processes result in a progressive decrease in glomerular capillary surface area and glomerular filtration rate.[50,52–54] However, because of loss of muscle mass, aging is not associated with an increase in serum creatinine. This physiologic, and often occult, aspect of senescence has practical implications in the perioperative period.

The old kidney has difficulty in maintaining circulating blood volume and sodium homeostasis in the perioperative period.[11,53–55] Sodium conservation and excretion are both impaired by aging. Additionally, fluid homeostasis is complicated by alterations in thirst mechanisms and antidiuretic hormone release that frequently result in dehydration.[53–56] During the perioperative period, metabolic acidosis is also relatively common because elderly patients are less efficient in the renal excretion of acid.[57]

Reductions in basal renal blood flow render the elderly kidney particularly susceptible to the deleterious effects of low cardiac output, hypotension, hypovolemia, and hemorrhage. Anesthetics, surgical stress, pain, sympathetic stimulation, and renal vasoconstrictive drugs all may compound subclinical renal insufficiency. The likelihood of acute renal insufficiency is especially great following aortic and intraabdominal operations. Finally, age-related decreases in glomerular filtration rate reduce the clearance of a number of drugs given in the perioperative period.

Aging, Pharmacokinetics, and Pharmacodynamics

Aging is associated with multiple physiologic changes that affect drug pharmacology.[58] Decreased lean body mass and total body water and an increased proportion of body fat alter the volume of distribution of drugs, their redistribution between body compartments, and, subsequently, their rates of clearance and elimination.[59–61] The effect of changes in body composition on drug distribution and action varies depending on the lipid or aqueous solubility of the drug. Water-soluble drugs have higher serum concentration and lower redistribution, whereas fat-soluble drugs tend to undergo wider distribution and accumulation, followed by delayed release.

While age-related changes in the proportions of different plasma proteins make predictions about pharmacokinetics complex in the elderly, for many drugs, decreased protein binding and increased free fraction have the potential to increase the pharmacologic effect of drugs administered in the perioperative period.[58] Potential alterations in cardiac output, renal, or hepatic clearance also may change effective plasma concentrations and duration of action.[62] Neuronal loss and decreased levels of neurotransmitters in the central nervous system increase sensitivity to anesthetic agents. The changes in pharmacokinetics that occur with aging make it difficult to identify an independent effect of aging on pharmacodynamics.[59,60] However, age-related changes in the central nervous system seem to increase the sensitivity to a variety of anesthetic agents (Figure 6-3).[63–65]

TABLE 6-1. Age and drug reactions.

Age of patients (years)	No. with reactions	Rate (%)
10–19	2	3.1
20–29	3	3.0
30–39	7	5.7
40–49	12	7.5
50–59	18	8.1
60–69	27	10.7
70–79	38	21.3
80–89	11	18.6
Total	118	10.2

Source: Modified with permission from Hurwitz.[66]

Pharmacokinetic changes, particularly decreased metabolism, plus drug interactions coupled with polypharmacy, conspire to make the elderly prone to adverse drug effects.[66,67] There is an almost linear increase in adverse drug reactions with age from below 10% at age 25 to above 20% at age 80.[68,69] The likelihood of adverse drug reactions increases with the number of drugs administered (Table 6-1).[66,67] Because many patients come to surgery already taking multiple medications, the addition of several drugs in the perioperative period makes adverse reactions likely.

Implications

It is clear from a review of normal changes in physiologic function with aging that even the fit elderly patient's ability to compensate for perioperative stress is compromised. The cardiac, pulmonary, neurologic, neuroendocrine, renal, and pharmacokinetic/pharmacodynamic changes that occur with aging make hypotension, low cardiac output, hypoxia, hypercarbia, disordered fluid regulation, and adverse drug effects more likely in the perioperative period. Additionally, because baseline cardiac, pulmonary, renal, and neurologic function are generally adequate, in the absence of acute challenges, it can be difficult to predict the effect of perioperative stress on the older patient.

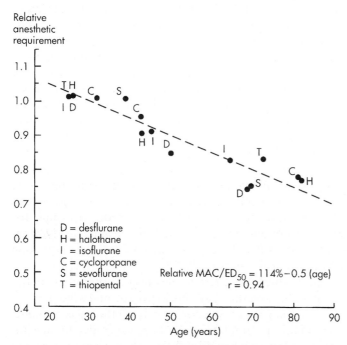

FIGURE 6-3. With advancing age, anesthetic requirement for unsedated human subjects expressed as relative median effective dose (ED_{50}) or its inhalational equivalent, minimum alveolar concentration (MAC), is progressively and consistently reduced. Anesthetic requirement declines both for inhalational (C, D, H, I, S) and for intravenous (T) anesthetics. (Reprinted with permission from Muravchick S. Geroanesthesia: Principles for Management of the Elderly Patient. St. Louis: Mosby-Year Book; 1997.)

Preoperative Assessment of the Elderly

The underlying health of the patient and the type and urgency of the procedure determine the extent of the preoperative assessment. The preoperative evaluation serves several purposes in most patients. Historically, it has served two primary functions: to alert the perioperative care providers to physiologic conditions that may alter perioperative management and to determine if medical intervention is indicated before proceeding. Two more contemporary uses of the preoperative assessment are to provide an index of risk, therefore contributing to decisions about the most appropriate intervention, and to provide baseline data on which the success of a surgical intervention might be judged.

Physiologic studies of aging and clinical experience with this population yield three important conclusions regarding preoperative assessment. First, there is tremendous heterogeneity in the geriatric population. As Muravchick[70] notes, humans are never so similar as at birth, and never so dissimilar as in old age. Second, whereas basal function in most elderly patients is sufficient to meet daily needs, under conditions of physiologic stress, impairment in functional reserve becomes evident (see above). Third, most older surgical patients have significant comorbidities. Up to 80% of elderly surgical patients have at least one comorbid condition and one third have three or more.[71,72]

Despite those concerns, even extreme age is not a contraindication to surgery. Acceptable outcomes are reported for operations even in very old patients.[73–77] What is less clear is how to identify which patients will do well and which will do poorly. Although this has been the subject of considerable research, no area of perioperative anesthetic care and management requires more investigation. The preoperative assessment of the patient is composed of four interrelated functions: risk stratification using population-based studies; history and physical examination of the individual patient; preoperative testing; and, in some cases, preoperative optimization. Each of these areas requires development and better definition for the geriatric surgical population.

Risk Stratification

Because age itself adds very little additional risk in the absence of comorbid disease,[78] most risk factor identification and risk predictive indexes have been disease oriented.[79–83] These investigations typically have studied a broad age range of patients and in multivariate analyses identified the relative contribution of age and comorbid conditions to surgical morbidity and mortality.[80,81,84–87] Others have examined the predictive value of the number of comorbid diseases independent of the operative condition or evaluated the impact of American Society of Anesthesiologists status, specific surgical factors, and intraoperative management.[81,87–92]

The applicability of many existing risk indices to the geriatric population is unclear. Because of the prevalence of comorbid conditions, it is difficult to stratify the older patient population into smaller subsets with better-defined risk. The paucity of population studies of perioperative risk and outcomes specifically in geriatric populations can make choosing the most suitable course of care difficult. Furthermore, elderly patients have unique perioperative risks. In addition to death, myocardial infarction, or congestive heart failure, older patients are unusually prone to postoperative delirium, aspiration, urosepsis, adverse drug interactions, pressure sores, malnutrition, falls, and failure to return to ambulation or to home. Therefore, preoperative assessment tools and the variables evaluated in outcomes trials require expansion for application to the geriatric surgical population. Population studies need to examine not only mortality and major cardiopulmonary morbidity, but also outcomes specific to the geriatric population. Once completed, epidemiologic studies that better stratify older patients would help define the preoperative assessment appropriate to older patients.

Functional Assessments

The efficacy of preoperative functional evaluation in elderly surgical patients requires investigation. This is important for several reasons. The evaluation of the "resting" patient does not indicate how the patient will respond to the cardiac, pulmonary, and metabolic demands of the perioperative period. This approach is emphasized in the American College of Cardiology/American Heart Association guidelines for preoperative cardiac evaluation in which the patient's activity level, expressed in metabolic units, is a primary determinant of the need for subsequent evaluation.[79] However, this concept must be expanded because the geriatric population has a unique need for functional evaluation in more areas than just cardiopulmonary capacity. Because of patient heterogeneity, functional assessments may be indicated to better characterize patient differences, whether it is for activities of daily living (ADL), instrumental ADL, cognitive and emotional status, or urologic function.[93,94] Scales such as the Medical Outcomes Study Short Form-36[95] have multiple domains that are particularly useful in the geriatric population. Although these metrics have been applied successfully in orthopedic and thoracic surgery[96–98] and can have predictive value for longer-term outcomes,[99–103] multidimensional assessment and perioperative functional assessment is largely lacking in the surgical literature.[97,104,105]

An example of their application is provided in the study of hip fracture patients by Keene and Anderson,[101] who scored patients preoperatively on the basis of physical condition, ambulation, ADL, preoperative living situation, and preexisting disabilities. The scoring system was then used to predict which patients would be discharged to nursing homes after surgery. The actual outcome after surgery was observed for 1 year and compared with the models' predictions (Table 6-2). Although the study is small, it serves as an example for the type of research needed in geriatric surgery.

In regard to preoperative functional assessment, cognitive and psychologic evaluation of the elderly surgical

TABLE 6-2. Predicted outcomes, actual outcomes, and average scores on functional rating scale of 39 patients discharged to nursing homes who were alive 1 year after hip fracture.

No. of patients	Residence before fracture	Nursing home placement (predicted outcome)	Actual outcome 1 year after fracture	Average score
10	Home	Temporary	Temporary	72
8	Home	Temporary	Permanent	52
6	Home	Permanent	Permanent	51
15	Nursing home	Permanent	Permanent	30

Source: Modified with permission from Keene and Anderson.[101]

patient deserves special comment. Although frank delirium or dementia at admission is very evident and clearly predicts poorer acute and long-term outcomes,[106,107] subtle forms of cognitive impairment are much more common in the elderly. In the absence of screening, preoperative cognitive deficits may not be evident until the postoperative period. Subtle forms of cognitive impairment can predict subsequent delirium in hospitalized medical patients[108] and worsened cognitive outcome in cardiac, orthopedic, and gastrointestinal surgery patients.[109–113] Therefore, preoperative mental status examination[114,115] should be considered in all geriatric surgical patients. Preoperative depression and alcohol abuse occur frequently and can affect postoperative outcomes in similar ways,[106,116–118] and, similar to mental status batteries, a variety of assessment tools for depression are available.[119,120] The impact of screening for mental status,

depression, and alcohol abuse on perioperative management of elderly patients is a huge potential area of investigation.

Preoperative functional assessment is also important because the goal should be to return the patient to at least their preoperative activity level. The success of surgery must be questioned if the procedure is technically adequate, but the patient suffers loss of independence. Multidimensional assessment may help redefine standards for success of surgery and reset therapeutic priorities.[96,97,121–123] Mangione and colleagues[97] applied this type of assessment by longitudinally measured quality of life indicators in patients undergoing hip, thoracic, and aortic surgery. A variety of metrics, including the Short Form-36, were used to measure physical, psychologic and social functions, and health perceptions preoperatively as well as 1, 6, and 12 months after surgery (Figure 6-4). Major morbidity and

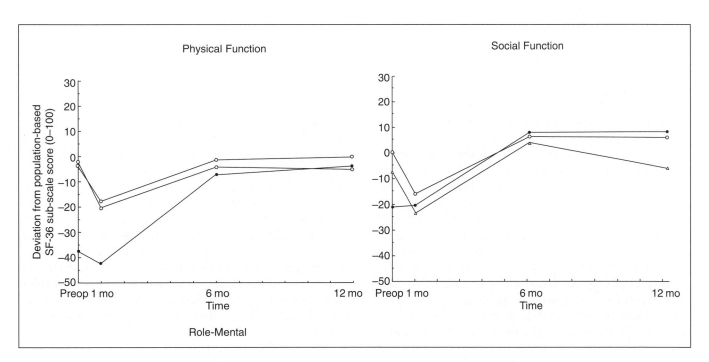

FIGURE 6-4. Deviation from age- and gender-adjusted population-based Short Form-36 subgroup scores by surgical procedure. Triangles indicate thoracic surgery for lung cancer; filled circles, total hip arthroplasty; open circles, abdominal aortic aneurysm; dotted line, age- and gender-adjusted population-based value. (Modified with permission from Mangione et al.[97] Published by Blackwell Publishing.)

mortality aside, these types of measures address what is fundamentally most important in the management of older patients: whether the surgical intervention improves functional status and well-being. These measures are of unique importance to the elderly because, unlike younger patients, the aged are at far greater risk for long-term functional compromise after surgery.

Preoperative Testing

The third area contributing to the preoperative evaluation of the elderly surgical patient is preoperative testing. Work in this area has been done for large populations of mixed age groups. However, it is not clear whether selected preoperative screening tests have a different yield in the elderly or, more likely, if specific testing is indicated for geriatric patients undergoing certain surgical procedures.

In the general population, there is agreement that the bulk of routine preoperative testing is not indicated.[124–127] In an evaluation of preoperative screening in 1010 individuals undergoing cholecystectomy, abnormal results were found in only 4.5% of tests.[124] In another investigation of 3131 patients aged 0–98 years who underwent 38,286 tests, unexpected abnormal results were found in 15% of patients.[125] However, only 3% had a change in their anesthetic or surgical plan based on those results. Unfortunately, in neither report were age-specific data provided, so it is unclear if the results can be translated to an older surgical population.

Smaller studies in elderly populations suggest a higher yield for specific tests. Seymour et al.[128] examined the value of routine chest X-ray (CXR) in 223 patients older than 65 years undergoing general surgery. Of these, 40% had an abnormality regarded as clinically significant, although in only 5% did the CXR affect the course of treatment. The same authors also examined the value of the electrocardiogram (ECG) in routine screening in 222 patients older than 65 years[129] and found that only 21% of patients had a normal ECG and that 53% had a major abnormality. They reported that, although only 1% of patients had abnormalities that delayed surgery, 30% developed new ECG abnormalities postoperatively. The authors concluded that the screening ECG has little or no value for predicting cardiac complications, but recommended preoperative ECG in all elderly patients to provide a basis for comparison and as a means of detecting patients for whom surgery should be deferred.[129]

In a small study of acutely ill elderly (mean age = 81 years) medical patients (50 admissions), Sewell and colleagues[130] examined the value of full blood count, sedimentation rate, urinalysis, electrolyte, liver, thyroid tests, and CXR. Six of 28 patients had abnormalities on CXR (21%), although management was only influenced in one. The most important finding in the screening battery was

the frequency of unknown urinary tract infections (16/50 patients, 32%). A retrospective analysis of 86 patients undergoing hip arthroplasty evaluated the impact of 24 laboratory tests on postoperative course.[131] In four patients (4.6%), care was altered, three of whom had urinary tract infections. A cost-benefit analysis justified routine urinary analysis to reduce hip infections in elderly patients undergoing total hip arthroplasties.

Assessment of nutritional status is useful in certain subpopulations of surgical patients. The 44-center Veterans Administration study found that serum albumin concentration was a better predictor of surgical outcomes than many other patient characteristics.[132,133] Although it can be difficult to separate the role of the disease process resulting in protein-calorie malnutrition from the effect of the malnutrition itself,[134] in elderly hospitalized nonsurgical patients, adverse outcomes can be attributed to malnutrition independent of greater acuity of illness or comorbidity.[135] Because of wide confidence limits, laboratory assessment of nutritional assessments may make their application to individual patients less useful than to populations.[134] Thus, it may prove useful to combine laboratory tests with anthropomorphic measurements, such as body mass index, limb circumferences, and weight loss.[136–139] The latter instruments are simple and inexpensive, but their clinical yield has not been determined. Nutritional assessment may have implications for preoperative management, and the timing of surgery as well as for risk stratification in certain types of surgery, but nutritional evaluation has not been adequately studied in elderly surgical patients.

A recent study of preoperative testing in 18,000 patients undergoing cataract procedures deserves comment. Patients were randomly assigned to undergo or not undergo routine testing (ECG, complete blood count, electrolytes, blood urea nitrogen, creatinine, and glucose).[140] The analysis was stratified by age and showed no benefit to routine testing for any group of patients. Similar conclusions were drawn in the recent study of 544 elderly noncardiac surgical patients by Dzankic et al.[141]

From these investigations, and a body of work in younger subjects, three themes are evident. First, routine screening in a general population of elderly patients does not add significantly to information obtained in the clinical history. Second, in a general population, the positive predictive value of abnormal findings on routine screening is limited. Third, positive results on screening tests have relatively little impact on the course of patient care. Despite those observations, further research is required.

Although the yield for routine screening is very low, it can be clinically valuable and cost-effective to develop guidelines for preoperative testing based on the type of surgery. Differing types of surgery impose different types and degrees of physiologic stress. As such, the results of the cataract trial will not be applicable to patients undergoing vascular surgery. Preoperative tests such as echocardiography and thallium scanning can have clinically relevant predictive value and potentially alter the course of care and outcomes if applied to specific populations at high risk for perioperative cardiac complications.[79,142,143] Similarly, nutritional assessment[133,144] might be useful before abdominal or major orthopedic surgery, but would be of much lower value before carotid endarterectomy. Screening for urinary tract infection before orthopedic surgery or pulmonary function testing before thoracic surgery are other examples. Because the interaction of the patient factors and the surgical insult determines outcome, specific testing might be equally indicated in a very physiologically challenged older patient undergoing minimally stressful surgery (e.g., hernia repair), and in the mildly compromised older patient undergoing surgery that imposes severe physiologic stress (e.g., aortic aneurysm surgery). Therefore, future studies in older patients will need to stratify patients as to the severity of their preexisting risk factors (low, intermediate, or high) and specifically examine their interaction with the specific surgical challenges most common in the elderly.

Preoperative Optimization

In addition to providing (1) an assessment of risk based on population studies, (2) functional data to help define surgical success, and (3) specific information to guide perioperative management, the fourth purpose of preoperative evaluation is to determine if medical intervention is indicated before proceeding. To some extent, this function has been lost with the foreshortening of the preoperative period, the "A.M. admit," and a progressive elimination of preoperative testing.

The research agenda for the care of elderly surgery patients must include preoperative optimization of medical status. This is an area in which relatively little work has been done. Again, in specific populations undergoing high-risk surgery, the value of preoperative optimization, particularly of cardiac and pulmonary status, can be demonstrated. Pulmonary toilet, antibiotics, and steroid therapy for some types of thoracic surgery, intervention for coronary disease before vascular surgery, and preoperative β-blockade for high-risk patients are areas in which the data are compelling.[142,143,145–149] Nevertheless, many areas have not been evaluated, particularly in the elderly. In addition to modifying cardiopulmonary risk, improving nutritional status before major elective surgery, preoperative hydration, and optimization of renal function in those with chronic or acute insufficiency could have broad impact. Preoperative management of antibiotic therapy, anticoagulation, antiplatelet therapy, and anemia are other obvious areas to examine. There are also suggestions that preoperative education, psychologic support, and physical therapy

might facilitate pain management and rehabilitation after some types of surgery,[150,151] but this area has not been adequately assessed.

In today's environment, it will be difficult to conduct studies on preoperative optimization. For example, in studies of preoperative nutritional optimization, it would be difficult to justify randomizing a clearly malnourished patient to a control group proceeding directly to the operating room without nutritional therapy when surgery could be delayed. Conversely, intervention and delay will add costs. However, limited studies in orthopedic and cardiac surgical patients suggest that appropriately applied preoperative care can be cost effective in that it shortens hospital stays and improves functional status after discharge.[151,152] Preoperative optimization will not be practical or necessary in many instances. However, much geriatric surgery is elective, so these studies can be conducted and, if positive, could influence the care and outcome of many patients.

Preoperative Research Agenda Items

- There is a need for epidemiologic studies describing outcomes, relatively unique to older surgical patients, for the most common types of surgery. The frequency is probably underestimated by retrospective analysis in much of the literature. With few exceptions, future studies will need to be prospective, cross-sectional studies. In the second phase, patient and surgery-specific risk factors for geriatric complications would be identified by multivariate analysis. These investigations would stratify surgical risk as low, intermediate, or high depending on type of surgery.

- The most pressing need for preoperative assessment is to develop better tools to predict which patients will do well and which will do poorly. The positive predictive value of these instruments would be first determined in prospective nonrandomized or prospective cohort trials. After that, prospective randomized trials would determine whether the application of these metrics could improve outcomes either by perioperative intervention or altering the surgical intervention based on the patient risk profile.

- The contribution of simple preoperative functional studies to surgical decision making has largely not been investigated. Prospective cohort or case-control studies would be required to determine if assessment of preoperative functional status changes surgical decision making (timing or type of surgery) or pre- or postoperative care strategies.

- The impact of screening for cognitive impairment, depression, and alcohol abuse on perioperative management of elderly patients is a huge potential area of investigation. Existing literature provides an incidence for these preexisting conditions, but an incomplete understanding of risk factors. Prospective cross-sectional or cohort studies will better identify association between these patient preexisting conditions and adverse geriatric outcomes by multivariate analysis. Subsequently, prospective randomized trials could determine the effect of pre- or postoperative interventions on adverse outcomes related to these risk factors.

- Assessment of preoperative nutritional status, hydration, and renal function may have implications for preoperative management and the timing of surgery as well as for risk stratification but this has not been adequately studied in the elderly. First, the positive or negative predictive value of instruments to evaluate nutrition and hydration would be tested in prospective studies. Second, prospective cohort or case-control studies would be used to determine if application of these metrics would change preoperative care, timing, or choice of surgery perioperative management and reduce complications.

Intraoperative Management

By its nature, anesthetic care is episodic, so most of the criteria to judge the success of anesthetic interventions are short term. Studies of anesthetic drugs and techniques typically address hemodynamic stability, time to awakening, extubation time, postoperative nausea and vomiting, recovery room time, and length of stay. Awareness of the physiologic and pharmacokinetic changes in the elderly has led investigators to examine the effects of a host of anesthetic agents and adjuncts in this population. The effects of intravenous induction agents, narcotics, benzodiazepines, volatile anesthetics, neuromuscular blocking agents, and various types of local anesthetics all have been evaluated in the elderly. Studies have included use of these agents for inpatient surgical procedures, outpatient procedures, premedication, sedation, and their administration by bolus and infusion techniques. Because there is a theoretical advantage to shortening recovery time in patients for whom awakening, ambulation, and discharge might otherwise be delayed (e.g., the elderly), much of the more recent work in the elderly has been devoted to the ultra–short-acting agents.

Some of these studies have identified age-related alterations in the pharmacokinetics, induction, awakening, or recovery room stay. However, perspective is needed. Although a drug may shorten extubation time by 10 minutes, recovery room time by 45 minutes, or total hospitalization in an outpatient procedure by 90 minutes, the clinical impact of these changes on patient outcomes is probably minimal. There is a role for this type of research in geriatric anesthesia, but in an era of limited time and research dollars, efforts should probably be directed elsewhere.

In addition to the numerous studies on the pharmacology and short-term recovery in aged surgical patients, a second major area of research effort has been to compare the risks and benefits of regional versus general anesthesia.

Regional Versus General Anesthesia

Because most general anesthetic agents depress cardiovascular and pulmonary function, as well as alter consciousness, regional anesthesia has been advocated in geriatric patients. Many of the most common procedures in the elderly can be performed with regional techniques, and many investigations have been conducted. Taken as a whole, these studies have broad implications for determining directions for research.

Anesthesiologists taking care of elderly patients undergoing orthopedic procedures have been the de facto leaders in research in geriatric anesthesia. The studies in this area have examined intraoperative cardiovascular stability in the elderly, cardiac, pulmonary and thrombotic complications, pain control, and cognitive outcomes. This subject was reviewed recently by Roy.[153]

A few early studies reported that regional anesthesia for hip surgery was associated with better outcomes.[154,155] Reduced mortality, higher postoperative PaO_2, and fewer mental changes have been reported in patients receiving regional anesthesia.[154,155] However, these studies were very small and their assessment of cognitive function would not meet current standards for reliability or validity.[156]

Subsequent investigations in elderly patients undergoing hip surgery found that intraoperative hypotension was more common with regional anesthesia, and although the incidence of deep vein thrombosis (DVT) and blood loss were typically lower with regional techniques, no difference in major morbidity or mortality could be identified.[84,157–162] Because most of these studies were underpowered for rare events, meta-analysis has been used to help address statistical limitations.

The benefit of regional or general anesthesia was addressed in a 1992 meta-analysis.[163] Sorenson and Pace examined 13 randomized controlled trials conducted between 1966 and 1991 that reported follow-up to at least 1 month. Meta-analysis endpoints were mortality, DVT, and blood loss. Other complications or adverse events were not evaluated because of inconsistencies in definitions or "the absence of systematic and unbiased application of diagnostic tests to record these events." Sorenson and Pace were unable to identify any statistically significant difference in mortality or blood loss by anesthetic technique, although there was a clearly reduced incidence of DVT in regional anesthesia groups. Much of the data

Outcome	T/P	Incidence (regional)	Incidence (general)	Peto OR (95% CI)	Peto OR (95% CI)
Mortality—1 month	7/1578	49/766 (6.4%)	76/812 (9.4%)		0.66 (0.47–0.96)
Mortality—3 months	6/1491	88/726 (12.1%)	98/765 (12.8%)		0.91 (0.67–1.24)
Mortality—6 months	3/1264	103/613 (16.8%)	105/651 (16.1%)		1.05 (0.78–1.41)
Mortality—12 months	2/726	80/354 (22.5%)	78/372 (21.0%)		1.10 (0.77–1.57)
Operative hypotension	7/873	146/426 (34.3%)	116/447 (26.0%)		1.51 (1.12–2.02)+ 1.21 (0.65–2.25)*
Patients receiving transfusion	3/228	63/108 (58.3%)	68/120 (56.7%)		1.02 (0.58–1.80)
Postoperative hypoxia	1/57	10/28 (35.7%)	14/29 (48.3%)		0.60 (0.21–1.71)
Pneumonia	8/1096	27/529 (5.1%)	31/567 (5.5%)		0.92 (0.53–1.59)
Myocardial infarction	4/888	4/431 (0.9%)	8/457 (1.8%)		0.51 (0.16–1.63)
Cerebrovascular accident	7/1085	10/529 (1.9%)	6/556 (1.1%)		1.72 (0.64–4.63)
Congestive cardiac failure	6/902	11/439 (2.5%)	12/463 (2.6%)		0.97 (0.42–2.23)
Renal failure	4/796	2/382 (0.5%)	3/414 (0.7%)		0.77 (0.13–4.50)
Acute confusional state	3/167	10/83 (12.0%)	19/84 (22.6%)		0.47 (0.21–1.06)
Urine retention	2/97	10/48 (20.8%)	10/49 (20.4%)		1.02 (0.39–2.71)
Nausea and vomiting	2/95	2/46 (4.3%)	3/49 (6.1%)		0.69 (0.12–4.13)
Deep vein thrombosis	4/259	39/129 (30.2%)	61/130 (46.9%)		0.41 (0.23–0.72)+
Pulmonary embolism	9/1184	8/575 (1.4%)	10/609 (1.6%)		0.84 (0.33–2.13)

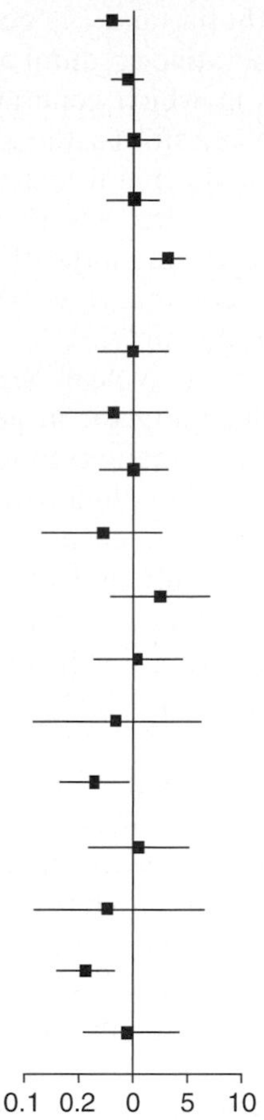

0.1 0.2 0 5 10

FIGURE 6-5. Comparison of outcome between regional and general anesthesia for dichotomous variables. All results were derived using fixed effects analysis except those marked with an asterisk, which were derived using random effects analysis. Statistically significant results are indicated by a plus sign. Results to the left of the vertical line indicate an advantage for regional anesthesia over general anesthesia. Results show the incidence of each outcome measure. T = number of trials, P = number of patients, OR = odds ratio, CI = confidence intervals. (Reprinted with permission from Urwin et al.[164])

in the study by Sorenson and Pace was recently reanalyzed in another meta-analysis with the addition of other trials.[164] Similar to Sorenson and Pace, the analysis by Urwin et al.[164] identified reduced DVT and 1-month mortality in 2162 hip fracture patients receiving regional anesthesia, although no other outcome measure reached statistical significance (Figure 6-5). The reduction in mortality was not evident at 3, 6, or 12 months when those data were available. Subsequent large single-center observational studies involving 741,[165] 1333,[166] and 9425[167] patients have also not identified meaningful differences in cardiopulmonary morbidity or mortality between regional and general anesthesia in hip surgery patients.

Another meta-analysis was conducted by Rodgers et al.[168] Those authors examined the effects of regional anesthesia in 141 randomized trials including 9559 patients. As in the report by Urwin et al., they describe reductions in 30-day mortality and DVT in the regional group, with the effect on mortality not evident beyond 1 month. They also describe reductions in pulmonary embolism, transfusion, respiratory depression, myocardial infarction, and renal failure. Although the results are enticing, the reporting of many outcomes was incomplete across studies so the analysis was based on smaller subsets of patients. Additionally, studies were not rated for quality, and data were included in the meta-analysis that were not reported in the published trials. Studies for general, obstetric and gynecologic, urologic, orthopedic, and "other" surgeries were combined, and no information about age is provided. Finally, it is difficult to make practice recommendations based on the results of this meta-analysis because all of the following treatment modalities were combined into the regional anesthesia group: (1) those receiving spinal anesthesia alone, (2) epidural anesthesia alone, (3) general anesthesia followed by postoperative regional anesthesia, (4) general anesthesia combined with intraoperative spinal anesthesia, and (5) general anesthesia combined with intraoperative epidural anesthesia. Additionally, in 22 studies in which general anesthesia was combined with regional anesthesia, the general anesthetic in the combined regional/general anesthesia group differed from that in the general anesthesia alone group. Thus, it is difficult to determine if the effects described in the meta-analysis are real and, if so, their origin or to which patients they would apply.

In addition to the more typical outcome measures, several of the studies in orthopedic surgery patients have examined the effect of anesthetic technique on cognitive or functional outcome, often following patients for 3 months or longer. Although each of the prospective studies is small, only the study by Hole et al.[155] has been able to identify any difference in cognitive outcome in elderly patients undergoing regional versus general anesthesia for hip or knee surgery. The bulk of investigations could identify no difference.[116,156,169-171]

In a well-designed, randomized prospective, double-blinded study, Norris and colleagues[172] examined the effect of general versus combined general/epidural anesthesia and intravenous patient-controlled opiate versus epidural analgesia in patients undergoing abdominal aortic aneurysm repair. There were no differences in length of stay, mortality, major morbidity, and pain scores.

Although not all studies are in agreement,[173,174] similar conclusions must be drawn for patients undergoing regional or general anesthesia for transurethral prostatectomy, and peripheral vascular surgery.[171,175-178] In carotid surgery, there is a suggestion of a better outcome with regional techniques; however, most investigations are retrospective or nonrandomized, so the effect of patient selection cannot be eliminated.[179-182] Additionally, in the multicenter North American Symptomatic Carotid Endarterectomy Trial, an independent effect of anesthetic technique (or intraoperative monitoring) on carotid surgical outcome could not be found.[183]

The difficulty in identifying clear and meaningful difference between regional and general anesthesia has tremendous implications for the conduct of research in geriatric anesthesia. Probably the most substantive difference in the choice of anesthetic is whether the patient undergoes a regional or a general anesthetic. The pharmacologic difference with that choice is far greater than the difference between different induction agents, narcotics, local anesthetics or muscle relaxants, or different doses of those medications. If little or no difference in outcome can be identified for elderly patients undergoing major procedures with general or regional anesthesia, then the yield for similar outcome studies on differing anesthetic agents is likely to be low.

Physiologic Management

In addition to establishing a surgical plane of anesthesia, the anesthesiologist maintains physiologic stability. Although numerous studies have examined the relationship between intraoperative physiologic management and outcome, outside of relatively rare catastrophic events, such as loss of the airway or uncontrolled hemorrhage, it seems that physiologic management has a modulatory rather than a primary role in outcomes. The best example is in cardiac surgery, for which the acute changes in blood pressure, hematocrit, and temperature typically exceed those seen with any other type of surgery. Additionally, most of the patients are older. Despite that, it has been difficult to demonstrate a direct relationship between physiologic management and outcome.[184-186] Rather, the primary determinants of outcome are technical issues during surgery and the comorbidities that the patent brings to the operating room.[187,188]

Although there is a role for specific studies related to physiologic or pharmacologic management in the elderly, those investigations are likely to have a smaller yield than risk stratification based on population studies and subsequent tailoring of the surgical procedure to the patient based on the preoperative assessment.

These conclusions are not an indictment on anesthetic practice or the role of the anesthesiologist in the operating room. Just the opposite is true. Over the past three decades, anesthesiology has made tremendous strides in patient safety, monitoring, drugs, and education that have made the intraoperative period extremely safe. Those advances have, and will continue, to expand what is possible surgically. At the same time, it is because the advances in intraoperative care have been so great that the greatest needs for research lie in the preoperative assessment and the postoperative management of patients.

There are also broad areas related to intraoperative management (rather than the specifics of anesthetic choice) in which research in the elderly would be productive. It is clear that anesthetics and alterations in autonomic function make it more difficult for older patients to maintain their body temperature and that postoperative hypothermia increases risk of adverse outcomes.[189-193] Thus, studies of temperature control in older patients could be expanded.

Perioperative β-adrenergic blockade reduces mortality and cardiac morbidity in high-risk patients.[194,195] Intraoperative β-blockade, per se, may also improve cardiac outcomes as well as improve early anesthetic recovery and decrease postoperative analgesic requirements.[147] In addition, perioperative clonidine may reduce cardiac morbidity and mortality.[196] Thus, the appropriate place for prophylactic β-blockade and central sympatholysis in elderly surgical patients needs to be examined. Similarly, studies need to address the appropriate roles for anti-platelet agents and H_2-blockers.

Recent data suggest that tight glucose control may improve perioperative outcomes. In a randomized, prospective trial involving critically ill, primarily surgical patients, van den Berghe et al.[197] found that using an insulin infusion to maintain blood glucose 80 and 110 mg/dL reduced intensive care unit (ICU) and in-hospital mortality as well as a variety of morbidities compared with treating only for blood glucose in excess of 215 mg/dL and a goal of 180–200 mg/dL. Further study is needed to determine applicability of this therapy in the elderly surgical patient and whether there is benefit to tight *intraoperative* glucose control.

Given that the immune response may be attenuated in the elderly and that infectious complications are very common, the appropriate dosage and scheduling for perioperative antibiotics may be a useful area of research. Furthermore, elderly patients receive most of the blood given in the perioperative period, so investigation into the immunosuppressive effects of homologous blood transfusion would be instructive. Older patients are also at increased risk for musculoskeletal and nerve injury as well as thrombotic complications. Therefore, documenting the relationship among patient positioning, nerve and skin injury, and thrombotic complications is indicated. Similarly, the timing of the preoperative fast, and its relationship to hypovolemia, and aspiration risk in the elderly would be an area of research with a large potential impact on practice and patient satisfaction.

In perspective, the lack of an independent effect of anesthetic choice or physiologic management on outcome is not surprising. Very large studies of perioperative morbidity and mortality indicate that the anesthetic episode per se seems to have little or no impact on 30-day outcomes apart from rare, catastrophic events.[88,91,198] And, although certain pathophysiologic processes may be initiated during the intraoperative period, with few exceptions, major morbidity and mortality in the operating room is rare.

Intraoperative Research Agenda Items

• Perioperative management of β-blockade, central sympatholysis, antiplatelet therapy, anticoagulation, and anemia are areas to examine in elderly patients. First, cross-sectional or retrospective case-control studies could be used to identify the incidence of adverse cardiac or thrombotic-embolic complications in elderly patients undergoing surgery with and without preoperative β-blockade, central sympatholysis, antithrombotic or antiplatelet therapy, or a hematocrit above a target value. These studies should be in surgeries identified as intermediate or high risk for related complications. Subsequently, prospective cohort, case-control or randomized studies would be used to determine if pre- or intraoperative therapies would reduce related complications in the elderly.

• A similar approach as above should be used to examine perioperative glucose control.

• The appropriate dosage and scheduling for perioperative antibiotics in prevention of perioperative infection in the elderly are important areas of research. As for β-blockade or antithrombotic strategies, initial studies would use retrospective or cross-sectional studies to identify any relationship between the use or timing of perioperative antibiotic therapy and postoperative pneumonia or wound infection. Differences, if any, between younger and older patients undergoing the same type of surgery could also be compared. Subsequently, prospective, nonrandomized studies would be used to determine if preoperative or postoperative antibiotic therapies can reduce infectious-related complications.

• Because elderly patients receive most blood given in the perioperative period, the immunosuppressive effects of homologous blood transfusion deserves further investigation in this population. Multicenter studies of a prospective case-control or prospective cohort design would examine the incidence of perioperative infection and immunosuppression in elderly patients receiving or not receiving blood in the perioperative period. Multivariate analysis would be required to separate the effect of homologous blood transfusion from the comorbid conditions, making transfusion more likely. If a significant independent effect of blood transfusion was identified, subsequent analysis would need to statistically compare the transfusion-associated risk with that of not receiving transfusion. Alternate strategies, such as delaying surgery or erythropoietin therapy, would need to be compared with blood transfusion in case-cohort or prospective, nonrandomized trials because a randomized trial could not be justified.

Appropriate preoperative fasting, its relationship to hypovolemia, and aspiration risk in the elderly would be a practical area of research. In prospective cohort or case-control studies, the incidence of perioperative hypotension, aspiration, and renal insufficiency should be compared in patients undergoing standard fasting orders before surgery with elderly patients who would be allowed clear liquids closer to the time of surgery. This study would need to be conducted in patients undergoing specific types of procedures:

• where liberalization of fluid intake is not contraindicated for surgical reasons,

• in patients undergoing procedures in which they are at greater risk for developing hypovolemia (bowel prep), and

- in instances in which preoperative hypovolemia may contribute to complications (angiographic procedures).

Postoperative Management

Most surgical morbidity and mortality occur in the postoperative period. Pedersen et al.[84] examined perioperative mortality in 7306 adult patients undergoing lower-risk surgery (no cardiac, thoracic, or neurosurgical procedures) and found that mortality during anesthesia was 0.05% (1:1800). In the first 24 hours, the mortality was twice as high, 0.1%, and increased fivefold over the next 6 days to 0.56%.[84] Morbidity, including myocardial ischemia and infarction, stroke, renal insufficiency, pneumonia, and delirium, is also most common postoperatively.[183,199,200]

Postoperative Respiratory Insufficiency

Respiratory morbidity is very common after noncardiac surgery. In the 84,000-patient Veterans Administration study (97% male, mean age of 60), 17% of patients experienced complications with pneumonia in 3.6%, ventilatory failure in 3.2%, and unplanned intubation in 2.4%.[87] In a study conducted by Seymour and Vaz[201] of 288 general surgical patients over age 65, 17% of patients had atelectasis, 12% acute bronchitis, and 10% developed pneumonia.

Although most elderly patients do not require invasive monitoring postoperatively, the appropriate use of pulse oximetry, ventilation monitoring, and O_2 therapy requires study.[202,203] As highlighted previously, elderly patients have an increased A-a gradient, reduced respiratory muscle strength, and decreased hypoxic and hypercarbic drives at baseline.[14,20,27] Additionally, aging is associated with a progressive loss of airway reflexes.[18] And apnea and periodic breathing following administration of narcotics are more common in older patients.[25,204] Postoperative pain, atelectasis, and fluid shifts further increase the likelihood of respiratory complications, as do shivering and reductions in cardiac output and hemoglobin concentration[191] The supine position during recovery increases the transpulmonary shunt and makes hypoxia more likely.[18] Finally, orthopedic and upper abdominal surgeries common in the elderly have an independent effect in increasing postoperative hypoxia and respiratory complications.[26,201,205] For these reasons, hypoxia may occur in 20%–60% of elderly surgical patients.[28,29]

Despite the frequency of postoperative hypoxia and hypercarbia in the elderly, clear guidelines for O_2 therapy, pulse oximetry, and capnography in older patients have not been developed. This issue is of pressing importance as "day surgery" becomes more common and continued efforts are made to abbreviate the time to discharge. Further, more and more patients, most of them elderly, undergo conscious sedation outside the operating room environment. Although the study by Bailey and colleagues[206] is more than 10 years old, its implications are unchanged. In a study of hypoxemia and apnea after sedation with fentanyl and midazolam, the authors describe deaths associated with the use of these drugs. Of 86 reported US deaths, "all but three . . . occurred outside the operating room . . . where patients are typically unattended by anesthesia personnel." Determination of the requirements for O_2 therapy, pulse oximetry, and capnography in elderly patients undergoing inpatient and outpatient surgery, as well as procedures with conscious sedation, are indicated.

The risk of postoperative aspiration in the elderly also requires attention. Because of alterations in pharyngeal function, diminished cough, and an increased incidence of gastroesophageal reflux, elderly patients are at increased risk of aspiration.[23,24] This risk is accentuated by the effect of anesthesia, sedatives, and narcotics as well as by endotracheal intubation, nasogastric tube placement, and upper abdominal or neck surgery.[30,207,208] Although the incidence of aspiration in the operative period is low and is uncommonly associated with clinically important pneumonitis or pneumonia,[209] the risk for aspiration extends well beyond the acute operative period.

It is likely that instrumentation of the pharynx, whether from an endotracheal tube,[30] nasogastric tube,[208] or a transesophageal echocardiography probe,[207] alters sensation, motor function, and the protective reflexes preventing aspiration. For patients with prolonged endotracheal intubation (>24 hours), this effect is persistent for at least 48 hours after extubation.[30] Nasogastric tubes may also contribute to aspiration by increasing the incompetence of the gastroesophageal junction. Although pharyngeal dysfunction and aspiration may be related to a greater acuity of illness, pharyngeal trespass itself has independent effects.

Given perioperative risk factors, the frequency of aspiration, and the incidence of postoperative respiratory morbidity, insufficient research has been directed to these issues in elderly surgical patients. Pharmacologic interventions to reduce gastric volume or increase pH have received attention in the anesthesia literature, but the investigation by Warner et al.[209] of aspiration occurring within 2 hours of surgery implies that research on aspiration and postoperative pneumonia must look beyond the immediate operative period.[210] More important research will focus on establishing appropriate use of nasogastric tubes, restoration of pharyngeal and tracheal reflexes and gastrointestinal motility, and advancement of feeding following surgery in the elderly. General studies as well as surgery-specific studies are indicated.

Acute Pain Management

The same questions that dominate research in pain management in the general population apply to the elderly. However, in many ways, the questions are more pressing in the elderly because they might receive the most potential harm as well as the greatest potential benefit from the treatment of postoperative pain. Because of ischemic heart disease, diminished pulmonary capacity, altered drug clearance, or increased drug sensitivity, the elderly patient is probably more vulnerable to the physiologic consequences of inadequate analgesia as well as the side effects related to analgesic use. Additionally, there is evidence in the literature indicating that in certain circumstances pain in the elderly may be less adequately treated.[48]

Pain and Adverse Outcomes

The perioperative period results in stress and inflammatory responses that peak postoperatively when cardiopulmonary and neurologic complications occur. Therefore, efforts have been made to link the adequacy of analgesia with the magnitude of the stress response. In particular, it has been proposed that inadequate postoperative analgesia may be associated with myocardial ischemia and pulmonary failure. Researchers have examined the effect of the intraoperative anesthetic[211–214] and postoperative epidural analgesia on plasma levels of cortisol, epinephrine, norepinephrine, leucocyte counts, and acute phase proteins and tried to relate these to cardiopulmonary outcomes.[173,211,215–219] Both negative and positive conclusions have been reached.

When this subject was reviewed by Liu et al.,[220] they concluded that intensive analgesia using regional techniques had a limited impact on cardiopulmonary outcomes or the stress response in a general population of surgical patients. They also concluded that pain and the stress response were not directly coupled because the neuroendocrine response was still demonstrated (although blunted) in the presence of intense surgical analgesia with local anesthetics or opioids.[220] However, studies in the highest-risk groups suggest a possible improvement in outcome with intense analgesia using regional techniques.[173,221] Intensive pain management strategies may be indicated in high-risk elderly patients or in low-risk elderly patients undergoing high-risk surgery. Defining the circumstances under which epidural analgesia or any other pain management strategy can improve outcomes is an important area for future research.

In addition to the stress response typically associated with the sympathetic-adrenal axis, most types of surgery initiate a significant catabolic state. Although an inhibitory effect of analgesia on protein wasting has been suggested,[222–224] a more pressing area for research is to understand postsurgical catabolism in the elderly. The relationship between preoperative nutritional status and postoperative catabolism must be better understood. Experience with some critically ill patients suggests that catabolism may become dissociated from the initial surgical stress. Because elderly patients have decreased nutritional and metabolic reserve, they are most challenged by the postoperative catabolic state. Basic investigation into postoperative catabolism in the elderly is fundamental as are investigations into interventions that might attenuate catabolism or facilitate the transition back to an anabolism.

Although the adequacy of postoperative analgesia does not seem to be an independent determinant of outcomes in the general population of surgical patients, a variety of other issues related to postoperative analgesia require attention. The relative benefit of patient-controlled analgesia (PCA)[225] versus a PRN or scheduled analgesic administration is of special importance in the elderly surgical patient. Because of the physiologic and psychologic heterogeneity in the geriatric population, it is unlikely that fixed formulae for age-appropriate drug dosing can be identified. Thus, administration of narcotics on a set schedule in the elderly is fraught with the potential for both over- and under-dosing. These considerations potentially make PCA analgesia an ideal choice. Nevertheless, the issue is complicated. The side-effect profile for PCA analgesics in the elderly has not been established.[226,227] It has also been suggested that many elderly patients may struggle with the technology. Similarly, the application of PCA for patients with altered mental status is problematic. Outcomes with PCA in the elderly must be compared with fixed and PRN dosing techniques as well as with postoperative pain control by regional blockade.

The same is true regarding route of administration for analgesic agents. Is there a clear advantage or disadvantage to the use of the intravenous, epidural, or intrathecal routes for analgesic administration in the elderly? The elderly are unusually susceptible to drug interactions and have an increased incidence of respiratory depression, urinary retention, ileus, constipation, and postoperative falls. These are influenced by choices in postoperative analgesia and may differ by route of administration.[226–229] As such, investigations into analgesic strategies for elderly surgical patients will need to determine not only quality of analgesia, but also a comprehensive examination of risks and benefits specific to that population. Additionally, because narcotics are associated with frequent side effects in the elderly, the use of analgesic adjuncts in postoperative pain management requires further investigation. Drugs such as ketorolac, clonidine, dexmedetomidine, and cyclooxygenase-2 inhibitors have the potential to achieve adequate analgesia with lower doses of opioids, potentially reducing side effects.[230–234]

A final reason why studies of acute pain management in the elderly are required is that acute pain management may bear on rehabilitation and subsequently on functional status on discharge.[235] This has been shown with analgesic programs for continuous passive motion machines used after knee replacement.[235–237] Research is required after other types of surgical procedures to determine whether facilitation of rehabilitation by acute pain management can improve other functional outcomes.

Another opportunity for research in the postoperative care of hospitalized patients is related to polypharmacy and adverse drug events in the elderly. There is a tendency for elderly patients to accumulate drug prescriptions over time, and there is a clear relationship between the number of drugs taken and the incidence of adverse drug-related events.[66–69] This problem will be compounded during the surgical period when additional medications are added.

A study by Cullen and colleagues[238] prospectively compared adverse drug events in ICU and non-ICU, surgical and medical, hospitalized patients and found that the rate of preventable and potential adverse drug events was related to the number of drugs administered rather than the type of care delivered (ICU or non-ICU, surgical or medical). An earlier report of the same data on 4031 adult hospital admissions identified, among other things, the incidence of adverse drug events, their preventability, and the classes of drugs that caused most events.[239] Those results have particular bearing for the perioperative care of the elderly.

In that investigation by Bates et al.,[239] analgesics were the class of drug associated with the most adverse drug events. Antibiotics caused the second-greatest number of adverse reactions. Analgesics were also the leading class of drug with preventable adverse drug events followed by sedatives and then antibiotics (Table 6-3). In the 20 adverse events related to analgesics, 40% were caused by overmedication.

There is a pressing need for research in pain management of the elderly surgical patient. There is also a compelling need for research into prevention of adverse drug events in hospitalized patients. The intersection of pain management and the incidence of preventable adverse events related to analgesics and sedatives places anesthesiologists squarely in a leadership role for research into appropriate analgesic and sedative strategies for the elderly.

In patients who are hospitalized, there is also a window of opportunity to review patient medications, in particular to examine redundancy in therapeutic profile and look for combinations that may make complications such as respiratory depression, aspiration, confusion, postural hypotension, urinary retention, and falls more likely. The development of pharmacy and electronic drug databases for this work would be appropriate and are more within the resources of hospitals than community practitioners. Although it would not be practical or appropriate to modify most patient chronic drug regimes in the postoperative period, the surgical hospitalization might provide an opportunity for drug review and recommendation in an effort to reduce iatrogenic complications in the elderly.

Delirium and Cognitive Decline

Postoperative delirium or cognitive decline affects 5%–50% of elderly patients; both have similar predisposing factors but the syndromes are not equivalent.[110,200,240–242] Disordered thinking and confusion that waxes and wanes characterize postoperative delirium. The onset is typically on the first to third postoperative day. It may be sustained for more than a week and is associated with other medical complications, prolonged hospitalization, and decreased functional status on discharge.[113,120,200,241,243–245] To date, much of the research on postoperative delirium has centered on the impact of regional versus general anesthesia in orthopedic surgery.[116,117,156,169–171,246] Postoperative cognitive dysfunction, a deterioration of psychomotor capacities such as memory, central processing time, and acquisition of new information, has been well described in both cardiac and noncardiac surgical patients.[247–250] It may be subtle or clinically obvious. The relationship between postoperative delirium and cognitive dysfunction has not been well studied.

The effect of differing anesthetics on postoperative delirium has been studied,[117,156,171,251–254] and a leading hypothesis has been that offending agents aggravate an age-associated central cholinergic insufficiency.[116,255,256] However, from review of the literature, it becomes evident that delirium can be triggered by many different perioperative events; no single cause is identifiable. Thus, no single intervention is likely to be successful.

In addition to being linked to opiates, sedatives, and anticholinergics, delirium has been associated with urinary tract infection, pneumonia, hypoxia or

TABLE 6-3. Adverse events by drug class.

Drug class	Adverse drug events No. (%) (n = 247)	Preventable adverse drug events No. (%) (n = 70)
Analgesics	73 (30)	20 (29)
Antibiotics	59 (24)	6 (9)
Sedatives	20 (8)	7 (10)
Antineoplastic	18 (7)	3 (4)
Cardiovascular	9 (4)	3 (4)
Anticoagulants	8 (3)	3 (4)
Antipsychotics	6 (2)	5 (7)
Diabetes	5 (2)	4 (6)
Electrolytes	3 (1)	3 (4)
Other	46 (19)	16 (23)

Source: Modified with permission from Bates et al.[239]

hypercarbia, fever, blood loss, and electrolyte disturbances.[200,240,241,257–259] Chronic patient factors such as preexisting frank or subclinical dementia, other organic brain disease, and vision and hearing loss are also predictors of postoperative delirium and cognitive decline.[102,110,113,200,240,260,261] Finally, pain, sleep deprivation, sensory deprivation, and an unfamiliar environment may contribute to delirium.[112,200,240,262,263]

Although most of the research in the anesthesia literature has focused on the effect of anesthetic and analgesic agents, the literature in medical patients suggests that the yield for those studies will be low. Studies of the type conducted by Inouye et al. might serve as a model for research in anesthesia.[103,108,259–261,264–266] Inouye describes a multifactorial model for delirium involving the interrelationship between a vulnerable patient and acute insults.[259,264] For example, a minor insult may result in delirium in highly vulnerable patients, whereas in less vulnerable patients, a major insult may be required to precipitate delirium. In a study of elderly medical patients, multivariate modeling identified four risk factors for developing hospitalization delirium: vision impairment, severe illness, preexisting cognitive impairment, and a blood urea nitrogen/creatinine ratio ≥18.[264,267] Patients were then divided into low-, intermediate-, and high-risk groups depending on the number of risk factors. In a subsequent validation cohort, the rates of delirium in the low-, intermediate-, and high-risk groups were 3%, 16%, and 32%, respectively (Table 6-4).[264] In those patients, the rate of death or nursing home placement was 3%, 14%, and 26%, respectively, an eightfold increase from the lowest to highest risk group.[267] Precipitating factors for delirium in hospitalized medical patients have also been described by Inouye and Charpentier.[259] Twenty-five factors occurring at least 24 hours before the onset of delirium were considered. Of those, a multivariate model identified five as predictive: use of physical restraints,

TABLE 6-4. In-hospital events and risk of delirium.

Risk group	No. of factors	Delirium rate, by person*	RR
Low	0	5/125 (4)†	1.0
Intermediate	1–2	31/156 (20)†	5.0
High	≥3	11/31 (35)†	8.9

Source: Modified with permission from Inouye.[264] Published by S. Karger AG, Basel.

RR = relative risk.

Each patient's risk group was determined by adding one point for each precipitating factor present: use of restraints, urinary catheter, more than three medications added, any iatrogenic event, and malnutrition. Figures in parentheses represent percentage.

*Corresponds with percentage of patients developing delirium per day.

†x^2 overall = 24.8, $p < 0.001$; x^2 trend = 24.8, $p < 0.001$.

Performance of the predictive model for delirium in medical patients in the validation cohort.

malnutrition, more than three medications added, use of a bladder catheter, and any iatrogenic event (volume overload, urinary tract infection, pressure ulcer, etc.).[259] Although the precipitating factors were independent of each other, the authors note that "... baseline and precipitating factors are highly interrelated and contribute to delirium in a cumulative fashion."[259]

In a subsequent publication, Inouye and colleagues[265] determined the effect of interventions based on their predictive model. Four hundred twenty-six elderly medical patients in an intervention group were matched to an equal number in a "usual care" group. In the intervention group, six risk factors for delirium were targeted for intervention: cognitive impairment, sleep deprivation, immobility, visual and hearing impairment, and dehydration. The group receiving intervention, by an interdisciplinary team, had a 9.9% incidence of delirium versus 15% in the usual care group (a 34% decline). Subdivision of patients into intermediate- or high-risk groups demonstrated that intervention reduced delirium in intermediate-risk patients, but the tendency to reduce delirium in the high-risk group was not statistically significant.[265]

These studies indicate that presence and severity of cognitive deficit are strong predictors of the likelihood of delirium during the hospitalization.[264] The same effect has been identified in surgical patients.[110–113] This brings us back to the recurring theme that subclinical decrements in functional status may become evident during the perioperative period. These findings are extended by the observation that postoperative delirium or cognitive decline may be a harbinger of a potentially permanent decrease in mental status.[247,268]

Together, the data on the predictive value of preoperative cognitive status[264] and the effect of that assessment on the success of intervention[265] provide a compelling rationale to conduct a simple, short mental status examination as part of the preoperative interview. Short functional scales have been designed which might be applicable in the preoperative interview.[115,269,270] The practicality of such metrics in elderly surgical patients must be established. After that, the incidence of preoperative cognitive impairment and its severity could be identified in populations of elderly patients undergoing different types of procedures. Research into the effectiveness of differing preventative strategies could follow. For example, pharmacologic prophylaxis of delirium shows promise.[271] Those investigations could also examine if reductions in delirium translate into reduced medical complications or improved functional status on discharge.

Chronic Pain

A significant proportion of the geriatric population suffers from chronic pain conditions.[46,47] Much of this is related to osteoarthritis, but many older patients have a variety of neuropathic pain disorders including herpes zoster, diabetic neuropathies, and complex regional pain syndromes.[272] Care of these patients is complex and for many of these painful conditions therapy is inadequate.

The factors limiting therapeutic success in chronic pain in the elderly are multiple. First, in contrast to acute postoperative pain, the conditions responsible for chronic pain are typically not reversible. Second, pain conditions may have a central nervous system component. Third, effective treatment of chronic pain is hampered by the side effects of medications and complications from polypharmacy. Fourth, depression and behavioral changes frequently complicate therapy.[273] Fifth, assessment of pain in older patients can be difficult.[46] And, finally, chronic pain in the elderly is often associated with unrelated comorbid conditions that may alter treatment plans.[43,274] Despite these limitations, geriatric patients benefit from chronic pain therapy in a manner similar to younger patients.[43,275,276]

Most pain syndromes can be classified into one of four types: nociceptive, neuropathic, mixed, or unspecified and psychogenic.[47] The usefulness of different classes of analgesic agents in these types of syndromes is reasonably well described. Nociceptive pain includes the pain typically associated with arthropathies, myalgias, and ischemic disorders; the mainstays of analgesia are initially acetaminophen and nonsteroidal antiinflammatory drugs, followed later by narcotics.[46,47,272] In contrast, narcotics are thought to have a lesser place in neuropathies such as diabetic neuropathy, postherpetic neuralgia (PHN), and complex regional pain syndromes.[272,277,278] Instead, the primary pharmacologic therapies are tricyclic antidepressants and anticonvulsant agents.[46,272,279–281] Antiarrhythmic drugs are second-tier agents for neuropathic conditions. Treatment of mixed or unspecified pain syndromes is challenging, because the mechanisms are unknown and treatment may require trials of differing analgesic approaches.[47] For patients whose pain has been classified as psychogenic, psychiatric intervention rather than analgesic agents is indicated.[47]

In addition to familiar analgesics and adjuncts, there is a clear need for a multidimensional approach to chronic pain in the elderly. Neuraxial opioids, local anesthetics, and steroids have a role in some patients, as do peripheral or central neuromodulatory techniques and a host of physical, physiatric, and cognitive-behavorial strategies.[43,46,47]

Defining research priorities for anesthesiologists in such a broad and complex area is difficult. The first priority is that chronic pain trials must have sufficient control groups and statistical power. As noted by Stanton-Hicks and colleagues,[280] studies of neuropathic pain conditions are typically small and anecdotal with few experimental findings and "without adequate predictors for the choice

of therapy, current practice is chaotic, and continues to use the trial-and-error approach."

After design issues are addressed, probably the most salient research recommendation for any of these types of pain conditions is that outcomes should emphasize functional status[276,282] rather than a change in a pain score, per se. This is superbly outlined in the Consensus Report on Complex Regional Pain Syndromes.[280] Although quantifying pain is relevant, ultimately, determination of which interventions facilitate rehabilitation, maintain or increase mobility, and support the activities of daily living is a priority.[276,282]

The second broad area requiring further investigation relates to prevention. One of the best examples is in PHN. Although the rash of acute herpes zoster is very common in the elderly, a lesser, but significant, percentage of those affected develop the chronic debilitating pain condition of PHN.[283] Because zoster is chronic and recurring, the percentage of the population affected with PHN increases with age.[283] Although PHN may develop in fewer than 5% of younger patients with zoster, it may develop in half of patients over age 60.[284] Once established, PHN is difficult to treat. Further research is indicated to determine whether antiviral, analgesic, antiinflammatory therapies during acute zoster can prevent the development of chronic PHN.[285–288] In addition, immunotherapeutic modalities show promise and deserve more study.[289–298] If a better understanding of precipitating events can be developed for other chronic pain conditions (as in PHN[299]), it might allow the introduction of preventive measures.

In addition to directing research efforts toward functional effects and trying to define opportunities for prevention of chronic pain conditions, for any strategy, it is important to examine the risk–benefit ratio, emphasizing adverse outcomes that are more likely to occur in a geriatric population. As in acute pain management, the effect of chronic therapy on the incidence of complications such as confusion, postural hypotension, falls, urinary retention, and constipation must be reported.

Finally, cognitive impairment is a continuum and in milder forms is very common. There is a two-way relationship: pain may impair cognition and cognitive impairment can interfere with the communication of pain.[46,300] Therefore, a further area of investigation relevant to the care of patients with chronic pain is its assessment in the cognitively impaired.

Postoperative Research Agenda Items

- Large cross-sectional studies describing analgesic practice and its complications in the elderly are needed. The effect of regional analgesic techniques, nonopioid adjunctive drugs, and nonpharmacologic interventions would be investigated in prospective cohort or case-control studies. These investigations must emphasize the type and incidence of adverse drug events in the elderly. After that, randomized controlled trials comparing outcomes with analgesic programs specific to types of surgery could be designed and conducted. Those prospective trials should determine if analgesic regimes designed for the elderly patient could reduce in-hospital morbidity or improve functional status on discharge.

- Prospective studies that better identify patient and procedural risk factors for respiratory failure, aspiration, and pneumonia are required. Randomized trials could then determine if respiratory monitoring, prophylactic antibiotics, changes in pharyngeal instrumentation, or the way feeding is advanced reduce respiratory failure, aspiration, and postoperative pneumonia.

- The relationship between postoperative nutritional support and functional outcome must be better understood. Cross-sectional studies that could identify if a relationship between nutritional support in high-risk surgery and functional status on discharge (chronic respiratory failure, ambulation, independent living, etc.) are the first step. Data from those investigations could then be used to design prospective-cohort or randomized controlled trials comparing feeding strategies in elderly patients at risk for malnutrition and muscle wasting following major surgery. In addition to protein and caloric support, interventions that might attenuate postoperative catabolism or facilitate the transition to an anabolism in the elderly could be compared with standard care.

- Practice governing stopping or resuming anticoagulation in the perioperative period is largely empiric. Studies determining the relationship between perioperative termination of anticoagulation and thromboembolic and bleeding risk are indicated. The effect of timing of termination and resumption as well as the temporizing use of antiplatelet agents should be compared in case-control or prospective cohort studies.

- The surgical hospitalization might provide an opportunity for drug review and recommendation in an effort to reduce iatrogenic complications in the elderly. Initially, a retrospective review could identify the incidence of polypharmacy with combinations of drugs that might contribute to geriatric complications (hypotension, bradycardia, falls, confusion, bleeding diathesis, constipation, and urinary retention). Subsequently, the presence or absence of an effect of simplifying drug regimens in hospital or the effect of communicating that information to primary care physicians could be identified in nonrandomized controlled trials.

- Using the models established in medical patients, evaluating prevention strategies for postoperative delirium must be tested. It should first be determined by cross-sectional studies, with multivariate analysis, if the risk factors for delirium in surgical patients are the same as those for medical patients. After that, prospective controlled trials in patients at moderate to high risk could determine the effect of preoperative or postoperative interventions on the incidence of delirium.

- The first priority in chronic pain trials is large cross-sectional studies that might identify any relationship between pain intervention and functional outcomes. After that, it must be determined prospectively if specific chronic pain therapies can improve functional outcomes in treatment groups relative to a historical or concurrent, nonrandomized control.

- Given the frequency of herpes zoster in the geriatric population, further prospective studies are needed to determine if antiviral, analgesic, or antiinflammatory therapies during acute zoster can reduce, relative to standard care, the development of chronic PHN.

- As in acute pain management, cross-sectional studies documenting the effect of chronic pain therapy on the incidence of complications such as confusion, postural hypotension, falls, urinary retention, and constipation in the elderly are indicated.

- Assessment and treatment of acute or chronic pain in the cognitively impaired is largely empiric. Cross-sectional studies that describe pain management in this population relative to a nonimpaired population are indicated. Additionally, pain assessment tools for the cognitively impaired must be compared prospectively to standard assessment methods. After that, prospective trials comparing different analgesic strategies with regard to clinical and functional endpoints could be conducted.

Summary and Conclusions

Perioperative care of the geriatric patient is complex. Age-related physiologic changes and disease limit functional reserve and render the elderly less able to tolerate the challenges of the perioperative period. Thus, they are at increased risk for a host of complications. Furthermore, it is probably easier to precipitate these complications than to directly prevent them.

Despite the unique challenges of the perioperative care of the elderly, existing literature offers clinicians insufficient guidance. Nevertheless, previous studies provide a framework to guide future research. Rather than focus attention on the choice of anesthetic technique or on short-term outcomes such as time to extubation or recovery room stay, improvement in patient outcomes will be better served by studies that yield better risk-stratification in the elderly. To some extent, pertinent patient risk factors will probably be surgery-specific. Subsequently, it can be determined if identified risk factors are amenable to therapy and whether such intervention improves outcome. An essential element of both types of investigations will be a focus on preoperative functional status and other pertinent geriatric outcomes rather than just major cardiopulmonary morbidity and mortality.

Surgical outcome is determined by the interaction of patient factors and the challenges introduced by an operation. Clearly, the surgical insult varies by procedure. Therefore, development of comprehensive care strategies for specific types of surgery common in the elderly is indicated. This approach is more likely to generate positive results and practical guidelines than pooling elderly patients undergoing differing types of surgery. Development of comprehensive clinical pathways specific to the care of the elderly patient undergoing specific types of surgeries is indicated because it would coordinate preoperative, intraoperative, and postoperative management in a particularly vulnerable population. This approach could improve outcomes and serve as a foundation for assessing alternative strategies. It might have particular value in postoperative care, including prevention of delirium, respiratory monitoring, and pain management.

The perioperative care of the elderly is a growing public health issue. Anesthesiologists are involved in the care of older surgical patients from the preoperative evaluation through the postoperative period. Because of this perspective, we offer unique insights into their care. Applying these to appropriately conceived studies will lead to improved perioperative outcomes and, ultimately, benefit society.

Highest Priority Research Questions in Geriatric Anesthesiology

1. What preoperative assessments are useful in developing patient management plans for surgeries common in the elderly?

Hypothesis-generating: Large, observational studies are needed to identify preoperative risk factors for adverse geriatric outcomes, such as decreased functional status or postoperative delirium, following common surgeries. These studies will identify both patient and surgery-dependent factors. Assessment tools for mental status, nutrition, hydration, thrombotic risk, and activities of daily living must be applied or developed when necessary. It then should be determined which risk factors are potentially modifiable.

Hypothesis-testing: Randomized controlled trials to determine if preoperative or postoperative intervention against modifiable risk factors will result in a decrease in perioperative geriatric complications. The adverse effects of such interventions, such as delay of surgery or postoperative bleeding, must be examined along with the potential benefits of the intervention. Examples for

which such interventions could be reasonably attempted include nutrition and hydration, postoperative delirium, pre- or postoperative rehabilitation programs for activities of daily living, and antiplatelet therapy for thrombotic and embolic complications.

2. Can postoperative analgesic techniques reduce postoperative morbidity or improve functional status at discharge?

Hypothesis-generating: Large prospective studies describing analgesic practice and its complications in the elderly are needed. The efficacy and complications of regional analgesic techniques, nonopioid adjunctive drugs, and physiatric interventions must be investigated. These investigations must emphasize the type and incidence of adverse drug events in the elderly.

Hypothesis-testing: Prospective randomized trials are needed to determine if perioperative intensive analgesic techniques (including traditional narcotic, regional, nonopioid adjunctive drugs, and physiatric interventions) designed for the elderly patient reduce in-hospital morbidity or improve functional status on discharge.

3. How can postoperative pulmonary complications in the elderly be reduced?

Hypothesis-generating: Cross-sectional or cohort studies that better identify high-risk procedures or perioperative periods of vulnerability for postoperative hypoxia, respiratory failure, and pneumonia in the elderly surgical patient are indicated. These investigations could identify both patient and procedure risk factors as well as their interaction for these complications.

Hypothesis-testing: Randomized trials to determine if respiratory monitoring, prophylactic antibiotics, changes in pharyngeal instrumentation, or the way feeding is advanced reduce respiratory failure, aspiration, and postoperative pneumonia.

References

1. Franklin SS, Gustin WT, Wong ND, et al. Hemodynamic patterns of age-related changes in blood pressure. The Framingham Heart Study. Circulation 1997;96:308–315.
2. Landahl S, Bengtsson C, Sigurdsson JA, Svanborg A, Svardsudd K. Age-related changes in blood pressure. Hypertension 1986;8:1044–1049.
3. Pan HY, Hoffman BB, Pershe RA, Blaschke TF. Decline in beta adrenergic receptor-mediated vascular relaxation with aging in man. J Pharmacol Exp Ther 1986;239:802–807.
4. Folkow B, Svanborg A. Physiology of cardiovascular aging. Physiol Rev 1993;73:725–764.
5. Falk RH. Etiology and complications of atrial fibrillation: insights from pathology studies. Am J Cardiol 1998;82:10N–17N.

6. Mackstaller LL, Alpert JS. Atrial fibrillation: a review of mechanism, etiology, and therapy. Clin Cardiol 1997;20: 640–650.

7. Lakatta EG. Age-related alterations in the cardiovascular response to adrenergic mediated stress. Fed Proc 1980; 39:3173–3177.

8. Rodeheffer RJ, Gerstenblith G, Becker LC, Fleg JL, Weisfeldt ML, Lakatta EG. Exercise cardiac output is maintained with advancing age in healthy human subjects: cardiac dilatation and increased stroke volume compensate for a diminished heart rate. Circulation 1984;69: 203–213.

9. Collins KJ, Exton-Smith AN, James MH, Oliver DJ. Functional changes in autonomic nervous responses with ageing. Age Ageing 1980;9:17–24.

10. McGarry K, Laher M, Fitzgerald D, Horgan J, O'Brien E, O'Malley K. Baroreflex function in elderly hypertensives. Hypertension 1983;5:763–766.

11. Phillips PA, Hodsman GP, Johnston CI. Neuroendocrine mechanisms and cardiovascular homeostasis in the elderly. Cardiovasc Drugs Ther 1991;4(Suppl 6):1209–1213.

12. Cleroux J, Giannattasio C, Bolla G, et al. Decreased cardiopulmonary reflexes with aging in normotensive humans. Am J Physiol 1989;257:H961–H968.

13. Rowe JW, Troen BR. Sympathetic nervous system and aging in man. Endocr Rev 1980;1:167–179.

14. Wahba WM. Influence of aging on lung function—clinical significance of changes from age twenty. Anesth Analg 1983;62:764–776.

15. Zaugg M, Lucchinetti E. Respiratory function in the elderly. Anesthesiol Clin North Am 2000;18:47–58, vi.

16. Fowler RW. Ageing and lung function. Age Ageing 1985; 14:209–215.

17. Tolep K, Kelsen SG. Effect of aging on respiratory skeletal muscles. Clin Chest Med 1993;14:363–378.

18. Pontoppidan H, Geffin B, Lowenstein E. Acute respiratory failure in the adult. 1. N Engl J Med 1972;287:690–698.

19. Kitamura H, Sawa T, Ikezono E. Postoperative hypoxemia: the contribution of age to the maldistribution of ventilation. Anesthesiology 1972;36:244–252.

20. Lynne-Davies P. Influence of age on the respiratory system. Geriatrics 1977;32:57–60.

21. Cerveri I, Zoia MC, Fanfulla F, et al. Reference values of arterial oxygen tension in the middle-aged and elderly. Am J Respir Crit Care Med 1995;152:934–941.

22. Kronenberg RS, Drage CW. Attenuation of the ventilatory and heart rate responses to hypoxia and hypercapnia with aging in normal men. J Clin Invest 1973;52:1812–1819.

23. Aviv JE. Effects of aging on sensitivity of the pharyngeal and supraglottic areas. Am J Med 1997;103:74S–76S.

24. Marik PE. Aspiration pneumonitis and aspiration pneumonia. N Engl J Med 2001;344:665–671.

25. Arunasalam K, Davenport HT, Painter S, Jones JG. Ventilatory response to morphine in young and old subjects. Anaesthesia 1983;38:529–533.

26. Sari A, Miyauchi Y, Yamashita S, Yokota K, Ogasahara H, Yonei A. The magnitude of hypoxemia in elderly patients with fractures of the femoral neck. Anesth Analg 1986; 65:892–894.

27. Kronenberg RS, Drage CW, Ponto RA, Williams LE. The effect of age on the distribution of ventilation and perfusion in the lung. Am Rev Respir Dis 1973;108:576–586.

28. Clayer M, Bruckner J. Occult hypoxia after femoral neck fracture and elective hip surgery. Clin Orthop 2000: 265–271.

29. Moller JT, Jensen PF, Johannessen NW, Espersen K. Hypoxaemia is reduced by pulse oximetry monitoring in the operating theatre and in the recovery room. Br J Anaesth 1992;68:146–150.

30. de Larminat V, Montravers P, Dureuil B, Desmonts JM. Alteration in swallowing reflex after extubation in intensive care unit patients. Crit Care Med 1995;23:486–490.

31. Morris JC, McManus DQ. The neurology of aging: normal versus pathologic change. Geriatrics 1991;46:47–48, 51–54.

32. Creasey H, Rapoport SI. The aging human brain. Ann Neurol 1985;17:2–10.

33. Morrison JH, Hof PR. Life and death of neurons in the aging brain. Science 1997;278:412–419.

34. Severson JA. Neurotransmitter receptors and aging. J Am Geriatr Soc 1984;32:24–27.

35. Wong DF, Wagner HN Jr, Dannals RF, et al. Effects of age on dopamine and serotonin receptors measured by positron tomography in the living human brain. Science 1984;226:1393–1396.

36. Muravchick S. Central nervous system. In: Geroanesthesia: Principles for Management of the Elderly Patient. St. Louis: Mosby-Year Book; 1997:78–113.

37. Peterson DD, Pack AI, Silage DA, Fishman AP. Effects of aging on ventilatory and occlusion pressure responses to hypoxia and hypercapnia. Am Rev Respir Dis 1981; 124:387–391.

38. Muravchick S. Peripheral and autonomic nervous system. In: Geroanesthesia: Principles for Management of the Elderly Patient. St. Louis: Mosby-Year Book; 1997: 114–148.

39. Gibson SJ, Helme RD. Age differences in pain perception and report: a review of physiological, psychological, laboratory and clinical studies. Pain Rev 1995;2:111–137.

40. Tucker MA, Andrew MF, Ogle SJ, Davison JG. Age-associated change in pain threshold measured by transcutaneous neuronal electrical stimulation. Age Ageing 1989;18:241–246.

41. Potvin AR, Syndulko K, Tourtellotte WW, Lemmon JA, Potvin JH. Human neurologic function and the aging process. J Am Geriatr Soc 1980;28:1–9.

42. Chakour MC, Gibson SJ, Bradbeer M, Helme RD. The effect of age on A delta- and C-fibre thermal pain perception. Pain 1996;64:143–152.

43. Helme RD, Gibson SJ. Pain in the elderly. In: Jensen TS, Turner JA, Wiesenfeld-Hallin Z, eds. Proceedings of the 8th World Congress on Pain. Parkville, Australia: IASP Press; 1997:919–944.

44. Harkins SW. Geriatric pain. Pain perceptions in the old. Clin Geriatr Med 1996;12:435–459.

45. Harkins SW, Davis MD, Bush FM, Kasberger J. Suppression of first pain and slow temporal summation of second pain in relation to age. J Gerontol A Biol Sci Med Sci 1996; 51:M260–M265.

46. Ferrell BA. Pain management in elderly people. J Am Geriatr Soc 1991;39:64–73.

47. Anonymous. The management of chronic pain in older persons: AGS Panel on Chronic Pain in Older Persons. American Geriatrics Society. J Am Geriatr Soc 1998;46: 635–651.

48. Jones JS, Johnson K, McNinch M. Age as a risk factor for inadequate emergency department analgesia. Am J Emerg Med 1996;14:157–160.

49. McLachlan MS. The ageing kidney. Lancet 1978;2:143–145.

50. Anderson S, Brenner BM. The aging kidney: structure, function, mechanisms, and therapeutic implications. J Am Geriatr Soc 1987;35:590–593.

51. Epstein M. Aging and the kidney. J Am Soc Nephrol 1996;7:1106–1122.

52. Anderson S, Brenner BM. Effects of aging on the renal glomerulus. Am J Med 1986;80:435–442.

53. Shannon RP, Minaker KL, Rowe JW. Aging and water balance in humans. Semin Nephrol 1984;4:346–353.

54. Miller M. Fluid and electrolyte balance in the elderly. Geriatrics 1987;42:65–76.

55. Phillips PA, Rolls BJ, Ledingham JG, et al. Reduced thirst after water deprivation in healthy elderly men. N Engl J Med 1984;311:753–759.

56. Rowe JW, Minaker KL, Sparrow D, Robertson GL. Age-related failure of volume-pressure-mediated vasopressin release. J Clin Endocrinol Metab 1982;54:661–664.

57. Kliger AS. The role of the kidney in fluid, electrolyte, and acid-base disorders. Int Anesthesiol Clin 1984;22:65–82.

58. Lamy PP, Wiser TH. Geriatric anesthesia. In: Katlic MR, ed. Pharmacotherapeutic Considerations in the Elderly Surgical Patient. Baltimore: Urban & Schwarzenberg; 1990:209–239.

59. Greenblatt DJ, Sellers EM, Shader RI. Drug therapy: drug disposition in old age. N Engl J Med 1982;306: 1081–1088.

60. Shafer SL. The pharmacology of anesthetic drugs in elderly patients. Anesthesiol Clin North Am 2000;18:1–29, v.

61. Matteo RS, Ornstein E. Pharmacokinetics and pharmaco-dynamics of injected drugs in the elderly. Adv Anesth 1988;5:25–52.

62. Silverstein JH, Bloom HG, Cassel CK. New challenges in anesthesia: new practice opportunities. Anesthesiol Clin North Am 1999;17:453–465.

63. Dundee JW, Robinson FP, McCollum JS, Patterson CC. Sensitivity to propofol in the elderly. Anaesthesia 1986; 41:482–485.

64. Jacobs JR, Reves JG, Marty J, White WD, Bai SA, Smith LR. Aging increases pharmacodynamic sensitivity to the hypnotic effects of midazolam. Anesth Analg 1995;80: 143–148.

65. Homer TD, Stanski DR. The effect of increasing age on thiopental disposition and anesthetic requirement. Anesthesiology 1985;62:714–724.

66. Hurwitz N. Predisposing factors in adverse reactions to drugs. Br Med J 1969;1:536–539.

67. Hurwitz N, Wade OL. Intensive hospital monitoring of adverse reactions to drugs. Br Med J 1969;1:531–536.

68. Patterson C. Iatrogenic disease in late life. Clin Geriatr Med 1986;2:121–136.

69. Williamson J, Chopin JM. Adverse reactions to prescribed drugs in the elderly: a multicentre investigation. Age Ageing 1980;9:73–80.

70. Muravchick S. The biology of aging and preoperative eval-uation. In: Geroanesthesia: Principles for Management of the Elderly Patient. St. Louis: Mosby-Year Book; 1997: 1–34.

71. Thomas DR, Ritchie CS. Preoperative assessment of older adults. J Am Geriatr Soc 1995;43:811–821.

72. Vaz FG, Seymour DG. A prospective study of elderly general surgical patients: I. Preoperative medical prob-lems. Age Ageing 1989;18:309–315.

73. Schneider JR, Droste JS, Schindler N, Golan JF. Carotid endarterectomy in octogenarians: comparison with patient characteristics and outcomes in younger patients. J Vasc Surg 2000;31:927–935.

74. Hoballah JJ, Nazzal MM, Jacobovicz C, Sharp WJ, Kresowik TF, Corson JD. Entering the ninth decade is not a contraindication for carotid endarterectomy. Angiology 1998;49:275–278.

75. Hosking MP, Warner MA, Lobdell CM, Offord KP, Melton LJd. Outcomes of surgery in patients 90 years of age and older [see comments]. JAMA 1989;261:1909–1915.

76. Warner MA, Saletel RA, Schroeder DR, Warner DO, Offord KP, Gray DT. Outcomes of anesthesia and surgery in people 100 years of age and older. J Am Geriatr Soc 1998;46:988–993.

77. Laskin RS. Total knee replacement in patients older than 85 years. Clin Orthop 1999:43–49.

78. Tiret L, Desmonts JM, Hatton F, Vourc'h G. Complications associated with anaesthesia—a prospective survey in France. Can Anaesth Soc J 1986;33:336–344.

79. Eagle KA, Brundage BH, Chaitman BR, et al. Guidelines for perioperative cardiovascular evaluation for noncardiac surgery. Report of the American College of Cardiology/ American Heart Association Task Force on Practice Guidelines. Committee on Perioperative Cardiovascular Evaluation for Noncardiac Surgery. Circulation 1996;93: 1278–1317.

80. Goldman L. Cardiac risks and complications of noncardiac surgery. Ann Intern Med 1983;98:504–513.

81. Liu LL, Leung JM. Predicting adverse postoperative outcomes in patients aged 80 years or older. J Am Geriatr Soc 2000;48:405–412.

82. Arvidsson S, Ouchterlony J, Sjostedt L, Svardsudd K. Predicting postoperative adverse events. Clinical efficiency of four general classification systems. The project peri-operative risk. Acta Anaesthesiol Scand 1996;40:783–791.

83. Detsky AS, Abrams HB, Forbath N, Scott JG, Hilliard JR. Cardiac assessment for patients undergoing noncardiac surgery. A multifactorial clinical risk index. Arch Intern Med 1986;146:2131–2134.

84. Pedersen T, Eliasen K, Henriksen E. A prospective study of risk factors and cardiopulmonary complications asso-ciated with anaesthesia and surgery: risk indicators of cardiopulmonary morbidity. Acta Anaesthesiol Scand 1990;34:144–155.

85. Pedersen T, Eliasen K, Henriksen E. A prospective study of mortality associated with anaesthesia and surgery: risk indicators of mortality in hospital. Acta Anaesthesiol Scand 1990;34:176–182.

86. Browner WS, Li J, Mangano DT. In-hospital and long-term mortality in male veterans following noncardiac surgery. The Study of Perioperative Ischemia Research Group. JAMA 1992;268:228–232.

87. Khuri SF, Daley J, Henderson W, et al. The National Veterans Administration Surgical Risk Study: risk adjustment for the comparative assessment of the quality of surgical care. J Am Coll Surg 1995;180:519–531.

88. Arvidsson S, Ouchterlony J, Nilsson S, Sjostedt L, Svardsudd K. The Gothenburg study of perioperative risk. I. Preoperative findings, postoperative complications. Acta Anaesthesiol Scand 1994;38:679–690.

89. Mohr DN. Estimation of surgical risk in the elderly: a correlative review. J Am Geriatr Soc 1983;31:99–102.

90. Cheng KW, Wang CH, Ho RT, Jawan B, Lee JH. Outcome of surgery and anesthesia in patients 80 years of age and older. Acta Anaesthesiol Sin 1994;32:37–43.

91. Cohen MM, Duncan PG, Tate RB. Does anesthesia contribute to operative mortality? JAMA 1988;260:2859–2863.

92. Cohen MM, Duncan PG. Physical status score and trends in anesthetic complications. J Clin Epidemiol 1988;41:83–90.

93. Goldman L, Hashimoto B, Cook EF, Loscalzo A. Comparative reproducibility and validity of systems for assessing cardiovascular functional class: advantages of a new specific activity scale. Circulation 1981;64:1227–1234.

94. Lawton MP, Brody EM. Assessment of older people: self-maintaining and instrumental activities of daily living. Gerontologist 1969;9:179–186.

95. Ware JE, Sherbourne CD. The MOS 36-item short-form health survey (SF-36). Med Care 1992;30:473–483.

96. Moy ML, Ingenito EP, Mentzer SJ, Evans RB, Reilly JJ Jr. Health-related quality of life improves following pulmonary rehabilitation and lung volume reduction surgery. Chest 1999;115:383–389.

97. Mangione CM, Goldman L, Orav EJ, et al. Health-related quality of life after elective surgery: measurement of longitudinal changes. J Gen Intern Med 1997;12:686–697.

98. Hannan EL, Magaziner J, Wang JJ, et al. Mortality and locomotion 6 months after hospitalization for hip fracture: risk factors and risk-adjusted hospital outcomes. JAMA 2001;285:2736–2742.

99. Tammela T, Kontturi M, Lukkarinen O. Postoperative urinary retention. I. Incidence and predisposing factors. Scand J Urol Nephrol 1986;20:197–201.

100. Duits AA, Boeke S, Taams MA, Passchier J, Erdman RA. Prediction of quality of life after coronary artery bypass graft surgery: a review and evaluation of multiple, recent studies. Psychosom Med 1997;59:257–268.

101. Keene JS, Anderson CA. Hip fractures in the elderly. Discharge predictions with a functional rating scale. JAMA 1982;248:564–567.

102. McCartney JR, Palmateer LM. Assessment of cognitive deficit in geriatric patients. A study of physician behavior. J Am Geriatr Soc 1985;33:467–471.

103. Inouye SK, Peduzzi PN, Robison JT, Hughes JS, Horwitz RI, Concato J. Importance of functional measures in predicting mortality among older hospitalized patients. JAMA 1998;279:1187–1193.

104. Raja SN, Haythornthwaite JA. Anesthetic management of the elderly: measuring function beyond the immediate perioperative horizon. Anesthesiology 1999;91:909–911.

105. Heyland DK, Guyatt G, Cook DJ, et al. Frequency and methodologic rigor of quality-of-life assessments in the critical care literature. Crit Care Med 1998;26:591–598.

106. Holmes J, House A. Psychiatric illness predicts poor outcome after surgery for hip fracture: a prospective cohort study. Psychol Med 2000;30:921–929.

107. Dolan MM, Hawkes WG, Zimmerman SI, et al. Delirium on hospital admission in aged hip fracture patients: prediction of mortality and 2-year functional outcomes. J Gerontol A Biol Sci Med Sci 2000;55:M527–M534.

108. Inouye SK, Schlesinger MJ, Lydon TJ. Delirium: a symptom of how hospital care is failing older persons and a window to improve quality of hospital care. Am J Med 1999;106:565–573.

109. Millar K, Asbury AJ, Murray GD. Pre-existing cognitive impairment as a factor influencing outcome after cardiac surgery. Br J Anaesth 2001;86:63–67.

110. Dyer CB, Ashton CM, Teasdale TA. Postoperative delirium. A review of 80 primary data-collection studies. Arch Intern Med 1995;155:461–465.

111. Ni Chonchubhair A, Valacio R, Kelly J, O'Keefe S. Use of the abbreviated mental test to detect postoperative delirium in elderly people. Br J Anaesth 1995;75:481–482.

112. Kaneko T, Takahashi S, Naka T, Hirooka Y, Inoue Y, Kaibara N. Postoperative delirium following gastrointestinal surgery in elderly patients. Surg Today 1997;27:107–111.

113. Gustafson Y, Berggren D, Brannstrom B, et al. Acute confusional states in elderly patients treated for femoral neck fracture. J Am Geriatr Soc 1988;36:525–530.

114. McDowell I, Kristjansson B, Hill GB, Hebert R. Community screening for dementia: the Mini Mental State Exam (MMSE) and Modified Mini-Mental State Exam (3MS) compared. J Clin Epidemiol 1997;50:377–383.

115. Folstein MF, Folstein SE, McHugh PR. "Mini-mental state." A practical method for grading the cognitive state of patients for the clinician. J Psychiatr Res 1975;12:189–198.

116. Berggren D, Gustafson Y, Eriksson B, et al. Postoperative confusion after anesthesia in elderly patients with femoral neck fractures. Anesth Analg 1987;66:497–504.

117. Williams-Russo P, Urquhart BL, Sharrock NE, Charlson ME. Post-operative delirium: predictors and prognosis in elderly orthopedic patients [see comments]. J Am Geriatr Soc 1992;40:759–767.

118. de Graeff A, de Leeuw JR, Ros WJ, Hordijk GJ, Blijham GH, Winnubst JA. Pretreatment factors predicting quality of life after treatment for head and neck cancer. Head Neck 2000;22:398–407.

119. Lyness JM, Noel TK, Cox C, King DA, Conwell Y, Caine ED. Screening for depression in elderly primary care patients. A comparison of the Center for Epidemiologic

Studies-Depression Scale and the Geriatric Depression Scale. Arch Intern Med 1997;157:449–454.

120. Roca R. Psychosocial aspects of surgical care in the elderly patient. Surg Clin North Am 1994;74:223–243.

121. Bradley EH, Bogardus ST Jr, van Doorn C, Williams CS, Cherlin E, Inouye SK. Goals in geriatric assessment: are we measuring the right outcomes? Gerontologist 2000; 40:191–196.

122. Heijmeriks JA, Pourrier S, Dassen P, Prenger K, Wellens HJ. Comparison of quality of life after coronary and/or valvular cardiac surgery in patients > or =75 years of age with younger patients. Am J Cardiol 1999;83:1129–1132, A9.

123. Katz S. Assessing self-maintenance: activities of daily living, mobility, and instrumental activities of daily living. J Am Geriatr Soc 1983;31:721–727.

124. Turnbull JM, Buck C. The value of preoperative screening investigations in otherwise healthy individuals. Arch Intern Med 1987;147:1101–1105.

125. Perez A, Planell J, Bacardaz C, et al. Value of routine preoperative tests: a multicentre study in four general hospitals. Br J Anaesth 1995;74:250–256.

126. Kaplan EB, Sheiner LB, Boeckmann AJ, et al. The usefulness of preoperative laboratory screening. JAMA 1985; 253:3576–3581.

127. Narr BJ, Warner ME, Schroeder DR, Warner MA. Outcomes of patients with no laboratory assessment before anesthesia and a surgical procedure. Mayo Clin Proc 1997; 72:505–509.

128. Seymour DG, Pringle R, Shaw JW. The role of the routine pre-operative chest X-ray in the elderly general surgical patient. Postgrad Med J 1982;58:741–745.

129. Seymour DG, Pringle R, MacLennan WJ. The role of the routine pre-operative electrocardiogram in the elderly surgical patient. Age Ageing 1983;12:97–104.

130. Sewell JM, Spooner LL, Dixon AK, Rubenstein D. Screening investigations in the elderly. Age Ageing 1981; 10:165–168.

131. Sanders DP, McKinney FW, Harris WH. Clinical evaluation and cost effectiveness of preoperative laboratory assessment on patients undergoing total hip arthroplasty. Orthopedics 1989;12:1449–1453.

132. Grimes CJ, Younathan MT, Lee WC. The effect of preoperative total parenteral nutrition on surgery outcomes. J Am Diet Assoc 1987;87:1202–1206.

133. Gibbs J, Cull W, Henderson W, Daley J, Hur K, Khuri SF. Preoperative serum albumin level as a predictor of operative mortality and morbidity: results from the National VA Surgical Risk Study. Arch Surg 1999;134:36–42.

134. Baker JP, Detsky AS, Wesson DE, et al. Nutritional assessment: a comparison of clinical judgement and objective measurements. N Engl J Med 1982;306:969–972.

135. Covinsky KE, Martin GE, Beyth RJ, Justice AC, Sehgal AR, Landefeld CS. The relationship between clinical assessments of nutritional status and adverse outcomes in older hospitalized medical patients. J Am Geriatr Soc 1999; 47:532–538.

136. Mazolewski P, Turner JF, Baker M, Kurtz T, Little AG. The impact of nutritional status on the outcome of lung volume reduction surgery: a prospective study. Chest 1999;116: 693–696.

137. Cohendy R, Gros T, Arnaud-Battandier F, Tran G, Plaze JM, Eledjam J. Preoperative nutritional evaluation of elderly patients: the Mini Nutritional Assessment as a practical tool. Clin Nutr 1999;18:345–348.

138. McClave SA, Snider HL, Spain DA. Preoperative issues in clinical nutrition. Chest 1999;115:64S–70S.

139. Moore AA, Siu AL. Screening for common problems in ambulatory elderly: clinical confirmation of a screening instrument. Am J Med 1996;100:438–443.

140. Schein OD, Katz J, Bass EB, et al. The value of routine preoperative medical testing before cataract surgery. Study of Medical Testing for Cataract Surgery. N Engl J Med 2000;342:168–175.

141. Dzankic S, Pastor D, Gonzalez C, Leung JM. The prevalence and predictive value of abnormal preoperative laboratory tests in elderly surgical patients. Anesth Analg 2001;93:301–308.

142. Berlauk JF, Abrams JH, Gilmour IJ, O'Connor SR, Knighton DR, Cerra FB. Preoperative optimization of cardiovascular hemodynamics improves outcome in peripheral vascular surgery. A prospective, randomized clinical trial. Ann Surg 1991;214:289–297;discussion 298–299.

143. Leppo JA. Preoperative cardiac risk assessment for noncardiac surgery. Am J Cardiol 1995;75:42D–51D.

144. Roubenoff R, Roubenoff RA, Preto J, Balke CW. Malnutrition among hospitalized patients. A problem of physician awareness. Arch Intern Med 1987;147:1462–1465.

145. Del Guercio LR, Cohn JD. Monitoring operative risk in the elderly. JAMA 1980;243:1350–1355.

146. Smith MS, Muir H, Hall R. Perioperative management of drug therapy, clinical considerations. Drugs 1996;51: 238–259.

147. Zaugg M, Tagliente T, Lucchinetti E, et al. Beneficial effects from beta-adrenergic blockade in elderly patients undergoing noncardiac surgery. Anesthesiology 1999;91: 1674–1686.

148. Yeager RA, Moneta GL, Edwards JM, Taylor LMJ, McConnell DB, Porter JM. Reducing perioperative myocardial infarction following vascular surgery: the potential role of beta-blockade. Arch Surg 1995;130:869–873.

149. Bisson A, Stern M, Caubarrere I. Preparation of high-risk patients for major thoracic surgery. Chest Surg Clin North Am 1998;8:541–555, viii.

150. Debigare R, Maltais F, Whittom F, Deslauriers J, LeBlanc P. Feasibility and efficacy of home exercise training before lung volume reduction. J Cardiopulm Rehabil 1999;19: 235–241.

151. Arthur HM, Daniels C, McKelvie R, Hirsh J, Rush B. Effect of a preoperative intervention on preoperative and postoperative outcomes in low-risk patients awaiting elective coronary artery bypass graft surgery. A randomized, controlled trial. Ann Intern Med 2000;133:253–262.

152. Fisher DA, Trimble S, Clapp B, Dorsett K. Effect of a patient management system on outcomes of total hip and knee arthroplasty. Clin Orthop 1997:155–160.

153. Roy RC. Choosing general versus regional anesthesia for the elderly. Anesthesiol Clin North Am 2000;18:91–104, vii.

154. McLaren AD, Stockwell MC, Reid VT. Anaesthetic techniques for surgical correction of fractured neck of femur.

A comparative study of spinal and general anaesthesia in the elderly. Anaesthesia 1978;33:10–14.

155. Hole A, Terjesen T, Breivik H. Epidural versus general anaesthesia for total hip arthroplasty in elderly patients. Acta Anaesthesiol Scand 1980;24:279–287.

156. Nielson WR, Gelb AW, Casey JE, Penny FJ, Merchant RN, Manninen PH. Long-term cognitive and social sequelae of general versus regional anesthesia during arthroplasty in the elderly. Anesthesiology 1990;73:1103–1109.

157. Davis FM, Woolner DF, Frampton C, et al. Prospective, multi-centre trial of mortality following general or spinal anaesthesia for hip fracture surgery in the elderly. Br J Anaesth 1987;59:1080–1088.

158. McKenzie PJ, Wishart HY, Dewar KM, Gray I, Smith G. Comparison of the effects of spinal anaesthesia and general anaesthesia on postoperative oxygenation and perioperative mortality. Br J Anaesth 1980;52:49–54.

159. McKenzie PJ, Wishart HY, Gray I, Smith G. Effects of anaesthetic technique on deep vein thrombosis. A comparison of subarachnoid and general anaesthesia. Br J Anaesth 1985;57:853–857.

160. Hendolin H, Mattila MA, Poikolainen E. The effect of lumbar epidural analgesia on the development of deep vein thrombosis of the legs after open prostatectomy. Acta Chir Scand 1981;147:425–429.

161. White PF. Anesthetic techniques for the elderly outpatient. Int Anesthesiol Clin 1988;26:105–111.

162. Valentin N, Lomholt B, Jensen JS, Hejgaard N, Kreiner S. Spinal or general anaesthesia for surgery of the fractured hip? A prospective study of mortality in 578 patients. Br J Anaesth 1986;58:284–291.

163. Sorenson RM, Pace NL. Anesthetic techniques during surgical repair of femoral neck fractures. A meta-analysis. Anesthesiology 1992;77:1095–1104.

164. Urwin SC, Parker MJ, Griffiths R. General versus regional anaesthesia for hip fracture surgery: a meta-analysis of randomized trials. Br J Anaesth 2000;84:450–455.

165. Gilbert TB, Hawkes WG, Hebel JR, et al. Spinal anesthesia versus general anesthesia for hip fracture repair: a longitudinal observation of 741 elderly patients during 2-year follow-up. Am J Orthop 2000;29:25–35.

166. Sutcliffe AJ, Parker M. Mortality after spinal and general anaesthesia for surgical fixation of hip fractures. Anaesthesia 1994;49:237–240.

167. O'Hara DA, Duff A, Berlin JA, et al. The effect of anesthetic technique on postoperative outcomes in hip fracture repair. Anesthesiology 2000;92:947–957.

168. Rodgers A, Walker N, Schug S, et al. Reduction of postoperative mortality and morbidity with epidural or spinal anaesthesia: results from overview of randomised trials. BMJ 2000;321:1493.

169. Riis J, Lomholt B, Haxholdt O, et al. Immediate and long-term mental recovery from general versus epidural anesthesia in elderly patients. Acta Anaesthesiol Scand 1983;27:44–49.

170. Bigler D, Adelhoj B, Petring OU, Pederson NO, Busch P, Kalhke P. Mental function and morbidity after acute hip surgery during spinal and general anaesthesia. Anaesthesia 1985;40:672–676.

171. Ghoneim MM, Hinrichs JV, O'Hara MW, et al. Comparison of psychologic and cognitive functions after general or regional anesthesia. Anesthesiology 1988;69:507–515.

172. Norris EJ, Beattie C, Perler BA, et al. Double-masked randomized trial comparing alternate combinations of intraoperative anesthesia and postoperative analgesia in abdominal aortic surgery. Anesthesiology 2001;95:1054–1067.

173. Yeager MP, Glass DD, Neff RK, Brinck-Johnsen T. Epidural anesthesia and analgesia in high-risk surgical patients. Anesthesiology 1987;66:729–736.

174. Chung F, Meier R, Lautenschlager E, Carmichael FJ, Chung A. General or spinal anesthesia: which is better in the elderly? Anesthesiology 1987;67:422–427.

175. Asbjorn J, Jakobsen BW, Pilegaard HK, Blom L, Ostergaard A, Brandt MR. Mental function in elderly men after surgery during epidural analgesia. Acta Anaesthesiol Scand 1989;33:369–373.

176. Edwards ND, Callaghan LC, White T, Reilly CS. Perioperative myocardial ischaemia in patients undergoing transurethral surgery: a pilot study comparing general with spinal anaesthesia. Br J Anaesth 1995;74:368–372.

177. Bode RH, Lewis KP, Zarich SW, et al. Cardiac outcome after peripheral vascular surgery. Comparison of general and regional anesthesia. Anesthesiology 1996;84:3–13.

178. Christopherson R, Beattie C, Frank SM, et al. Perioperative morbidity in patients randomized to epidural or general anesthesia for lower extremity vascular surgery. Perioperative Ischemia Randomized Anesthesia Trial Study Group. Anesthesiology 1993;79:422–434.

179. Corson JD, Chang BB, Shah DM, Leather RP, DeLeo BM, Karmody AM. The influence of anesthetic choice on carotid endarterectomy outcome. Arch Surg 1987;122:807–812.

180. Papavasiliou AK, Magnadottir HB, Gonda T, Franz D, Harbaugh RE. Clinical outcomes after carotid endarterectomy: comparison of the use of regional and general anesthetics. J Neurosurg 2000;92:291–296.

181. Fiorani P, Sbarigia E, Speziale F, et al. General anaesthesia versus cervical block and perioperative complications in carotid artery surgery. Eur J Vasc Endovasc Surg 1997;13:37–42.

182. Bowyer MW, Zierold D, Loftus JP, Egan JC, Inglis KJ, Halow KD. Carotid endarterectomy: a comparison of regional versus general anesthesia in 500 operations. Ann Vasc Surg 2000;14:145–151.

183. Ferguson GG, Eliasziw M, Barr HW, et al. The North American Symptomatic Carotid Endarterectomy Trial: surgical results in 1415 patients [see comments]. Stroke 1999;30:1751–1758.

184. Slogoff S, Reul GJ, Keats AS, et al. Role of perfusion pressure and flow in major organ dysfunction after cardiopulmonary bypass. Ann Thorac Surg 1990;50:911–918.

185. Wong BI, McLean RF, Naylor CD, et al. Central-nervous-system dysfunction after warm or hypothermic cardiopulmonary bypass. Lancet 1992;339:1383–1384.

186. Gold JP, Charlson ME, Williams-Russo P, et al. Improvement of outcomes after coronary artery bypass. A randomized trial comparing intraoperative high versus low mean arterial pressure. J Thorac Cardiovasc Surg 1995;110:1302–1311; discussion 1311–1314.

187. Roach GW, Kanchuger M, Mangano CM, et al. Adverse cerebral outcomes after coronary bypass surgery. Multicenter Study of Perioperative Ischemia Research Group and the Ischemia Research and Education Foundation Investigators. N Engl J Med 1996;335:1857–1863.

188. Cook DJ. Neurologic effects. In: Gravlee GP, Davis RF, Kurusz M, Utley JR, eds. Cardiopulmonary Bypass: Principles and Practice. 2nd ed. Philadelphia: Lippincott Williams & Wilkins; 2000:403–431.

189. Frank SM, Beattie C, Christopherson R, et al. Unintentional hypothermia is associated with postoperative myocardial ischemia. The Perioperative Ischemia Randomized Anesthesia Trial Study Group. Anesthesiology 1993;78:468–476.

190. Frank SM, El-Rahmany HK, Cattaneo CG, Barnes RA. Predictors of hypothermia during spinal anesthesia. Anesthesiology 2000;92:1330–1334.

191. Frank SM, Fleisher LA, Breslow MJ, et al. Perioperative maintenance of normothermia reduces the incidence of morbid cardiac events. A randomized clinical trial. JAMA 1997;277:1127–1134.

192. Frank SM, Fleisher LA, Olson KF, et al. Multivariate determinants of early postoperative oxygen consumption in elderly patients. Effects of shivering, body temperature, and gender. Anesthesiology 1995;83:241–249.

193. Frank SM, Higgins MS, Breslow MJ, et al. The catecholamine, cortisol, and hemodynamic responses to mild perioperative hypothermia. A randomized clinical trial. Anesthesiology 1995;82:83–93.

194. Mangano DT, Layug EL, Wallace A, Tateo I. Effect of atenolol on mortality and cardiovascular morbidity after noncardiac surgery. Multicenter Study of Perioperative Ischemia Research Group. N Engl J Med 1996;335:1713–1720.

195. Poldermans D, Boersma E, Bax JJ, et al. The effect of bisoprolol on perioperative mortality and myocardial infarction in high-risk patients undergoing vascular surgery. Dutch Echocardiographic Cardiac Risk Evaluation Applying Stress Echocardiography Study Group. N Engl J Med 1999;341:1789–1794.

196. Nishina K, Mikawa K, Uesugi T, et al. Efficacy of clonidine for prevention of perioperative myocardial ischemia: a critical appraisal and meta-analysis of the literature. Anesthesiology 2002;96:323–329.

197. van den Berghe G, Wouters P, Weekers F, et al. Intensive insulin therapy in the critically ill patients. N Engl J Med 2001;345:1359–1367.

198. Cohen MM, Duncan PG, Tweed WA, et al. The Canadian four-centre study of anaesthetic outcomes: I. Description of methods and populations. Can J Anaesth 1992;39:420–429.

199. Rao TL, Jacobs KH, El-Etr AA. Reinfarction following anesthesia in patients with myocardial infarction. Anesthesiology 1983;59:499–505.

200. O'Keeffe ST, Ni Chonchubhair A. Postoperative delirium in the elderly. Br J Anaesth 1994;73:673–687.

201. Seymour DG, Vaz FG. A prospective study of elderly general surgical patients: II. Post-operative complications. Age Ageing 1989;18:316–326.

202. Moller JT, Johannessen NW, Espersen K, et al. Randomized evaluation of pulse oximetry in 20,802 patients: II. Perioperative events and postoperative complications. Anesthesiology 1993;78:445–453.

203. Moller JT, Svennild I, Johannessen NW, et al. Perioperative monitoring with pulse oximetry and late postoperative cognitive dysfunction. Br J Anaesth 1993;71:340–347.

204. Pontoppidan H, Beecher HK. Progressive loss of protective reflexes in the airway with the advance of age. JAMA 1960;174:2209–2213.

205. Pedersen T, Viby-Mogensen J, Ringsted C. Anaesthetic practice and postoperative pulmonary complications. Acta Anaesthesiol Scand 1992;36:812–818.

206. Bailey PL, Pace NL, Ashburn MA, Moll JW, East KA, Stanley TH. Frequent hypoxemia and apnea after sedation with midazolam and fentanyl. Anesthesiology 1990;73:826–830.

207. Hogue CW Jr, Lappas GD, Creswell LL, et al. Swallowing dysfunction after cardiac operations. Associated adverse outcomes and risk factors including intraoperative transesophageal echocardiography. J Thorac Cardiovasc Surg 1995;110:517–522.

208. Mitchell CK, Smoger SH, Pfeifer MP, et al. Multivariate analysis of factors associated with postoperative pulmonary complications following general elective surgery. Arch Surg 1998;133:194–198.

209. Warner MA, Warner ME, Weber JG. Clinical significance of pulmonary aspiration during the perioperative period. Anesthesiology 1993;78:56–62.

210. Roberts JR, Shyr Y, Christian KR, Drinkwater D, Merrill W. Preemptive gastrointestinal tract management reduces aspiration and respiratory failure after thoracic operations. J Thorac Cardiovasc Surg 2000;119:449–452.

211. Breslow MJ, Parker SD, Frank SM, et al. Determinants of catecholamine and cortisol responses to lower extremity revascularization. The PIRAT Study Group. Anesthesiology 1993;79:1202–1209.

212. Rem J, Nielsen OS, Brandt MR, Kehlet H. Release mechanisms of postoperative changes in various acute phase proteins and immunoglobulins. Acta Chir Scand Suppl 1980;502:51–56.

213. Kilickan L, Toker K. The effects of preemptive intravenous versus preemptive epidural morphine on postoperative analgesia and surgical stress response after orthopaedic procedures. Minerva Anestesiol 2000;66:649–655.

214. Schulze S, Schierbeck J, Sparso BH, Bisgaard M, Kehlet H. Influence of neural blockade and indomethacin on leucocyte, temperature, and acute-phase protein response to surgery. Acta Chir Scand 1987;153:255–259.

215. Klasen JA, Opitz SA, Melzer C, Thiel A, Hempelmann G. Intraarticular, epidural, and intravenous analgesia after total knee arthroplasty. Acta Anaesthesiol Scand 1999;43:1021–1026.

216. Schulze S, Sommer P, Bigler D, et al. Effect of combined prednisolone, epidural analgesia, and indomethacin on the systemic response after colonic surgery. Arch Surg 1992;127:325–331.

217. Rem J, Brandt MR, Kehlet H. Prevention of postoperative lymphopenia and granulocytosis by epidural analgesia. Lancet 1980;1:283–284.

218. Hjortso NC, Andersen T, Frosig F, Neumann P, Rogon E, Kehlet H. Failure of epidural analgesia to modify postop-

erative depression of delayed hypersensitivity. Acta Anaesthesiol Scand 1984;28:128–131.

219. Rutberg H, Hakanson E, Anderberg B, Jorfeldt L, Martensson J, Schildt B. Effects of the extradural administration of morphine, or bupivacaine, on the endocrine response to upper abdominal surgery. Br J Anaesth 1984; 56:233–237.

220. Liu S, Carpenter RL, Neal JM. Epidural anesthesia and analgesia. Their role in postoperative outcome. Anesthesiology 1995;82:1474–1506.

221. Tuman KJ, McCarthy RJ, March RJ, DeLaria GA, Patel RV, Ivankovich AD. Effects of epidural anesthesia and analgesia on coagulation and outcome after major vascular surgery. Anesth Analg 1991;73:696–704.

222. Giesecke K, Klingstedt C, Ljungqvist O, Hagenfeldt L. The modifying influence of anaesthesia on postoperative protein catabolism. Br J Anaesth 1994;72:697–699.

223. Heindorff H, Schulze S, Mogensen T, Almdal T, Kehlet H, Vilstrup H. Hormonal and neural blockade prevents the postoperative increase in amino acid clearance and urea synthesis. Surgery 1992;111:543–550.

224. Carli F, Halliday D. Continuous epidural blockade arrests the postoperative decrease in muscle protein fractional synthetic rate in surgical patients. Anesthesiology 1997; 86:1033–1040.

225. Wasylak TJ, Abbott FV, English MJ, Jeans ME. Reduction of postoperative morbidity following patient-controlled morphine. Can J Anaesth 1990;37:726–731.

226. Petros JG, Alameddine F, Testa E, Rimm EB, Robillard RJ. Patient-controlled analgesia and postoperative urinary retention after hysterectomy for benign disease. J Am Coll Surg 1994;179:663–667.

227. Petros JG, Mallen JK, Howe K, Rimm EB, Robillard RJ. Patient-controlled analgesia and postoperative urinary retention after open appendectomy. Surg Gynecol Obstet 1993;177:172–175.

228. Carpenter RL, Abram SE, Bromage PR, Rauck RL. Consensus statement on acute pain management. Reg Anesth 1996;21:152–156.

229. Carpenter RL. Gastrointestinal benefits of regional anesthesia/analgesia. Reg Anesth 1996;21:13–17.

230. Kumar A, Bose S, Bhattacharya A, Tandon OP, Kundra P. Oral clonidine premedication for elderly patients undergoing intraocular surgery. Acta Anaesthesiol Scand 1992; 36:159–164.

231. Singelyn FJ, Gouverneur JM. Extended "three-in-one" block after total knee arthroplasty: continuous versus patient-controlled techniques. Anesth Analg 2000;91:176–180.

232. De Kock MF, Pichon G, Scholtes JL. Intraoperative clonidine enhances postoperative morphine patient-controlled analgesia. Can J Anaesth 1992;39:537–544.

233. Wong HY, Carpenter RL, Kopacz DJ, et al. A randomized, double-blind evaluation of ketorolac tromethamine for postoperative analgesia in ambulatory surgery patients. Anesthesiology 1993;78:6–14.

234. Milligan KR, Convery PN, Weir P, Quinn P, Connolly D. The efficacy and safety of epidural infusions of levobupivacaine with and without clonidine for postoperative pain relief in patients undergoing total hip replacement. Anesth Analg 2000;91:393–397.

235. Capdevila X, Barthelet Y, Biboulet P, Ryckwaert Y, Rubenovitch J, d'Athis F. Effects of perioperative analgesic technique on the surgical outcome and duration of rehabilitation after major knee surgery. Anesthesiology 1999;91:8–15.

236. Mahoney OM, Noble PC, Davidson J, Tullos HS. The effect of continuous epidural analgesia on postoperative pain, rehabilitation, and duration of hospitalization in total knee arthroplasty. Clin Orthop 1990:30–37.

237. Williams-Russo P, Sharrock NE, Haas SB, et al. Randomized trial of epidural versus general anesthesia: outcomes after primary total knee replacement. Clin Orthop 1996: 199–208.

238. Cullen DJ, Sweitzer BJ, Bates DW, Burdick E, Edmondson A, Leape LL. Preventable adverse drug events in hospitalized patients: a comparative study of intensive care and general care units. Crit Care Med 1997;25:1289–1297.

239. Bates DW, Cullen DJ, Laird N, et al. Incidence of adverse drug events and potential adverse drug events. Implications for prevention. ADE Prevention Study Group. JAMA 1995;274:29–34.

240. Parikh SS, Chung F. Postoperative delirium in the elderly. Anesth Analg 1995;80:1223–1232.

241. Ritchie K, Polge C, de Roquefeuil G, Djakovic M, Ledesert B. Impact of anesthesia on the cognitive functioning of the elderly. Int Psychogeriatr 1997;9:309–326.

242. Grichnik KP, Ijsselmuiden AJ, D'Amico TA, et al. Cognitive decline after major noncardiac operations: a preliminary prospective study. Ann Thorac Surg 1999;68: 1786–1791.

243. Billig N, Stockton P, Cohen-Mansfield J. Cognitive and affective changes after cataract surgery in an elderly population. Am J Geriatr Psychiatry 1995;4:29–38.

244. Goldstein MZ, Young BL, Fogel BS, Benedict RH. Occurrence and predictors of short-term mental and functional changes in older adults undergoing elective surgery under general anesthesia. Am J Geriatr Psychiatry 1998;6: 42–52.

245. Rogers MP, Liang MH, Daltroy LH, et al. Delirium after elective orthopedic surgery: risk factors and natural history. Int J Psychiatry Med 1989;19:109–121.

246. Williams-Russo P, Sharrock NE, Mattis S, Szatrowski TP, Charlson ME. Cognitive effects after epidural vs general anesthesia in older adults. A randomized trial. JAMA 1995;274:44–50.

247. Moller JT, Cluitmans P, Rasmussen LS, et al. Long-term postoperative cognitive dysfunction in the elderly ISPOCD1 study. (ISPOCD investigators. International Study of Post-Operative Cognitive Dysfunction). Lancet 1998;351:857–861.

248. McKhann GM, Goldsborough MA, Borowicz LM Jr, et al. Cognitive outcome after coronary artery bypass: a one-year prospective study. Ann Thorac Surg 1997;63: 510–515.

249. Newman MF, Kramer D, Croughwell ND, et al. Differential age effects of mean arterial pressure and rewarming on cognitive dysfunction after cardiac surgery. Anesth Analg 1995;81:236–242.

250. Selnes OA, Goldsborough MA, Borowicz LM, Enger C, Quaskey SA, McKhann GM. Determinants of cognitive change after coronary artery bypass surgery: a multifactorial problem. Ann Thorac Surg 1999;67:1669–1676.

251. Chung FF, Chung A, Meier RH, Lautenschlaeger E, Seyone C. Comparison of perioperative mental function after general anaesthesia and spinal anaesthesia with intravenous sedation. Can J Anaesth 1989;36:382–387.

252. Marcantonio ER, Juarez G, Goldman L, et al. The relationship of postoperative delirium with psychoactive medications. JAMA 1994;272:1518–1522.

253. Herrick IA, Ganapathy S, Komar W, et al. Postoperative cognitive impairment in the elderly. Choice of patient-controlled analgesic opioid. Anaesthesia 1996;51:356–360.

254. Crul BJ, Hulstijn W, Burger IC. Influence of the type of anaesthesia on post-operative subjective physical well-being and mental function in elderly patients. Acta Anaesthesiol Scand 1992;36:615–620.

255. Tune LE, Damlouji NF, Holland A, Gardner TJ, Folstein MF, Coyle JT. Association of postoperative delirium with raised serum levels of anticholinergic drugs. Lancet 1981; 2:651–653.

256. Brebner J, Hadley L. Experiences with physostigmine in the reversal of adverse post-anaesthetic effects. Can Anaesth Soc J 1976;23:574–581.

257. Marcantonio ER, Goldman L, Orav EJ, Cook EF, Lee TH. The association of intraoperative factors with the development of postoperative delirium. Am J Med 1998;105: 380–384.

258. Dodds C, Allison J. Postoperative cognitive deficit in the elderly surgical patient. Br J Anaesth 1998;81:449–462.

259. Inouye SK, Charpentier PA. Precipitating factors for delirium in hospitalized elderly persons. Predictive model and interrelationship with baseline vulnerability. JAMA 1996; 275:852–857.

260. Inouye SK. Delirium in hospitalized older patients: recognition and risk factors. J Geriatr Psychiatry Neurol 1998; 11:118–125; discussion 157–158.

261. Inouye SK. Delirium in hospitalized older patients. Clin Geriatr Med 1998;14:745–764.

262. Lynch EP, Lazor MA, Gellis JE, Orav J, Goldman L, Marcantonio ER. The impact of postoperative pain on the development of postoperative delirium. Anesth Analg 1998;86:781–785.

263. Koenig HG, George LK, Stangl D, Tweed DL. Hospital stressors experienced by elderly medical inpatients: developing a Hospital Stress Index. Int J Psychiatry Med 1995; 25:103–122.

264. Inouye SK. Predisposing and precipitating factors for delirium in hospitalized older patients. Dement Geriatr Cogn Disord 1999;10:393–400.

265. Inouye SK, Bogardus ST Jr, Charpentier PA, et al. A multicomponent intervention to prevent delirium in hospitalized older patients [see comments]. N Engl J Med 1999; 340:669–676.

266. Inouye SK, Rushing JT, Foreman MD, Palmer RM, Pompei P. Does delirium contribute to poor hospital outcomes? A three-site epidemiologic study. J Gen Intern Med 1998; 13:234–242.

267. Inouye SK, Viscoli CM, Horwitz RI, Hurst LD, Tinetti ME. A predictive model for delirium in hospitalized elderly medical patients based on admission characteristics. Ann Intern Med 1993;119:474–481.

268. Goldstein MZ. Cognitive change after elective surgery in nondemented older adults. Am J Geriatr Psychiatry 1993; 1:118–125.

269. McDowell I, Newell C. Measuring Health: a Guide to Rating Scales and Questionnaires. 2nd ed. New York: Oxford University Press; 1996.

270. Froehlich TE, Robison JT, Inouye SK. Screening for dementia in the outpatient setting: the time and change test [see comments]. J Am Geriatr Soc 1998;46:1506–1511.

271. Kalisvaart KJ, de Jonghe JF, Bogaards MJ, et al. Haloperidol prophylaxis for elderly hip-surgery patients at risk for delirium: a randomized placebo-controlled study. J Am Geriatr Soc 2005;53:1658–1666.

272. Freedman GM, Peruvemba R. Geriatric pain management. The anesthesiologist's perspective. Anesthesiol Clin North Am 2000;18:123–141, vii.

273. Parmelee PA, Katz IR, Lawton MP. The relation of pain to depression among institutionalized aged. J Gerontol 1991;46:15–21.

274. Farrell MJ, Gerontol M, Gibson SJ, Helme RD. The effect of medical status on the activity level of older pain clinic patients. J Am Geriatr Soc 1995;43:102–107.

275. Sorkin BA, Rudy TE, Hanlon RB, Turk DC, Stieg RL. Chronic pain in old and young patients: differences appear less important than similarities. J Gerontol 1990;45: 64–68.

276. Cutler RB, Fishbain DA, Rosomoff RS, Rosomoff HL. Outcomes in treatment of pain in geriatric and younger age groups. Arch Phys Med Rehabil 1994;75:457–464.

277. Lipman AG. Analgesic drugs for neuropathic and sympathetically maintained pain. Clin Geriatr Med 1996;12: 501–515.

278. Arner S, Meyerson BA. Lack of analgesic effect of opioids on neuropathic and idiopathic forms of pain. Pain 1988; 33:11–23.

279. Swerdlow M. Anticonvulsants in the therapy of neuralgic pain. Pain Clinic 1986;1:9–19.

280. Stanton-Hicks M, Baron R, Boas R, et al. Complex regional pain syndromes: guidelines for therapy. Clin J Pain 1998; 14:155–166.

281. Max MB, Kishore-Kumar R, Schafer SC, et al. Efficacy of desipramine in painful diabetic neuropathy: a placebo-controlled trial. Pain 1991;45:3–9; discussion 1–2.

282. Cutler RB, Fishbain DA, Lu Y, Rosomoff RS, Rosomoff HL. Prediction of pain center treatment outcome for geriatric chronic pain patients. Clin J Pain 1994;10: 10–17.

283. Carmichael JK. Treatment of herpes zoster and postherpeutic neuralgia. Am Fam Physician 1991;44:203–210.

284. Watson CP, Evans RJ, Watt VR. Post-herpetic neuralgia and topical capsaicin. Pain 1988;33:333–340.

285. Hwang SM, Kang YC, Lee YB, Yoon KB, Ahn SK, Choi EH. The effects of epidural blockade on the acute pain in herpes zoster. Arch Dermatol 1999;135:1359–1364.

286. Chiarello SE. Tumescent infiltration of corticosteroids, lidocaine, and epinephrine into dermatomes of acute her-

petic pain or postherpetic neuralgia. Arch Dermatol 1998;
134:279–281.

287. Alper BS, Lewis PR. Does treatment of acute herpes zoster prevent or shorten postherpetic neuralgia? J Fam Pract 2000;49:255–264.

288. Kost RG, Straus SE. Postherpetic neuralgia. Predicting and preventing risk. Arch Intern Med 1997;157:1166–1167.

289. Weller TH. Varicella and herpes zoster. Changing concepts of the natural history, control, and importance of a not-so-benign virus. N Engl J Med 1983;309:1434–1440.

290. Ragozzino MW, Melton LJ 3rd, Kurland LT, Chu CP, Perry HO. Population-based study of herpes zoster and its sequelae. Medicine (Baltimore) 1982;61:310–316.

291. Donahue JG, Choo PW, Manson JE, Platt R. The incidence of herpes zoster. Arch Intern Med 1995;155:1605–1609.

292. Choo PW, Galil K, Donahue JG, Walker AM, Spiegelman D, Platt R. Risk factors for postherpetic neuralgia. Arch Intern Med 1997;157:1217–1224.

293. Galil K, Choo PW, Donahue JG, Platt R. The sequelae of herpes zoster. Arch Intern Med 1997;157:1209–1213.

294. Miller AE. Selective decline in cellular immune response to varicella-zoster in the elderly. Neurology 1980;30:582–587.

295. Berger R, Florent G, Just M. Decrease of the lymphoproliferative response to varicella-zoster virus antigen in the aged. Infect Immun 1981;32:24–27.

296. Burke BL, Steele RW, Beard OW, Wood JS, Cain TD, Marmer DJ. Immune responses to varicella-zoster in the aged. Arch Intern Med 1982;142:291–293.

297. Levin MJ, Murray M, Rotbart HA, Zerbe GO, White CJ, Hayward AR. Immune response of elderly individuals to a live attenuated varicella vaccine. J Infect Dis 1992;166:253–259.

298. Oxman MN, Levin MJ, Johnson GR, et al. A vaccine to prevent herpes zoster and postherpetic neuralgia in older adults. N Engl J Med 2005;352:2271–2284.

299. Byrd JC, McGrail LH, Hospenthal DR, Howard RS, Dow NA, Diehl LF. Herpes virus infections occur frequently following treatment with fludarabine: results of a prospective natural history study. Br J Haematol 1999;105:445–447.

300. Sengstaken EA, King SA. The problems of pain and its detection among geriatric nursing home residents. J Am Geriatr Soc 1993;41:541–544.

Part II
Cardinal Manifestations of Aging and Disease in the Elderly

Part II
Cardinal Manifestations of Aging and Disease in the Elderly

7
Alterations in Metabolic Functions and Electrolytes

Michael C. Lewis

Aging has been characterized as a comprehensive, progressive, and irreversible biologic process resulting in the maintenance of life but with a diminishing capability for adaptation.[1,2] In fact, it has been estimated that after the age of 30 years, organ systems lose approximately 1% of their function per annum.[3] Implied in this description are the concepts of increased biologic entropy, functional deterioration, loss of viability, and an augmented likelihood of death.[4]

The aging population is rapidly growing[5-7] and utilizes a growing proportion of medical resources,[8-10] including surgery.[11-14] However, because of factors such as decreased functional reserve, existing comorbidity, and polypharmacy, older patients have higher morbidity[15] and mortality,[16] especially when the surgery is emergent.[17,18] Their medical management is becoming one of the greatest challenges to anesthesiologists. Yet, despite this reality, little time is spent on formal training in geriatrics during anesthesia residency training.[19]

The Concept of Functional Reserve

Organ function in the elderly is usually well maintained under basal conditions. One measure of "health" in the aged is their ability to tolerate increased physiologic loads. When an individual can maintain a steady state in the face of increased physiologic demand, they are said to demonstrate a good functional reserve. In contrast, when there is latent disease and diminished ability to maintain function in the face of stressors, there is said to be decreased functional reserve. Age leads to a gradual reduction in functional reserve (Figure 7-1). Consequently, when stress exceeds functional reserve, imbalance within systems will likely develop and result in a breakdown of homeostatic compensation.

Aging per se is typified by a decreased performance of many biologic regulatory processes in the face of biologic stress. Because these regulatory mechanisms provide functional integration between cells and organ systems, growing old may be associated with a failure to maintain homeostatic functions. This impaired capability affects diverse regulatory systems uniquely in aged subjects and may at least partly explain the increased interindividual variability in functional reserve that occurs as people get older. The decline in functional reserve is inconsistent among individuals, with the variability in deterioration rooted within lifestyle choices, environmental factors, genetics, and the presence of age-related disease. A decline in functional reserve may precipitate a serious decline in performance when the elderly patient is exposed to stress such as those of surgery and anesthesia, and thereby increases the risk of age-related disease.

Aims

This chapter will function primarily as an introduction to the complex area of metabolic changes in the elderly. In addition, issues concerning the fluid and electrolyte status of the elderly patient will be touched upon. Within each of its sections, the impact of these changes on the anesthetic management of these patients will be examined, and the concept of reduced functional reserve and its consequences will be continually reemphasized.

Basal Metabolic Rate

Mitochondria, being the powerhouse of biologic processes, underlie all of the metabolic functions of the body. These organelles provide the power that fuels metabolic functions.

The energy required to maintain basic cellular functions is termed basal metabolic rate (BMR) and it is generally accepted that it decreases with advancing age. It decreases by approximately 1%–2% per decade from the ages of 20–80 years,[20-22] and additive declines in BMR have been shown to decrease the rate of drug metabolism.[23]

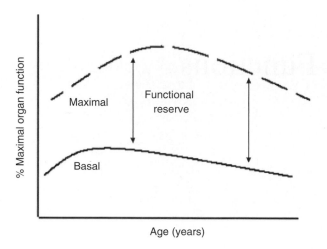

FIGURE 7-1. The functional reserve is the difference between basal function (solid line) and maximal function (broken line). Even in healthy elderly individuals, this functional reserve will be reduced. (Modified from Muravchick S. Geroanesthesia: Principles for Management of the Elderly Patient. St. Louis: Mosby-Year Book; 1997. Copyright © 1997 with permission from Elsevier.)

This decreased BMR is associated with increased levels of circulating epinephrine[24,25] and reduced β-receptor sensitivity.[26] These receptors are involved in sympathetically mediated thermogenesis, hence, the fact that the β-response becomes blunted has been used to explain a predisposition to obesity.[21] Such a tendency to obesity in the elderly may contribute to the observed increase in incidence of both Type 2 diabetes[27] and cardiac disease.[28] Moreover, this diminution of β-receptor sensitivity in the elderly results in a decreased ability to cope with physiologic stressors.

Impaired thermogenesis and reduced BMR predispose the elderly to more severe postoperative hypothermia and a protracted recovery from this phenomenon.[29] Slowness to recover from hypothermia is also partly attributable to the reduced amount of shivering compared with younger patients[30] with total body oxygen consumption increasing only about 38% in the elderly.[31] Such vulnerability to hypothermia increases the risk of adverse physiologic outcomes such as increased risk of wound infections[32] and myocardial ischemia.[33]

In summary, changes in BMR in the elderly are characterized by:

- Gradual decline in BMR even allowing for changes in body composition
- Increase in circulating catecholamines, together with decreased β-receptor sensitivity, increasing the predisposition to obesity
- Impaired ability to protect against and recover from hypothermia exposing the geriatric patient to increased intra- and postoperative complications

Body Composition

The changes in body structure with aging are typified by an increase in the percentage of body fat,[34] a loss of protein,[35] and intracellular dehydration.[36] These changes in body composition have been shown to be even greater in women.[18]

Changes in Body Fat

Age-related accumulation of body fat increases the deposition of lipid-soluble drugs including anesthetics.[37] Consequently, the larger concentration of these agents in fat tissue results in a longer time for redistribution and a slower elimination time thereby prolonging anesthetic effects.[38,39]

Loss of Protein

There is a significant loss of body protein with aging.[40] The following section will describe the sources of this protein loss.

Muscle Mass

The majority of the age-related loss of body protein is accounted for by the up to 20% decrease of skeletal muscle mass[41] of unknown etiology[42] and is termed sarcopenia.[43] This occurs even in the fit adult and is associated with a loss of strength. For a person in their second decade, muscle comprises up to 60% of the lean body mass, and yet at 70 years of age, this decreases to less than 40%. Although the decrease in muscle tissue begins around the age of 50 years, it becomes more dramatic beyond the 60th year of life.[44] This decline can be partially reversed using resistance exercises.[45]

Despite this degree of muscle loss, there is no difference in sensitivity of the elderly to muscle relaxants.[46] The pharmacokinetics of such agents are characterized by decreased elimination. The initial administration of such drugs may not have to be reduced,[47] but the total dose administered should be generally reduced.[48] However, because of decreased elimination, their effect should be carefully monitored using a component of neuromuscular function such as the train-of-four tests.

Transport Proteins

Intravenous anesthetic induction agents are transported through the body bound to plasma proteins. Any agent attached to such proteins is not capable of crossing biologic membranes to produce the desired drug effect. Conversely, the segment that remains free in plasma is able to cross these lipid membranes, including the blood–brain barrier, and in the case of induction agents produces the preferred effect.

Albumin

This is the primary transport carrier[49] and is responsible for transporting most of the acidic drugs in the plasma. Its synthesis represents a major component of the proteins produced by the liver. Increasing age is associated with a slight decrease in the concentration of albumin[50] by 0.54 g/L per decade. The decrease amounts to a total reduction in plasma albumin concentration of around 10% in older people.[51] This reduction in albumin plasma level has been shown to reduce the unbound fraction of certain drugs.[52] On average, the unbound fraction of drugs increases by approximately 10%, paralleling the age-related decrease in albumin.[18,53] Theoretically, the net effect is that anesthetic drugs that bind to albumin, such as thiopental, should have their dose decreased. However, overall age-related effects on protein binding do not produce clinical differences.[54] Because of the polypharmacy often seen in the geriatric patient, concomitant diseases, and the reduced circulating albumin level, there may be a greater opportunity for displacement reactions between drugs.

Renal failure has been associated with decreased levels of circulating albumin.[55] As a result, the pharmacokinetics of anesthetic agents can be altered.[56,57] However, those patients with global hypoproteinemia, not just decreased albumin, will have decreased binding of both acidic and basic drugs.[58]

Alpha₁ Acid Glycoprotein

Alpha$_1$ Acid Glycoprotein

Whereas acidic drugs are primarily bound to albumin, basic drugs tend to be bound to alpha$_1$ acid glycoprotein. Data suggest that this transport protein is either not affected by aging[59] or even slightly increased,[54] probably reflecting the age-associated increases in inflammatory disease.[11] The binding and consequent dosage of basic anesthetic drugs, such as lidocaine, is therefore unaffected by aging.

Changes in Total Body Water

Changes in Total Body Water

A 20%–30% reduction in blood volume occurs by age 75 with total body water (TBW), plasma volume and intracellular water content all decreasing.[60] Consequently, intravenous administration of an anesthetic drug will be distributed in a reduced blood volume producing a higher than expected initial plasma drug concentration. Such changes can have very important implications on the action of anesthetic agents.[61] For example, a patient who is relatively dehydrated and is given a bolus of an induction agent, will distribute this drug into a reduced circu-

lating volume. Anesthetic and hemodynamic effects of the drug will be exaggerated. This resultant exaggerated pharmacologic effect could give the impression of an augmented sensitivity to the agent. Such changes in the distribution and half-life of a particular anesthetic agent will depend on its relative lipid and water solubility as well as the degree of protein binding.

In summary, changes in body composition in the elderly are characterized by:

- A decrease in protein content, mostly in the form of muscle loss, but also in carrier proteins
- Adipose tissue comprising an increased proportion of body mass
- A decrease in TBW, with this reduction manifest mostly in the intracellular component but somewhat in the extracellular compartment also

Hepatic Function in the Elderly

The effects of maturation on drug clearance by the liver have been examined extensively[62,63] and the contentious question of whether or not liver function is compromised in the aged has still not been clearly determined. As is the general pattern with most aging organs, the decline in function is gradual and minimal. Senescence is only experienced when the normal homeostatic mechanisms fail. Decline in biochemical functions are slow and negligible and are reflected in assays of liver function such as total bilirubin and liver enzymes.[64]

Morphologic Changes

Gross Changes

The aging liver develops a classic gross anatomic appearance termed "brown atrophy."[65,66] This discoloration is attributed to hepatocyte accumulation of the pigment lipofuscin, but it is not clear whether these morphologic changes are associated with alteration in function.[67,68]

Hepatic blood flow decreases with increasing age.[69–71] Most of this reduction is associated with a 35% decrease in liver mass.[72–76] The reduction in hepatic blood flow is probably slightly greater than can be explained by the decrease in liver mass,[51] resulting in a 10% decrease in blood flow per unit mass of liver.[51] However, the large size of the aging liver provides a large measure of functional reserve therefore conserving its function relatively well.[51,54,55]

Microscopic Changes

Age-related subcellular changes in the liver are slight.[26,77] Hepatocyte volume increases, probably as a function of intracellular swelling.[78] There are some characteristic age-related organelle changes. For example, it has been shown that the number and the density of the mitochondria decrease with increasing age.[79,80] In addition, there is a decline in the amount of both rough and smooth endoplasmic reticulum.[81] The reduction in the amount of rough endoplasmic reticulum may be a reflection of a reduced ability to synthesize proteins. However, the decrease in the quantity of smooth endoplasmic reticulum may correlate with the decline in the yield of microsomal protein.[82]

Physiologic Changes

Drug Metabolism

Although there is variability in published reports concerning hepatic clearance,[83] it is clear that the hepatic metabolism of anesthetic agents is affected by the reduced hepatic blood flow. This is probably a reflection of the confounding variables already discussed in this chapter, such as differences in functional reserve, the effects of comorbid conditions, polypharmacy, and numerous environmental factors.

Minimal changes have been noted in the mixed function oxidase activity. However, the total capability of the liver to metabolize many drugs by these enzymes may be reduced[84,85] with aging. This decline is erratic and unpredictable,[84,86,87] varying from drug to drug and from individual to individual.

The liver converts lipid-soluble drugs into inactive and water-soluble metabolites by a number of processes that can be divided into two distinct phases, both of which are not radically altered[88,89] in the elderly patient:

- **Phase 1** renders functionally reactive chemical locations inactive. These reactions consist of oxidation, reduction, and hydrolysis, which seem to be the most changed with aging. Although the levels of drug-metabolizing enzymes in the cytochrome P-450 systems do not decline significantly with age, overall hepatic metabolism of some drugs by these enzymes is diminished. Such changes in phase I reactions, however, are probably less significant than the effects of alcohol, tobacco,[90] and environmental factors on liver function.[91–93]
- **Phase 2** reactions involve the addition of a polar group, rendering the altered molecule more water-soluble. These reactions include glucuronidation, methylation, sulfation, and acylation.

Compounds with a suitable reactive site may skip Phase 1 conversion and pass straight into Phase 2. This is the case with acetaminophen[94] which contains a hydroxyl group and is, for the most part, directly glucuronidated and sulfated.

The decrease in liver mass may have a role in the decline[66] in hepatic drug metabolism. As described before, total hepatic blood flow is reduced in elderly subjects and this may affect drug clearance.[63,64] Also, the reduction in hepatic first-pass metabolism of highly extracted drugs in the elderly (extraction ratio >0.8 such as morphine[11]) results in increased plasma drug concentrations and a propensity to dose-dependent adverse effects.

Laboratory Tests

Routine clinical tests of liver function do not change significantly with age. The aminotransferases and the serum bilirubin levels remain normal in the elderly. It has been postulated that a correlation exists between age-associated impairment of cell metabolism and specific changes in mitochondrial function and structure.

In summary, hepatic metabolic function in the elderly is characterized by:

- Decrease in hepatic blood flow
- Decrease in liver size by 35%
- No clinically significant change in routine tests of function
- Phase I and II metabolism not significantly impaired

Renal Function

In both human and animal models, the aging process results in structural and functional renal changes[95–98] that diminish functional reserve. This creates homeostatic limitations on the kidney's capability to respond properly to either volume excess or deficit.

Renal Blood Flow

This function progressively decreases by about 10% per decade after the age of 50.[99] The elderly often have associated medical conditions such as hypertension, vascular disease, diabetes, and heart disease that may exacerbate the effects of these renal abnormalities. Such reductions in flow, paired with a reduced response to vasodilatory stimuli,[100–103] render the elderly kidney particularly susceptible to the harmful effects of reduced cardiac output, hypotension, hypovolemia, and hemorrhage. Anesthetic and surgical stress, pain, sympathetic stimulation, and renal vasoconstrictive drugs may contribute to perioperative renal dysfunction.

Renal Mass

The decrease in blood flow as in the case of the liver is accompanied by a reduction in renal parenchyma.[104,105] Primarily there is a loss of about 20%–25% of the renal cortical mass between the age of 30 and 80 years. At the light microscopic level, the aging human kidney is characterized by increased fibrosis, tubular atrophy, and arteriosclerosis.[106,107] The presence of small vessel pathology in older people without apparent renal disease or hypertension, suggests that even in healthy elderly individuals, renal changes may be secondary to vascular disease and altered vascular responsiveness.

Changes in Glomerular Filtration Rate

A microscopic assessment confirms the loss of the kidney's functional units with increasing age.[108,109] As many as half of the glomeruli present in a young adult may be gone or rendered nonfunctional by 80 years of age. Although the number of glomeruli is decreased, the remaining ones are relatively large in size. The reductions in cortical mass are accompanied by progressive sclerosis of the kidney's functional units and by the eighth decade 10%–30% of the remaining nephrons are sclerotic. The net result of these changes is that there is a gradual decline in the surface area available for filtration and a steady reduction of the glomerular filtration rate (GFR). Age-related decline in GFR is often considered the most important pharmacokinetic change in old age. GFR, normally about 125 mL/min in a young adult, decreases to approximately 80 mL/min at 60 years of age, and to about 60 mL/min at 80 years.

Because GFR decreases less than renal plasma flow, the filtration fraction increases to a state of hyperfiltration. This compensates to a certain extent for the decreased number of functional glomeruli. As a result, the pressure within the glomerulus increases, possibly accelerating glomerulosclerosis.

Creatinine Clearance

Because of the decrease in muscle mass with aging, the decrease in GFR does not result in an increase in serum creatinine. However, creatinine clearance can be used for the approximation of GFR.[110] Although the structural and functional changes seem to have minimal consequences under normal circumstances, they attain clinical significance when the remaining renal function is challenged by the imposition of acute physiologic stress. When GFR decreases below 80 mL/min, dose adjustments should be made to renally excreted drugs. Dosing periods for medications that are renally excreted, such as aminoglycoside antibiotics and pancuronium need to be adjusted, and where indicated, drug levels closely watched. Logic dictates that nephrotoxic drugs should be avoided. Creatinine clearance decreases by approximately 1 mL/min/year after the age of 40 years. Renal changes with aging also result in very tangible problems in the perioperative period. Drugs that depend on renal function for

clearance may accumulate in the elderly, an effect that may be exaggerated by preexisting renal disease. In addition, the elderly are prone to fluid and electrolyte abnormalities and drug-induced renal failure.[108]

Tubular Function

Fluid and electrolyte status should be carefully monitored in the elderly patient during the perioperative period. In the absence of disease, and under normal "non-stress" conditions, the concentrations of electrolytes in the extracellular fluid are within the normal range. In the face of physiologic stress, however, the aging kidney has difficulty maintaining electrolyte balance and circulating volume,[111] because both sodium conservation and excretion become more limited with age.

Under normal conditions, age has no effect on the ability of the individual to maintain extracellular fluid volume. However, the adaptive systems responsible for controlling fluid balance are impaired in the elderly and the aging kidney has a decreased ability to dilute and concentrate urine. Studies show that tubular function is generally decreased in the elderly,[108,112] limiting the degree to which urine can be concentrated in response to water deprivation. Similarly, the rate at which a salt load can be excreted becomes more impaired with age. Additionally, the elderly cannot maximally suppress antidiuretic hormone secretion when serum osmolarity is reduced. These observations, together with decreased efficiency of the renin-angiotensin system, means that elderly patients' failure to retain sodium effectively under conditions of plasma volume contraction is not solely attributable to reductions in the GFR.

Concentration capacity is an additional sensitive indicator of renal function. When fluid is restricted, the aged patient shows a reduced capability to concentrate the urine. The activity of the renin-angiotensin system declines with age,[113] and above 40 years of age there is a decline in both plasma renin aldosterone activity, and the kidney is less efficient at retaining salt with restricted intake.

Sick patients, especially very elderly ill individuals, have a tendency to inadequately regulate their intake of nutrients and water,[114] and have impaired release of antidiuretic hormone.[106] Therefore, in the perioperative period, inadequate electrolyte (via food) and water ingestion may result in dehydration plus net sodium loss from obligatory sodium excretion. It has been reported that 11% of acutely ill, aged patients have hyponatremia. This figure increases to 22% in those patients in chronic care institutions.[115] Often, the characteristics of their fluid administration are poorly documented and this contributes to the less-than-adequate management.[116]

Low sodium plasma levels may lead to disturbed cardiac electrophysiologic function.[117] In addition, the age-related reduction in muscle mass decreases total body potassium content. However, serum electrolytes are generally maintained within the same range as is found in younger adults,[54,118] until situations of surgical stress abnormalities develop. The relationship between abnormal preoperative potassium levels and arrhythmias is unclear.[119] Yet, if the surgery is significant, it may be worthwhile to replenish very low levels.[103]

The aging kidney is able to maintain acid-base homeostasis when functioning under baseline conditions.[120] However, the impaired tubular ability of the elderly kidney to excrete an acid load as compared with that of the younger patient contributes to the higher incidence of metabolic acidosis in the elderly.[121]

Among elderly surgical patients, acute renal failure is responsible for up to one-fifth of all perioperative deaths.[122] Following thoracic surgery, perioperative renal failure may be as much as 30%[123] with an associated mortality of 20%–90%.[124,125] Fifty percent of all patients requiring acute dialysis do so because of perioperative renal failure. The cause of renal failure leading to dialysis is not clearly understood. However, most cases are attributable to acute tubular necrosis.

In summary, renal metabolic function in the elderly is characterized by:

- Decreases in renal blood flow
- Decreases in kidney size
- Morphologic changes include a decrease in the number of glomeruli, compensatory increase in the size of the remaining nephrons, and significant glomerulosclerosis
- No clinically significant changes in routine laboratory tests, but decreases in creatinine clearance, maximum sodium concentrating ability, and free water excretion
- Decreases in tubular function, including impaired ability to handle an acid load, as well as impaired renin-angiotensin and antidiuretic hormone systems
- Decreased thirst response

Implications for Anesthesiology Practice

In light of the previous discussion, it is clear that aging results in important changes in drug pharmacokinetics, including anesthetic medications.[126,127] These changes are summarized in Table 7-1.

In What Way Does This Affect Our Practice?

Age-related alterations in the pharmacokinetics of administered anesthetic agents give rise to changes in the magnitude of effect of anesthetic agents. Reduced lean body mass and TBW, and increased percentage of body fat alter the volume of distribution of anesthetic agents. Altered renal and liver function reduces drug clearance from the body. Such changes account for differences between younger adult patients and their older contemporaries. This has been demonstrated in studies that have been performed in the adult population with ages that range from 20 to 80 years of age.[14,19] This phenomenon affects drugs not usually thought of when considering age-related decreases in metabolism. For example, it has been shown that the rate of propofol elimination declines with age above 60 years of age.[128]

However, much of the information concerning the pharmacology of anesthetic or any other agent in the elderly is lacking because the aged are often methodically excluded from drug trials.[129] Because many drugs are tested and formulated for younger adults, consideration must be given to the changes described above when determining proper dosages for their use in the geriatric population. Conclusions are often drawn from inference. Although some models of practice have been accepted, there remain some contentious issues with regard to aging effects. Failure to recognize such reductions in both metabolism and excretion will result in adverse drug effects.[130]

TABLE 7-1. Physiologic changes in the elderly and their effect on pharmacokinetics.

Pharmacologic factor	Change with aging	Importance
Absorption	↑ Gastric pH	
	↓ Gastric emptying	↓ Absorption
	↓ Absorptive surface	
	↓ Splanchnic blood flow	
Distribution	↑ Body fat	↑ VD_L, lipophilic drugs
	↑ α_1 glycoprotein	↓ Free fraction of basic drugs
	↓ Albumin	↑ Free fraction of acidic drugs
	↓ Body water	↑ Concentration of polar drugs
Metabolism	↓ Hepatic metabolism	↓ Biotransformation
Elimination	↓ Glomerular filtration rate	↓ Elimination fluid, pH, and electrolyte disturbance
	↓ Renal tubular function	

Adverse Drug Reactions and Aging

Not surprisingly, the older patient is at risk of adverse drug reactions from chronic medications. Pharmacokinetic changes, polypharmacy, and drug interactions summate to make adverse drug interactions more likely.[131,132] Drug elimination is decreased in the aged, leading to higher blood concentrations and hence a higher possibility of a type A adverse reaction (exaggerated or excessive but otherwise normal pharmacologic action of a drug).[133,134] In fact, there is an almost linear increase of adverse drug reactions with age.[135] Geriatric patients are up to three times more likely to experience adverse drug reactions.[136] In addition, the risk of adverse drug reactions increases with the number of medications given. Thus, the addition of several drugs, even short-acting ones, in the perioperative period makes adverse reactions more likely.[137] This situation is further complicated by the fact that advanced age is accompanied by comorbidity and the consequent polypharmacy for treatment of these disease states.[138,139] If we, as perioperative physicians of the elderly, are going to use these drugs in a rational and safe manner, it is incumbent upon us to acquire an understanding of how such age-dependent change occurs. An example of how this information may be useful is seen with hypertension. This disease is highly prevalent in the elderly and often requires multiple medications for its management. Concomitant medications, such as β-adrenergic blocking drugs and diuretics might further impair reflex heart rate and cardiac output increases. The use of a volatile anesthetic in these patients may give rise to exaggerated decreases in blood pressure, especially if the patient is hypovolemic.

Summary

The perioperative care of the elderly patient is challenging. Aging progressively diminishes functional reserve, and therefore diminishes the patient's ability to handle stress. As illustrated in this chapter, a global understanding of the metabolic alterations that take place with aging helps us to better manage and respond to pharmacokinetic and pharmacodynamic reactions within this patient population. Such knowledge will aid us in providing an optimal anesthetic for each elderly patient. Part of our role as perioperative physicians may well include the detection and possible correction of metabolic abnormalities. We, as anesthesiologists, should act as "homeostasis in absentia." This may help to preserve existing function, and avoid adverse outcomes.

References

1. Travis KW, Mihevc NT, Orkin FK, Zeitlin GL. Age and anesthetic practice: a regional perspective. J Clin Anesthesiol 1999;11:175–186.
2. Gibson JR, Mendenhall MK, Axel NJ. Geriatric anesthesia: minimizing the risk. Clin Geriatr Med 1985;1:313–321.
3. Medawar P. An unsolved problem of biology. An inaugural lecture delivered at University College London, 6 December 1951. London: H.K. Lewis; 1952.
4. Sehl ME, Yates FE. Kinetics of human aging: I. Rates of senescence between ages 30 and 70 years in healthy people. J Gerontol A Biol Sci Med Sci 2001;56:198–208.
5. Clergue F, Auroy Y, Pequignot F, Jougla E, Lienhart A, Lexenaire MC. French survey of anesthesia in 1996. Anesthesiology 1999;91:1509–1520.
6. US Census Bureau: population projections program. Population Division. Projections of the total resident population by 5-year age groups, and sex with special age categories: middle series, 2025 to 2045. Washington, DC; 2000.
7. http://factfinder.census.gov/jsp/saff/SAFFInfo.jsp?_pageId=tp2_aging. Accessed August 15, 2007.
8. Sloan RW. Principles of drug therapy in geriatric patients. Am Fam Physician 1992;45:2709–2718.
9. Ergina P, Gold S, Meakins J. Perioperative care of the elderly patient. World J Surg 1993;17:192–198.
10. Klopfenstein CE, Herrmann FR, Michel JP, et al. The influence of an aging surgical population on the anesthesia workload: a ten-year survey. Anesth Analg 1998;86:1165–1170.
11. Hosking MP, Warner MA, Lobdell CM, et al. Outcomes of surgery in patients 90 years of age and older. JAMA 1989;261:1909–1915.
12. Ackerman RJ, Vogel RL, Johnson LA, et al. Surgery in nonagenarians: morbidity, mortality and functional outcomes. J Fam Pract 1996;40:129–135.
13. Warner MA, Saletel DR, Schroeder DR, Warner DO, Offord KP, Gray DT. Outcomes of anesthesia and surgery in people 100 years of age and older. J Am Geriatr Soc 1998;46:988–993.
14. Graves EJ, Gillum BS. Advance Data from Vital and Health Statistics [1994 Summary: National Hospital Discharge Survey]. Atlanta: Centers for Disease Control and Prevention; 1996:278.
15. Seymour DG, Vaz FG. A prospective study of elderly general surgical patients. Post-operative complications. Age Aging 1989;18:316–326.
16. Linn BS, Linn MW, Wallen N. Evaluation of results of surgical procedures in the elderly. Ann Surg 1982;195:90.
17. Pofahl WE, Pories WJ. Current status and future directions of geriatric general surgery. J Am Geriatr Soc 2003;51:S351–S354.
18. Palmberg S, Hirsjarvi E. Mortality in geriatric surgery. With special reference to the type of surgery, anaesthesia, complicating diseases, and prophylaxis of thrombosis. Gerontology 1979;25:103–112.
19. Silverstein JH, Bloom HG, Cassel CK. Geriatrics and anesthesia. Anesthesiol Clin North Am 1999;17:453–465.
20. Roberts SB, Fuss P, Heyman MB, Young VR. Influence of age on energy requirements. Am J Clin Nutr 1995;62:1053S–1058S.
21. Fukagawa NK, Bandini LG, Young JB. Effect of age on body composition and resting metabolic rate. Am J Physiol 1990;259:E233–E238.

22. Henry CJK. Mechanisms of changes in basal metabolism during ageing. Eur J Clin Nutr 2000;54:77–91.
23. Muravchick S. The aging process: anesthetic implications. Acta Anaesthesiol Belg 1998;49:85–90.
24. Schwartz RS, Jaeger LF, Veith RC. The importance of body composition to the increase in plasma norepinephrine appearance rate in elderly men. J Gerontol 1987;42:546–551.
25. Daniëlle AJ, Kerckhoffs M, Blaak EE, Van Baak MA, Saris WHM. Effect of aging on β-adrenergically mediated thermogenesis in men. Am J Physiol Endocrinol Metab 1998;274:E1075–E1079.
26. Zeeh J, Platt D. The aging liver: structural and functional changes and their consequences for drug treatment in old age. Gerontology 2002;48:121–127.
27. Busby-Whitehead J. The epidemic in your waiting room. Geriatrics 2004;59:6–7.
28. Straus SE. Geriatric medicine. Clinical review. BMJ 2001;322:86–89.
29. Vaughan MS, Vaughan RW, Cork RC. Postoperative hypothermia in adults: relationship of age, anesthesia, and shivering to rewarming. Anest Analg 1981;60:746–751.
30. Frank SM, Fleisher LA, Olson KF, et al. Multivariate determinants of early postoperative oxygen consumption in elderly patients. Effects of shivering, body temperature, and gender. Anesthesiology 1995;83:241–249.
31. El-Gamal N, El-Kassabany N, Frank SM, et al. Age-related thermoregulatory differences in a warm operating room environment (approximately 26 degrees C). Anesth Analg 2000;90:694–698.
32. Sessler DI, Kurz A, Lenhardt R. Re: Hypothermia reduces resistance to surgical wound infections. Am Surg 1999;65:1193–1196.
33. Frank SM, Beattie C, Christopherson R, et al. Unintentional hypothermia is associated with postoperative myocardial ischemia. The Perioperative Ischemia Randomized Anesthesia Trial Study Group. Anesthesiology 1993;78:468–476.
34. Leslie K, Sessler DI. The implications of hypothermia for early tracheal extubation following cardiac surgery. J Cardiothorac Vasc Anesth 1998;12:30–34.
35. Beaufrere B, Morio B. Fat and protein redistribution with aging: metabolic considerations. Eur J Clin Nutr 2000;54:S48–S53.
36. Forbes GB, Reina JC. Adult lean body mass declines with age: some longitudinal observations. Metabolism 1970;19:653–663.
37. Muravchick S. Current concepts: anesthetic pharmacology in the geriatric patient. Prog Anesthesiol 1987;1:2.
38. Greenblatt DJ, Abernethy DR, Locniskar A, Harmatz JS, Limjuco RA, Shader RI. Effect of age, gender, and obesity on midazolam kinetics. Anesthesiology 1984;61:27–35.
39. Saraiva RA, Lunn JN, Mapleson WW, Willis BA, France JM. Adiposity and the pharmacokinetics of halothane. The effect of adiposity on the maintenance of and recovery from halothane anaesthesia. Anaesthesia 1977;32:240–246.
40. Pierson RN Jr. Body composition in aging: a biological perspective. Curr Opin Clin Nutr Metab Care 2003;6:15–20.
41. Doherty TJ. Invited review: aging and sarcopenia. J Appl Physiol 2003;95:1717–1727.
42. Roubenoff R. Sarcopenia and its implications for the elderly. Eur J Clin Nutr 2000;54:S40–S47.
43. Rosenberg IH. Summary comments. Am J Clin Nutr 1989;50:1231–1233.
44. Deschenes MR. Effects of aging on muscle fibre type and size. Sports Med 2004;34:809–824.
45. Short KR, Vittone JL, Bigelow ML, Proctor DN, Nair KS. Age and aerobic exercise training effects on whole body and muscle protein metabolism. Am J Physiol Endocrinol Metab 2004;286:E92–101.
46. Ornstein E, Matteo RS, Schwartz AE, Jamdar SC, Diaz J. Pharmacokinetics and pharmacodynamics of pipecuronium bromide (Arduan) in elderly surgical patients. Anesth Analg 1992;74:841–844.
47. Lauven PM, Nadstawek J, Albrecht S. The safe use of anaesthetics and muscle relaxants in older surgical patients. Drugs Aging 1993;3:502–509.
48. Rupp SM, Castagnoli KP, Fisher DM, Miller RD. Pancuronium and vecuronium pharmacokinetics and pharmacodynamics in younger and elderly adults. Anesthesiology 1987;67:45–49.
49. Koch-Weser J, Sellers EM. Binding of drugs to serum albumin. N Engl J Med 1976;294:311–316.
50. Greenblatt DJ, Sellers EM, Shader RI. Drug therapy: drug disposition in old age. N Engl J Med 1982;306:1081–1088.
51. Campion EW, deLabry LO, Glynn RJ. The effect of age on serum albumin in healthy males: report from the Normative Aging Study. J Gerontol 1988;43:M18–20.
52. Greenblatt DJ. Reduced serum albumin concentration in the elderly: a report from the Boston Collaborative Drug Surveillance Program. J Am Geriatr Soc 1979;27:20–22.
53. Boudinot SG, Funderburg ED, Boudinot FD. Effects of age on the pharmacokinetics of piroxicam in rats. J Pharm Sci 1993;82:254–257.
54. Grandison MK, Boudinot FD. Age-related changes in protein binding of drugs: implications for therapy. Clin Pharmacokinet 2000;38:271–290.
55. Bernus I, Dickinson RG, Hooper WD, Eadie MJ. Anticonvulsant therapy in aged patients. Clinical pharmacokinetic considerations. Drugs Aging 1997;10:278–289.
56. Grossman SB, Yap SH, Shafritz DA. Influence of chronic renal failure on protein synthesis and albumin metabolism in rat liver. J Clin Invest 1977;59:869–887.
57. Christensen JH, Andreasen F, Jansen J. Pharmacokinetics and pharmacodynamics of thiopental in patients undergoing renal transplantation. Acta Anaesthesiol Scand 1983;27:513–518.
58. Riant P, Barre J, Albengres E, Lemaire M, Tillement JP. Plasma binding of drugs in chronic renal failure. Nephrologie 1986;7:89–93.
59. Veering BT, Burm AG, Souverijn JH, Serree JM, Spierdijk J. The effect of age on serum concentrations of albumin and alpha 1-acid glycoprotein. Br J Clin Pharmacol 1990;29:201–206.
60. Lamy PP. Comparative pharmacokinetic changes and drug therapy in an older population. J Am Geriatr Soc 1982;30:S11–S19.

61. Matteo RS, Ornstein E, Schwartz AE, Ostapkovich N, Stone JG. Pharmacokinetics and pharmacodynamics of rocuronium (Org 9426) in elderly surgical patients. Anesth Analg 1993;77:1193–1197.
62. LeCouteur DG, McLean AJ. The aging liver: drug clearance and an oxygen diffusion barrier hypothesis. Clin Pharmacokinet 1998;34:359–373.
63. Schmucker DL. Liver function and phase I drug metabolism in the elderly: a paradox. Drugs Aging 2001;18: 837–851.
64. Tietz NW, Shuey DF, Wekstein DR. Laboratory values in fit aging individuals—sexagenarians through centenarians. Clin Chem 1992;38:1167–1185.
65. Zeeh J, Platt D. Age related changes in the liver. Consequences for drug therapy. Fortschr Med 1990;108:651–653.
66. Wynne HA, James OFW. The aging liver. Age Ageing 1990;19:1–3.
67. Ettore GM, Sommacale D, Farges O, et al. Postoperative liver function after elective right hepatectomy in elderly patients. Br J Surg 2001;88:73–76.
68. Marchesini G, Bua V, Brunori A, et al. Galactose elimination capacity and liver volume in aging man. Hepatology 1988;8:1079–1083.
69. Schmucker DL. Aging and the liver: an update. J Gerontol Biol Sci 1998;53A:B315–320.
70. Vestal RE. Drug use in the elderly. A review of problems and special consideration. Drugs 1978;16:358–382.
71. Muravchick S. The aging patient and age related disease. ASA Annual Refresher Course Lecture #151. Park Ridge, IL: American Society of Anesthesiologists; 1987.
72. Vestal RE. Aging and determinants of hepatic drug clearance. Hepatology 1989;9:331–334.
73. Vestal RE. Pharmacology and aging. J Am Geriatr Soc 1982;30:191–200.
74. Woodhouse KW, James OFW. Hepatic drug metabolism and aging. Br Med Bull 1980;46:22–35.
75. Wynne HA, Cope E, Mutch E, Rawlins MD, Woodhouse KW, James OF. The effects of age upon liver volume and apparent liver blood flow in healthy man. Hepatology 1989;9:297–301.
76. Zoli M, Magalotti D, Bianchi G, et al. Total and functional hepatic blood flow decrease in parallel with aging. Age Aging 1999;28:29–33.
77. Seaman DS. Adult living donor transplantation: current status. J Clin Gastroenterol 2001;33:97–106.
78. LeCouteur DG, McLean AJ. The aging liver. Drug clearance and an oxygen diffusion barrier hypothesis. Clin Pharmacokinet 1998;34:359–373.
79. Pieri C, Zs-Nagy I, Mazzufferi G, Giuli C. The aging of rat liver as revealed by electron microscopic morphometry. I. Basic parameters. Exp Gerontol 1975;10:291–304.
80. Sastre J, Pallardo FV, Pla R, et al. Aging of the liver: age-associated mitochondrial damage in intact hepatocytes. Hepatology 1996;24:1199–1205.
81. Schmucker DL, Wang RK. Age related changes in the hepatic endoplasmic reticulum: a quantitative analysis. Science 1977;197:1005–1008.
82. Wynne H, Mutch E, James OF, Rawlins MD, Woodhouse KW. The effect of age on mono-oxygenase enzyme kinetics in rat liver microsomes. Age Ageing 1987;16:153–158.
83. Sheweita SA. Drug-metabolizing enzymes: mechanisms and functions. Curr Drug Metab 2000;1:107–132.
84. Kato R, Vassanelli P, Frontino G. Variation in the activity of liver microsomal drug metabolizing enzymes in rats in relation to age. Biochem Pharmacol 1964;12:1037–1051.
85. Sutter MA, Wood WG, Williamson LS, Strong R, Pickham K, Richardson A. Comparison of the hepatic mixed function oxidase system of young, adult, and old non-human primates (Macaca nemestrina). Biochem Pharmacol 1985;34:2983–2987.
86. Williams RT. Comparative patterns of drug metabolism. Fed Proc 1967;26:1029–1039.
87. Crooks J, O'Malley K, Stevenson LH. Pharmacokinetics in the elderly. Clin Pharmacokinet 1976;1:280–296.
88. Seifalian AM, Stansby GP, Hobbs KE, Hawkes DJ, Colchester AC. Measurement of liver blood flow: a review. HPB Surg 1991;4:171–186.
89. Hunt CM, Westerkam WR, Stave GM. Effects of age and gender on the activity of human hepatic CYP3A. Biochem Pharmacol 1992;44:275–283.
90. Vestal RE, Wood AJ. Influence of age and smoking on drug kinetics in man. Clin Pharmacokinet 1980;5:309–318.
91. Sellers EM, Frecker RC, Romach MK. Drug metabolism in the elderly: confounding of age, smoking and ethanol effects. Drug Metab Rev 1983;14:225–250.
92. Kinirons MT, O'Mahony MS. Drug metabolism and ageing. Br J Clin Pharmacol 2004;57:540–544.
93. Herd B, Wynne H, Wright P, James O, Woodhouse K. The effect of age on glucuronidation and sulphation of paracetamol by human liver fractions. Br J Clin Pharmacol 1991;32:768–770.
94. Bessems JG, Vermeulen NP. Paracetamol (acetaminophen)-induced toxicity: molecular and biochemical mechanisms, analogues and protective approaches. Crit Rev Toxicol 2001;31:55–138.
95. Anderson S, Brenner BM. Effects of aging on the renal glomerulus. Am J Med 1986;80:435–442.
96. Kaysen GA, Myers BD. The aging kidney. Clin Geriatr Med 1985;1:207–222.
97. Goldstein RS, Tarloff JB, Hook JB. Age related nephropathy in laboratory rats. FASEB J 1988;2:2241–2251.
98. Tauchi H, Tsuboi K, Okutomi J. Age changes in the human kidney of different races. Gerontologica 1971;17:87–97.
99. Epstein M. Aging and the kidney. J Am Soc Nephrol 1996;7:1106–1122.
100. Nyengaard JR, Bendtsen TF. Glomerular number and size in relation to age, kidney weight and body surface in normal man. Anat Rec 1992;232:194–201.
101. Baylis C, Fredericks M, Wilson C, Munger K, Colins R. Renal vasodilatory response to intravenous glycine in the aging rat kidney. Am J Kidney Dis 1990;15:244–251.
102. Fuiano G, Sund S, Mazza G, et al. Renal hemodynamic response to maximal vasodilating stimulus in healthy older subjects. Kidney Int 2001;59:1052–1058.
103. Fliser D, Ritz E. Renal hemodynamics in the elderly. Nephrol Dial Transplant 1996;11(Suppl 9):2–8.
104. Beck LH. Changes in renal function with aging. Clin Geriatr Med 1998;14:199–209.

105. Neugarten J, Gallo G, Silbiger S, Kasiske B. Glomerulo-sclerosis in aging humans is not influenced by gender. Am J Kidney Dis 1999;34:884–888.

106. Goyal VK. Changes with age in the human kidney. Exp Gerontol 1982;17:321–331.

107. Corman B, Barrault MB, Klinger C, et al. Renin gene expression in the aging kidney: effect of sodium restriction. Mech Ageing Dev 1995;84:1–13.

108. Muhlberg W, Platt D. Age-dependent changes of the kidneys: pharmacological implications. Gerontology 1999; 45:243–253.

109. Kaplan C, Pasternack B, Shah H, Gallo G. Age-related incidence of sclerotic glomeruli in human kidneys. Am J Pathol 1975;80:227–234.

110. Miller M. Fluid and electrolyte balance in the elderly. Geriatrics 1987;42:65–76.

111. Sunderam SG, Mankikar GD. Hyponatremia in the elderly. Age Ageing 1983;12:77–80.

112. Dontas AS, Marketos S, Papanayiotou P. Mechanisms of renal tubular defects in old age. Postgrad Med J 1972; 48:295–303.

113. Phillips PA, Hodsman GP, Johnson CI. Neuroendo-crine mechanisms and cardiovascular homeostasis in the elderly. Cardiovasc Drugs Ther 1991;4(Suppl 6):1209–1213.

114. Kleinfeld M, Casmir M, Borra S. Hyponatremia as observed in a chronic disease facility. J Am Geriatric Soc 1979;29: 156–161.

115. O'Neill PA, Faragher DS, Davies I, Wears R, McLean KA, Fairweather DS. Reduced survival with increased plasma osmolality in elderly continued care patients. Age Ageing 1990;19:68–71.

116. National confidential enquiry into patient outcome and death (1999). Available at: http://www.ncepod.org.uk/pdf/1999/99eld.pdf.

117. Amar D, Hao Z, Leung DHY, Roistacher N, Kadish AH. Older age is the strongest predictor of postoperative atrial fibrillation. Anesthesiology 2002;96:352–356.

118. Morimoto S, Ogihara T. Physiological and pathological aging and electrolyte metabolism. Nippon Ronen Igakkai Zasshi 1991;28:325–330.

119. Wahr JA, Parks R, Boisvert D, Comunale M, Fabian J, Mangano DT. Preoperative serum potassium levels and perioperative outcomes in cardiac surgery patients. Multi-centre study of Perioperative Ischemia Research Group. JAMA 1999;281:2203–2210.

120. Frasseto L, Sebastian A. Age and systemic acid-base equilibrium: analysis of published data. J Gerontol A Biol Sci Med Sci 1996;51:B91–99.

121. Okusawa S, Aikawa N, Abe O. Postoperative metabolic alkalosis following general surgery: its incidence and possible etiology. Jpn J Surg 1989;19:312–318.

122. Aronson S. Renal function monitoring. In: Miller RD, ed. Anesthesia. 4th ed. New York: Churchill Livingstone; 1994:1293–1317.

123. Cowan JA Jr, Dimick JB, Wainess RM, Henke PK, Stanley JC, Upchurch GR Jr. Ruptured thoracoabdominal aortic aneurysm treatment in the United States: 1988 to 1998. J Vasc Surg 2003;38:319–322.

124. Wilkes BM, Mailloux LU. Acute renal failure: pathogenesis and prevention. Am J Med 1986;80:1129–1136.

125. Carmichael P, Carmichael AR. Acute renal failure in the surgical setting. ANZ J Surg 2003;73:144–153.

126. Shafer SL. Pharmacokinetics and pharmacodynamics of the elderly. In: McLesky CH, ed. Geriatric Anesthesiology. Baltimore: Williams & Wilkins; 1997:123–142.

127. Crome P. What's different about older people? Toxicology 2003;192:49–54.

128. Schuttler J, Ihmsen H. Population pharmacokinetics of propofol: a multicenter study. Anesthesiology 2000;92:727–738.

129. Cheitlin MD, Gerstenblith G, Hazzard WR, et al. Database Conference January 27–30, 2000, Washington D.C.: Do existing databases answer clinical questions about geriatric cardiovascular disease and stroke? Am J Geriatr Cardiol 2001;10:207–223.

130. Vancura EJ. Guard against unpredictable drug responses in the aging. Geriatrics 1979;34:63–65, 69–70, 73.

131. Hurwitz N. Predisposing factors in adverse reactions to drugs. Br Med J 1969;1:536–539.

132. Hurwitz N, Wade OL. Intensive hospital monitoring of adverse reactions to drugs. Br Med J 1969;1:531–536.

133. Editorial: medications for the elderly. J R Coll Phys Lond 1984;18:7–17.

134. Schmucker DL. Age related changes in drug disposition. Pharmacol Rev 1979;30:445–456.

135. Paterson C. Iatrogenic disease in late life. Clin Geriatr Med 1986;2:121–136.

136. Woodhouse KW, Mortimer O, Wilhom BE. Hepatic adverse drug reactions. In: Kitani K, ed. The Effects of Age in Liver and Ageing. Amsterdam: Elsevier; 1986:75–80.

137. Williamson J, Chopin JM. Adverse reactions to prescribed drugs in the elderly: a multicenter investigation. Age Ageing 1980;9:73–80.

138. Hughes SG. Prescribing for the elderly patient: why do we need to exercise caution? Br J Clin Pharmacol 1998;46: 531–533.

139. Turnheim K. Drug dosage in the elderly. Is it rational? Drugs Aging 1998;13:357–379.

8
Perioperative Thermoregulation

Daniel I. Sessler

Perioperative thermal disturbances are common and there is considerable evidence that disturbances are especially frequent in the elderly. The most common perioperative thermal disturbance—hypothermia—is both more likely and more severe in the elderly than in younger patients. Anesthetic drugs impair thermoregulation in all patients, and delayed or insufficient thermoregulatory defenses are the primary causes of hypothermia in most patients. Excessive hypothermia in the elderly results largely because central and efferent thermoregulatory controls are particularly disturbed in these patients.

Perioperative hypothermia has long been associated with complications including decreased drug metabolism and postoperative shivering. In recent years, mild hypothermia has been shown to significantly alter patient outcomes by increasing the incidence of myocardial ischemia, augmenting blood loss, decreasing resistance to surgical wound infections, and prolonging hospitalization. There is no reason to believe that the elderly are resistant to complications associated with hypothermia. Instead, they are especially susceptible to many of them because of normal age-related changes in organ function and because many have substantial underlying diseases. In contrast, thermal management in the elderly does not differ importantly from that in younger patients.

Normal Thermoregulation

Core body temperature is among the most jealously guarded physiologic parameters and is justifiably considered one of the "vital signs." The major thermoregulatory defenses are behavior,[1,2] sweating,[3] precapillary vasodilation,[4] arteriovenous shunt vasoconstriction,[5] nonshivering thermogenesis,[6] and shivering.[7] Each can be

characterized by its threshold (triggering core temperature), gain (intensity increase with further core-temperature deviation), and maximum intensity.[8] Temperatures between the first autonomic warm response (sweating) and the first autonomic cold defense (vasoconstriction) define the interthreshold range; these temperatures do not trigger autonomic thermoregulatory defenses.[9]

Precise control of core temperature is maintained by a powerful thermoregulatory system incorporating afferent inputs, central control, and efferent defenses.[10] Efferent defenses can be broadly divided into autonomic responses (i.e., sweating and shivering) and behavioral responses (i.e., closing a window, putting on a sweater). Autonomic responses depend largely on core temperature and are mostly mediated by the anterior hypothalamus. In contrast, behavioral responses are mostly determined by skin temperature and are controlled by the posterior hypothalamus[11] (Figure 8-1).

Afferent Input

Warm afferent signals are conveyed by unmyelinated C-fibers, as is pain. In contrast, cold signals traverse myelinated A-delta fibers, both of which are widely distributed.[12] Most thermal input is conducted along the spinothalamic tracts, although both afferent and efferent thermal signals are diffusely distributed within the neuraxis.[13]

The central thermoregulatory control system accepts thermal input from tissues all over the body. The relative contributions of most tissues have yet to be determined in humans. However, animal studies suggest that the hypothalamus, other portions of the brain, the spinal cord, and deep thoracic and abdominal tissues each contribute very roughly 20%.[8,14–16]

Mean skin temperature contributes 5%-20% as much as core temperature (deep central tissues and brain) to control of sweating and active vasodilation; furthermore, the relation between mean skin and core temperatures at response thresholds is linear.[4,17–20] That is, a 1°C increase

The author does not consult for, accept honoraria from, or own stock or stock options in any company related to products discussed in this chapter.

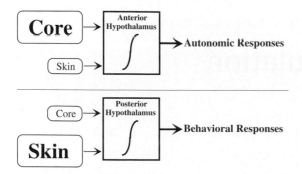

FIGURE 8-1. Control of autonomic and behavioral thermoregulatory defenses. Efferent defenses can be broadly divided into autonomic responses (e.g., sweating and shivering) and behavioral responses (e.g., closing a window, putting on a sweater). Autonomic responses depend largely on core temperature and are mediated largely by the anterior hypothalamus. In contrast, behavioral responses are mostly determined by skin temperature and are controlled by the posterior hypothalamus.

in skin temperature reduces the sweating and active capillary vasodilation thresholds (expressed in terms of core temperature) by 0.05–0.2°C. Arithmetically, this relation takes the form

$$\text{Thres}_{MBT} = \beta T_{skin} + (1 - \beta)T_{core},$$

where Thres_{MBT} is the sweating or vasodilation threshold in terms of physiologic (rather than anatomic) mean body temperature, T_{skin} is mean skin temperature, and T_{core} is core temperature, all in degrees centigrade.

The proportionality constant, β, in this case is 0.05–0.2. The skin surface contributes 20% ± 6% to control of vasoconstriction and 19% ± 8% to control of shivering, and the contribution in linear[16] (Figure 8-2). Regional sensory contributions to thermoregulatory control have not been specifically evaluated in the elderly. However, there is little reason to believe that temperature sensation fails in the elderly or that integration differs markedly.

Central Control

Thermal afferent signals are integrated at numerous levels within the neuraxis, including the spinal cord and brainstem. The dominant controller in mammals, however, is the hypothalamus. (Interestingly, the spinal cord dominates in birds.) Although core temperature varies with a daily circadian rhythm,[21] body temperature is normally controlled to within a few tenths of a degree centigrade almost irrespective of the environment.[22] Such precise control is maintained by a powerful thermoregulatory system incorporating afferent inputs, central control, and efferent defenses.

The thresholds triggering thermoregulatory defenses are uniformly about 0.3°C greater during the follicular

phase in women than in men,[22] and would be an additional ≈10.5°C greater during the luteal phase.[23] However, men and women regulate core body temperature with comparable precision, usually maintaining core temperature within a few tenths of a °C of the target temperature (Figure 8-3).

The major autonomic warm defenses, sweating and active vasodilation, are triggered at about the same temperature and seem to operate synchronously.[24] In contrast, vasoconstriction is the first autonomic response to cold.[22] Only when vasoconstriction is insufficient to maintain core temperature (in a given environment), is nonshivering thermogenesis or shivering initiated. In humans, nonshivering thermogenesis is restricted to infancy, and infants use this defense in preference to shivering.[25] In contrast, nonshivering thermogenesis is of little importance in adult humans,[26–28] although it is the most important cold defense in small animals.

When one efferent response is inadequate to maintain core temperature in a given environment, others are acti-

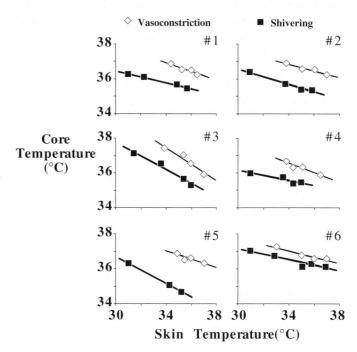

FIGURE 8-2. The relative contribution of mean skin temperature to control of thermoregulatory vasoconstriction and shivering in six men. The threshold (triggering core temperature) for each response is plotted vertically against mean skin temperature. Core and skin temperatures at the vasoconstriction and shivering thresholds were linearly related. The extent to which mean skin temperature contributed to central thermoregulatory control (β) was calculated from the slopes (S) of the skin-temperature versus core-temperature regressions, using the formula: $\beta = S/(S - 1)$. Cutaneous contribution to vasoconstriction averaged 20% ± 6%, which did not differ significantly from the contribution to shivering: 19% ± 8%. (Reprinted with permission from Cheng et al.[16] Copyright © Lippincott Williams & Wilkins.)

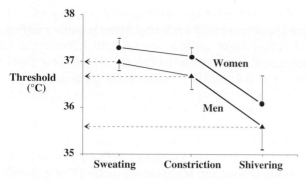

FIGURE 8-3. The thresholds (triggering core temperatures) for the three major autonomic thermoregulatory defenses: sweating, vasoconstriction, and shivering. Temperatures between the sweating and vasoconstriction threshold define the interthreshold range, temperatures *not* triggering autonomic responses. The thresholds are uniformly about 0.3°C greater during the follicular phase in women than in men, and would be an additional ≈0.5°C greater during the luteal phase. However, men and women regulate core body temperature with comparable precision. Results are presented as means ± SD. (Reprinted with permission from Lopez et al.[22] Copyright © Lippincott Williams & Wilkins.)

vated. Similarly, secondary defenses compensate for those working poorly. For example, when arteriovenous shunt vasoconstriction is defeated by administration of a vasodilating drug, core hypothermia will initiate shivering. Because autonomic responses are to some extent compromised in the elderly, behavioral responses are probably more important in this population—although this theory has yet to be formally evaluated.

Efferent Responses

Sweating is mediated by postganglionic, cholinergic nerves that terminate on sweat follicles.[29] These follicles apparently have no purpose other than thermoregulation. In this regard, they differ from most other thermoregulatory effectors which seem to have been co-opted by the thermoregulatory system but continue to have important roles, for example vasomotion in blood pressure control or skeletal muscles in postural maintenance.

Heat exposure can increase cutaneous water loss from trivial amounts to 500 mL/h. Losses in trained athletes can even exceed 1 L/h. In a dry, convective environment, sweating can dissipate enormous amounts of heat—perhaps to 10 times the basal metabolic rate. Sweating is the only thermoregulatory defense that continues to dissipate heat when environmental temperature exceeds core temperature.

Active precapillary vasodilation is mediated by a yet-to-be-identified factor released from sweat glands, and thus occurs synchronously with sweating. Although origi-

nally thought to be bradykinin,[30] recent evidence supports nitric oxide as the mediator.[31,32] Active dilation can increase cutaneous capillary flow enormously, perhaps to as much as 7.5 L/min.[33] The purpose of this dilation, presumably, is to transport heat from muscles and the core to the skin surface where it can be dissipated to the environment by evaporation of sweat.

Active arteriovenous shunt vasoconstriction is adrenergically mediated. The shunts are 100-μm–diameter vessels that convey 10,000 times as much blood as a comparable length of 10-μm capillary.[5] Anatomically, they are restricted to the fingers, toes, nose, and nipples. Despite this restriction, shunt vasoconstriction is among the most frequently used and important thermoregulatory defenses. The reason is that the blood traversing shunts in the extremities must flow through the arms and legs, thus altering heat content of these relatively large tissue masses.

Shivering is an involuntary, thermogenic tonic tremor.[7] Typically, it doubles metabolic rate,[34,35] although greater increases can be sustained briefly. The shivering threshold is normally ≈1°C less than the vasoconstriction threshold, suggesting that it is activated only under critical conditions and is not the preferred means of maintaining core temperature. One reason may be that shivering is a relatively inefficient response. Although shivering effectively transfers metabolic energy sources into heat, the heat is largely produced in the periphery where the largest muscles are located. Loss of the peripherally produced heat to a cold environment is further accentuated by the metabolic needs of shivering muscle and the resulting vasodilation.

Impaired Thermoregulation in the Elderly

There is considerable epidemiologic evidence that the elderly often fail to adequately regulate body temperature. Accidental hypothermia is especially likely in three populations: drug abusers (especially alcoholics), people suffering extreme exposure (such as cold-water immersion), and the elderly.[36] While extreme—and usually prolonged—cold exposure is required to produce clinical hypothermia in young, healthy individuals, serious hypothermia is common among alcohol abusers even with mild exposure.[37] Hypothermia in these patients presumably results from drug-induced inhibition of thermoregulatory defenses. The extent to which alcohol impairs autonomic defenses remains controversial[38–41]; however, alcohol at the very least significantly impairs appropriate behavioral responses to cold exposure.

Hypothermia in the elderly can occur in only moderately cold environments and is typically not associated with drug use.[36,37] This observation suggests that hypo-

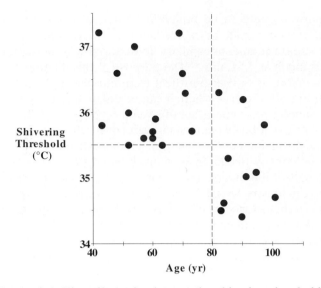

FIGURE 8-4. The effect of aging on the shivering threshold. Fifteen patients aged <80 years (58 ± 10 years) (mean ± SD) shivered at 36.1 ± 0.6°C; in contrast, 10 patients aged ≥80 years (89 ± 7 years) shivered at a significantly lower mean temperature, 35.2 ± 0.8°C (p < 0.001). The shivering thresholds in 7 of the 10 patients aged more than 80 years was <35.5°C, whereas the threshold equaled or exceeded this value in all the younger patients. (Reprinted with permission from Vassilieff et al.[50] Copyright © Lippincott Williams & Wilkins.)

thermia in the elderly may result from age-induced thermoregulatory failure. Supporting this thesis is the work of MacMillan et al.[42] who demonstrated in 1967 that elderly victims of accidental hypothermia responded abnormally to cold challenge. Subsequent study has demonstrated that cold exposure produces more hypothermia in the elderly than in younger subjects.[43,44] Cold tolerance is also poor in elderly rats.[45]

Excessive hypothermia in the elderly presumably results from inadequate activation or efficacy of thermoregulatory defenses. Consistent with this theory, several features of thermoregulatory control in the elderly are known to differ from those in younger subjects. Sweating thresholds remain normal to the age of ≈70 years; however, sweating rate is reduced in the elderly. Age-relative reduction in the sweating rate seems to depend on fitness level[46]—although fitness level may itself depend on overall health. Decreased gain resulted from reduced sweat production per activated gland, rather than recruitment of fewer glands.[47] Sweating is also less effective in children than in adolescents.[48] Other studies, however, failed to identify age-related differences in sweating.[49]

Vasoconstriction in response to cold exposure is reduced,[43] and it is likely that this is a clinically important observation because vasoconstriction is the primary autonomic response to cold exposure. Similarly, the shivering threshold is significantly reduced in the elderly.[50] Interestingly, abnormally reduced thresholds were not apparent in subjects younger than 80 years of age, and even then were apparent in only a fraction of the population (Figure 8-4). These data suggest age-related thermoregulatory impairment may not be common at ages less than 80 years. The data further suggest that impairment is not a linear function of age, but instead occurs unpredictably in a fraction of the elderly population.

Altogether, there are surprisingly few studies evaluating age-related thermoregulatory changes in humans, especially in subjects exceeding 80 years of age. Even fewer are recent and use modern methods of controlling (or compensating) for changes in skin temperature. Most also do not distinguish altered thresholds from reduced gain or maximum response intensity. The ethical and practical difficulties of conducting controlled physiologic evaluations in the elderly are apparent, and these difficulties are magnified in extremely old subjects who are most likely to have impaired responses. Nonetheless, as a large fraction of the United States population enters this age bracket, greater understanding of age-dependent thermoregulatory inhibition is clearly required.

Thermoregulation During Anesthesia

Thermoregulatory Defenses During Anesthesia

All general anesthetics and most sedatives increase the threshold for warm-defense responses. These drugs also decrease cold-response thresholds, thus increasing the interthreshold range 10- to 20-fold to ≈4°C at typical doses of the usual anesthetics. Because temperatures within this range do not trigger autonomic thermoregulatory defenses (by definition) and because behavioral compensations are unavailable in anesthetized patients, body-temperature perturbations are common during anesthesia.

The first major thermal problem associated with surgery was hyperthermia.[51] Hyperthermia resulted in part from the frequent use of ether, a drug associated with substantial sympathetic nervous system activation and, thus, peripheral vasoconstriction. More importantly, however, hyperthermia resulted when anesthetic-induced thermoregulatory impairment was combined with a warm operating environment. This mechanism continues to produce clinically important hyperthermia in some developing countries, although ether has largely been supplanted by halothane. Hyperthermia in developed countries gave way to hypothermia, however, with the introduction of air conditioning. Hypothermia is now by far the most common perioperative thermal disturbance, and results from anesthetic-induced inhibition of thermoregulatory defenses combined with a cold surgical environment.

Sedatives and general anesthetics, with the exception of midazolam[52] and buspirone,[53] markedly impair thermoregulatory control. For example, the sweating threshold is linearly increased by propofol,[54] alfentanil,[55] isoflurane,[24] and desflurane.[56] Reduction of the vasoconstriction and shivering thresholds is also a linear function of propofol,[54] dexmedetomidine,[57] meperidine,[58] and alfentanil[55] concentrations. Desflurane and isoflurane, however, produce a nonlinear reduction in the major cold-response thresholds, reducing the vasoconstriction and shivering thresholds disproportionately at higher anesthetic concentrations[56] (Figure 8-5). The result is that clinical doses of all anesthetics markedly increase the interthreshold range, substantially impairing thermoregulatory defenses.

Anesthetic-Induced Thermoregulatory Impairment in the Elderly

Intraoperative hypothermia is more common and more severe in the elderly than in younger patients.[59] Because a major cause of intraoperative hypothermia is anesthetic-induced inhibition of thermoregulatory responses, these two observations suggest that anesthetics impair thermoregulation more in elderly than in young patients. This thesis is supported by the observation that the vasoconstriction threshold is approximately 1°C lower in elderly surgical patients than in younger ones[60] (Figure 8-6).

Intraoperative hypothermia is not only more common in the elderly, but lasts longer postoperatively.[61] It is associated with less shivering than in younger patients,[59,62] and what shivering does occur is at a low intensity.[63] Pro-

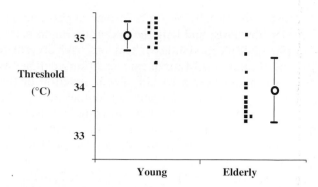

FIGURE 8-6. The effect of aging on thermoregulatory vasoconstriction during general anesthesia. The vasoconstriction threshold was significantly less in the elderly (33.9 ± 0.6°C, mean ± SD) than in younger patients (35.1 ± 0.3°C) (p < 0.01). Filled squares indicate the vasoconstriction threshold in each patient; the open circles show the mean and standard deviations in each group. (Reprinted with permission from Kurz et al.[60] Copyright © Lippincott Williams & Wilkins.)

longed hypothermia without shivering suggests that thermoregulatory defenses are not being activated, which is consistent with reduced perioperative vasoconstriction[60] and shivering[50] thresholds in the elderly.

An additional factor to consider is the age-dependent effects of anesthetic drugs. Renal and hepatic function is often reduced in the elderly. Consequently, clinically important plasma concentrations are likely to persist at high levels for longer in the elderly. Equally important, any given plasma concentrations of many drugs produce a greater effect in the elderly. The minimum alveolar concentration of volatile anesthetics, for example, decreases about 25% in the elderly.[64,65] Similarly, the effect of midazolam is markedly age-dependent.[66] Combined pharmacokinetic and pharmacodynamic augmentation of anesthetic drug effects is thus likely to further impair thermoregulation in the elderly.

Perioperative Heat Balance

Both physical and physiologic factors contribute to perioperative hypothermia. Hypothermia would be unlikely without anesthetic-induced inhibition of thermoregulatory control because thermoregulatory defenses would normally be sufficient to prevent core-temperature perturbations even in a cool operating room environment. However, all anesthetics so far tested markedly increase the range of temperatures *not* triggering thermoregulatory defenses.[67] Within this interthreshold range, body-temperature changes are determined by patients' physical interactions with their immediate environments. Larger operations and colder rooms are thus associated with greater hypothermia. Once triggered, however (in patients becoming sufficiently hypothermic), thermoregulatory

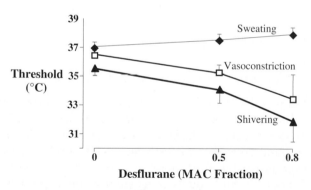

FIGURE 8-5. Thermoregulatory response thresholds during desflurane anesthesia. The sweating threshold increased linearly, but slightly, during desflurane anesthesia. Desflurane markedly—although nonlinearly—reduced the vasoconstriction threshold. Consequently, the interthreshold range (temperatures *not* triggering autonomic thermoregulatory defenses) increased enormously during desflurane administration. In contrast, the vasoconstriction-to-shivering range remained essentially unchanged. Results are presented as means ± SD. MAC = minimal anesthetic concentration. (Reprinted with permission from Annadata et al.[56] Copyright © Lippincott Williams & Wilkins.)

vasoconstriction usually prevents further hypothermia—no matter how large and long the operation might be.[68]

Despite multiple modalities of heat loss, each described by different (and mostly nonlinear) equations, cutaneous heat loss in patients is a roughly linear function of the difference between skin and ambient temperatures. The physical laws and equations characterizing heat transfer are comparably valid for all animate and inanimate substances and, of course, apply equally in young and elderly patients.

Mechanisms of Heat Transfer

There are four types of heat transfer: radiation, convection, conduction, and evaporation.[69] Among these, radiation and convection are by far the most important in patients, together accounting for approximately 85% of the total loss.[70] Fractional losses via each route are, however, determined by numerous physical and physiologic factors including incision size, amount of administered (cold) intravenous fluid, and thermoregulatory vasoconstriction.

Radiative losses are mediated by photons and do not depend on any intervening media. Losses via this mechanism are related to surface properties (emissivity) and the difference of the fourth power of exposed skin and wall temperature (in degrees Kelvin). Radiative losses are thus not directly influenced by ambient temperature, although ambient temperature indirectly influences both wall and skin temperature. Radiation probably contributes about 60% to total heat loss.[70,71]

Conduction is defined by direct transfer of heat energy between opposing surfaces. It is related only to the insulating properties of the surfaces (or of an intervening layer) and the temperature difference between the surfaces. It is unlikely that conduction contributes more than about 5% to overall heat loss in the perioperative period. The reason conduction contributes so little is that only a small fraction of the body surface area is in direct contact with another solid surface, and that surface is likely to be the operating table mattress which is a good insulator. Body heat required to warm cold intravenous fluids is probably best considered as a conductive loss. Loss via this route usually far exceeds conventional surface-to-surface heat transfer.

Convection, which is often termed "facilitated conduction," contributes considerably more than conduction, perhaps about 25% of the total loss. Normally there is essentially no conduction into air because still air is an excellent insulator and because a small layer of still air is maintained adjacent to the skin surface. When warm air next to the skin is moved away, however, it is replaced by cool air from the surrounding environment. This air is itself warmed by extracting heat from the skin, only in turn to be replaced by additional cool air. The equation describing convection is similar to that characterizing conduction, with addition of a factor for the square root of air speed.

The heat of vaporization of water is among the highest of any substances: 0.58 kcal/g. Evaporation of large amounts of water thus absorbs enormous amounts of heat, which is why sweating is such an effective defense against heat stress. Except in infants though, insensible cutaneous water loss is negligible[72,73] and evaporative heat loss a tiny fraction of the total. Evaporative loss contributes to surgical hypothermia during skin preparation when the skin surface is scrubbed with water- or alcohol-based solution that is subsequently allowed to evaporate. Because skin preparation is usually restricted to a relatively small area and because evaporation is permitted for only a brief time, total heat loss is generally relatively small.[74]

Water is also vaporized and lost from the lungs when they are ventilated with dry, cold gases. Numerous clinical studies[75,76] and thermodynamic calculations[77] indicate that respiratory heat loss in adults is less than 10% of the total. Other studies identify effects of airway heating and humidification on core temperature that seem difficult to reconcile with thermodynamic calculations of heat transfer[78–80]; in some cases, these aberrant results are attributable to study design flaws. (In contrast, respiratory losses are somewhat more important in infants and children than in adults.[81,82]) And finally, heat is lost when water evaporates from exposed surfaces within surgical incisions. The extent of this loss in humans remains unknown, although clinical experience suggests that it may be substantial because patients undergoing large operations become considerably more hypothermic than those having smaller procedures. Evaporative loss from within large incisions can may be up to half of the total heat loss in animals,[83] although this ratio is likely less in humans.

Distribution of Heat Within the Body

Intraoperative hypothermia develops with a characteristic three-phase pattern. The first is a rapid, 1–1.5°C decrease in core temperature occurring during the first hour after induction of anesthesia.[84] This is followed by a slower, nearly linear decrease in core temperature lasting 2–3 hours.[85] And finally, core temperature reaches a plateau and does not decrease further.[68] Each portion of this curve has a different etiology.

The initial, rapid decrease in core temperature after induction of general anesthesia results from a core-to-peripheral redistribution of body heat. Redistribution results when anesthetic-induced inhibition of tonic thermoregulatory vasoconstriction allows heat to flow from the relatively warm core thermal compartment to cooler peripheral tissues. (Surprisingly, anesthetic-induced vasodilation increases cutaneous heat loss only slightly.[86]) Although redistribution, by definition, does not alter body-heat content, it does markedly decrease core tem-

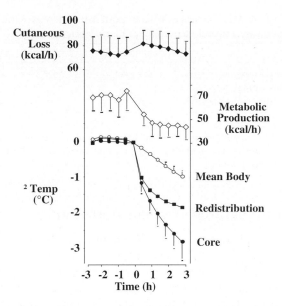

FIGURE 8-7. Changes in body-heat content and distribution of heat within the body during induction of general anesthesia. Heat loss and metabolic heat production were initially similar. Overall heat balance was thus near zero before induction of anesthesia (at elapsed time zero), but subsequently decreased ≈31 kcal/h. The contributions of decreased overall heat balance and internal redistribution of body heat to the decrease in core temperature were separated by multiplying the change in overall heat balance by body weight and the specific heat of humans. The resulting change in mean body temperature ("mean body") was subtracted from the change in core temperature ("core"), leaving the core hypothermia specifically resulting from redistribution ("redistribution"). After 1 hour of anesthesia, core temperature had decreased 1.6 ± 0.3°C, with redistribution contributing 81% to the decrease. During the subsequent 2 hours of anesthesia, core temperature decreased an additional 1.1 ± 0.3°C, with redistribution contributing only 43%. Redistribution thus contributed 65% to the entire 2.8 ± 0.5°C decrease in core temperature during the 3 hours of anesthesia. All results are shown as means ± SD. (Reprinted with permission from Matsukawa et al.[87] Copyright © Lippincott Williams & Wilkins.)

perature. Internal redistribution of body heat is a major cause of core hypothermia in most patients[84] (Figure 8-7). Redistribution is also a major cause of hypothermia during epidural anesthesia.[87]

The 2- to 3-hour-long linear decrease in core temperature results simply from heat loss exceeding heat production.[75] In part, this results from an ≈30% reduction in metabolic heat production during general anesthesia.[84] The slope of this curve thus depends on the difference between metabolic heat production and cutaneous and respiratory heat loss. Metabolic heat production is nearly constant during anesthesia and minimally influenced by anesthetic technique.[68,88] Respiratory heat (even with a nonrebreathing circuit and unwarmed, dry gases) loss is simply a linear function of metabolic rate. In contrast,

cutaneous heat loss is determined largely by surface insulation and ambient temperature, and can therefore be altered by anesthetic management.

After 3–4 hours of anesthesia, core temperature usually reaches a plateau and does not decrease further. This plateau is generally associated with arteriovenous shunt vasoconstriction. Vasoconstriction contributes to the plateau via two distinct mechanisms. The first is simply decreasing cutaneous heat loss.[89] The second is by constraining metabolic heat to the core thermal compartment, thus re-forming the normal core-to-peripheral temperature gradient that was obliterated by the initial redistribution hypothermia. Because heat loss may continue to exceed heat production during the core-temperature plateau, body-heat content often continues to decrease during this period—even though core temperature is constant[68] (Figure 8-8). For a detailed discussion

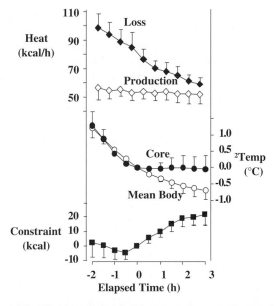

FIGURE 8-8. Changes in body-heat content and distribution of heat within the body during the core-temperature plateau in anesthetized subjects. Vasoconstriction decreased cutaneous heat loss ≈25 kcal/h. However, heat loss exceeded heat production throughout the study. Consequently, mean body temperature, which decreased at a rate of ≈0.6°C/h before vasoconstriction, subsequently decreased at a rate of ≈0.2°C/h. Core temperature also decreased at a rate of ≈0.6°C before vasoconstriction, but remained virtually constant during the subsequent 3 hours. Because mean body temperature and body-heat content continued to decrease, constraint of metabolic heat to the core thermal compartment contributed to the core-temperature plateau. That is, vasoconstriction reestablished the normal core-to-peripheral temperature gradient by preventing metabolic heat (which is largely generated in the core) from escaping to peripheral tissues. Constrained heat is presented cumulatively, referenced to the onset of intense vasoconstriction defined as time zero; data are expressed as means ± SD. (Reprinted with permission from Kurz et al.[68] Copyright © Lippincott Williams & Wilkins.)

of perioperative heat balance, readers are referred to a recent review.[89]

Benefits of Mild Hypothermia

Severe hypothermia (i.e., core temperatures near 28°C) has been known for decades to be protective against cerebral ischemia.[90] The basis for this protection was thought to be a decrease in the cerebral metabolic rate to about half of normal levels.[91] Although decreased metabolic rate surely contributes to hypothermic protection, there is increasing evidence that other mechanisms contribute as much or more. These include decreased release of excitatory amino acids (such as glutamate) and free fatty acids,[92,93] inhibition of calcium/calmodulin-dependent protein kinase II,[94] preservation of the blood–brain barrier,[95,96] reduced synthesis of nitric oxide[97] and ubiquitin.[98]

More than 100 animal studies in virtually every ischemic model demonstrate that just 1–3°C brain hypothermia provides substantial protection against ischemia.[93,99–102] In each case, the protection seems to far exceed that resulting simply from reduced metabolic rate. There is also evidence that mild hypothermia also protects the spinal cord and liver against ischemia.[103] Furthermore, mild hypothermia seems protective during spinal cord ischemia[104] and is beneficial during hypoxia and shock.

The benefits of mild hypothermia in ameliorating cerebral ischemia in humans have only been demonstrated after cardiac arrest.[105,106] Many neuroanesthesiologists nonetheless allow patients undergoing neurosurgery to become at least slightly hypothermic (i.e., ≈34°C) even though a major trial of hypothermia for intracranial aneurysm surgery failed to identify a benefit from therapeutic hypothermia.[107] The elderly are probably at greater risk of ischemia because of age-related vascular compromise while simultaneously being at greater risk of hypothermia-related complications.

Complications of Mild Hypothermia

Although once considered the major complication associated with hypothermia, shivering is now known to be a relatively unimportant response that is easily treated using a variety of techniques. Furthermore, shivering is now less common than it was previously, perhaps because the use of opioids and propofol has increased. Postoperative shivering is especially uncommon in the elderly, and its intensity modest in any case. In contrast, recent years have seen publication of numerous studies documenting other major complications of hypothermia, some of which have been shown to alter patient outcome.

TABLE 8-1. Mild intraoperative hypothermia increases the incidence of myocardial ischemia in elderly patients.

	Normothermic	Hypothermic	p Value
Initial postoperative core temperature (°C)	35.9 ± 0.1	34.2 ± 0.1	<0.01
Myocardial ischemia (%)	13	36	<0.01

Source: Frank et al.[108]
Note: Mild hypothermia (<2°C) in elderly patients undergoing vascular surgery tripled the incidence of myocardial ischemia in the first 24 postoperative hours.

Myocardial Ischemia and Arrhythmias

Myocardial infarction remains one of the leading causes of perioperative mortality. The incidence of myocardial ischemia within 24 hours of surgery is tripled by ≈2°C core hypothermia in elderly patients undergoing vascular surgery[108] (Table 8–1). Surprisingly, ischemia is *not* related to postoperative shivering and the mechanism by which hypothermia triggers ischemia remains unknown. One factor may be significantly increased concentrations of circulating norepinephrine, with concomitant arterial hypertension.[109] Perhaps related to increased catecholamine concentrations, the incidence of ventricular tachycardia is significantly increased by mild hypothermia.[110] Hypothermia thus increases the risk of morbid perioperative cardiac outcomes, but may be therapeutically useful for preserving myocardium once an infarction has occurred.

Perioperative ischemia presumably requires underlying coronary artery disease, a predisposition that would be unusual in young patients but is typical in the elderly. It is thus the elderly that are most susceptible to perioperative ischemia and have most to benefit from maintenance of perioperative normothermia.

Coagulopathy and Allogeneic Transfusion Requirement

Hypothermia decreases platelet function,[111] apparently by decreasing release of thromboxane A$_2$.[112] These effects of hypothermia on platelet function seem to be entirely related to local, rather than core, temperature. (This is a factor that should be considered when interpreting a bleeding time.) Hypothermia also directly inhibits the enzymes of the coagulation cascade.[113,114] The effects of hypothermia on bleeding have not generally been appreciated by clinicians, in large part because coagulation tests are performed at 37°C, irrespective of patients' actual temperatures.

Hip arthroplasty is among the more common operations in the elderly, and it is a procedure associated with substantial blood loss. Just 2°C core hypothermia substantially increases perioperative blood loss during total hip arthroplasty, and also increases the requirement for

TABLE 8-2. Mild intraoperative hypothermia increases blood loss during hip arthroplasty.

	Normothermic	Hypothermic	p Value
Final intraoperative core temperature (°C)	36.6 ± 0.4	35.0 ± 0.5	<0.001
Blood loss (L)	1.7 ± 0.4	2.2 ± 0.6	<0.001
Allogeneic blood (mL/patient)	10 ± 55	80 ± 154	<0.02

Source: Schmied et al.[115]
Note: Mild hypothermia (<2°C) significantly increased blood loss and the requirement for allogeneic blood transfusion in patients undergoing total hip arthroplasty. As is typical for this procedure, the patients were elderly, averaging 63 ± 10 years of age.

allogeneic blood transfusion, as shown in some[115,116] but not all[117] studies (Table 8-2).

Surgical Wound Infections and Duration of Hospitalization

Wound infections are common and serious complications of anesthesia and surgery. In patients undergoing colon surgery, for example, the risk of wound infection ranges from 3% to 22%.[118] Infections typically prolong hospitalization by 5–20 days per infection and substantially increase cost.[119,120] Hypothermia facilitates perioperative wound infections in two ways: First, sufficient intraoperative hypothermia triggers thermoregulatory vasoconstriction[121] and postoperative vasoconstriction is universal in hypothermic patients.[122] Vasoconstriction decreases tissue oxygen partial pressure which reduces resistance to infection.[123,124] Second, mild core hypothermia directly impairs numerous immune functions.[125,126]

Finally, vasoconstriction-induced tissue hypoxia also decreases wound strength independently of its effect on resistance to infection. Scar formation requires proline and lysine hydroxylation, permitting the crosslinking between collagen strands that provides wound tensile strength.[127] The hydroxylases catalyzing this reaction are oxygen tension-dependent.[128] Collagen deposition is thus proportional to arterial PO_2 in animals[129] and to wound tissue oxygen tension in humans.[130]

Consistent with these in vitro data, mild hypothermia during anesthesia reduces resistance to *Escherichia coli* and *Staphylococcus aureus* inoculations in guinea pigs.[131,132] Furthermore, just 2°C core hypothermia triples the incidence of wound infection in patients undergoing colon surgery. Hypothermic patients also require significantly longer hospitalizations[133] (Table 8-3).

Postoperative Shivering

It is common in reviews and book chapters to include the following logic: (1) shivering increases metabolic rate "up to 400%"; and (2) increased metabolic rate could be detrimental to elderly patients having cardiovascular disease.[134,135] However, postoperative shivering in elderly patients is relatively rare,[63] and usually of low intensity when it does occur. On the average, postoperative shivering in young patients doubles oxygen consumption (although higher values may occasionally be sustained),[136,137] whereas metabolic rate increases only ≈20% in the elderly.[63] Furthermore, although intraoperative hypothermia is associated with postoperative ischemia, there is no apparent association between shivering and ischemia.[108] There thus seems to be little support for the theory that elderly patients allowed to become hypothermic subsequently develop myocardial ischemia because of shivering.

Some patients, nonetheless, shiver during recovery from general anesthesia. At the very least, shivering is uncomfortable and remembered by many patients as one of the worst aspects of their surgical experience. Most postoperative shivering-like tremor is thermoregulatory,[122] and therefore can be completely prevented by maintaining intraoperative normothermia.[138] However, there is a small incidence of low-intensity tremor that is not thermoregulatory,[139] a tremor that correlates with inadequate treatment of surgical pain.[140] A similar non-thermoregulatory shivering-like tremor can be observed during epidural analgesia for labor.[141]

Shivering can be treated using a variety of techniques. The least invasive is skin-surface warming. Because mean skin temperature contributes ≈20% to control of shivering,[16] cutaneous warming decreases the shivering

TABLE 8-3. Mild intraoperative hypothermia increases the incidence of surgical wound infections and the duration of hospitalization.

	Normothermic	Hypothermic	p Value
Final intraoperative core temperature (°C)	36.6 ± 0.5	34.7 ± 0.6	<0.001
Infections/number of patients	6/105	18/95	<0.01
Duration of hospitalization (days)	11 ± 4	14 ± 4	<0.01

Source: Kurz et al.[133]
Note: Mild hypothermia (<2°C) tripled the incidence of surgical wound infections and prolonged hospitalization 25% in patients undergoing elective colon resection.

threshold proportionately. A typical forced-air warmer increases mean skin temperature ≈3°C, thereby reducing the shivering threshold ≈0.6°C. If a shivering patient's core temperature is within 0.6°C of the shivering threshold, cutaneous warming can thus increase the threshold sufficiently to stop shivering.[142]

Numerous drugs have also been proven effective for the treatment of postoperative shivering. The prototypical drug for this purpose is meperidine, which is far more effective than equianalgesic doses of other opioids.[136] For example, meperidine reduces the shivering threshold twice as much as equianalgesic concentrations of alfentanil.[55] Furthermore, meperidine markedly reduces the gain of shivering, whereas alfentanil does not.[143] The special antishivering activity of meperidine was thought to result from its kappa-receptor activity,[144] but kappa-opioids do not share disproportionately to reduce the shivering threshold.[145] Meperidine's central anticholinergic activity also fails to explain this drug's special antishivering activity.[145] Clonidine[146–148] and ketanserin[148] are also effective treatments for postoperative shivering, as are magnesium[149] and doxapram.[150–152] The efficacy of various antishivering treatments has been the subject of a recent meta-analysis.[153] For a detailed discussion of perioperative shivering, readers are referred to a recent review.[154]

Impaired Drug Metabolism

The pharmacokinetic effects of mild hypothermia are poorly documented. Nonetheless, the duration of action of vecuronium, for example, is doubled by just 2°C core hypothermia.[155] Hypothermia prolongs the duration of action of atracurium less, ≈70% with 3°C reduction in core temperature,[156] perhaps because Hoffman elimination is relatively temperature-insensitive compared with enzymatic degradation. Antagonism of the neuromuscular block is not compromised with either drug.[155,156] And finally, steady-state plasma concentrations of propofol (during a constant-rate infusion) were increased ≈30% by 3°C core hypothermia.[156]

Whether the pharmacokinetic effects of hypothermia are aggravated in the elderly has yet to be studied. However, drug metabolism in the elderly is often already compromised. It thus seems likely that hypothermia-induced prolongation of drug action, combined with age-related deficiencies in drug metabolism, may result in anesthetic drugs lasting unexpectedly long times in elderly, hypothermic patients. These pharmacokinetic effects will, in many cases, be confounded by pharmacodynamic ones. Although the magnitude of these effects has yet to be quantified, it would seem prudent to prevent hypothermia in the elderly and use minimum required drug doses to minimize drug-induced thermoregulatory impairment.

Thermal Management

The combination of anesthetic-induced inhibition of thermoregulatory defenses and cold exposure makes most unwarmed surgical patients hypothermic. Hypothermia produces complications in both young and elderly patients, and the severity of these complications seems worse in the elderly. Consequently, active thermal management is especially important in elderly patients. The physical principles of heat transfer, however, apply equally in all patients. Thus, the same warming techniques proven effective in the general surgical population will also be useful in the elderly. For a detailed discussion of patient warming techniques, readers are referred to a recent review.[157]

Ambient Temperature, Passive Insulation, and Cutaneous Warming

Heat loss is a (very) roughly linear function of the difference between skin and environmental temperature. Typical intraoperative skin temperature is near 34°C, which is ≈14°C above ambient temperature. Consequently, each 1°C increase in ambient temperature reduces heat loss ≈7%. Patients become hypothermic most rapidly during the initial 30 minutes after induction of anesthesia, and this is the period when patients are most likely to be undraped. However, core hypothermia during this period results from internal redistribution of body heat, not primarily from heat loss to the environment.[84] Increasing ambient temperature for the brief period before and after induction of anesthesia therefore has little impact on patient temperature.[158]

A single layer of passive insulation decreases cutaneous heat loss ≈30%. However, the type of insulation makes little difference, with the efficacy of cotton blankets, plastic bags, cloth or paper surgical drapes, and "space blankets" all being comparable[159] (Figure 8-9). Patients who remain normothermic during surgery while covered only with a single layer of insulation require no additional thermal management. But surprisingly, increasing the number of layers makes relatively little difference, reducing loss by a total of only 50%; furthermore, warm and cold blankets provide similar insulation.[160] It is thus unlikely that progressive intraoperative hypothermia will be successfully treated simply by providing additional layers of insulation. Instead, active cutaneous warming will be required.

Circulating-water mattresses remain a common method of thermal management, despite evidence that these devices are nearly ineffective[161] and cause pressure-heat necrosis ("burns").[162,163] The efficacy of circulating water is restricted because relatively little heat is lost

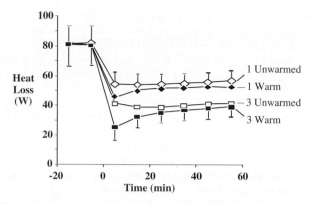

FIGURE 8-9. Mean cutaneous heat loss during the control period (−20 to 0 elapsed minutes) and when the volunteers were covered with a single warmed or unwarmed blanket ("1 Warm" or "1 Unwarmed") or three warmed or unwarmed blankets ("3 Warm" or "3 Unwarmed"). There was no clinically important difference between warmed and unwarmed blankets. Increasing the number of layers from one to three slightly decreased heat loss, but the decrease was unlikely to be sufficient to prevent further intraoperative hypothermia. (Reprinted with permission from Sessler and Schroeder.[160] Copyright © Lippincott Williams & Wilkins.)

from patients' backs into the foam insulation covering most operating tables.[75] Instead, most heat is lost by radiation and convection from patients' anterior surfaces, loss that cannot be prevented by a water mattress. Forced-air warming is far more effective than circulating water, and is safer.[161] However, recently developed circulating water garments transfer even more heat than forced-air.[164–167]

Fluid Warming

It is not possible to warm patients by warming intravenous fluids. Fluid warming alone is thus unlikely to maintain perioperative normothermia because it will not compensate for redistribution hypothermia, much less heat loss from the skin and from within surgical incisions. However, it is certainly possible to cool patients by administering fluids much below body temperature. The amount of cooling is easy to calculate: in a typically sized adult, 1 L of fluid at ambient temperature decreases mean body temperature 0.25°C. One unit of blood at refrigerator temperatures causes a similar decrease in body temperature.[168] Fluid warming should thus be restricted to patients who are already being warmed with some effective surface technique such as forced-air *and* in whom large amounts of fluid (>1 L/h) is being given. Cooling of fluid in tubing between warmers and patients is clinically unimportant except in the occasional neonate who requires large amounts of fluid.[169]

Prewarming

Internal core-to-peripheral redistribution of body heat is among the most important causes of hypothermia in most patients.[84] Because the internal flow of heat is large, it has proven difficult to treat with surface warming.[75] An alternative is to prevent redistribution. One method of minimizing redistribution is to produce drug-induced peripheral vasodilation well before induction of anesthesia. Because central thermoregulatory control remains normal before induction of anesthesia, behavioral compensation protects core temperature. The result is a constant core temperature, accompanied by increased peripheral tissue temperature. Because heat flows only down a temperature gradient, induction of anesthesia is associated with little redistribution because the core-to-peripheral temperature gradient is small. This concept has been demonstrated using nifedipine,[170] phenylephrine,[171] and ketamine,[172] all of which support the importance of redistribution hypothermia.

An alternative method of minimizing redistribution hypothermia is to actively warm peripheral tissues before induction of anesthesia. Even just 30 minutes of forced-air "prewarming" increases peripheral tissue heat content ≈69 kcal, and 1 hour of prewarming transfers nearly 136 kcal.[173] Either amount should be sufficient to minimize redistribution. The benefits of prewarming have been demonstrated in both volunteers[174] and surgical patients[138,175,176] (Figure 8-10). Assuming intraoperative forced-air warming is anticipated, there is no additional patient cost to prewarming because the same disposable cover can be used before and during surgery.

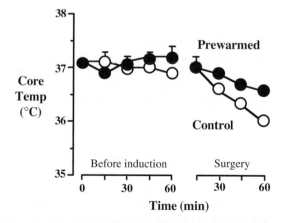

FIGURE 8-10. Core temperatures during the preinduction period did not change significantly in the control group (open circles) or patients prewarmed with forced-air (solid circles). After induction of anesthesia, core temperature in the control group decreased at nearly twice the rate of that in the prewarmed patients. After 1 hour of anesthesia, core temperatures were 0.6°C greater in the prewarmed patients than in the control group. Results presented as means ± SEM. (Reprinted with permission from Camus et al.[175] Copyright © 1995 Elsevier.)

Summary

Normal thermoregulatory control is impaired in the elderly, as is thermoregulation during general anesthesia. A major factor influencing intraoperative core-temperature changes is internal core-to-peripheral redistribution of body heat that results from anesthetic-induced inhibition of thermoregulatory control. Many of the identified complications of mild perioperative hypothermia are likely to be more common or more severe in the elderly. Similarly, the core-temperature plateau results from reemergence of thermoregulatory control, which may be impaired in the elderly. In contrast, the physical factors influencing heat loss do not differ much in young and elderly patients and thermal management strategies are similar in young and elderly patients.

References

1. Cabanac M, Dib B. Behavioural responses to hypothalamic cooling and heating in the rat. Brain Res 1983;264:79–87.
2. Satinoff E, McEwen GN Jr, Williams BA. Behavioral fever in newborn rabbits. Science 1976;193:1139–1140.
3. Nadel ER, Pandolf KB, Roberts MF, Stolwijk JAJ. Mechanisms of thermal acclimation to exercise and heat. J Appl Physiol 1974;37:515–520.
4. Nadel ER, Cafarelli E, Roberts MF, Wenger CB. Circulatory regulation during exercise in different ambient temperatures. J Appl Physiol 1979;46:430–437.
5. Hales JRS. Skin arteriovenous anastomoses, their control and role in thermoregulation. In: Johansen K, Burggren W, eds. Cardiovascular Shunts: Phylogenetic, Ontogenetic and Clinical Aspects. Copenhagen: Munksgaard; 1985:433–451.
6. Nedergaard J, Cannon B. The uncoupling protein thermogenin and mitochondrial thermogenesis. New Comp Biochem 1992;23:385–420.
7. Israel DJ, Pozos RS. Synchronized slow-amplitude modulations in the electromyograms of shivering muscles. J Appl Physiol 1989;66:2358–2363.
8. Jessen C, Mayer ET. Spinal cord and hypothalamus as core sensors of temperature in the conscious dog. I. Equivalence of responses. Pflügers Arch 1971;324:189–204.
9. Sessler DI. Perianesthetic thermoregulation and heat balance in humans. FASEB J 1993;7:638–644.
10. Satinoff E. Neural organization and evolution of thermal regulation in mammals—several hierarchically arranged integrating systems may have evolved to achieve precise thermoregulation. Science 1978;201:16–22.
11. Satinoff E, Rutstein J. Behavioral thermoregulation in rats with anterior hypothalamic lesions. J Comp Physiol Psychol 1970;71:77–82.
12. Poulos DA. Central processing of cutaneous temperature information. Fed Proc 1981;40:2825–2829.
13. Kosaka M, Simon E, Walther O-E, Thauer R. Response of respiration to selective heating of the spinal cord below partial transection. Experientia 1969;25:36–37.
14. Jessen C. Independent clamps of peripheral and central temperatures and their effects on heat production in the goat. J Physiol (Lond) 1981;311:11–22.
15. Jessen C, Feistkorn G. Some characteristics of core temperature signals in the conscious goat. Am J Physiol 1984;247:R456–R464.
16. Cheng C, Matsukawa T, Sessler DI, et al. Increasing mean skin temperature linearly reduces the core-temperature thresholds for vasoconstriction and shivering in humans. Anesthesiology 1995;82:1160–1168.
17. Wyss CR, Brengelmann GL, Johnson JM, et al. Altered control of skin blood flow at high skin and core temperatures. J Appl Physiol 1975;38:839–845.
18. Nadel ER, Mitchell JW, Stolwijk JAJ. Control of local and total sweating during exercise transients. Int J Biometeorol 1971;15:201–206.
19. Tam H-S, Darling RC, Cheh H-Y, Downey JA. The dead zone of thermoregulation in normal and paraplegic man. Can J Physiol Pharmacol 1978;56:976–983.
20. Wenger CB, Roberts MF, Stolwijk JJA, Nadel ER. Forearm blood flow during body temperature transients produced by leg exercise. J Appl Physiol 1975;38:58–63.
21. Mistlberger T, Rusak B. Mechanisms and models of the circadian time keeping system. In: Kryger MH, Dement WC, eds. Principles and Practice of Sleep Medicine. Philadelphia: WB Saunders; 1989:141–152.
22. Lopez M, Sessler DI, Walter K, et al. Rate and gender dependence of the sweating, vasoconstriction, and shivering thresholds in humans. Anesthesiology 1994;80:780–788.
23. Stephenson LA, Kolka MA. Menstrual cycle phase and time of day alter reference signal controlling arm blood flow and sweating. Am J Physiol 1985;249:R186–R191.
24. Washington D, Sessler DI, Moayeri A, et al. Thermoregulatory responses to hyperthermia during isoflurane anesthesia in humans. J Appl Physiol 1993;74:82–87.
25. Mestyan J, Jarai I, Bata G, Fekete M. The significance of facial skin temperature in the chemical heat regulation of premature infants. Biol Neonat 1964;7:243–254.
26. Jessen K. An assessment of human regulatory nonshivering thermogenesis. Acta Anaesthesiol Scand 1980;24:138–143.
27. Jessen K, Rabøl A, Winkler K. Total body and splanchnic thermogenesis in curarized man during a short exposure to cold. Acta Anaesthesiol Scand 1980;24:339–344.
28. Joy RJT, Matone JC, Newcomb GW, Bradford WC. Responses of cold-acclimatized men to infused norepinephrine. J Appl Physiol 1963;18:1209–1212.
29. Brück K. Thermoregulation: control mechanisms and neural processes. In: Sinclair JC, ed. Temperature Regulation and Energy Metabolism in the Newborn. New York: Grune & Stratton; 1978:157–185.
30. Fox RH, Hilton SM. Bradykinin formation in human skin as a factor of heat vasodilatation. J Physiol 1958;142:219–232.
31. Warren JB. Nitric oxide and human skin blood flow responses to acetylcholine and ultraviolet light. FASEB J 1994;8:247–251.
32. Hall DM, Buettner GR, Matthes RD, Gisolfi CV. Hyperthermia stimulates nitric oxide formation: electron

paramagnetic resonance detection of .NO-heme in blood. J Appl Physiol 1994;77:548–553.

33. Detry J-MR, Brengelmann GL, Rowell LB, Wyss C. Skin and muscle components of forearm blood flow in directly heated resting man. J Appl Physiol 1972;32:506–511.

34. Giesbrecht GG, Sessler DI, Mekjavic IB, et al. Treatment of immersion hypothermia by direct body-to-body contact. J Appl Physiol 1994;76:2373–2379.

35. Horvath SM, Spurr GB, Hutt BK, Hamilton LH. Metabolic cost of shivering. J Appl Physiol 1956;8:595–602.

36. Danzl DF, Pozos RS. Accidental hypothermia. N Engl J Med 1994;331:1756–1760.

37. Lønning PE, Skulberg A, Abyholm F. Accidental hypothermia: review of the literature. Acta Anaesthesiol Scand 1986;30:601–613.

38. Kalant H, Le AD. Effects of ethanol on thermoregulation. Pharmacol Ther 1984;23:313–364.

39. Fellows I, Bennett T, Macdonald IA. Influence of environmental temperature on the thermoregulatory responses to ethanol. In: Hales JRS, ed. Thermal Physiology. New York: Raven Press; 1984:221–223.

40. Fox GR, Hayward JS, Hobson GN. Effect of alcohol on thermal balance of man in cold water. Can J Physiol Pharmacol 1979;57:860–865.

41. Hobson GN, Collis ML. The effects of alcohol upon cooling rates of humans immersed in 7.5° C water. Can J Physiol Pharmacol 1977;55:744–746.

42. MacMillan AL, Corbett JL, Johnson RH, et al. Temperature regulation in survivors of accidental hypothermia of the elderly. Lancet 1967;2:165–169.

43. Khan F, Spence VA, Belch JJF. Cutaneous vascular responses and thermoregulation in relation to age. Clin Sci 1992;82:521–528.

44. Wagner JA, Robinson S, Marino RP. Age and temperature regulation of humans in neutral and cold environments. J Appl Physiol 1974;37:562–565.

45. McDonald RB, Day C, Carlson K, et al. Effect of age and gender on thermoregulation. Am J Physiol 1989;257:R700–R704.

46. Tankersley CG, Smolander J, Kenney WL, Fortney SM. Sweating and skin blood flow during exercise: effects of age and maximal oxygen uptake. J Appl Physiol 1991;71:236–242.

47. Inoue Y, Nakao M, Araki T, Murakami H. Regional differences in the sweating responses of older and younger men. J Appl Physiol 1991;71:2453–2459.

48. Falk B, Bar-Or O, Macdougall JD, et al. Sweat lactate in exercising children and adolescents of varying physical maturity. J Appl Physiol 1991;71:1735–1740.

49. Yousef MK, Dill DB, Vitez TS, et al. Thermoregulatory responses to desert heat: age, race and sex. J Gerontol 1984;39:406–414.

50. Vassilieff N, Rosencher N, Sessler DI, Conseiller C. The shivering threshold during spinal anesthesia is reduced in the elderly. Anesthesiology 1995;83:1162–1166.

51. Clark RE, Orkin LR, Rovenstine EA. Body temperature studies in anesthetized man: effect of environmental temperature, humidity, and anesthesia system. JAMA 1954;154:311–319.

52. Kurz A, Sessler DI, Annadata R, et al. Midazolam minimally impairs thermoregulatory control. Anesth Analg 1995;81:393–398.

53. Mokhtarani M, Mahgob AN, Morioka N, et al. Buspirone and meperidine synergistically reduce the shivering threshold. Anesth Analg 2001;93:1233–1239.

54. Matsukawa T, Kurz A, Sessler DI, et al. Propofol linearly reduces the vasoconstriction and shivering thresholds. Anesthesiology 1995;82:1169–1180.

55. Kurz A, Go JC, Sessler DI, et al. Alfentanil slightly increases the sweating threshold and markedly reduces the vasoconstriction and shivering thresholds. Anesthesiology 1995;83:293–299.

56. Annadata RS, Sessler DI, Tayefeh F, et al. Desflurane slightly increases the sweating threshold, but produces marked, non-linear decreases in the vasoconstriction and shivering thresholds. Anesthesiology 1995;83:1205–1211.

57. Talke P, Li J, Jain U, et al. Effects of perioperative dexmedetomidine infusion in patients undergoing vascular surgery. Anesthesiology 1995;82:620–633.

58. Kurz A, Ikeda T, Sessler DI, et al. Meperidine decreases the shivering threshold twice as much as the vasoconstriction threshold. Anesthesiology 1997;86:1046–1054.

59. Vaughan MS, Vaughan RW, Cork RC. Postoperative hypothermia in adults: relationship of age, anesthesia, and shivering to rewarming. Anesth Analg 1981;60:746–751.

60. Kurz A, Plattner O, Sessler DI, et al. The threshold for thermoregulatory vasoconstriction during nitrous oxide/isoflurane anesthesia is lower in elderly than young patients. Anesthesiology 1993;79:465–469.

61. Frank SM, Beattie C, Christopherson R, et al. Epidural versus general anesthesia, ambient operating room temperature, and patient age as predictors of inadvertent hypothermia. Anesthesiology 1992;77:252–257.

62. Roe CF, Goldberg MJ, Blair CS, Kinney JM. The influence of body temperature on early postoperative oxygen consumption. Surgery 1966;60:85–92.

63. Frank SM, Fleisher LA, Olson KF, et al. Multivariate determinants of early postoperative oxygen consumption in elderly patients. Anesthesiology 1995;83:241–249.

64. Nakajima R, Nakajima Y, Ikeda K. Minimum alveolar concentration of sevoflurane in elderly patients. Br J Anaesth 1993;70:273–275.

65. Stevens WC, Dolan WM, Gibbons RT, et al. Minimum alveolar concentrations (MAC) of isoflurane with and without nitrous oxide in patients of various ages. Anesthesiology 1975;42:197–200.

66. Jacobs JR, Reves JG, Marty J, et al. Aging increases pharmacodynamic sensitivity to the hypnotic effects of midazolam. Anesth Analg 1995;80:143–148.

67. Sessler DI. Perioperative hypothermia. N Engl J Med 1997;336:1730–1737.

68. Kurz A, Sessler DI, Christensen R, Dechert M. Heat balance and distribution during the core-temperature plateau in anesthetized humans. Anesthesiology 1995;83:491–499.

69. English MJM, Farmer C, Scott WAC. Heat loss in exposed volunteers. J Trauma 1990;30:422–425.

70. Robins HI, Grossman J, Davis TE, et al. Preclinical trial of a radiant heat device for whole-body hyperthermia using a porcine model. Cancer Res 1983;43:2018–2022.

71. Hardy JD, Milhorat AT, DuBois EF. Basal metabolism and heat loss of young women at temperatures from 22 degrees C to 35 degrees C. J Nutr 1941;21:383–403.

72. Baumgart S. Radiant energy and insensible water loss in the premature newborn infant nursed under a radiant warmer. Clin Perinatol 1982;9:483–503.

73. Hammarlund K, Sedin G. Transepidermal water loss in newborn infants. III. Relation to gestational age. Acta Paediatr Scand 1979;68:795–801.

74. Sessler DI, Sessler AM, Hudson S, Moayeri A. Heat loss during surgical skin preparation. Anesthesiology 1993;78: 1055–1064.

75. Hynson J, Sessler DI. Intraoperative warming therapies: a comparison of three devices. J Clin Anesth 1992;4: 194–199.

76. Deriaz H, Fiez N, Lienhart A. Influence d'un filtre hygrophobe ou d'un humidificateur-réchauffeur sur l'hypothermie peropératoire. Ann Fr Anesth Réanim 1992;11:145–149.

77. Hendrickx HHL, Trahey GE, Argentieri MP. Paradoxical inhibition of decreases in body temperature by use of heated and humidified gases [letter]. Anesth Analg 1982; 61:393–394.

78. Ip Yam PC, Carli F. Maintenance of body temperature in elderly patients who have joint replacement surgery. Anesthesia 1990;45:563–565.

79. Goldberg MI, Epstein R, Rosenblum F, et al. Do heated humidifiers or heat and moisture exchangers prevent temperature drop during lower abdominal surgery? J Clin Anesth 1992;4:16–20.

80. Stone DR, Downs JB, Paul WL, Perkins HM. Adult body temperature and heated humidification of anesthetic gases during general anesthesia. Anesth Analg 1981;60: 736–741.

81. Bissonnette B, Sessler DI. Passive or active inspired gas humidification in infants and children. Anesthesiology 1989;71:381–384.

82. Bissonnette B, Sessler DI. Passive or active inspired gas humidification increases thermal steady-state temperatures in anesthetized infants. Anesth Analg 1989;69:783–787.

83. Roe CF. Effect of bowel exposure on body temperature during surgical operations. Am J Surg 1971;122:13–15.

84. Matsukawa T, Sessler DI, Sessler AM, et al. Heat flow and distribution during induction of general anesthesia. Anesthesiology 1995;82:662–673.

85. Kurz A, Sessler DI, Narzt E, Lenhart R. Morphometric influences on intraoperative core temperature changes. Anesth Analg 1995;80:562–567.

86. Sessler DI, McGuire J, Moayeri A, Hynson J. Isoflurane-induced vasodilation minimally increases cutaneous heat loss. Anesthesiology 1991;74:226–232.

87. Matsukawa T, Sessler DI, Christensen R, et al. Heat flow and distribution during epidural anesthesia. Anesthesiology 1995;83:961–967.

88. Stevens WC, Cromwell TH, Halsey MJ, et al. The cardiovascular effects of a new inhalation anesthetic, Forane, in human volunteers at constant arterial carbon dioxide tension. Anesthesiology 1971;35:8–16.

89. Sessler DI. Perioperative heat balance. Anesthesiology 2000;92:578–596.

90. Todd MM, Warner DS. A comfortable hypothesis reevaluated: cerebral metabolic depression and brain protection during ischemia [editorial]. Anesthesiology 1992;76: 161–164.

91. Hagerdal M, Harp JR, Nilsson L, Siesjo BK. The effect of induced hypothermia upon oxygen consumption in the rat brain. J Neurochem 1975;24:311–316.

92. Busto R, Globus MY-T, Dietrich WD, et al. Effect of mild hypothermia on ischemia-induced release of neurotransmitters and free fatty acids in rat brain. Stroke 1989; 20:904–910.

93. Illievich UM, Zornow MH, Choi KT, et al. Effects of hypothermia or anesthetics on hippocampal glutamate and glycine concentrations after repeated transient global cerebral ischemia. Anesthesiology 1994;80:177–186.

94. Churn SB, Taft WC, Billingsley MS, et al. Temperature modulation of ischemic neuronal death and inhibition of calcium/calmodulin-dependent protein kinase II in gerbils. Stroke 1990;21:1715–1721.

95. Dietrich WD, Busto R, Halley M, Valdes I. The importance of brain temperature in alterations of the blood-brain barrier following cerebral ischemia. J Neuropathol Exp Neurol 1990;49:486–497.

96. Jurkovich GJ, Pitt RM, Curreri PW, Granger DN. Hypothermia prevents increased capillary permeability following ischemia-reperfusion injury. J Surg Res 1988;44:514–521.

97. Kader A, Frazzini VI, Baker CJ, et al. Effect of mild hypothermia on nitric oxide synthesis during focal cerebral ischemia. Neurosurgery 1994;35:272–277.

98. Yamashita I, Eguchi Y, Kajiwara K, Ito H. Mild hypothermia ameliorates ubiquitin synthesis and prevents delayed neuronal death in the gerbil hippocampus. Stroke 1991;22: 1574–1581.

99. Busto R, Dietrich WD, Globus MY-T, Ginsberg MD. Postischemic moderate hypothermia inhibits CA1 hippocampal ischemic neuronal injury. Neurosci Lett 1989;101: 299–304.

100. Minamisawa H, Smith M-L, Siesjo BK. The effect of mild hyperthermia and hypothermia on brain damage following 5, 10, and 15 minutes of forebrain ischemia. Ann Neurol 1990;28:26–33.

101. Sakai F, Amaha K. The effects of hypothermia on a cloned human brain glutamate transporter (hGLT-1) expressed in Chinese hamster ovary cells: –[3H]L-glutamate uptake study. Anesth Analg 1999;89:1546–1550.

102. Popovic R, Liniger R, Bickler PE. Anesthetics and mild hypothermia similarly prevent hippocampal neuron death in an in vitro model of cerebral ischemia. Anesthesiology 2000;92:1343–1349.

103. Vacanti RX, Ames A III. Mild hypothermia and Mg^{++} protect against irreversible damage during CNS ischemia. Stroke 1984;15:695–698.

104. Pontius RG, Brockman HL, Hardy EG, et al. The use of hypothermia in the prevention of paraplegia following temporary aortic occlusion: experimental observations. Surgery 1954;36:33–38.

105. Bernard SA, Gray TW, Buist MD, et al. Treatment of comatose survivors of out-of-hospital cardiac arrest with induced hypothermia. N Engl J Med 2002;346:557–563.

106. Hypothermia after Cardiac Arrest Study Group. Mild therapeutic hypothermia to improve the neurologic outcome after cardiac arrest. N Engl J Med 2002;346: 549–556.

107. Todd MM, Hindman BJ, Clarke WR, Torner JC. Mild intraoperative hypothermia during surgery for intracranial aneurysm. N Engl J Med 2005;352:135–145.

108. Frank SM, Beattie C, Christopherson R, et al. Unintentional hypothermia is associated with postoperative myocardial ischemia. Anesthesiology 1993;78:468–476.

109. Frank SM, Higgins MS, Breslow MJ, et al. The catecholamine, cortisol, and hemodynamic responses to mild perioperative hypothermia. Anesthesiology 1995;82:83–93.

110. Frank SM, Fleisher LA, Breslow MJ, et al. Perioperative maintenance of normothermia reduces the incidence of morbid cardiac events: a randomized clinical trial. JAMA 1997;277:1127–1134.

111. Michelson AD, MacGregor H, Barnard MR, et al. Reversible inhibition of human platelet activation by hypothermia in vivo and in vitro. Thromb Haemost 1994;71: 633–640.

112. Valeri CR, Khabbaz K, Khuri SF, et al. Effect of skin temperature on platelet function in patients undergoing extracorporeal bypass. J Thorac Cardiovasc Surg 1992;104: 108–116.

113. Reed L, Johnston TD, Hudson JD, Fischer RP. The disparity between hypothermic coagulopathy and clotting studies. J Trauma 1992;33:465–470.

114. Rohrer M, Natale A. Effect of hypothermia on the coagulation cascade. Crit Care Med 1992;20:1402–1405.

115. Schmied H, Kurz A, Sessler DI, et al. Mild intraoperative hypothermia increases blood loss and allogeneic transfusion requirements during total hip arthroplasty. Lancet 1996;347:289–292.

116. Winkler M, Akça O, Birkenberg B, et al. Aggressive warming reduces blood loss during hip arthroplasty. Anesth Analg 2000;91:978–984.

117. Johansson T, Lisander B, Ivarsson I. Mild hypothermia does not increase blood loss during total hip arthroplasty. Acta Anaesthesiol Scand 1999;43:1005–1010.

118. Culver DH, Horan TC, Gaynes RP, et al. Surgical wound infection rates by wound class, operative procedure, and patient risk index. National Nosocomial Infections Surveillance System. Am J Med 1991;91:152S–157S.

119. Bremmelgaard A, Raahave D, Beir-Holgersen R, et al. Computer-aided surveillance of surgical infections and identification of risk factors. J Hosp Infect 1989;13: 1–18.

120. Haley RW, Culver DH, Morgan WM, et al. Identifying patients at high risk of surgical wound infection: a simple multivariate index of patient susceptibility and wound contamination. Am J Epidemiol 1985;121:206–215.

121. Leslie K, Sessler DI, Bjorksten A, et al. Propofol causes a dose-dependent decrease in the thermoregulatory threshold for vasoconstriction, but has little effect on sweating. Anesthesiology 1994;81:353–360.

122. Sessler DI, Rubinstein EH, Moayeri A. Physiological responses to mild perianesthetic hypothermia in humans. Anesthesiology 1991;75:594–610.

123. Chang N, Mathes SJ. Comparison of the effect of bacterial inoculation in musculocutaneous and random-pattern flaps. Plast Reconstr Surg 1982;70:1–10.

124. Jonsson K, Hunt TK, Mathes SJ. Oxygen as an isolated variable influences resistance to infection. Ann Surg 1988; 208:783–787.

125. van Oss CJ, Absolom DR, Moore LL, et al. Effect of temperature on the chemotaxis, phagocytic engulfment, digestion and O_2 consumption of human polymorphonuclear leukocytes. J Reticuloendothel Soc 1980;27:561–565.

126. Leijh CJ, Van den Barselaar MT, Van Zwet TL, et al. Kinetics of phagocytosis of Staphylococcus aureus and Escherichia coli by human granulocytes. Immunology 1979;37:453–465.

127. Prockop DJ, Kivirikko KI, Tuderman L, Guzman NA. The biosynthesis of collagen and its disorders: part one. N Engl J Med 1979;301:13–23.

128. De Jong L, Kemp A. Stoichiometry and kinetics of the prolyl 4-hydroxylase partial reaction. Biochim Biophys Acta 1984;787:105–111.

129. Hunt TK, Pai MP. Effect of varying ambient oxygen tensions on wound metabolism and collagen synthesis. Surg Gynecol Obstet 1972;135:257–260.

130. Jönsson K, Jensen JA, Goodson WH, et al. Tissue oxygenation, anemia, and perfusion in relation to wound healing in surgical patients. Ann Surg 1991;214:605–613.

131. Sheffield CW, Sessler DI, Hunt TK. Mild hypothermia during isoflurane anesthesia decreases resistance to E. coli dermal infection in guinea pigs. Acta Anaesthesiol Scand 1994;38:201–205.

132. Sheffield CW, Sessler DI, Hunt TK, Scheuenstuhl H. Mild hypothermia during halothane anesthesia decreases resistance to S. aureus dermal infection in guinea pigs. Wound Repair Regen 1994;2:48–56.

133. Kurz A, Sessler DI, Lenhardt RA. Study of wound infections and temperature group. Perioperative normothermia to reduce the incidence of surgical-wound infection and shorten hospitalization. N Engl J Med 1996;334: 1209–1215.

134. Flacke JW, Flacke WE. Inadvertent hypothermia: frequent, insidious, and often serious. Semin Anesth 1983;2:183–196.

135. Flacke W. Temperature regulation and anesthesia. Int Anesthesiol Clin 1963;2:43–54.

136. Guffin A, Girard D, Kaplan JA. Shivering following cardiac surgery: hemodynamic changes and reversal. J Cardiothorac Vasc Anesth 1987;1:24–28.

137. Just B, Delva E, Camus Y, Lienhart A. Oxygen uptake during recovery following naloxone. Anesthesiology 1992; 76:60–64.

138. Just B, Trévien V, Delva E, Lienhart A. Prevention of intraoperative hypothermia by preoperative skin-surface warming. Anesthesiology 1993;79:214–218.

139. Horn E-P, Sessler DI, Standl T, et al. Non-thermoregulatory shivering in patients recovering from isoflurane or desflurane anesthesia. Anesthesiology 1998; 89:878–886.

140. Horn E-P, Schroeder F, Wilhelm S, et al. Postoperative pain facilitates non-thermoregulatory tremor. Anesthesiology 1999;91:979–984.

141. Panzer O, Ghazanfari N, Sessler DI, et al. Shivering and shivering-like tremor during labor with and without epidural analgesia. Anesthesiology 1999;90:1609–1616.

142. Sharkey A, Lipton JM, Murphy MT, Giesecke AH. Inhibition of postanesthetic shivering with radiant heat. Anesthesiology 1987;66:249–252.

143. Ikeda T, Sessler DI, Tayefeh F, et al. Meperidine and alfentanil do not reduce the gain or maximum intensity of shivering. Anesthesiology 1998;88:858–865.

144. Kurz M, Belani K, Sessler DI, et al. Naloxone, meperidine, and shivering. Anesthesiology 1993;79:1193–1201.

145. Greif R, Laciny S, Rajek AM, et al. Neither nalbuphine nor atropine possess special antishivering activity. Anesth Analg 2001;93:620–627.

146. Delaunay L, Bonnet F, Duvaldestin P. Clonidine decreases postoperative oxygen consumption in patients recovering from general anaesthesia. Br J Anaesth 1991; 67:397–401.

147. Delaunay L, Bonnet F, Liu N, et al. Clonidine comparably decreases the thermoregulatory thresholds for vasoconstriction and shivering in humans. Anesthesiology 1993; 79:470–474.

148. Joris J, Banache M, Bonnet F, et al. Clonidine and ketanserin both are effective treatments for postanesthetic shivering. Anesthesiology 1993;79:532–539.

149. Kizilirmak S, Karakas SE, Akça O, et al. Magnesium sulfate stops postanesthetic shivering. Ann NY Acad Sci 1997; 813:799–806.

150. Singh P, Dimitriou V, Mahajan RP, Crossley AW. Double-blind comparison between doxapram and pethidine in the treatment of postanaesthetic shivering. Br J Anaesth 1993; 71:685–688.

151. Gautier H. Doxapram and shivering. Anaesthesia 1991; 46:1092–1093.

152. Sarma V, Fry EN. Doxapram after general anaesthesia. Its role in stopping shivering during recovery. Anaesthesia 1991;46:460–461.

153. Kranke P, Eberhart LH, Roewer N, Tramer MR. Pharmacological treatment of postoperative shivering: a quantitative systematic review of randomized controlled trials. Anesth Analg 2002;94:453–460.

154. De Witte J, Sessler DI. Perioperative shivering: physiology and pharmacology. Anesthesiology 2002;96:467–484.

155. Heier T, Caldwell JE, Sessler DI, Miller RD. Mild intraoperative hypothermia increases duration of action and spontaneous recovery of vecuronium blockade during nitrous oxide-isoflurane anesthesia in humans. Anesthesiology 1991;74:815–819.

156. Leslie K, Sessler DI, Bjorksten AR, Moayeri A. Mild hypothermia alters propofol pharmacokinetics and increases the duration of action of atracurium. Anesth Analg 1995;80:1007–1014.

157. Sessler DI. Complications and treatment of mild hypothermia. Anesthesiology 2001;95:531–543.

158. Roizen MF, Sohn YJ, L'Hommedieu CS, et al. Operating room temperature prior to surgical draping: effect on patient temperature in recovery room. Anesth Analg 1980;59:852–855.

159. Sessler DI, McGuire J, Sessler AM. Perioperative thermal insulation. Anesthesiology 1991;74:875–879.

160. Sessler DI, Schroeder M. Heat loss in humans covered with cotton hospital blankets. Anesth Analg 1993;77: 73–77.

161. Kurz A, Kurz M, Poeschl G, et al. Forced-air warming maintains intraoperative normothermia better than circulating-water mattresses. Anesth Analg 1993;77:89–95.

162. Gendron F. "Burns" occurring during lengthy surgical procedures. J Clin Eng 1980;5:20–26.

163. Gendron FG. Unexplained Patient Burns: Investigating Iatrogenic Injuries. Brea, CA: Quest Publishing; 1988.

164. Nesher N, Zisman E, Wolf T, et al. Strict thermoregulation attenuates myocardial injury during coronary artery bypass graft surgery as reflected by reduced levels of cardiac-specific troponin I. Anesth Analg 2003;96:328–335.

165. Hofer CK, Worn M, Tavakoli R, et al. Influence of body core temperature on blood loss and transfusion requirements during off-pump coronary artery bypass grafting: a comparison of 3 warming systems. J Thorac Cardiovasc Surg 2005;129:838–843.

166. Motta P, Mossad E, Toscana D, et al. Effectiveness of a circulating-water warming garment in rewarming after pediatric cardiac surgery using hypothermic cardiopulmonary bypass. J Cardiothorac Vasc Anesth 2004;18: 148–151.

167. Taguchi A, Ratnaraj J, Kabon B, et al. Effects of a circulating-water garment and forced-air warming on body heat content and core temperature. Anesthesiology 2004;100: 1058–1064.

168. Sessler DI. Consequences and treatment of perioperative hypothermia. Anesth Clin North Am 1994;12:425–456.

169. Presson RGJ, Bezruczko AP, Hillier SC, McNiece WL. Evaluation of a new fluid warmer effective at low to moderate flow rates. Anesthesiology 1993;78:974–980.

170. Vassilieff N, Rosencher N, Deriaz H, et al. Effect of premedication by nifedipine on intraoperative hypothermia. Ann Fr Anesth Réanim 1992;11:484–487.

171. Ikeda T, Ozaki M, Sessler DI, et al. Intraoperative phenylephrine infusion decreases the magnitude of redistribution hypothermia. Anesth Analg 1999;89:462–465.

172. Ikeda T, Kazama T, Sessler DI, et al. Induction of anesthesia with ketamine reduces the magnitude of redistribution hypothermia. Anesth Analg 2001;93:934–938.

173. Sessler DI, Schroeder M, Merrifield B, et al. Optimal duration and temperature of pre-warming. Anesthesiology 1995;82:674–681.

174. Hynson JM, Sessler DI, Moayeri A, et al. The effects of pre-induction warming on temperature and blood pressure during propofol/nitrous oxide anesthesia. Anesthesiology 1993;79:219–228.

175. Camus Y, Celva E, Sessler DI, Lienhart A. Pre-induction skin-surface warming minimizes intraoperative core hypothermia. J Clin Anesth 1995;7:384–388.

176. Horn EP, Schroeder F, Gottschalk A, et al. Active warming during cesarean delivery. Anesth Analg 2002;94: 409–414.

9
Postoperative Central Nervous System Dysfunction

Deborah J. Culley, Terri G. Monk, and Gregory Crosby

This chapter reviews common forms and causes of central nervous system (CNS) morbidity in the elderly after routine surgery and anesthesia. These include, in order of descending prevalence, delirium, prolonged postoperative cognitive dysfunction (POCD), and perioperative stroke. Although these same conditions are also common during and after cardiac surgery, we will not deal with those situations here because the contributing factors are somewhat different and cognitive morbidity after cardiac surgery is a topic unto itself. We begin with a brief overview of how the brain changes during healthy and pathologic aging because aging of the CNS is a prominent factor in determining susceptibility to cognitive and neurologic morbidity after surgery and anesthesia.

Central Nervous System Changes of Aging

Normal Aging

Healthy aging is associated with significant changes in the morphology, physiology, and biochemistry of the brain (Table 9-1). Brain size and weight inevitably decline with age. These changes begin in young adulthood but accelerate after age 60, resulting in a 15% decrease in the ratio of brain/skull volume in nonarians whereas ventricular volume triples.[1] There are also age-associated decreases in neuronal size, loss of complexity of the dendritic tree, and a reduced number of synapses.[2] In contrast, the physiology of the cerebral circulation appears to be remarkably normal in the healthy aged. Global cerebral blood flow (CBF) is decreased 10%–20% with advanced age, not because of "hardening of the arteries," but rather because there is less brain mass to perfuse.[3] Therefore, the lower CBF seems to be a consequence of reduced metabolic demand, not a cause of it. Hence, although CBF and cerebral metabolic rate decline progressively with age, they remain tightly coupled.[4] Similarly, cerebral

autoregulation and responsiveness to carbon dioxide/hypoxemia are reasonably well preserved.[5] Neurotransmitters do not fare as well. The range of neurotransmitter systems affected by aging is extensive; dopamine uptake sites, transporters, and levels are reduced, as are cortical serotonergic, α_2 and β_1, and +-aminobutyric acid binding sites, among others.[6] Markers of central cholinergic activity also decrease, which is a finding of particular significance because failure of cholinergic neurotransmission is a central feature of Alzheimer's disease.[7] Moreover, beginning at age 40 and continuing into late old age, there is reduced expression in the human brain of genes involved in learning and memory and neuronal survival.[8] Nevertheless, not all the news is bad. Dendritic complexity and growth can increase in cognitively normal octogenarians, suggesting that neuronal mechanisms involved in neural plasticity crucial for learning and memory are retained in the aged but healthy CNS.[2] Furthermore, consistent with this concept but counter to what many of us learned in medical school, the adult brain makes new neurons and this capability is preserved, albeit at reduced levels, into old age.[9,10] Thus, although it loses some of its capacity for plasticity, the healthy brain continues to adapt and mold to its environment into old age.

The real issue, however, is the degree to which these changes in brain morphology, physiology, and biochemistry affect brain function. Intellectual decline does not invariably accompany aging but it is common and there are some consistently observed changes.[11] Both reaction time and cognitive processing slow with age such that there is an inverse relationship between age and speed of motor performance, which becomes exaggerated with increasing task complexity.[12] In addition, "fluid" intelligence (i.e., the ability to dynamically evaluate, accommodate, and respond to novel environmental events) deteriorates. In contrast, vocabulary, math, and comprehension skills are reasonably well maintained, as is "crystallized" intelligence (i.e., accumulated knowledge), at least into the seventh decade of life. Not surprisingly,

TABLE 9-1. Neurobiologic changes of aging.

- **Decreased brain weight/volume**
  Cell shrinkage and loss
- **Decreased neurotransmitter system function**
  Acetylcholine, 5-hydroxytryptamine, dopamine, serotonin,
  γ aminobutyric acid, adrenergic, glutamate
- **Decreased neuronal gene expression**
- **Alzheimer-type changes**
  Amyloid plaques and neurofibrillary tangles

short-term memory dysfunction is reported by 30% to 50% of elders.[13] Much of this impairment is in working memory—which requires not only retention but also manipulation of information.[14] Thus, the ability to store recently processed information while simultaneously acquiring new data is compromised in the otherwise healthy aged brain.

Pathologic Aging

Unfortunately, not all brain aging is healthy or normal. With advanced age, the prevalence of dementia increases rapidly from 10% to 15% in persons aged 65 to nearly 50% at age 85.[11] Dementia is always a disease process and is characterized by a chronic, progressive decline in cognitive performance that interferes with all cognitive domains. Although pathologic brain aging can be caused by a number of systemic and neurologic disorders (e.g., stroke, Parkinson's disease), Alzheimer's disease is the most common.[15] The histopathologic hallmarks of Alzheimer's disease—neurofibrillary tangles, extracellular amyloid deposits, and neuritic plaques—are also seen in normal aging, albeit to a markedly lesser degree.[6,16] In the Alzheimer's brain, loss of brain mass occurs at 2.5 times the rate observed in healthy aging and neurotransmitter hypofunction is likewise more pronounced.[17] Accordingly, Alzheimer's dementia should be considered a major CNS and systemic illness; consistent with this perspective, the average lifespan from diagnosis to death is 3–4 years.[18]

From the perspective of CNS aging, therefore, the "take home" message is that the elderly are heterogeneous. There is no such thing as a "typical" older person and chronologic age is often not a predictor of cognitive capability. This makes studies of this population difficult and means that any attempt to evaluate changes in cognition should include evaluation of baseline cognitive performance.

Postoperative Central Nervous System Dysfunction

Delirium

Delirium is the most common form of cognitive impairment in hospitalized patients. It is an acute transient

organic brain syndrome characterized by disturbances of consciousness and cognition that develop over a relatively short period of time (hours to days) and fluctuate over the course of the day. Delirium can nonetheless be subtle enough that it is frequently underdiagnosed by health care providers. The diagnosis is based on Diagnostic and Statistical Manual-IV diagnostic criteria, which include disturbance of consciousness with altered awareness of the environment; reduced ability to focus, sustain or shift attention; and a change in cognition or development of perceptual disturbances that are not better accounted for by a preexisting, established, or evolving dementia.[19] Delirium is generally divided into three types: hyperactive, hypoactive, and mixed. Agitation, irritability, restlessness, and aggression characterize the hyperactive form whereas hypoactive delirium is typified by somnolence, latency in reaction and response to verbal stimulation, and psychomotor slowing. As noted above, the diagnosis can be difficult for nonpsychiatrists to make, meaning many cases go undetected. To aid medical personnel without psychiatric training in this regard, a simple, standardized assessment tool has been developed. That tool, the Confusion Assessment Method (CAM), is the most widely used instrument for diagnosing delirium because it has the benefits of ease, speed, reliability, and validity (Table 9-2).[20] A variant of the CAM, the CAM-ICU, has been validated for delirium assessment of intubated, nonverbal patients in an intensive care unit.[21]

Delirium is common in hospitalized elderly patients regardless of whether the hospitalization is for medical

TABLE 9-2. Confusion assessment method.*

1. Acute onset and fluctuating course
Is there evidence of an acute change in mental status from the patient's baseline?

AND

Did this behavior tend to come and go or increase and decrease in severity during the past day?

2. Inattention
Does the patient have difficulty focusing attention (i.e., easily distractible or having difficulty keeping track of what is being said)?

3. Disorganized thinking
Is the patient's speech disorganized or incoherent (rambling or irrelevant conversations, unclear or illogical flow of ideas, or unpredictable switching from subject to subject)?

4. Altered level of consciousness
Is the patient's level of consciousness alert (normal), vigilant (hyperalert), lethargic (drowsy, easily aroused), stuporous (difficult to arouse), or comatose (unarousable)?

Source: Adapted with permission from Inouye et al.[20]
*The diagnosis of delirium requires features 1 and 2 plus either 3 or 4.

or surgical reasons. It occurs as a comorbidity in 40% of elderly, hospitalized medical patients.[22] Postoperative delirium is also quite common in surgical patients but the reported incidence varies from 9% to 74%, probably reflecting differences in the study population, diagnostic criteria, and the methods of surveillance.[23–27] Delirium usually presents during postoperative days 1–4, often following a lucid interval. Postoperative delirium has traditionally been considered a temporary or transient phenomenon but it can last for days to weeks after the surgical procedure, extend hospital stay, increase costs, and may even be a marker for subsequent cognitive deterioration and predictor of higher mortality.

Conditions contributing to delirium can be divided into nonmodifiable and modifiable factors and there are clinical prediction algorithms that take these into account.[28] Among the former, age greater than 70 years, preexisting cognitive impairment, a history of delirium, depression, multiple comorbidities, and poor functional status are positive predictors for the development of postoperative delirium.[25,28–31] Also included in this category is the type of surgical procedure; organ transplantation, orthopedic, cardiac, thoracic, major vascular, and emergency surgery carry the greatest risk.[23] The duration of surgery, however, does not seem to be a risk factor.

The modifiable factors are more interesting because of the potential to intervene. Among the more obvious of these is the type of anesthesia but, surprisingly, the anesthetic technique does not seem to affect delirium risk.[23,27] Specifically, there is no benefit of regional anesthesia. However, certain anesthetic adjuvants such as benzodiazepines and anticholinergic drugs may increase the risk of postoperative delirium perhaps, at least in the latter case, by reducing further cholinergic neurotransmission in the already compromised elderly brain.[26,32,33] Thus, regardless of whether an elderly patient requires regional or general anesthesia, one should choose anesthetic adjuvants carefully and consider using an anticholinergic agent that does not readily cross the blood–brain barrier (e.g., glycopyrrolate) if such an agent is needed. The roles of perfusion pressure and oxygen delivery have also been investigated. Intraoperative hypotension may contribute to the development of postoperative delirium but not all studies agree.[23,34,35] For example, in elderly patients having knee surgery under epidural anesthesia, those randomly assigned to a mean arterial blood pressure (MAP) of 45–55 mm Hg were no more or less likely to develop postoperative delirium than those whose MAP was maintained between 55–70 mm Hg.[35] In a similar vein, there is evidence that low perioperative hematocrit is associated with development of postoperative delirium.[23] However, no studies have investigated whether blood transfusion decreases the incidence.[23] Hypoxia may in subtle ways also be a factor. That is, delirium may be a delayed manifestation of hypoxia, with nocturnal oxygen desaturation

by pulse oximetry on postoperative day 2 correlating with altered mental status on day 3.[36,37] Whether enhancing oxygen delivery with supplemental oxygen or blood transfusion reduces the incidence of delirium is another matter but hypoxemia is best avoided or treated.

Pain can be an important contributor to delirium in the postoperative period. Elderly, cognitively intact patients with undertreated postoperative pain are nine times more likely to develop delirium than those whose pain is adequately treated.[38] In fact, the specifics of pain treatment are less important so long as the pain is controlled.[26,39] Thus, in a study comparing intravenous fentanyl with epidural analgesia for management of postoperative pain after bilateral total knee replacement surgery, the incidence of postoperative delirium was similar.[26] Indeed, in the postoperative period, low but not high narcotic utilization is a factor in the development of delirium.[26,32,38] This is relevant because studies show that cognitively impaired patients receive only 30%–50% as much narcotic as cognitively intact patients. This suggests that suboptimal pain management in demented and delirious patients may contribute further to their cognitive deterioration.[38,40] Meperidine is an exception to this rule and should probably be avoided in geriatric patients because it has been associated with the development of postoperative delirium, presumably attributable either to accumulation of toxic metabolites or its anticholinergic activity.[32,38]

Perhaps the most important way to mitigate the risk of postoperative delirium is with attentive, careful medical management. This is because numerous medical complications including hypoxemia, sepsis, electrolyte and metabolic disturbances, cardiopulmonary events such as myocardial ischemia or pneumonia, and inadequate nutrition can trigger delirium.[37] As such, one should expeditiously identify and treat these complications. Medications can be another problem. More than six medications or three new inpatient medications have been shown to be precipitating factors for delirium, as have drugs with anticholinergic properties that cross the blood–brain barrier (i.e., atropine, scopolamine).[33,41,42] Hence, eliminating unnecessary or potentially toxic medications may be helpful. Another potentially beneficial intervention is ambulation. This is best studied in orthopedic surgical patients but, given evidence that even minimal exercise preserves cognition, is likely to be worthwhile for any bedridden hospitalized elderly person.[43–45] Accordingly, early ambulation may be an important and simple way to prevent postoperative delirium.

Delirium and Adverse Outcomes

Postoperative delirium is associated with significant morbidity and mortality.[25,28,31,46] The cost of care increases because of longer hospitalization and, reflecting a decline in activities of daily living, the patient must often be placed in a long-term care facility. Postoperative delirium may also be a predictor of subsequent dementia; in one small study of cognitively intact elderly patients, nearly 70% of those who developed postoperative delirium were demented 5 years later whereas only 20% of those who did not experience delirium became demented.[34] Moreover, 5-year mortality was 70% in the patients that had postoperative delirium whereas it was 35% in those who remained cognitively intact postoperatively.[34] Although it is unclear whether delirium triggers a dementing process or is simply a marker for preclinical dementia, it is apparent that postoperative delirium has important short- and long-term implications for the elderly patient.

Treatment/Prevention

Effective prevention and treatment of delirium is hampered by the fact that some risk factors (e.g., advanced age, preexisting cognitive impairment, type of surgical procedure) are not modifiable and by poor understanding of how the aged brain responds to the rigors of surgery, anesthesia, and hospitalization. Thus, the mainstay of treatment remains prompt diagnosis and treatment of the underlying medical conditions and/or discontinuation of unnecessary or toxic medications. Once this is done, attention should be directed toward creating a calm, quiet environment populated with the familiar faces of the patient's family and friends. Although scientific rationale for this recommendation is lacking, there is a growing body of evidence that a broad spectrum of preventative interventions may be modestly effective. Specifically, pre- and postoperative geriatric consultation decreases the incidence of delirium by as much as 30%, offering hope that relatively simple measures may be useful in decreasing the incidence and/or severity of postoperative delirium.[46,47] That said, there is no evidence that such programs improve the outcome of patients who still become delirious.

The role of medications in treating perioperative delirium is a controversial topic, with some experts arguing that pharmacologic intervention prolongs the delirious phase. Low-dose haloperidol is still considered the standard for treatment of hyperactive delirium but evidence for its efficacy is not as strong as one might like and atypical antipsychotics such as risperidone and olanzapine, although gaining in popularity, lack evidence from well-designed clinical studies to demonstrate superiority.[48,49] Before embarking on a course of pharmacotherapy, however, one should be aware of the unique pharmacology of psychoactive agents in the elderly. First, as mentioned previously, three or more new inpatient medications is an independent precipitating factor for delirium in hospitalized elderly persons.[42] This suggests that sometimes discontinuing medications is the best course of

action. Second, certain frequently used sedatives can actually increase delirium risk. Diphenhydramine, often prescribed for sleep or sedation in elderly hospitalized patients, nearly doubles the risk of delirium.[50] Meperidine, but not other opiates, nearly triples the risk.[32] Third, given the paucity of sound clinical evidence to guide the choice of pharmacologic agents for treating delirium in elderly postoperative patients and their greater susceptibility to psychoactive medications, some drugs are used inappropriately. Even atypical antipsychotics such as haloperidol, the mainstay of pharmacologic treatment of agitated delirium, are often given in dosages higher than those recommended for elderly patients and have a high incidence of extrapyramidal and anticholinergic side effects.[51] Lorazepam and other benzodiazepines, used for sedation or anxiolysis, have themselves been implicated in the development of delirium and can produce a paradoxic reaction of agitation and disinhibition.[51] Thus, pharmacotherapy has a place in the management in agitated delirium in the elderly postsurgical patient but one should resort to it only after seeking and treating remediable medical or pharmacologic causes of delirium and abiding by the geriatrician's adage to "start low and go slow."

Postoperative Cognitive Dysfunction

It has been suspected for more than 50 years that general anesthesia and surgery lead to cognitive dysfunction in the elderly.[52] Interest in the topic is increasing, driven partially by patients (or their family members) who often complain that the ability to think and concentrate is impaired for months after surgery and anesthesia.[53] Recent work justifies concern but we are still far from sure about the etiology of the problem.[54,55] What is clear is that the structural and functional changes associated with normal aging render the elderly more vulnerable to the development of mild POCD.[56]

Since Bedford, in a retrospective chart review, first reported in 1955 that general anesthesia produces long-term cognitive dysfunction in the elderly, there have been numerous subsequent studies of the problem.[52–54] Most are flawed or inconclusive because they lack a control group, did not perform formal neuropsychometric testing, or were small and retrospective. That changed in 1998 with publication of a large, prospective, controlled international study. The International Study of Postoperative Cognitive Dysfunction (ISPOCD1) included 1218 patients aged 60 years or older from 13 hospitals in eight European countries and the United States who underwent a variety of noncardiac, nonneurosurgical procedures plus 176 United Kingdom and 145 nonhospitalized, community controls.[57] Cognitive performance was assessed with a battery of neuropsychometric tests completed before surgery as well as 1 week and approximately 3 months after surgery. Using this design, nearly a quarter of elderly

TABLE 9-3. Incidence of cognitive dysfunction after surgery and general anesthesia in the elderly.

	Control (321)	Surgery and anesthesia (1218)
1 week postoperatively	3.4%	25.8%*
3 months postoperatively	2.8%	9.9%†

Source: Moller et al.[57]
*p < 0.01.
†p < 0.0001.

patients had cognitive deficits the first week after surgery and general anesthesia and, more remarkably, almost 10% were still impaired 3 months postoperatively (Table 9-3).[57] In contrast, only about 3% of the age-matched community controls were impaired.[57] A subsequent study of middle-aged patients (40–60 years) using similar methods and criteria for impairment found a slightly lower incidence of cognitive impairment during the first postoperative week (19%) but no residual deficit by objective testing at 3 months postoperatively (Table 9-4).[58] However, 29% of the patients felt subjectively impaired at 3 months, associated in many cases with depression. Together, these studies convincingly demonstrate that middle-aged and elderly patients experience short-term cognitive dysfunction after surgery and general anesthesia but that, judging by objective criteria, the elderly are uniquely vulnerable to persistent cognitive impairment. Further substantiating the age-dependence of POCD is the fact that incidence is highest among patients 75 years of age or older, with nearly 15% impaired at 3 months postoperatively.[57]

The natural history of POCD in the elderly has not been thoroughly studied but there is some encouraging news. The only follow-up study reevaluated 336 older adults and 47 controls from the English and Danish sites of the original ISPOCD1 study and found that 35 of the 336 tested (10.4%) still had cognitive dysfunction 1–2 years later.[59] However, among the 47 controls who had not been hospitalized, 10.6% (n = 5) also met criteria for POCD—an incidence similar to that of the surgery patients. Thus, in elderly persons, cognitive changes occur over time even when surgery is not performed. This emphasizes the importance of a control group in studies

TABLE 9-4. Incidence of cognitive dysfunction after surgery and general anesthesia in middle-aged patients.

	Control (183)	Surgery and anesthesia (463)
1 week postoperatively	4.0%	19.2%*
3 months postoperatively	4.1%	6.2%

Source: Johnson et al.[58]
*p < 0.001.

TABLE 9-5. Potential risk factors for postoperative cognitive dysfunction.

- **Patient**
  Age
  Educational level
  Mental health status
  Preoperative alcohol, benzodiazepine use
  Comorbidities
- **Physiology**
  Inadequate oxygen delivery (hypoxia, hypotension, hypocarbia, anemia)
- **Surgery**
  Inpatient versus outpatient
  Duration
  Type (cardiac/thoracic, orthopedic, major abdominal)
  Stress
  Immobility
- **Anesthesia**

investigating POCD and suggests that POCD is a reversible condition in the majority of elderly patients undergoing general surgery. That said, the small size of the study prevents firm conclusions and other considerations give reason for concern. First, of the 318 surgery patients who completed cognitive testing at each of the three time points postoperatively (discharge, 3 months, 1–2 years), three met criteria for POCD at every one. The likelihood that the same subject would meet criteria for POCD at all three times by chance is remote (1:64,000 or 0.0002%), making it probable that POCD is permanent in some persons. Second, 2-year follow-up may not be sufficient. In a prospective but uncontrolled study of cardiac surgery patients, for instance, the incidence of cognitive impairment decreased from 53% at hospital discharge to 24% at 6 months postoperatively but increased again to 42% by 5 years postoperatively.[60] Such longer-term follow-up of noncardiac patients with POCD is not yet available.

The search for causes of POCD and ways it might be prevented or treated is under way but is complicated by the fact that it is likely to be a complicated entity with numerous contributing factors. For the purposes of this review, we will group them into patient, surgical, physiologic, and anesthetic conditions (Table 9-5).

Patient Factors

Advanced age is the most consistent and least controversial risk factor for POCD in both cardiac and noncardiac surgery.[55,57,58,61] The close association between age and POCD implies that the normal and pathologic changes of brain aging contribute in an important way. The association between age and POCD is most clearly demonstrated by the ISPOCD investigations discussed above. The key difference between elderly and middle-aged patients in this regard is that objective impairment persists for at least 3 months in the former but not the latter.[57,58] Thus, POCD may be problematic for many adult patients early during recuperation, but it is primarily older patients who experience subtle cognitive dysfunction for a longer period of time.

Other putative patient-related risk factors include years of education, mental health, comorbid diseases, gender, and genetics. A low level of education predicts cognitive decline at 3 months after noncardiac surgery and, conversely, education seems to protect against cognitive decline after surgery involving cardiopulmonary bypass.[57,61] The reasons for this protective effect of formal education are unknown, but possibilities include greater "cognitive reserve," better test-taking abilities in the better educated, and known interrelationships between educational advancement, social support, and quality of medical care. The roles of preexisting mental health status and comorbid conditions in POCD are difficult to ascertain. In the ISPOCD studies, there was no association between functional status, as defined by American Society of Anesthesiologists physical status classification, and the development of POCD in elderly patients whereas it was a predictor of early POCD in middle-aged patients.[57,58] Similarly, whereas presurgical depression is associated with POCD in middle-aged patients, its contribution to POCD in the elderly has not been systematically evaluated.[58] The main reason data on these subjects are limited is that most studies of POCD exclude individuals who have major depression or anxiety disorders, multiple systemic disease, severe systemic illness, or perform below a certain cognitive level on screening measures.[57,58,62] Indeed, even when comorbidity is entered into the final multivariate analyses as a possible predictor, the indices and score range (e.g., Charlson Comorbidity Index) may be too insensitive to serve as a viable predictor of POCD.[63] The role of gender in POCD is also unresolved because the ISPOCD1 study found no differences in the incidence of POCD by gender[57] but evidence from cardiac surgery hints that it could be a factor under some circumstances. Thus, although the frequency of cognitive impairment after cardiac surgery is statistically equivalent between genders, women decline on tasks believed to depend more on the frontal lobes and right hemisphere and have worse functional outcome and decreased quality of life than men.[64,65] Likewise, women have a higher risk for perioperative neurologic deficits than men after cardiac surgery.[66] Finally, largely unexplored are genetic factors. The only gene investigated thus far is the apolipoprotein ε4 (apoE4) allele, a gene that has been associated with greater vulnerability of the brain to various insults such as Alzheimer's disease and head trauma.[67–69] Although no link with POCD risk was identified, more studies of this nature should be forthcoming because it is likely that certain patients are predisposed to POCD by virtue of their unique genetic profile.

Preoperative drug usage—particularly for alcohol and benzodiazepines—is another potentially important risk factor for POCD.[58] Here again, the data are mixed. In the elderly undergoing a major surgical procedure, there is no association between moderate preoperative alcohol consumption and susceptibility to POCD but, curiously, lack of preoperative alcohol consumption predicts early POCD in middle-aged patients and aged patients undergoing minor surgical procedures.[57,58,70] With respect to benzodiazepines, there was a favorable association between preoperative usage and protection against POCD 3 months postoperatively,[57] but this is likely attributable to a change in use of benzodiazepines postoperatively. Nearly half of the patients using benzodiazepines preoperatively in that study were no longer taking them 3 months postoperatively; among these, none met POCD criteria. In contrast, those patients still taking benzodiazepines 3 months postoperatively had an incidence of POCD similar to the study population as a whole. The most reasonable interpretation of these data is that discontinuation of benzodiazepines postoperatively, not preoperative usage, improves cognitive performance. The fact that there is also no correlation between blood concentration of benzodiazepines and POCD 1 week postoperatively[71] supports this conclusion.

Surgery/Illness Factors

Not surprisingly, the type, duration, and complexity of surgery seem to contribute to the risk of POCD. Thus, elderly patients undergoing minor surgical procedures have a lower incidence of both early and late POCD than those undergoing major procedures[57,70] and, even when controlling for the nature and duration of the surgical procedure, the incidence of early POCD is lowest in patients cared for on an outpatient versus inpatient basis.[70] This suggests that for minor surgical procedures, an outpatient setting may benefit the elderly and that postoperative hospitalization contributes importantly to development of POCD. Similarly, the duration of the procedure (and hence the anesthetic) has repeatedly been associated with development of POCD, such that risk is greater with longer procedures.[57,58]

The type of operation also matters, at least in middle-aged persons. In elderly patients, the incidence of POCD at either 1 week or 3 months postoperatively does not correlate with the type of surgical procedure but in middle-aged adults the incidence at 1 week is highest after upper abdominal (33%) and orthopedic surgery (20%).[57,58] The reasons for these associations are not known but proposed mechanisms include endotoxin release and cerebral emboli. Interleukin-6 and -8 increase during major abdominal surgery, perhaps because of bowel hypoperfusion or manipulation.[72] Interleukins, which act on the CNS, are peptide mediators of the systemic inflammatory cascade and are stimulated by endotoxin, a component of the gram-negative bacterial cell wall.[73] Although no studies have directly investigated the role of interleukins in POCD in general surgical patients, evidence from cardiac surgery shows that a low preoperative level of an antiendotoxin core antibody is associated with POCD.[73] This suggests that a reduced immune response to endotoxin may contribute to development of POCD. In the case of POCD after orthopedic surgery, indirect evidence suggests cerebral microemboli could be a culprit. Fatty emboli are common during certain orthopedic procedures (e.g., total knee replacement) and many reach the brain via paradoxical embolization through a patent foramen ovale or the pulmonary vasculature.[74,75] Although a plausible mechanism for cognitive decline in these patients, the hypothesis has not yet been systematically tested.

Surgery, and the associated illness requiring it, may also contribute to POCD indirectly. Surgery involves stress, loss of mobility, and oftentimes social isolation, each of which has been associated with cognitive deterioration in the elderly. For instance, chronically elevated plasma cortisol is associated with hippocampal atrophy and impaired cognitive performance.[76] Similarly, given substantial evidence that modest physical exercise and social involvement improves cognitive performance in both the healthy and cognitively impaired elderly,[43,44,77] it is easy to see how a stressed, relatively immobile, socially isolated elderly surgical patient may suffer cognitive consequences.

Physiologic Factors

Perhaps the oldest and most intuitive hypothesis is that perioperative hypoxia or hypotension has a role in the development of POCD. Unfortunately, POCD does not seem to be that simple. In particular, in the large international study, there was no correlation between perioperative hypotension (MAP <60% for ≥30 minutes) or hypoxia (SpO$_2$ ≤80 for >2 minutes) and POCD in the elderly.[57] Moreover, another study of elderly patients having knee arthroplasty under epidural anesthesia found no difference in cognitive outcome between those maintained at a MAP of 45–55 versus 55–70 mm Hg.[35] This is not to say that perioperative hypoxia or hypotension cannot cause significant CNS impairment—because we know it can—but rather that variations of the magnitude and duration that characterize routine, uncomplicated anesthesia do not seem to be responsible for the subtle but persistent perioperative cognitive changes that define POCD.

Other physiologic conditions that influence cerebral oxygenation have also been implicated but, again, with limited evidence. Anemia is one such factor. Anemia obviously occurs sometimes during surgery and is associated with changes in CBF and oxygenation in animals.[78]

Nevertheless, support for a link to cognitive dysfunction is indirect, coming mainly from evidence that isovolemic anemia to a hemoglobin concentration of 5–6 g/dL in healthy adults is associated with subtle changes in cognitive functioning and that normalizing hematocrit with erythropoietin in chronic renal failure patients improves cognitive performance.[79,80] For similar reasons (i.e., reduced cerebral oxygen delivery), there has been concern about inadvertent hyperventilation. Studies that have looked at this are too small to be conclusive but fail to identify an adverse effect of hyperventilation on cognition and even suggest that mild hypoventilation is worse in this regard than mild hyperventilation.[81]

Anesthetic Factors

Despite the fact that general anesthesia is obviously a form of profound CNS dysfunction, its role in prolonged cognitive impairment has received surprisingly little attention. There is clinical evidence that general anesthesia contributes to early POCD, with one study showing a higher incidence after general, as opposed to regional, anesthesia 1 week postoperatively[82] and several demonstrating an association between POCD and the duration of anesthesia.[57,58] Prolonged POCD is another matter. Some studies show that the risk of POCD is similar with regional or general anesthesia. For instance, the frequency of cognitive impairment 6 months postoperatively was similar (4%–6%) between epidural and general anesthesia in elderly patients undergoing total knee replacement, but the study lacked a concurrent control.[62] Moreover, intravenous sedation is often used to supplement regional anesthetic techniques, making it difficult to isolate the influence of anesthesia itself in most, but not all, such studies.[62,82] To complicate matters further, there is a strong association of supplementary epidural anesthesia/analgesia and POCD 1 week postoperatively in middle-aged patients.[58] Whether this is a feature of intraoperative use of the epidural or accumulation of local anesthetic in the blood or cerebrospinal fluid because of continuous postoperative epidural infusion is unclear, but it emphasizes the sensitivity of the brain to even seemingly minor pharmacologic interventions.

The only studies that have examined the long-term effects of general anesthesia without surgery on learning and memory have been performed in animals. Most, but not all of them, demonstrate long-lasting impairment. One recent study in aged mice found no persistent memory impairment after isoflurane anesthesia but they were also unable to detect well-known differences between young and old animals in this regard, indicating the behavioral paradigm used was probably not capable of detecting more subtle anesthesia-induced changes.[83] In contrast, several studies in aged rats with isoflurane–nitrous oxide and isoflurane alone, demonstrate spatial learning impairment for weeks after general anesthesia without surgery.[84–86] This was true for a task that was partially learned beforehand as well as for one testing acquisition of entirely new memory. These results may have implications for understanding POCD. Because the agents are long cleared from the brain by the time behavioral testing was begun 48 h to 2 weeks after anesthesia, the data imply that general anesthesia alters the brain in some lasting way. There is some biochemical support for this notion; the profile of protein expression in the brain is changed for at least 72 hours after general anesthesia in rats.[87] There is also emerging evidence that some general anesthetics (e.g., ketamine, nitrous oxide) can be toxic to the brain during certain phases of the lifespan, including old age, producing vacuolation, swelling, and programmed cell death of neurons.[88–91] Additionally, based on recent work in cell culture, it seems that some general anesthetics may increase the cytotoxicity of β-amyloid, a protein implicated in the pathogenesis of Alzheimer's disease but also present in the normally aging brain.[92] Although the relevance of this information to the genesis of POCD is the subject of debate, it is conceivable—but not yet firmly established—that general anesthetics may contribute to lingering postoperative cognitive impairment in the elderly.[90,93]

In summary, one can say that POCD occurs commonly during the early weeks and months after surgery and anesthesia. The etiology of POCD is likely to be multifactorial and the relative contributions of age- and disease-related processes, surgery, physiologic perturbations, anesthesia, and hospitalization are still unclear. Longitudinal studies using age- and disease-matched control groups will be necessary to clarify the long-term impact of surgery on patients' ultimate cognitive health and such investigations will best be accomplished through collaborative efforts of anesthesiologists, surgeons, neuropsychologists, and geriatricians. Until then, because the fundamental mechanisms are uncertain, it is difficult to identify prevention or treatment strategies. In particular, there is presently no scientific basis for recommending (or avoiding) a specific anesthetic agent or technique in this regard. This will change as further research is conducted on this common, subtle, and troubling complication. In the meantime, it is reassuring that the prognosis for recovery from POCD seems to be good.

Perioperative Stroke

The development of a stroke after routine surgery is uncommon and seldom expected. Although the elderly represent a high-risk group for this devastating adverse perioperative outcome, questions remain as to whether perioperative stroke is a random event or one provoked by perioperative management or altered physiology.

TABLE 9-6. Risk factors for perioperative stroke.

- Age
- Cardiac disease
- Peripheral vascular disease
- Hypertension
- Smoking
- Previous cerebrovascular insult

There is a growing body of evidence indicating that the risk of stroke increases in the perioperative period but that the etiology is often unknown. One large retrospective, case-control study reported that the risk of ischemic stroke during the first 30 days after routine anesthesia and surgery is three times that of nonsurgical controls.[94] Several smaller studies report similar data, with most placing the elderly at substantially greater risk.[95–97] In one retrospective study involving patients undergoing general surgical procedures, the overall incidence of perioperative stroke was 0.07% but the risk was 0.22% when only patients over age 65 were considered.[95] The greater risk of perioperative stroke in the elderly is presumably explained by the prevalence of age-related risk factors for stroke such as a history of stroke, hypertension, smoking, peripheral vascular and cardiac disease, and aspirin or anticoagulant use (Table 9-6).[97,98–101] Nonetheless, whereas the risk of stroke seems to be greater in the perioperative period, conditions that predispose elderly surgical patients to it are not obvious.[95,96]

Factors that have been considered include preexisting cerebrovascular disease, hypotension, and thromboembolic events. As for cerebrovascular disease, there is good agreement that an asymptomatic carotid bruit, which is present in 14% of surgical patients 55 years or older and 20% of vascular surgical patients, is not itself a risk factor for perioperative stroke.[102–104] Hence, elective general surgical procedures probably need not be delayed in individuals without symptoms of focal cerebral ischemia but such individuals should be referred for subsequent evaluation because carotid endarterectomy may reduce long-term stroke risk.[98,105–107] Relationships between symptomatic cerebrovascular disease and perioperative stroke are controversial. There has been disagreement as to whether transient ischemic events, which are predictors of stroke in the general patient population, are also associated with a higher incidence of perioperative stroke.[108,109] However, it is often recommended that patients undergoing elective general surgical procedures with symptomatic carotid stenosis and a greater than 70% arterial narrowing be evaluated preoperatively for possible carotid endarterectomy or stenting.[106] At the other extreme, prior stroke does increase the risk of perioperative cerebral reinfarction. In a small study, stroke was 5–10 times more common in those patients with a history of stroke.[96] The reasons for greater vulnerability to perioperative reinfarction after a previous stroke are unknown but may relate to a prolonged period of altered cerebrovascular reactivity after a stroke and known alterations in cerebral autoregulation and carbon dioxide reactivity in vessels distal to a carotid stenosis.[110,111] After an acute cerebral ischemic event, the clinical and radiographic picture evolves over days to weeks, indicating that stroke is not a static event and suggesting that there may be an interval of special vulnerability to physiologic perturbations. Perhaps for this reason, it may be prudent to defer elective surgery after a stroke but there is no demonstrated benefit of doing so and no consensus on the optimal timing of elective surgery in patients with a recent ischemic stroke.[104]

Hypotension is another potential cause of perioperative stroke. Certainly there is no question that hypotension can produce cerebral ischemia and infarction if it is severe and prolonged.[112] That said, retrospective analyses indicate that most patients who had a stroke postoperatively experienced hypotension intraoperatively and yet emerged from anesthesia without a neurologic deficit.[95,98] Furthermore, in cases in which perioperative hypotension is proposed as an inciting event, there may be a long asymptomatic interval between the hypotensive episode and the stroke.[101] Thus, at levels of hypotension frequently encountered in routine clinical situations, a cause-and-effect relationship between hypotension and stroke is often difficult to establish, in part because the consequences may be delayed and occur by as yet unknown mechanisms.

Further confusing the story of hypotension and cerebral ischemia are results of an old underpowered study that deliberately exposed conscious patients with transient ischemic attacks to as much as a 60% decrease in systolic blood pressure.[113] Despite such profound, transient hypotension, no patient had a stroke and only one had a true transient ischemic attack, even though most developed unrelated focal signs or evidence of global cerebral ischemia. Also, as described earlier, induced hypotension (MAP 45–55 versus 55–70 mm Hg) during epidural anesthesia in elderly patients was not associated with either stroke or a higher incidence of cognitive impairment.[35] Although underpowered for a rare event such as stroke, assuming that cerebral infarction occurs at lower levels of perfusion than deterioration in cognitive performance, the data support the idea that the aged brain tolerates a moderate and transient reduction in perfusion pressure relatively well. However, in hypertensive patients, strokes have been precipitated by a rapid, pharmacologically induced, moderate blood pressure reduction, suggesting that there may be a vulnerable patient population that has not been clearly defined.[114] Accordingly, although it is difficult to prove that transient intraoperative hypotension is benign, there is also little evidence to establish a cause-and-effect relationship

between transient intraoperative hypotension and perioperative stroke.

Indeed, in most cases, perioperative stroke is attributable to thrombotic or embolic events.[101] The risk of this type of stroke may be related to common perioperative complications including cardiac arrhythmias, withholding antithrombotic therapy, and hypercoagulability related to surgery and anesthesia. Dissection and/or thrombosis of the carotid or vertebral arteries have been reported perioperatively, ostensibly in conjunction with malpositioning of the neck.[99] Similar neurologic catastrophes are also reported after common activities such as coughing or sneezing, however, so the relationship to positioning is speculative at best. With respect to embolic events, one retrospective review found that cardiogenic embolism accounted for 40% of perioperative strokes and the majority of these occurred postoperatively.[95] An antecedent myocardial infarction was present in 17% of the patients and 33% were in atrial fibrillation at the time of the stroke. Moreover, perioperative embolic phenomena may be more common than previously appreciated, at least in certain procedures. Tourniquet deflation during total knee replacement is associated with venous and cerebral embolization in a large percentage of patients even if they do not have a patent foramen ovale or atrial or ventricular septal defect.[74,75] Perioperative changes in coagulation are also theorized to have a role because alterations in plasma concentrations of coagulation factors, platelet number and function, and altered fibrinolysis are well documented and may produce a hypercoagulable state.[100]

Neurologic consultation and additional diagnostic procedures should be sought expediently if a new and persistent focal neurologic deficit is identified in the perioperative period. Early detection becomes important as promising new therapeutic modalities to reverse or minimize the permanent consequences of injury are tested. Accordingly, the history should be carefully reviewed and a through neurologic examination performed. In view of the high incidence of embolic stroke, an echocardiogram can be diagnostically useful. Precordial echocardiograms are not reliable for detecting a patent foramen ovale and passage of surgical debris through the pulmonary veins is well documented.[74] Hence, a negative study does not eliminate the possibility of a perioperative paradoxical embolism.[95,115,116] Computed tomography and magnetic resonance imaging have long been used to provide information about infarct type, size, and location but until recently ischemic areas were not identifiable radiographically for hours to days after an event. This has changed with newer diagnostic modalities such as perfusion and diffusion weighted magnetic resonance imaging, which permit the detection of cerebral ischemia within a few hours after the onset of neurologic symptoms.[117]

If an acute stroke is diagnosed, care should conform to guidelines recently established by the American Heart Association.[118,119] Defining the type of stroke (ischemic versus hemorrhagic) is essential because certain aspects of management are quite different.[118,119] The emphasis in both cases is on good physiologic management because more specific "protective" measures have proven ineffective.[120–122] Thus, the ABCs (airway, breathing, circulation) of basic life support, including supplemental oxygen until the diagnosis is confirmed and/or endotracheal intubation as necessary for hypoxia, hypercarbia, or prevention of aspiration, are crucial.[118,119] The guidelines for blood pressure management differ markedly for patients with hemorrhagic and ischemic stroke.[118,119] In the former, assuming a history of hypertension, it is recommended that MAP be maintained between 90–130 mm Hg.[119] In contrast, a more cautious approach is recommended for patients with ischemic stroke, with antihypertensives given only when systolic blood pressure is >220 mm Hg or diastolic pressure is >120 mm Hg.[118] Likewise, if intracranial pressure monitoring is available, cerebral perfusion pressure should be maintained above 70 mm Hg with osmotherapy, hyperventilation ($PaCO_2$ 30–35 mm Hg), sedatives, and neuromuscular blocking agents as needed. Fever should be treated with antipyretics and hypovolemia and hyperglycemia avoided.[118,119] As already noted, although the search for an effective stroke treatment has been extensive, no neuroprotective agent has proven effective.[123] Thus, none is recommended for treatment of acute stroke. However, there is a correlation between administration of benzodiazepines, dopamine antagonists, α-2 agonists, α-1 antagonists, and phenytoin or phenobarbital in the first 28 days after stroke and adverse neurologic outcome.[124] Although use of such drugs may be a marker for illness severity, these data caution that common drugs may have unanticipated neurologic consequences among patients with cerebral ischemia and that unnecessary pharmacotherapy should be avoided.

The greatest advance in stroke management in recent years is the realization that stroke can be treated. Whereas treatment of stroke was simply supportive and rehabilitative in the past (with the exception of hyperbaric therapy for treatment of air emboli), today stroke is considered a medical emergency.[125] The main impetus for this important change in thinking is the success of low-molecular-weight heparin and thrombolytics for acute ischemic stroke.[126] Several studies demonstrate that tissue plasminogen activator administered within 3 hours improves overall neurologic outcome.[127] Although the safety of thrombolytics and heparins in the treatment of the surgical patient with acute stroke has not been established and the risk of hemorrhage remains a concern, there are reports of safe and successful administration of these agents in the acute postoperative setting.[128] Thus, although stroke is a rare and unpredictable complication

of anesthesia and surgery, it is important to make the diagnosis expediently because, for the first time, there is real potential for effective treatment and promptness of treatment is an important factor.

Conclusion

The aged brain is different from the young brain in many respects, making elders more vulnerable to common perioperative complications such as POCD, delirium, and stroke. With the population aging, the challenge for the decades ahead is to better understand the role of surgery and anesthesia in causation of these complications so that perioperative physicians can tailor care for the elderly patient with the aged brain in mind.

References

1. Coffey CE, Wilkinson WE, Parashos IA, et al. Quantitative cerebral anatomy of the aging human brain: a cross-sectional study using magnetic resonance imaging. Neurology 1992;42(3 Pt 1):527–536.
2. Selkoe DJ. Aging brain, aging mind. Sci Am 1992;267(3): 134–142.
3. Davis SM, Ackerman RH, Correia JA, et al. Cerebral blood flow and cerebrovascular CO_2 reactivity in stroke-age normal controls. Neurology 1983;33(4):391–399.
4. Bentourkia M, Bol A, Ivanoiu A, et al. Comparison of regional cerebral blood flow and glucose metabolism in the normal brain: effect of aging. J Neurol Sci 2000; 181(1–2):19–28.
5. Carey BJ, Panerai RB, Potter JF. Effect of aging on dynamic cerebral autoregulation during head-up tilt. Stroke 2003; 34(8):1871–1875.
6. Mrak RE, Griffin ST, Graham DI. Aging-associated changes in human brain. J Neuropathol Exp Neurol 1997; 56(12):1269–1275.
7. Francis PT, Palmer AM, Snape M, Wilcock GK. The cholinergic hypothesis of Alzheimer's disease: a review of progress. J Neurol Neurosurg Psychiatry 1999;66(2):\137–147.
8. Lu T, Pan Y, Kao SY, et al. Gene regulation and DNA damage in the ageing human brain. Nature 2004;429(6994): 883–891.
9. Eriksson PS, Perfilieva E, Bjork-Eriksson T, et al. Neurogenesis in the adult human hippocampus. Nat Med 1998; 4(11):1313–1317.
10. Shors TJ, Miesegaes G, Beylin A, Zhao M, Rydel T, Gould E. Neurogenesis in the adult is involved in the formation of trace memories. Nature 2001;410(6826):372–376.
11. Keefover RW. Aging and cognition. Neurol Clin 1998; 16(3):635–648.
12. Morris JC, McManus DQ. The neurology of aging: normal versus pathologic change. Geriatrics 1991;46(8):47–54.
13. Compton DM, Bachman LD, Brand D, Avet TL. Age associated changes in cognitive function in highly educated adults: emerging myths and realities. Int J Geriatr Psychiatry 2000;15(1):75–85.

14. Gilbert DK, Rogers WA. Age-related differences in the acquisition, utilization, and extension of a spatial mental model. J Gerontol B Psychol Sci Soc Sci 1999;54(4):246–255.

15. Richards SS, Hendrie HC. Diagnosis, management, and treatment of Alzheimer disease: a guide for the internist. Arch Intern Med 1999;159(8):789–798.

16. Growdon JH. Biomarkers of Alzheimer disease. Arch Neurol 1999;56(3):281–283.

17. Jack CR Jr, Petersen RC, Xu Y, et al. Rate of medial temporal lobe atrophy in typical aging and Alzheimer's disease. Neurology 1998;51(4):993–999.

18. Wolfson C, Wolfson DB, Asgharian M, et al. A reevaluation of the duration of survival after the onset of dementia. N Engl J Med 2001;344(15):1111–1116.

19. Diagnostics and Statistical Manual of Mental Disorders—Text Revision. Washington, DC: American Psychiatric Association; 2000.

20. Inouye SK, van Dyck CH, Alessi CA, Balkin S, Siegal AP, Horwitz RI. Clarifying confusion: the confusion assessment method. A new method for detection of delirium. Ann Intern Med 1990;113(12):941–948.

21. Ely EW, Inouye SK, Bernard GR, et al. Delirium in mechanically ventilated patients: validity and reliability of the confusion assessment method for the intensive care unit (CAM-ICU). JAMA 2001;286(21):2703–2710.

22. Sandberg O, Gustafson Y, Brannstrom B, Bucht G. Clinical profile of delirium in older patients. J Am Geriatr Soc 1999;47(11):1300–1306.

23. Marcantonio ER, Goldman L, Orav EJ, Cook EF, Lee TH. The association of intraoperative factors with the development of postoperative delirium. Am J Med 1998;105(5):380–384.

24. Zakriya K, Sieber FE, Christmas C, Wenz JF Sr, Franckowiak S. Brief postoperative delirium in hip fracture patients affects functional outcome at three months. Anesth Analg 2004;98(6):1798–1802.

25. Litaker D, Locala J, Franco K, Bronson DL, Tannous Z. Preoperative risk factors for postoperative delirium. Gen Hosp Psychiatry 2001;23(2):84–89.

26. Williams-Russo P, Urquhart BL, Sharrock NE, Charlson ME. Post-operative delirium: predictors and prognosis in elderly orthopedic patients. J Am Geriatr Soc 1992;40(8):759–767.

27. Dyer CB, Ashton CM, Teasdale TA. Postoperative delirium. A review of 80 primary data-collection studies. Arch Intern Med 1995;155(5):461–465.

28. Marcantonio ER, Goldman L, Mangione CM, et al. A clinical prediction rule for delirium after elective noncardiac surgery. JAMA 1994;271(2):134–139.

29. Galanakis P, Bickel H, Gradinger R, Von GS, Forstl H. Acute confusional state in the elderly following hip surgery: incidence, risk factors and complications. Int J Geriatr Psychiatry 2001;16(4):349–355.

30. Zakriya KJ, Christmas C, Wenz JF Sr, Franckowiak S, Anderson R, Sieber FE. Preoperative factors associated with postoperative change in confusion assessment method score in hip fracture patients. Anesth Analg 2002;94(6):1628–1632.

31. Weed HG, Lutman CV, Young DC, Schuller DE. Preoperative identification of patients at risk for delirium after major head and neck cancer surgery. Laryngoscope 1995;105(10):1066–1068.

32. Marcantonio ER, Juarez G, Goldman L, et al. The relationship of postoperative delirium with psychoactive medications. JAMA 1994;272(19):1518–1522.

33. Tune L, Carr S, Cooper T, Klug B, Golinger RC. Association of anticholinergic activity of prescribed medications with postoperative delirium. J Neuropsychiatry Clin Neurosci 1993;5(2):208–210.

34. Lundstrom M, Edlund A, Bucht G, Karlsson S, Gustafson Y. Dementia after delirium in patients with femoral neck fractures. J Am Geriatr Soc 2003;51(7):1002–1006.

35. Williams-Russo P, Sharrock NE, Mattis S, et al. Randomized trial of hypotensive epidural anesthesia in older adults. Anesthesiology 1999;91(4):926–935.

36. Rosenberg J, Kehlet H. Postoperative mental confusion—association with postoperative hypoxemia. Surgery 1993;114(1):76–81.

37. Aakerlund LP, Rosenberg J. Postoperative delirium: treatment with supplementary oxygen. Br J Anaesth 1994;72(3):286–290.

38. Morrison RS, Magaziner J, Gilbert M, et al. Relationship between pain and opioid analgesics on the development of delirium following hip fracture. J Gerontol A Biol Sci Med Sci 2003;58(1):76–81.

39. Lynch EP, Lazor MA, Gellis JE, Orav J, Goldman L, Marcantonio ER. The impact of postoperative pain on the development of postoperative delirium. Anesth Analg 1998;86(4):781–785.

40. Adunsky A, Levy R, Mizrahi E, Arad M. Exposure to opioid analgesia in cognitively impaired and delirious elderly hip fracture patients. Arch Gerontol Geriatr 2002;35(3):245–251.

41. Han L, McCusker J, Cole M, Abrahamowicz M, Primeau F, Elie M. Use of medications with anticholinergic effect predicts clinical severity of delirium symptoms in older medical inpatients. Arch Intern Med 2001;161(8):1099–1105.

42. Inouye SK, Charpentier PA. Precipitating factors for delirium in hospitalized elderly persons. Predictive model and interrelationship with baseline vulnerability. JAMA 1996;275(11):852–857.

43. Weuve J, Kang JH, Manson JE, Breteler MM, Ware JH, Grodstein F. Physical activity, including walking, and cognitive function in older women. JAMA 2004;292(12):1454–1461.

44. Heyn P, Abreu BC, Ottenbacher KJ. The effects of exercise training on elderly persons with cognitive impairment and dementia: a meta-analysis. Arch Phys Med Rehabil 2004;85(10):1694–1704.

45. Kamel HK, Iqbal MA, Mogallapu R, Maas D, Hoffmann RG. Time to ambulation after hip fracture surgery: relation to hospitalization outcomes. J Gerontol A Biol Sci Med Sci 2003;58(11):1042–1045.

46. Marcantonio ER, Flacker JM, Michaels M, Resnick NM. Delirium is independently associated with poor functional recovery after hip fracture. J Am Geriatr Soc 2000;48(6):618–624.

47. Marcantonio ER, Flacker JM, Wright RJ, Resnick NM. Reducing delirium after hip fracture: a randomized trial. J Am Geriatr Soc 2001;49(5):516–522.
48. Mittal D, Jimerson NA, Neely EP, et al. Risperidone in the treatment of delirium: results from a prospective open-label trial. J Clin Psychiatry 2004;65(5):662–667.
49. Han CS, Kim YK. A double-blind trial of risperidone and haloperidol for the treatment of delirium. Psychosomatics 2004;45(4):297–301.
50. Agostini JV, Leo-Summers LS, Inouye SK. Cognitive and other adverse effects of diphenhydramine use in hospitalized older patients. Arch Intern Med 2001;161(17): 2091–2097.
51. Carnes M, Howell T, Rosenberg M, Francis J, Hildebrand C, Knuppel J. Physicians vary in approaches to the clinical management of delirium. J Am Geriatr Soc 2003;51(2): 234–239.
52. Bedford PD. Adverse cerebral effects of anaesthesia on old people. Lancet 1955;269:259–263.
53. Dijkstra JB, Jolles J. Postoperative cognitive dysfunction versus complaints: a discrepancy in long-term findings. Neuropsychol Rev 2002;12(1):1–14.
54. Dodds C, Allison J. Postoperative cognitive deficit in the elderly surgical patient. Br J Anaesth 1998;81(3):449–462.
55. Rasmussen LS, Siersma VD. Postoperative cognitive dysfunction: true deterioration versus random variation. Acta Anaesthesiol Scand 2004;48(9):1137–1143.
56. Crosby G, Culley DJ. Anesthesia, the aging brain, and the surgical patient. Can J Anaesth 2003;50:R1–R5.
57. Moller JT, Cluitmans P, Rasmussen LS, et al. Long-term postoperative cognitive dysfunction in the elderly ISPOCD1 study. ISPOCD investigators. International Study of Post-Operative Cognitive Dysfunction. Lancet 1998;351(9106):857–861.
58. Johnson T, Monk T, Rasmussen LS, et al. Postoperative cognitive dysfunction in middle-aged patients. Anesthesiology 2002;96(6):1351–1357.
59. Abildstrom H, Rasmussen LS, Rentowl P, et al. Cognitive dysfunction 1–2 years after non-cardiac surgery in the elderly. ISPOCD group. International Study of Post-Operative Cognitive Dysfunction. Acta Anaesthesiol Scand 2000;44(10):1246–1251.
60. Newman MF, Kirchner JL, Phillips-Bute B, et al. Longitudinal assessment of neurocognitive function after coronary-artery bypass surgery. N Engl J Med 2001;344(6): 395–402.
61. Newman MF, Croughwell ND, Blumenthal JA, et al. Predictors of cognitive decline after cardiac operation. Ann Thorac Surg 1995;59:1326–1330.
62. Williams-Russo P, Sharrock NE, Mattis S, Szatrowski TP, Charlson ME. Cognitive effects after epidural vs general anesthesia in older adults. A randomized trial. JAMA 1995;274(1):44–50.
63. Charlson ME, Pompei P, Ales KL, MacKenzie CR. A new method of classifying prognostic comorbidity in longitudinal studies: development and validation. J Chronic Dis 1987;40(5):373–383.
64. Hogue CW, Lillie R, Hershey T, et al. Gender influence on cognitive function after cardiac operation. Ann Thorac Surg 2003;76(4):1119–1125.
65. Phillips BB, Mathew J, Blumenthal JA, et al. Female gender is associated with impaired quality of life 1 year after coronary artery bypass surgery. Psychosom Med 2003;65(6): 944–951.
66. Hogue CW Jr, Sundt T III, Barzilai B, Schecthman KB, Vila-Roman VG. Cardiac and neurologic complications identify risks for mortality for both men and women undergoing coronary artery bypass graft surgery. Anesthesiology 2001;95(5):1074–1078.
67. Bennett DA, Wilson RS, Schneider JA, et al. Apolipoprotein E epsilon4 allele, AD pathology, and the clinical expression of Alzheimer's disease. Neurology 2003;60(2): 246–252.
68. Sundstrom A, Marklund P, Nilsson LG, et al. APOE influences on neuropsychological function after mild head injury: within-person comparisons. Neurology 2004;62(11): 1963–1966.
69. Abildstrom H, Christiansen M, Siersma VD, Rasmussen LS. Apolipoprotein E genotype and cognitive dysfunction after noncardiac surgery. Anesthesiology 2004;101(4):855–861.
70. Canet J, Raeder J, Rasmussen LS, et al. Cognitive dysfunction after minor surgery in the elderly. Acta Anaesthesiol Scand 2003;47(10):1204–1210.
71. Rasmussen LS, Steentoft A, Rasmussen H, Kristensen PA, Moller JT. Benzodiazepines and postoperative cognitive dysfunction in the elderly. ISPOCD Group. International Study of Postoperative Cognitive Dysfunction. Br J Anaesth 1999;83(4):585–589.
72. Lu CH, Chao PC, Borel CO, et al. Preincisional intravenous pentoxifylline attenuating perioperative cytokine response, reducing morphine consumption, and improving recovery of bowel function in patients undergoing colorectal cancer surgery. Anesth Analg 2004;99(5): 1465–1471.
73. Hindman BJ. Emboli, inflammation, and CNS impairment: an overview. Heart Surg Forum 2002;5(3):249–253.
74. Sulek CA, Davies LK, Enneking FK, Gearen PA, Lobato EB. Cerebral microembolism diagnosed by transcranial Doppler during total knee arthroplasty: correlation with transesophageal echocardiography. Anesthesiology 1999; 91(3):672–676.
75. Ogino Y, Tatsuoka Y, Matsuoka R, et al. Cerebral infarction after deflation of a pneumatic tourniquet during total knee replacement. Anesthesiology 1999;90(1):297–298.
76. Lupien SJ, de Leon M, de Santi S, et al. Cortisol levels during human aging predict hippocampal atrophy and memory deficits. Nat Neurosci 1998;1(1):69–73.
77. Bassuk SS, Glass TA, Berkman LF. Social disengagement and incident cognitive decline in community-dwelling elderly persons. Ann Intern Med 1999;131(3):165–173.
78. Morimoto Y, Mathru M, Martinez-Tica JF, Zornow MH. Effects of profound anemia on brain tissue oxygen tension, carbon dioxide tension, and pH in rabbits. J Neurosurg Anesthesiol 2001;13(1):33–39.
79. Weiskopf RB, Kramer JH, Viele M, et al. Acute severe isovolemic anemia impairs cognitive function and memory in humans. Anesthesiology 2000;92(6):1646–1652.
80. Pickett JL, Theberge DC, Brown WS, Schweitzer SU, Nissenson AR. Normalizing hematocrit in dialysis patients

improves brain function. Am J Kidney Dis 1999;33(6): 1122–1130.

81. Linstedt U, Meyer O, Berkau A, Kropp P, Zenz M, Maier C. Does intraoperative hyperventilation improve neurological functions of older patients after general anaesthesia? Anaesthesist 2002;51(6):457–462.

82. Rasmussen LS, Johnson T, Kuipers HM, et al. Does anaesthesia cause postoperative cognitive dysfunction? A randomised study of regional versus general anaesthesia in 438 elderly patients. Acta Anaesthesiol Scand 2003;47(3): 260–266.

83. Butterfield NN, Graf P, Ries CR, MacLeod BA. The effect of repeated isoflurane anesthesia on spatial and psychomotor performance in young and aged mice. Anesth Analg 2004;98(5):1305–1311.

84. Culley DJ, Yukhananov R, Baxter MG, Crosby G. The memory effects of general anesthesia persist for weeks in young and aged rats. Anesth Analg 2003;96(4):1004–1009.

85. Culley DJ, Yukhananov R, Baxter MG, Crosby G. Long-term impairment of acquisition of a spatial memory task following isoflurane-nitrous oxide anesthesia in rats. Anesthesiology 2004;100:309–314.

86. Culley DJ, Yukhananov R, Baxter MG, Crosby G. Impaired acquisition of spatial memory two weeks after isoflurane and isoflurane-nitrous oxide anesthesia in aged rats. Anesth Analg 2004;99:1393–1397.

87. Futterer CD, Maurer MH, Schmitt A, Feldmann RE Jr, Kuschinsky W, Waschke KF. Alterations in rat brain proteins after desflurane anesthesia. Anesthesiology 2004; 100(2):302–308.

88. Jevtovic-Todorovic V, Beals J, Benshoff N, Olney JW. Prolonged exposure to inhalational anesthetic nitrous oxide kills neurons in adult rat brain. Neuroscience 2003; 122(3):609–616.

89. Jevtovic-Todorovic V, Hartman RE, Izumi Y, et al. Early exposure to common anesthetic agents causes widespread neurodegeneration in the developing rat brain and persistent learning deficits. J Neurosci 2003;23(3):876–882.

90. Anand KJ, Soriano SG. Anesthetic agents and the immature brain: are these toxic or therapeutic? Anesthesiology 2004;101(2):527–530.

91. Olney JW, Young C, Wozniak DF, Ikonomidou C, Jevtovic-Todorovic V. Anesthesia-induced developmental neuroapoptosis. Does it happen in humans? Anesthesiology 2004;101(2):273–275.

92. Eckenhoff RG, Johansson JS, Wei H, et al. Inhaled anesthetic enhancement of amyloid-beta oligomerization and cytotoxicity. Anesthesiology 2004;101(3):703–709.

93. Todd MM. Anesthetic neurotoxicity: the collision between laboratory neuroscience and clinical medicine. Anesthesiology 2004;101(2):272–273.

94. Wong GY, Warner DO, Schroeder DR, et al. Risk of surgery and anesthesia for ischemic stroke. Anesthesiology 2000; 92(2):425–432.

95. Hart R, Hindman B. Mechanisms of perioperative cerebral infarction. Stroke 1982;13(6):766–773.

96. Landercasper J, Merz BJ, Cogbill TH, et al. Perioperative stroke risk in 173 consecutive patients with a past history of stroke. Arch Surg 1990;125:986–989.

97. Larsen SF, Zaric D, Boysen G. Postoperative cerebrovascular accidents in general surgery. Acta Anaesthesiol Scand 1988;32(8):698–701.

98. Parikh S, Cohen JR. Perioperative stroke after general surgical procedures. NY State J Med 1993;93(3):162–165.

99. Kim J, Gelb AW. Predicting perioperative stroke. J Neurosurg Anesthesiol 1995;7(3):211–215.

100. Kam PC, Calcroft RM. Peri-operative stroke in general surgical patients. Anaesthesia 1997;52(9):879–883.

101. Limburg M, Wijdicks EF, Li H. Ischemic stroke after surgical procedures: clinical features, neuroimaging, and risk factors. Neurology 1998;50(4):895–901.

102. Shorr RI, Johnson KC, Wan JY, et al. The prognostic significance of asymptomatic carotid bruits in the elderly. J Gen Intern Med 1998;13(2):86–90.

103. Ropper AH, Wechsler LR, Wilson LS. Carotid bruit and the risk of stroke in elective surgery. N Engl J Med 1982; 307:1388–1390.

104. Blacker DJ, Flemming KD, Link MJ, Brown RD Jr. The preoperative cerebrovascular consultation: common cerebrovascular questions before general or cardiac surgery. Mayo Clin Proc 2004;79(2):223–229.

105. Dodick DW, Meissner I, Meyer FB, Cloft HJ. Evaluation and management of asymptomatic carotid artery stenosis. Mayo Clin Proc 2004;79(7):937–944.

106. Barnett HJ, Taylor DW, Eliasziw M, et al. Benefit of carotid endarterectomy in patients with symptomatic moderate or severe stenosis. North American Symptomatic Carotid Endarterectomy Trial Collaborators. N Engl J Med 1998; 339(20):1415–1425.

107. Halliday A, Mansfield A, Marro J, et al. Prevention of disabling and fatal strokes by successful carotid endarterectomy in patients without recent neurological symptoms: randomised controlled trial. Lancet 2004;363(9420):1491–1502.

108. Turnipseed WD, Berkoff HA, Belzer FO. Postoperative stroke in cardiac and peripheral vascular disease. Ann Surg 1980;192(3):365–368.

109. Evans BA, Wijdicks EF. High-grade carotid stenosis detected before general surgery: is endarterectomy indicated? Neurology 2001;57(7):1328–1330.

110. Widder B, Kleiser B, Krapf H. Course of cerebrovascular reactivity in patients with carotid artery occlusions. Stroke 1994;25(10):1963–1967.

111. White RP, Markus HS. Impaired dynamic cerebral autoregulation in carotid artery stenosis. Stroke 1997;28(7): 1340–1344.

112. Blacker DJ, Flemming KD, Wijdicks EF. Risk of ischemic stroke in patients with symptomatic vertebrobasilar stenosis undergoing surgical procedures. Stroke 2003;34(11): 2659–2663.

113. Kendell RE, Marshall J. Role of hypotension in the genesis of transient focal cerebral ischaemic attacks. Br Med J 1963;2:344–348.

114. Fischberg GM, Lozano E, Rajamani K, Ameriso S, Fisher MJ. Stroke precipitated by moderate blood pressure reduction. J Emerg Med 2000;19(4):339–346.

115. Oliver S, Cucchiara RF, Nishimura R, Michenfelder JD. Parameters affecting the occurrence of paradoxical air embolism. Anesthesiology 1987;(3A).

116. Black S, Muzzi DA, Nishimura RA, Cucchiara RF. Preoperative and intraoperative echocardiography to detect right-to-left shunt in patients undergoing neurosurgical procedures in the sitting position. Anesthesiology 1990; 72(3):436–438.

117. Bonaffini N, Altieri M, Rocco A, Di Piero V. Functional neuroimaging in acute stroke. Clin Exp Hypertens 2002; 24(7–8):647–657.

118. Adams HP Jr, Adams RJ, Brott T, et al. Guidelines for the early management of patients with ischemic stroke: a scientific statement from the Stroke Council of the American Stroke Association. Stroke 2003;34(4):1056–1083.

119. Broderick JP, Adams HP Jr, Barsan W, et al. Guidelines for the management of spontaneous intracerebral hemorrhage: a statement for healthcare professionals from a special writing group of the Stroke Council, American Heart Association. Stroke 1999;30(4):905–915.

120. Warner DS. Perioperative neuroprotection: are we asking the right questions? Anesth Analg 2004;98(3):563–565.

121. Patel P. No magic bullets: the ephemeral nature of anesthetic-mediated neuroprotection. Anesthesiology 2004; 100(5):1049–1051.

122. Auer RN. Non-pharmacologic (physiologic) neuroprotection in the treatment of brain ischemia. Ann NY Acad Sci 2001;939:271–282.

123. De Keyser J, Sulter G, Luiten PG. Clinical trials with neuroprotective drugs in acute ischaemic stroke: are we doing the right thing? Trends Neurosci 1999;22(12):535–540.

124. Goldstein LB. Common drugs may influence motor recovery after stroke. The Sygen In Acute Stroke Study Investigators. Neurology 1995;45(5):865–871.

125. Shank ES, Muth CM. Decompression illness, iatrogenic gas embolism, and carbon monoxide poisoning: the role of hyperbaric oxygen therapy. Int Anesthesiol Clin 2000;38(1): 111–138.

126. Warlow C, Wardlaw J. Therapeutic thrombolysis for acute ischaemic stroke. BMJ 2003;326(7383):233–234.

127. Albers GW, Amarenco P, Easton JD, Sacco RL, Teal P. Antithrombotic and Thrombolytic Therapy for Ischemic Stroke: The Seventh ACCP Conference on Antithrombotic and Thrombolytic Therapy. Chest 2004;126(3 Suppl): 483S–512S.

128. Moazami N, Smedira NG, McCarthy PM, et al. Safety and efficacy of intraarterial thrombolysis for perioperative stroke after cardiac operation. Ann Thorac Surg 2001;72(6): 1933–1937.

10
Alterations in Circulatory Function

Thomas J. Ebert and G. Alec Rooke

According to a 2006 statistical update published by the American Heart Association, 37.3% of all deaths in the United States in 2003 were attributable to cardiovascular disease (CVD).[1] About 83% of the deaths related to CVD occur in people age 65 and older. The prevalence of CVD in American men and women aged 65–74 are 68.5% and 75%, respectively. For those aged 75+, prevalence is 77.8% and 86.4%, respectively. These numbers demonstrate the strong association between adverse cardiac events and the aging process.

With advancing age, the frequency of concurrent disease processes increases in a nearly exponential manner, such that many of the CVDs in the elderly have been considered an expected process of aging. We now recognize that preventing or delaying these disease processes through good nutrition and an active lifestyle can achieve "healthy or successful" aging. It is also recognized that preoperative "medical fitness" (a synonym for "successful aging"), rather than chronologic age, is an important determinant of postoperative outcome in the elderly surgical patient[2] (Figure 10-1).

Even in the absence of the confounding influences of disease and lifestyle, the rate of functional aging on an organ or system, such as the cardiovascular system, varies from individual to individual. To better understand the expected effects of the "usual" aging process on the cardiovascular system, we must appreciate the net effect of the multiple, interdependent variables of heart rate, coronary blood flow, afterload or impedance, preload or diastolic filling, and inotropic state in describing cardiac function. All show age-dependent changes. The autonomic nervous system (ANS) modulates each of these variables through both sympathetic and parasympathetic mechanisms, and aging of the ANS further contributes to modifying cardiovascular function in the elderly.

Although there is a general bias that age weakens the heart, in fact, this is not the case. Several functional adaptations of the heart help maintain resting and exercise cardiovascular physiology.[3] However, some of these adaptations account for problematic physiology in the elderly that adversely affects anesthetic management. This chapter will identify the critical changes in the cardiovascular system related to the aging process and the consequent modifications to the clinical management of the elderly undergoing anesthesia and surgery.

Heart and Vessel Structural Alterations

As the human body ages, it undergoes a variety of changes. Some of these changes are relatively benign. However, there are alterations that influence and even impair the overall health of the aging person. An example of such a detrimental digression accompanying increasing age is the increased stiffness of the heart and vascular tree.

Many factors contribute to stiffening of the vascular tree. Aging can radically transform the endothelial layers via changes in extracellular matrix compositions. Elasticity in connective tissues depends primarily on the properties of its constituent collagen and elastin. Both connective tissue proteins are long-lived but slow in their production. By the age of 25, production of elastin has essentially ceased, and the rate of turnover of collagen decreases with increasing age. The consequent increase in the collagen-to-elastin ratio, plus an accumulating damage to collagen by glycation and free radicals, results in progressive connective tissue stiffness. Thus arteries, veins, and myocardium become less compliant over time.

Nonenzymatic glycation is a reaction between reducing sugars and proteins on the vascular endothelium. Over time, these glycation sites cause tight crosslinking of proteins called advanced glycation end-products (AGE). This AGE formation leads to changes in the physiochemical properties of endothelial tissues. AGE crosslinking structurally results in vessels with less elasticity and

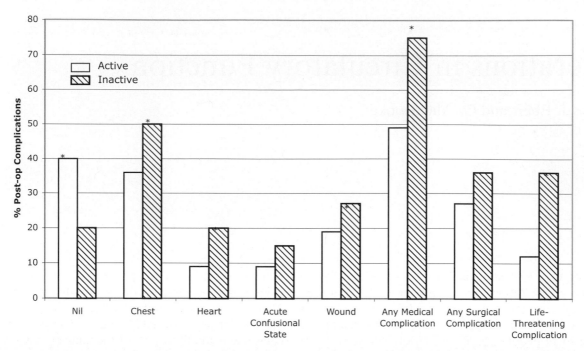

FIGURE 10-1. Preoperative activity level and percent occurrence of postoperative complications. Active = patients who normally left their home without assistance, at least two times per week. *p < 0.05. (Adapted with permission from Seymour DG, Pringle R. Post-operative complications in the elderly surgical patient. Gerontology 1983;29(4):262–270. Basel, Switzerland: S. Karger.)

compliance.[4] Furthermore, the interaction of AGE with receptors for AGE (RAGE) on endothelial cells has been implicated as an initiating event in atherogenesis. In smooth muscle cells, binding of AGE-modified proteins to RAGE is associated with increased cellular proliferation of smooth muscle cells. This interaction also causes an increase in vascular cell adhesion molecule-1, which enhances binding of macrophages to the endothelial surface. This induces oxidative stress on the vascular endothelium and contributes to vascular stiffness.[5]

Several studies have shown that the nitric oxide pathway deteriorates with age. This has implications on vascular compliance. Nitric oxide suppresses key events in atherosclerotic development such as vascular smooth muscle proliferation and migration. It also inhibits the adhesion of monocytes and leukocytes in the endothelium, as well as platelet–vessel interaction. Furthermore, nitric oxide is known to regulate endothelial permeability, reducing the flux of lipoproteins into the vessel wall.[6] The reduced effects of nitric oxide on all of these pathways may contribute to vascular stiffness in aging.

The above mechanisms serve to explain the pathogenesis of vascular stiffness associated with aging. As arterial walls stiffen, blood vessel compliance is reduced, leading to an increase in systolic blood pressure and pulse wave velocity (Figure 10-2). The reflected waves return earlier

to the thoracic aorta, arriving by late ejection instead of early diastole. Thus, the left ventricle must pump against a higher pressure in late ejection than under normal circumstances. This additional afterload places an increased

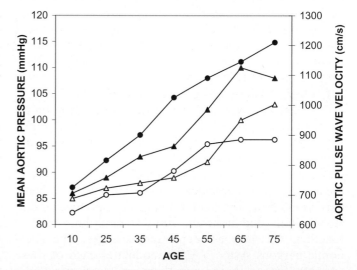

FIGURE 10-2. Mean aortic pressure (triangles) and pulse wave velocity (circles) in two Chinese populations: rural Guanzhou (unfilled symbols) and urban Beijing (filled symbols). (Adapted with permission from Avolio AP, Chen SG, Wang RP, Zhang CL, Li MF, O'Rourke MF. Effects of aging on changing arterial compliance and left ventricular load in a northern Chinese urban community. Circulation 1983;68:50–58.)

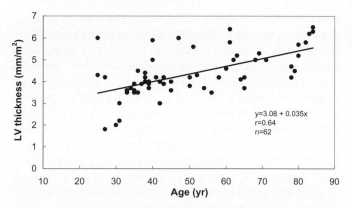

FIGURE 10-3. Left ventricular (LV) posterior wall thickness (mm/m²) in normotensive men as a function of age (years). (Adapted with permission from Gerstenblith G, Frederiksen J, Yin FC, Fortuin NJ, Lakatta EG, Weisfeldt ML. Echocardiographic assessment of a normal adult aging population. Circulation 1977;56:273–278.)

burden on the heart, particularly because it occurs late in systole when the myocardial muscle is normally losing its strength, and therefore provides a significant stimulus for cardiac hypertrophy (Figure 10-3).

The cardiac muscle hypertrophy that develops secondary to the increased late systolic afterload also leads to myocardial stiffening and diastolic dysfunction. Diastolic dysfunction is defined as impairment in the relaxation phase of the ventricles. The aging heart contains AGE crosslinked collagen, which has the same effect on stiffness as it does in the peripheral vascular system. It is implicated in the signaling of macrophage recruitment in hypertensive myocardial fibrosis that contributes to deteriorating diastolic function.[4]

In diastolic dysfunction, there also is a functional component to the impairment of relaxation. It has been proposed that alterations in the myocyte calcium-handling proteins disturb the calcium transient in failing hearts. Calcium uptake in the sarcoplasmic reticulum declines with heart failure because of reduced expression of certain calcium channel enzymes.[7] This contributes to delayed relaxation of the myocardial muscle fibers, and the stiff ventricles have less ability to "spring open" in early diastole.

As a consequence, there is a progressive decrease in the early diastolic filling period between the ages of 20 and 80. At its worst, the diastolic filling period is reduced by 50% compared with younger controls. With increased stiffness, there also is a decline in the diastolic filling rate (Figure 10-4). However, resting end-diastolic volume does not change with increasing age. Because the passive early ventricular filling is impaired with age, the heart is increasingly dependent on an adequate atrial filling pressure and the atrial contraction (Figure 10-5). The atrial

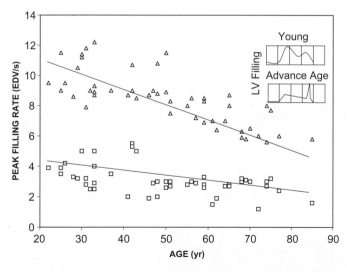

FIGURE 10-4. Changes in early diastolic left ventricular filling and the atrial contribution to filling associated with increased age. Age and peak filling rate relationship was obtained at rest (squares) and maximum workload (triangles). Inset: top image = left ventricular filling, young; bottom image = left ventricular filling, advanced age. (Adapted with permission from Lakatta EG. Cardiovascular aging in health. Clin Geriatr Med 2000;16(3):419–444. Copyright © 2000 Elsevier.)

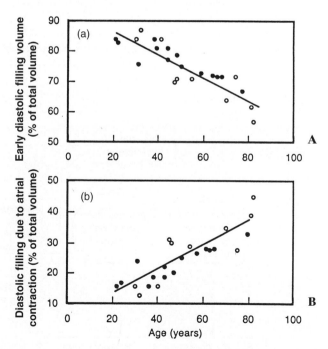

FIGURE 10-5. Echo-Doppler evaluation of diastolic filling in healthy men and women as a function of age. **A:** Early diastolic filling volume (% of total volume). **B:** Diastolic filling caused by atrial contraction (% of total volume). (Adapted with permission from Lakatta.[3])

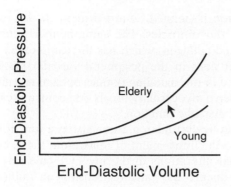

FIGURE 10-6. The increased ventricular stiffness associated with age requires an increased atrial pressure to achieve the same end-diastolic volume. (Adapted with permission from Dauchot PJ, Cascorbi H, Fleisher LA, Prough DS, eds. Problems in Anesthesia: Management of the Elderly Surgical Patient. Vol. 9, No. 4. Philadelphia: Lippincott-Raven; 1997:482–497.)

pressures must rise to maintain the end-diastolic volume in the presence of stiffened ventricles. The increased atrial pressure can result in increased pulmonary blood pressures and ultimately lead to congestion in the sys-

temic venous circulation. The cumulative effect of these alterations results in diastolic dysfunction (Figure 10-6). About half of heart failure in the elderly population (older than 75 years) is associated with impaired left ventricular diastolic function, but preserved left ventricular systolic function.[8] Unfortunately, patients with isolated left ventricular diastolic dysfunction are not as likely to present with the traditional physical manifestations of heart failure. Instead, they are frequently asymptomatic or present with only mild pulmonary congestion, exertional dyspnea, and orthopnea. These symptoms may be aggravated by systemic stressors such as fever, exercise, tachycardia, or anemia. As a result, prevention and detection of diastolic heart failure may be difficult since it is often recognized only by echocardiography.

Systolic function of the heart also is affected by the aging process. From a functional standpoint, the prolonged myocardial contraction maintains the flow delivered to the stiffened arterial tree, thereby maintaining cardiac output (Figure 10-7). The functional adaptation to vascular stiffening and afterload is able to maintain

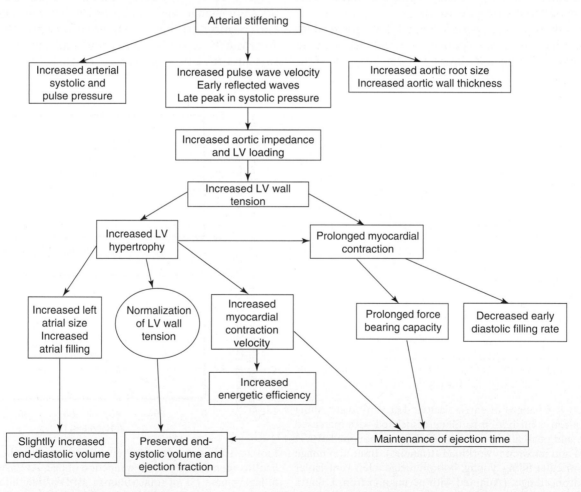

FIGURE 10-7. A cascade of functional adaptations to vascular stiffening in the elderly. LV = left ventricular. (Adapted with permission from Lakatta EG. Cardiovascular aging in health. Clin Geriatr Med 2000;16(3):419–444. Copyright © 2000 Elsevier.)

cardiac output at rest; however, an age-related decline in systolic function may be unmasked in the presence of exercise or sympathetic stimulation. For example, administration of an α-adrenergic agonist such as phenylephrine will acutely increase afterload to the heart, increasing left ventricular wall stress during systole, unmasking an age-related decrease in contractile reserve.[9]

Further studies have shown that there is abnormal systolic function in many patients who have hypertension-induced concentric hypertrophy with a normal ejection fraction. Reduced midwall shortening in relation to stress is clearly evident in patients with greater relative wall thickness. This translates to abnormal pump function and reduced cardiac output. Subtle systolic dysfunction may be present even if patients have seemingly normal ejection fractions and are without clinical heart failure, and it would be incorrect to equate a normal ejection fraction with normal systolic function.[10]

Reduced vascular compliance, diastolic dysfunction, and systolic dysfunction in the elderly are all interconnected. It is reasonable to assume that these are not separate pathologies and in fact develop in parallel. Reduced vascular compliance resulting in hypertension, increased afterload, and eventual cardiac remodeling is an extremely common finding in the aging population. In a large portion of this group, this inevitably results in some evidence of diastolic dysfunction. Furthermore, the above concepts demonstrate that some systolic dysfunction exists in many of these same hypertensive elderly patients.

The interrelationships among vascular stiffening, hypertension, diastolic dysfunction, and even systolic dysfunction in the absence of overt cardiac disease have led to a reexamination of our concepts of hypertension and its management. Conventional wisdom suggests that patients who have hypertension can sometimes be classified as "systolic" hypertension or "diastolic" hypertension if their hypertension is limited to their systolic or diastolic pressure, respectively. However, an emerging concept is of "pulse pressure" hypertension and is characterized by a large difference between systolic and diastolic pressure, for example, 80 mm Hg or greater.[11]

A relatively high systolic pressure in comparison to diastolic is harmful for several reasons. First, a high pulse pressure indicates that the patient's arterial conduit system is stiff. Low compliance means that a high systolic pressure is required in order to distend the aorta and other large arteries as the stroke volume is received. Even though this increase in pressure occurs relatively early in ejection, it still forces the ventricle to pump against a high pressure and stimulates hypertrophy that, in turn, increases myocardial stiffness and further impairs diastolic relaxation. Indeed, there is a strong correlation between the severity of reduced arterial compliance and the severity of diastolic dysfunction.[12] Second, when the diastolic pressure is low compared with systolic pressure, there is an immediate predisposition to an imbalance of myocardial oxygen supply and demand. Demand correlates most closely to systolic pressure,[13] whereas coronary blood flow occurs mostly during diastole, making supply highly dependent on diastolic pressure. With rapid transit of reflected arterial waves, there is loss of the accentuated pressure in early diastole. This lowering of aortic pressure during diastole potentially diminishes coronary perfusion. In patients with coronary stenoses, this imbalance could result in subendocardial ischemia, thereby worsening diastolic relaxation and increasing atrial pressure.

Because of the consequences of arterial stiffening, arterial compliance has been suggested as a better measure of biologic age, as opposed to chronologic age.[14] And it is not surprising that there is great interest in strategies to reduce or even reverse arterial stiffening in the hope of preventing CVD. Current human therapy primarily involves drugs that relax smooth muscle tone.[15] Statins not only inhibit myocardial remodeling but may reduce vascular stiffness. Angiotensin blockers and aldosterone seem to lessen fibrosis. In recent studies that have largely been limited to animals, drugs have been used to break the stiffening links in connective tissue proteins caused by glycosylation.[15,16] In the meantime, exercise slows vascular stiffening and remains a useful therapy for all ages.

Reflex Control Mechanisms and Aging

The aging process affects autonomic cardiovascular control mechanisms in a nonuniform manner. Attenuated respiratory sinus arrhythmia in older individuals suggests that parasympathetic control of sinus node function declines with age. Because the reflex regulation of heart rate in humans is primarily dependent on cardiac vagal activity, it is correct to assume that the impaired baroreflex regulation of heart rate is related to deficient parasympathetic mechanisms (Figure 10-8). Although the parasympathetic component of the arterial baroreflex becomes diminished in the aging population, the baroreflex control of sympathetic outflow and the vascular response to sympathetic stimulation are well maintained in moderately old, active individuals.[17] It is well established that basal levels of plasma catecholamines and sympathetic nerve activity increase with age. Plasma noradrenaline levels increase 10%–15% per decade.[18] In addition, there is an age-dependent reduction in activity of the cardiac neuronal noradrenaline reuptake mechanism, resulting in higher concentrations of noradrenaline at β_1-receptor sites in the heart.[19]

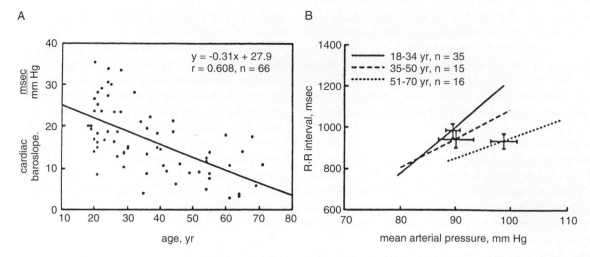

FIGURE 10-8. **A:** Individual cardiac baroreflex sensitivities versus age. Regression revealed a significant ($p < 0.05$) inverse relationship between reflex sensitivity and age. **B:** Mean regression lines describing relationship between mean arterial pressure and corresponding R-R interval for each of the three age groups. Regression line slopes were smaller in older and middle-aged subjects than in younger subjects. Baseline values (mean ± SE) are superimposed on regression lines. (Adapted with permission from Ebert et al.[17])

Adrenergic Receptor Activity and Aging

Aging has been associated with a decrease in the response to stimulation of β-receptors. This is noted in the peripheral circulation by a reduced arterial and venous dilation response to the β-agonist, isoproterenol, and the mixed agonist, epinephrine, in the elderly (Figure 10-9). In cardiac muscle, there is a reduction in the inotropic response to exercise and to the administration of catecholamines in the aging patient.[20] In isolated cardiac myocytes, it has been shown that the EC_{50} for isoprenaline (a $β_1$- and $β_2$-agonist) is nearly twice as high in the elderly.[18] A result of the decreased contractile response to β-adrenergic stimulation in the elderly is a greater dependency on the Frank-Starling (length-tension) mechanism of contraction to maintain cardiac output.

Although multiple studies indicate that the heart rate increase to β-stimulation of the heart is attenuated with age, recent data question the age-related attenuated chronotropic response.[20] Studies also provide conflicting results regarding age-related changes in myocardial β-adrenoceptor density. The mechanism for decreased cardiac inotropic response to sympathetic stimulation is more likely attributable to changes in the second messenger system. Impaired coupling of the β-adrenoceptor to the Gs protein and to the catalytic unit of adenylyl cyclase is consistently observed in the elderly myocardium. Furthermore, an increase in Gi protein levels observed in aged myocardial tissue indicates a reduction in the catalytic subunit of adenylyl cyclase.[21] Both of these mechanisms will attenuate adenosine 3′,5′-cyclic monophosphate (cAMP) formation and subsequent β-adrenoceptor response. This desensitization of the intracellular processing of receptor signaling is likely a compensatory adaptation to an increase in endogenous norepinephrine resulting from age-related increases in sympathetic activity and reduced neuronal uptake of norepinephrine.

This attenuated β-adrenoceptor response as a result of changes in second messenger function has implications in

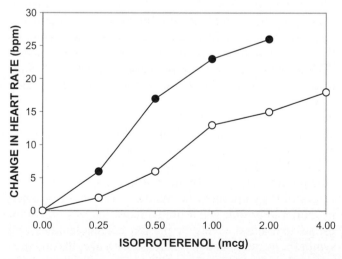

FIGURE 10-9. The effect of intravenous isoproterenol infusions on increasing heart rate in healthy young (filled circles) and older (unfilled circles) men at rest. (Adapted with permission from Lakatta EG. Cardiovascular aging in health. Clin Geriatr Med 2000;16(3):419–444. Copyright © 2000 Elsevier.)

the peripheral vascular system. Vasorelaxation is accomplished in vascular smooth muscle cells via cAMP. cAMP activates protein kinase A (PKA) that then lowers cytosolic calcium levels, causing vasorelaxation. Decreased generation of cAMP in the vasculature leads to impairment of this pathway. This may be a contributing factor for hypertension in the elderly. And because cAMP is an antiproliferative agent, this deficiency may be associated with the progression of atherosclerosis.[21]

Genetic variation in β-adrenoceptors is now documented and may have a significant role in CVD heterogeneity among individuals. There are many known polymorphisms of both β_1- and β_2-adrenoceptor subtypes. These variants may have differing effects on the cardiovascular system with age. The most common polymorphism, whose allele frequency is 60%, causes enhanced down regulation of β_2-adrenoceptors. Because peripheral β_2-receptors cause vasodilation and a reduction in blood pressure, individuals with this polymorphism are more prone to hypertension with increasing age. This fact has been confirmed in familial studies, which show increased prevalence of this allele in families with a history of essential hypertension. Another β-adrenoceptor polymorphism with important implications in cardiac disease is one that causes blunted agonist responsiveness. Studies have shown that in heart failure patients, this variant carries a relative risk of death or transplant of 4.8 compared with the normal allele. There also exists a particular polymorphism that tends to improve survival in those with heart failure. The existence of β-receptor polymorphisms may have additional implications for the efficacy of β-blockade. However, at this time, little is known about their particular impact on patient therapy.[22]

It would seem logical to expect a down regulation of α-adrenergic receptors with age, but surprisingly the number of α_1-receptors remains well preserved. Interestingly, in normotensive older subjects, an increased rate of infusion of an α-agonist is required to achieve the same degree of vasoconstriction compared with young subjects.[8] Animal studies have shown that maximal binding of vascular α_1-receptors is significantly reduced with age.[23] The α_2-receptors appear to show some age-related decline. Normally, α_2-receptors predominate in the venous side of the circulation, suggesting that a compromised venoconstrictor response to the upright posture, secondary to α_2-receptor loss, might contribute to orthostatic intolerance in the elderly.[17] The evidence of adrenergic receptor desensitization with age has further implications as hypertension develops in the elderly. In normotensive elderly subjects, the decrease in responsiveness of α-adrenergic receptors seems to be a regulated compensatory effect of the heightened level of sympathetic nervous system activity in the elderly. Despite some evidence of diminished α-adrenergic responsiveness, it seems that the overall baroreflex control of vasoconstriction is well pre-

served with age and might be heightened compared with young adults.[7,24]

As with β-adrenoceptors, polymorphisms in α-adrenergic receptors may have implications on hypertension and cardiac disease in the elderly. It has been proposed that individuals with a particular α_{2B}-adrenergic receptor polymorphism may be at greater risk for acute coronary events and sudden cardiac death.[25] The in vivo effect of the α_2-agonist dexmedetomidine on patients with this polymorphism has been investigated and there is a trend toward an increased systolic blood pressure response to dexmedetomidine in patients with this polymorphism.[25]

Vagal Activity and Aging

Baroreflex control of heart rate is known to be diminished in older individuals. Indeed, there clearly is an attenuated respiratory sinus arrhythmia suggesting either reduced vagal outflow or reduced intracellular responses to muscarinic receptor activation with age.[26] Both changes seem to be present in the elderly. Lower resting vagal tone in the elderly has been implicated in the diminished heart rate increase in response to a large dose of atropine compared with younger controls.[8] Studies have shown that right atrial muscarinic receptor density is significantly and negatively correlated with age. Furthermore, it has also been shown that muscarinic receptor function declines in the elderly population. This is evident by a reduction in carbachol-induced inhibition of forskolin-activated adenylyl cyclase in muscarinic receptors of aged myocardium.[27] All of these mechanisms, taken together, contribute to reduced vagal activity in the elderly. Finally, autoantibodies to M_2-muscarinic receptors exist in the sera of normal individuals, and are found in high levels in those with idiopathic dilated cardiomyopathy. The prevalence of these autoantibodies is significantly increased in the elderly.[28] The implications of these findings on muscarinic receptor function and cardiac performance have yet to be determined.

Renin and Vasopressin Activity

As already described, there are many vascular changes associated with aging. These changes contribute to renal damage and functionally result in decreased glomerular filtration rate and renal blood flow. Aging also affects sodium balance in the kidney. This results in decreased ability to conserve sodium in the face of sodium restriction as well as a decreased sodium excretion in the presence of increased sodium load. Despite the increased sympathetic activity accompanying old age, the elderly experience a decrease in plasma and renal levels of renin.

Plasma renin activity is diminished in the supine position, and physiologic stimuli such as hemorrhage, sodium restriction, and orthostasis are followed by attenuated increases in renin release and consequently lower concentrations of angiotensin in the circulation.[29] Although renin-angiotensin levels are decreased in the elderly, the aging population shows an enhanced vasoconstriction in response to angiotensin I and angiotensin II. The above finding helps to explain the key role that angiotensin-converting enzyme inhibitors and angiotensin II receptor blockers have in improving renal structure and function in the elderly.[30]

In the elderly, there seems to be an elevation in plasma vasopressin levels under basal conditions and a heightened response to an osmotic challenge such as water deprivation. Surprisingly, after a water restriction period, older subjects had a relatively low spontaneous fluid consumption as well as diminished thirst.[29] In addition, by age 80, the total body water content has declined to 50% of body mass from the average content of 60% in younger persons.[31] Such decreases in thirst mechanism, total body water, and fluid consumption in combination with an age-related decrease in glomerular function cause older persons to be increasingly vulnerable to water imbalance.

Arrhythmias

Several changes with aging predispose the older patient to arrhythmias. Sinus node dysfunction develops with the progressive loss of pacemaker cells, and contributes to the risk of sick sinus syndrome and/or bradycardia.[32] Bradycardia promotes atrial fibrillation as does age-related atrial fibrosis and atrial enlargement. The incidence of atrial fibrillation increases with age such that it is present in 10% of those over 80. This predisposition to atrial fibrillation undoubtedly contributes to the relatively high incidence of new onset atrial fibrillation (and supraventricular tachycardia) not only after thoracic and cardiac surgery, but after most major surgical procedures. Patients presenting for surgery who are found to have previously undiagnosed atrial fibrillation should be evaluated before surgery, including an echocardiogram to rule out structural abnormality. Perioperatively, the management of new onset atrial fibrillation is initially rate control, with restoration of sinus rhythm within 24 hours as the next goal in order to reduce the risk of clot formation and thromboembolus.[33] For patients with chronic atrial fibrillation, early anticoagulation after surgery may be important, especially if the patient is at high risk for thromboembolism.

Heart block and ventricular ectopy are examples of other arrhythmias prevalent in older patients.[34] Heart block below the atrioventricular node most often occurs secondary to idiopathic degeneration of the conduction system, but is not likely to carry adverse consequences unless there is concomitant cardiac disease.

Ischemic Preconditioning

An episode of myocardial ischemia reduces the severity of myocardial damage associated with a subsequent, more prolonged ischemic event. This phenomenon, known as ischemic preconditioning, exists in both an immediate (minutes to a few hours) and delayed (many hours to days) form.[35] Clinically, ischemic preconditioning is likely involved with warm-up angina in which patients who exert to the onset of angina, rest, and exert again can then achieve higher levels of exertion before developing the second bout of angina.[36] Patients who suffer a myocardial infarction are much less likely to die or develop heart failure if they experienced angina within 48 hours of their myocardial infarction.[37] Exposure to volatile anesthetics yields a preconditioning effect as well.[35]

Unfortunately, aging is associated with the loss of ischemic preconditioning. Warm-up angina is nonexistent beyond age 75[38] and in patients older than 65, myocardial infarction with or without antecedent angina is associated with the same high rates of death and heart failure as younger subjects who did not have prior angina.[37] At least in an animal model, anesthetic cardioprotection from preconditioning is essentially abolished in aged rats.[39,40]

Implications in Anesthesia

Although normal aging affects virtually all components of the cardiovascular system, perhaps the most important changes that influence anesthetic management in the elderly are the stiffened cardiac and vascular system, the diminished β-adrenergic receptor response, and the impaired autonomic reflex control of heart rate. Compounding these age-related changes are the well-described effects of the intravenous and volatile anesthetics on the myocardium, vascular tone, and the ANS.

Many of the elderly patients coming to the operating room are in a relatively volume-depleted state because of NPO guidelines, reduced thirst mechanisms, and diminished renal capacity to conserve water and salt. Additionally, increases in heart rate and contractility during volume loss are limited by diminished reflex control systems and by reduced β-receptor responses. Consequently, further hypovolemia, e.g., intraoperative blood loss, can result in substantial hypotension. This volume sensitivity of the elderly has been demonstrated in the laboratory during head-up tilt testing after subjects had been made hypovolemic with diuretics and low salt intake. The older subjects had greater decreases in blood pressure during upright tilting than both the younger hypovolemic control subjects and the older normovolemic control subjects.[41] Impaired responses to hypovolemia are further confounded by volatile anesthetics and the sedative-hypnotics that impair baroreflex control mechanisms.[42,43] Healthy or preserved baroreflex control mechanisms clearly minimize the cardiovascular changes that result from anesthetics. For example, diabetic patients with preserved autonomic reflexes had a lower incidence of hypotension during induction and maintenance of anesthesia than patients with impaired reflexes.[44] Thus, the net effect of physiologic changes with adult aging compounded by anesthetic effects should be more frequent and more significant blood pressure changes in the elderly. Such blood pressure lability has been observed in older patients.[45,46]

In the aged patient, the relative hypovolemic state has many important clinical implications. The elderly heart is heavily dependent on an adequate end-diastolic volume to maintain stroke volume, and cardiac filling is in turn dependent on higher atrial filling pressures because of a stiffened ventricle and possible diastolic dysfunction. As a result, the elderly are very sensitive to hypovolemia. In this setting, decreased systemic blood pressure should generally be treated with intravenous fluids rather than vasopressors to maintain proper diastolic function. One study has shown that volatile anesthetics do not impair diastolic function whereas propofol has some negative effects.[47]

As important as maintenance of an adequate cardiac preload is to an older patient, it is equally important to avoid excess fluid administration. There are two ways in which one can be misled into administration of excess volume. First, with anesthetic-induced relaxation of vascular smooth muscle and/or sympathectomy comes venodilation and increased venous pooling of blood. Restoration of preload would therefore seem to require significant volume administration just to compensate for the effects of the anesthetic. However, once the anesthetic is worn off, vascular smooth muscle relaxation lessens and sympathetic tone is not only restored, but quite possibly heightened because of pain or recovery from the surgical trauma. Restoration of normal to increased venous tone will then shift that excess volume back to the heart and potentially lead to pulmonary and cardiac dysfunction as the elderly heart copes with what now is volume overload.

The second mechanism that can mislead practitioners into giving excess volume occurs when cardiac filling and cardiac output are not diminished, but the patient is still hypotensive from arterial vasodilation. The natural reaction to hypotension is to assume the patient is hypovolemic and therefore give more volume. That treatment may not be appropriate with older patients. Young, healthy patients have minimal sympathetic tone when supine and at rest. Thus, anesthesia is likely to decrease blood pres-

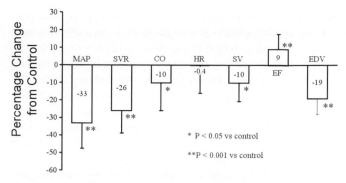

FIGURE 10-10. Hemodynamic response to high spinal anesthesia in older men with a history of cardiac disease. MAP = mean arterial pressure, SVR = systemic vascular resistance, CO = cardiac output, HR = heart rate, SV = stroke volume, EF = ejection fraction, EDV = left ventricular end-diastolic volume. (Adapted with permission from Rooke et al.[48])

sure in young patients more by the direct effects of the anesthetic on blood vessels than by removal of sympathetic tone. Elderly patients, however, often have high levels of sympathetic tone[17] and removal of that tone can produce more than just an apparent hypovolemia. In a study of older men with varying degrees of cardiac disease, high spinal anesthesia produced an average decrease in blood pressure of 33% (Figure 10-10).[48] Even though pooling of blood in the abdomen and legs caused a 19% decrease in left ventricular end-diastolic volume, cardiac output only decreased by 10%, largely because the decrease in blood pressure (afterload reduction) allowed the ejection fraction to increase. The primary mechanism for hypotension, however, was the 26% decrease in systemic vascular resistance. It is physically impossible to increase end-diastolic volume indefinitely and fully compensate for such a significant decrease in vascular resistance. In fact, it could be argued that the attempt would merely predispose the patient to volume overload, especially on emergence as discussed above. Increased left ventricular end-diastolic pressures from excessive volume could also precipitate or aggravate myocardial ischemia by creating high left ventricular subendocardial wall stress.[49]

In all but the sickest of older patients, therefore, the most likely mechanism of intraoperative hypotension is either decreased vascular resistance or hypovolemia. Should bradycardia be a limiting factor, it is easily detected and treated. What should be done, then, to manage the patient who is hypotensive with a stable heart rate even after adequate volume deficits are replaced? Vasopressors are the likely treatment of choice, with ephedrine and phenylephrine being the most frequently used agents. Phenylephrine has the advantage over ephedrine in that it does not exhibit tachyphylaxis and will not promote tachycardia. Furthermore, α-receptor activation generally results in venoconstriction in addition to vasoconstriction, thereby shifting blood from the periphery back to the heart and alleviating the anesthetic-induced peripheral pooling.[50] As with all drugs, adverse consequences can occur. Coronary vasoconstriction, decreased cardiac output, imbalance in the distribution of the cardiac output, and wall motion abnormalities are all potential undesired effects. The key to the rational use of pressors such as phenylephrine is to minimize hypovolemia, and not feel obliged to return overall vascular resistance back to pre-anesthetic levels. In other words, tolerate a mild decrease in blood pressure. The cardiac dysfunction that has been observed with the use of phenylephrine typically occurs when blood pressure is increased to levels above the patient's awake baseline,[9] or under unusual loading conditions such as excessive anesthesia.[51]

How can we foresee, prevent, or treat the elderly patient who has not successfully aged such that he has a decreased cardiovascular reserve and is to be exposed to anesthetic and surgical stresses? A pulmonary artery catheter and/or transesophageal echocardiography to monitor cardiac filling pressures/volumes along with invasive blood pressure monitoring are the obvious answers that would permit very tight control of preload and afterload. However, this approach should be reserved for the elderly patient with significant limitation of cardiac performance related to coexisting CVD (e.g., coronary artery disease, congestive heart failure, or documented significant myocardial injury). The need for such extensive monitoring also must be weighed against the risks for blood loss and stress associated with the planned surgical intervention. A more realistic approach is to obtain a careful history and chart review to get a reasonably good idea of the biologic age of the patient. The importance of determining the biologic age or "medical fitness" of the elderly patient has been emphasized by a prospective study demonstrating a significant relationship between coexisting diseases in the elderly patient and postoperative morbidity and mortality[52] (Figure 10-11). In addition, the preoperative level of physical activity proved to be a sensitive predictor of postoperative morbidity.

In a patient who has aged "successfully," routine monitoring with close attention to fluid status and a more gradual titration and thoughtful selection of anesthetics may be sufficient to minimize the nearly unavoidable hypotension. A useful approach in the anesthetic management of the elderly is to replace NPO deficits before anesthetic induction and to induce anesthesia with etomidate. It has been demonstrated that there is a good preservation of sympathetic outflow and autonomic reflexes with this sedative/hypnotic.[53] However, opioids or esmolol must be given to avoid the reflex response to tracheal intubation that is poorly attenuated by etomidate. Benzodiazepines should be minimized or avoided because

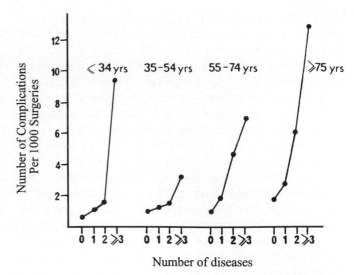

FIGURE 10-11. The influence of age and comorbid disease on major perioperative complications. Increased comorbid disease is associated with increased risk of complications, regardless of age. In patients free of disease, age has a minimal effect on risk. In patients with multiple diseases, however, the effect of age is substantial. (Adapted with permission from Tiret et al.[52])

they interact with opioids to produce sympatho-inhibition and hypotension.

The goal of anesthesia in the elderly is cardiac stability. Volatile agents are direct vasodilators and are known to depress baroreflex responses. Furthermore, volatile anesthetics can produce myocardial depression and nodal rhythms that are poorly tolerated in patients with cardiac abnormalities such as aortic stenosis, mitral stenosis, or hypertrophic obstructive cardiomyopathy.[54] A preference might be given to the new, less soluble, volatile anesthetics because they can be titrated up or down quickly, and emergence times as well as time to orientation are remarkably better than with the older volatile anesthetics.[55] Maintenance can include nitrous oxide when appropriate, because it helps to maintain sympathetic outflow and lessens the need for higher concentrations of the potent volatile anesthetics.

Hypertension and tachycardia should be recognized as undesirable events in the elderly because of the increased myocardial oxygen demand and the reduced time for atrial filling and coronary flow. Esmolol can be given (0.5–1.0 mg/kg) to attenuate the intubation response and avoid excessive increases in heart rate. α2-Agonists such as clonidine or dexmedetomidine also are effective in reducing the sympathetic response to laryngoscopy and intubation, but add to intraoperative hypotension because of their long half-lives. Additionally, adequate analgesia is an important aspect of heart rate and blood pressure control. Fentanyl can be titrated (1–3 μg/kg) before intubation to attenuate the sympathetic response. Naloxone should be avoided or used with extreme caution in the elderly, because large doses can cause pain, leading to an acute increase in catecholamine levels. This may result in life-threatening complications such as pulmonary edema, myocardial ischemia, arrhythmias, and cardiac arrest.[54]

In patients at higher risk of coronary ischemia and undergoing noncardiac surgery, prophylactic, perioperative β-blockade should be considered. Many studies have shown a decreased incidence of myocardial ischemia, as well as an overall survival benefit when β-blockers are administered perioperatively,[56] although optimal duration of β-blockade both pre- and postoperatively remains uncertain. β-Blockade may induce protective effects via many mechanisms. It may reduce the neuroendocrine stress response with surgery, it may reduce the incidence of acute coronary plaque rupture by reducing shear stress, and it may decrease the incidence of cardiac arrhythmias.[54] For those patients receiving chronic β-blocker therapy, it should be continued in the perioperative period. In fact, an increase in the dosage may be prudent.[49]

Postoperatively, the older patient will be at risk for developing pulmonary congestion when significant third spaced fluid becomes mobilized. Patients with no history of heart failure, but who have borderline diastolic dysfunction, stiff vessels, and/or poor renal function, may experience significant increases in atrial pressure with even modest increases in blood volume. Careful and frequent bedside examination of the patient during the first several postoperative days may permit timely use of diuretics; avoiding fluid overload may prevent progression to more serious complications such as hypoxia, respiratory failure, cardiac dysfunction, or myocardial infarction.

Summary

A stiffened heart and vascular system, impaired autonomic control mechanisms, and altered β-receptor function characterize an aging cardiovascular system. These alterations make the aged heart more sensitive to volume changes in the face of minimal ability to compensate via the ANS. When biologic age ("medical fitness") exceeds chronologic age, these changes are likely worsened. The addition of volatile anesthetics or propofol causes further changes in the ANS and increases the risk of hemodynamic fluctuations. Finally, compounding biologic age and anesthetics with surgical stress and blood loss could lead to substantial hemodynamic instability. It is only with a clear understanding of these additive factors (age, fitness, anesthesia, and surgical events) that the anesthesia provider can effectively predict and manage blood pressure and cardiac function during the perioperative period.

References

1. Thom T, Haase N, Rosamond W, et al. Heart disease and stroke statistics—2006 update: a report from the American Heart Association Statistics Committee and Stroke Statistics Subcommittee. Circulation 2006;113:85–151.
2. Seymour DG, Vaz FG. A prospective study of elderly general surgical patients: II. Post-operative complications. Age Ageing 1989;18:316–326.
3. Lakatta EG. Changes in cardiovascular function with aging. Eur Heart J 1990;11:22–29.
4. Bakris GL, Bank AJ, Kass DA, et al. Advanced glycation end-product cross-link breakers. A novel approach to cardiovascular pathologies related to the aging process. Am J Hypertens 2004;17:23S–30S.
5. Aronson D, Rayfield EJ. How hyperglycemia promotes atherosclerosis: molecular mechanisms. Cardiovasc Diabetol 2002;1:1–10.
6. Yu BP, Chung HY. Oxidative stress and vascular aging. Diabetes Res Clin Pract 2001;54:S73–80.
7. Kass DA, Bronzwaer JGF, Paulus WJ. What mechanisms underlie diastolic dysfunction in heart failure? Circ Res 2004;94:1533–1542.
8. Rooke GA. Cardiovascular aging and anesthetic implications. J Cardiothorac Vasc Anesth 2003;17:512–523.
9. Turner MJ, Mier CM, Spina RJ, et al. Effects of age and gender on cardiovascular responses to phenylephrine. J Gerontol Med Sci 1999;54A:M17–24.
10. Vinch CS, Aurigemma GP, Simon HU, et al. Analysis of left ventricular systolic function using midwall mechanics in patients >60 years of age with hypertensive heart disease and heart failure. Am J Cardiol 2005;96:1299–1303.
11. Aronson S, Fontes ML. Hypertension: a new look at an old problem. Curr Opin Anaesthesiol 2006;19:59–64.
12. Mottram PM, Haluska BA, Leano R, et al. Relation of arterial stiffness to diastolic dysfunction in hypertensive heart disease. Heart 2005;91:1551–1556.
13. Rooke GA, Feigl EO. Work as a correlate of canine left ventricular oxygen consumption, and the problem of catecholamine oxygen wasting. Circ Res 1982;50:273–286.
14. Bulpitt CJ, Rajkumar C, Cameron JD. Vascular compliance as a measure of biological age. J Am Geriatr Soc 1999;47:657–663.
15. Kass DA. Ventricular arterial stiffening—integrating the pathophysiology. Hypertension 2005;46:185–193.
16. Najjar SS, Scuteri A, Lakatta EG. Arterial aging—is it an immutable cardiovascular risk factor? Hypertension 2005;46:454–462.
17. Ebert TJ, Morgan BJ, Barney JA, et al. Effects of aging on baroreflex regulation of sympathetic activity in humans. Am J Physiol 1992;263:H798–H803.
18. Brodde O-E, Leineweber K. Autonomic receptor systems in the failing and aging human heart: similarities and differences. Eur J Pharmacol 2004;500:167–176.
19. Leineweber K, Wangemann T, Giessler C, et al. Age-dependent changes of cardiac neuronal noradrenaline reuptake transport (uptake₁) in the human heart. J Am Coll Cardiol 2002;40:1459–1465.
20. Hees PS, Fleg JL, Mirza ZA, et al. Effects of normal aging on left ventricular lusitropic, inotropic, and chronotropic

responses to dobutamine. J Am Coll Cardiol 2006;47: 1440–1447.

21. Alemany R, Perona JS, Sánchez-Dominguez JM, et al. G protein-coupled receptor systems and their lipid environment in health disorders during aging. Biochim Biophys Acta 2007;1768(4):964–975.

22. McNamara DM, MacGowan GA, London B. Clinical importance of beta-adrenoceptor polymorphisms in cardiovascular disease. Am J Pharmacogenomics 2002;2:73–78.

23. Passmore JC, Rowell PP, Joshua IG, et al. Alpha 1 adrenergic receptor control of renal blood vessels during aging. Can J Physiol Pharmacol 2005;83:335–342.

24. Folkow B, Svanborg A. Physiology of cardiovascular aging. Physiol Rev 1993;73:725–764.

25. Talke P, Stapelfeldt C, Lobo E, et al. Effect of α_{2b}-adrenoceptor polymorphism on peripheral vasoconstriction in healthy volunteers. Anesthesiology 2005;102:536–542.

26. Mancia G, Mark AL. Arterial baroreflexes in humans. In: Shepherd JT, ed. The Cardiovascular System. Bethesda, MD: American Physiological Society; 1983:755–793.

27. Brodde O-E, Konschak U, Becker K, et al. Cardiac muscarinic receptors decrease with age. In vitro and in vivo studies. J Clin Invest 1998;101:471–478.

28. Liu HR, Zhao RR, Zhi JM, et al. Screening of serum autoantibodies to cardiac beta$_1$-adrenoceptors and M$_2$-muscarinic acetylcholine receptors in 408 healthy subjects of varying ages. Autoimmunity 1999;29:43–51.

29. Ferrari AU. Modifications of the cardiovascular system with aging. Am J Geriatr Cardiol 2002;11:30–43.

30. Long DA, Mu W, Price KL, et al. Blood vessels and the aging kidney. Nephron Exp Nephrol 2005;101:e95–99.

31. Kugler JP, Hustead T. Hyponatremia and hypernatremia in the elderly. Am Fam Physician 2000;15:3623–3630.

32. Podrid PJ. Atrial fibrillation in the elderly. Cardiol Clin 1999;17:173–188.

33. Amar D. Perioperative atrial tachyarrhythmias. Anesthesiology 2002;97:1618–1623.

34. Gupta AK, Maheshwari A, Tresch DD, et al. Cardiac arrhythmias in the elderly. Card Electrophysiol Rev 2002; 6:120–128.

35. Riess ML, Stowe DF, Warltier DC. Cardiac pharmacological preconditioning with volatile anesthetics: from bench to bedside? Am J Physiol 2004;286:H1603–1607.

36. Maybaum S, Ilan M, Mogilevsky J, et al. Improvement in ischemic parameters during repeated exercise testing: a possible model for myocardial preconditioning. Am J Cardiol 1996;78:1087–1091.

37. Abete P, Ferrara N, Cacciatore F, et al. Angina-induced protection against myocardial infarction in adult and elderly patients: a loss of preconditioning mechanism in the aging heart? J Am Coll Cardiol 1997;30:947–954.

38. Longobardi G, Abete P, Ferrara N, et al. "Warm-up" phenomenon in adult and elderly patients with coronary artery disease: further evidence of the loss of "ischemic preconditioning" in the aging heart. J Gerontol 2000;55A: M124–129.

39. Sniecinski R, Liu H. Reduced efficacy of volatile anesthetic preconditioning with advanced age in isolated rat myocardium. Anesthesiology 2004;100:589–597.

40. Riess ML, Camara AK, Rhodes SS, et al. Increasing heart size and age attenuate anesthetic preconditioning in guinea pig isolated hearts. Anesth Analg 2005;101:1572–1576.

41. Shannon RP, Wei JY, Rosa RM, et al. The effect of age and sodium depletion on cardiovascular response to orthostasis. Hypertension 1986;8:438–443.

42. Ebert TJ, Harkin CP, Muzi M. Cardiovascular responses to sevoflurane: a review. Anesth Analg 1995;81:S11–S22.

43. Ebert TJ, Muzi M. Propofol and autonomic reflex function in humans. Anesth Analg 1994;78:369–375.

44. Burgos LG, Ebert TJ, Asiddao C, et al. Increased intraoperative cardiovascular morbidity in diabetics with autonomic neuropathy. Anesthesiology 1989;70:591–597.

45. Forrest JB, Rehder K, Cahalan MK, et al. Multicenter study of general anesthesia. III. Predictors of severe perioperative adverse outcomes. Anesthesiology 1992;76: 3–15.

46. Carpenter RL, Caplan RA, Brown DL, et al. Incidence and risk factors for side effects of spinal anesthesia. Anesthesiology 1992;76:906–916.

47. Filipovic M, Wang J, Michaux I, et al. Effects of halothane, sevoflurane and propofol on left ventricular diastolic function in humans during spontaneous and mechanical ventilation. Br J Anaesth 2005;94:186–192.

48. Rooke GA, Freund PR, Jacobson AF. Hemodynamic response and change in organ blood volume during spinal anesthesia in elderly men with cardiac disease. Anesth Analg 1997;85:99–105.

49. Levine WC, Mehta V, Landesberg G. Anesthesia for the elderly: selected topics. Curr Opin Anaesthesiol 2006;19: 320–324.

50. Stanton-Hicks M, Hock A, Stuhmeier K-D, et al. Venoconstrictor agents mobilize blood from different sources and increase intrathoracic filling during epidural anesthesia in supine humans. Anesthesiology 1987;66:317–322.

51. Smith JS, Roizen MF, Cahalan MK, et al. Does anesthetic technique make a difference? Augmentation of systolic blood pressure during carotid endarterectomy: effects of phenylephrine versus light anesthesia and of isoflurane versus halothane on the incidence of myocardial ischemia. Anesthesiology 1988;69:846–853.

52. Tiret L, Desmonts JM, Hatton F, et al. Complications associated with anaesthesia—a prospective survey in France. Can Anaesth Soc J 1986;33:336–344.

53. Ebert TJ, Muzi M, Berens R, et al. Sympathetic responses to induction of anesthesia in humans with propofol or etomidate. Anesthesiology 1992;76:725–733.

54. Sear JW, Higham H. Issues in the perioperative management of the elderly patient with cardiovascular disease. Drugs Aging 2002;19:429–451.

55. Ebert TJ, Robinson BJ, Uhrich TD, et al. Recovery from sevoflurane anesthesia: a comparison to isoflurane and propofol anesthesia. Anesthesiology 1998;89:1524–1531.

56. Mangano DT, Layug EL, Wallace A, et al. Effect of atenolol on mortality and cardiovascular morbidity after noncardiac surgery. N Engl J Med 1996;335:1713–1720.

11
The Aging Respiratory System: Anesthetic Strategies to Minimize Perioperative Pulmonary Complications

Rodrigo Cartin-Ceba, Juraj Sprung, Ognjen Gajic, and David O. Warner

Because of increased life expectancy, the number of elderly individuals over the age of 65 is increasing all over the world, especially in developed countries. Although respiratory function is relatively well preserved in resting elderly patients, reduced respiratory reserve may lead to problems in the setting of acute illness or surgery. To anticipate and prevent potential problems that may result from reduced respiratory reserve, it is important to understand the effects of aging on respiratory function. Such changes may have particular significance during the perioperative period when numerous anesthetic and surgical factors, such as body positioning, residual effects of anesthetics on control of respiration, structural and functional disruption of respiratory muscles, and perioperative changes in lung fluid balance, may impose additional burdens on elderly patients with diminished pulmonary reserve. Indeed, postoperative respiratory complications account for approximately 40% of the perioperative deaths in patients over 65 years of age.[1] In this chapter, we review the effects of aging on pulmonary function and the effects of anesthesia and surgery on this function. Particular emphasis is directed to the surgical and anesthetic factors that stress the respiratory system of the elderly and how these factors increase the risk of postoperative pulmonary complications, such as respiratory failure.

The Physiology of the Aging Lung

Cellular Mechanisms

Lung function gradually deteriorates with age even in healthy individuals who attempt to maintain aerobic capacity.[2,3] Aging is a complex process that begins at the cellular level. Normal cells undergo senescence as a result of multiple mechanisms such as telomere shortening during continuous proliferation, oxidative stress, DNA damage, and aberrant oncogene activation.[4] Normal mitochondrial respiration is associated with oxidative stress for the cell because of a continuous production of superoxide and hydrogen peroxide, inevitably resulting in minor macromolecular damage. Damaged cellular components are not completely recycled by autophagy and other cellular repair systems, leading to a progressive age-related accumulation of biologic "waste" material, including defective mitochondria, cytoplasmic protein aggregates, and an intralysosomal undegradable material called lipofuscin.[5] At the physiologic level, aging is associated with multiple changes in the respiratory system, including structural changes in both the lungs and chest wall, leading to alteration in measurable mechanical properties of the respiratory system, interference with gas exchange, and impaired response to hypoxia and hypercapnia.

The respiratory system is a network of organs and tissues that exchanges gases between the individual and the environment, delivering oxygen to venous blood in exchange for carbon dioxide.[6] The lungs continue to develop throughout life with the maximal number of alveoli attained before 12 years of age. The maximal function of the respiratory system, defined as a maximal ability to exchange gas, is achieved at approximately the mid-third decade of life.[7]

The three most important physiologic changes associated with aging are: a decrease in strength of respiratory muscles, a decrease in the elastic recoil[8] (Figure 11-1) of the lung, and a decrease in the compliance of the chest wall.[7]

Age-Related Changes in Mechanics of Breathing

Chest Wall and Respiratory Muscles

The chest wall progressively stiffens with aging because of structural changes of the intercostal muscles, intercos-

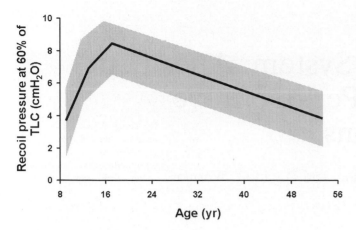

FIGURE 11-1. Static elastic recoil decreases throughout life starting around the age of 20. TLC = total lung capacity. Shaded area represents mean ± 1 SD. (Reprinted with permission from Janssens et al.[7]; publisher: *European Respiratory Journal*; and adapted with permission from Turner et al.[8]; publisher: *American Physiological Society*.)

tal joints, and rib-vertebral articulations, leading to a decrease in static chest wall compliance.[8,9] The increase in the rigidity of the rib cage with age is secondary to multiple factors, including changes in rib-vertebral articulations, changes in the shape of the chest (mainly because of osteoporosis that increases both dorsal kyphosis and anteroposterior chest diameter), costal cartilage calcification, and narrowing in the intervertebral disk spaces.[7,9]

The changes in the chest wall geometry with aging result in flattening of the diaphragm curvature (Figure 11-2),[1] which has a negative effect on the maximal transdiaphragmatic pressure.[1,7] Associated reduction in muscle mass contributes to a decrease in the force produced by respiratory muscles. In a 70-year-old individual, maximal skeletal muscle electromyographic activity is reduced by approximately 50%.[10] Respiratory muscle strength may be further affected by nutritional status, which may be deficient in the elderly.[11,12] The main consequence of the reduction in the maximal transdiaphragmatic pressure is predisposition of the diaphragm to fatigue in the presence of increased ventilatory load,[13] which may lead to difficulty in weaning an elderly patient from the ventilator.

Lung Parenchyma

Lung compliance increases with aging primarily because of the loss in parenchymal elasticity (Table 11-1).[7,8] As a result, elastic recoil pressure of the lungs decreases with aging (Figure 11-1).[7,8,14] A presumed mechanism of decrease in elasticity is attributed to changes in the spatial arrangement and/or crosslinking of the elastic fiber network.[9] The changes in lung parenchyma become more pronounced after 50 years of age, resulting in a homoge-

neous enlargement of air spaces causing the reduction of alveolar surface area from $75\,m^2$ at age 30 to $60\,m^2$ at age 70.[9] Because these changes functionally resemble emphysema, they are sometimes referred to as "senile emphysema.'"[6,15]

Spirometry: Static and Dynamic Tests and Underlying Physiology

All lung volumes increase from birth until somatic growth stops. Total lung capacity (TLC) decreases slightly with age. However, TLC is correlated with height, and, given the fact that height diminishes with age (because of flattening of the intervertebral disks), TLC, normalized for height, remains unchanged (Figure 11-3).[7,16,17] Furthermore, the overall effect of loss of inward elastic recoil of the lung with aging is somewhat balanced by the decline in the chest wall outward force such that the TLC remains unchanged.[9] Because TLC remains unchanged, an increase in residual volume (RV) of 5%–10% per decade results in a decrease in vital capacity (VC); after age 20, VC decreases 20–30 mL per year.[18] The RV/TLC ratio increases from 25% at 20 years to 40% in a 70-year-old subject. Functional residual capacity (FRC) is determined by the balance between the inward recoil of the lungs and the outward recoil of the chest wall. FRC increases by 1%–3% per decade (Figure 11-3) because at relaxed end-expiration, the rate of decrease in lung recoil with aging exceeds that of the rate of increase in chest wall stiffness.[18,19]

Forced expiratory volume in 1 second (FEV_1) and forced VC (FVC) increase up to 20 years of age in females and up to 27 years of age in males, followed by gradual decrease (up to 30 mL per year) (Figure 11-4).[9,20,21] After

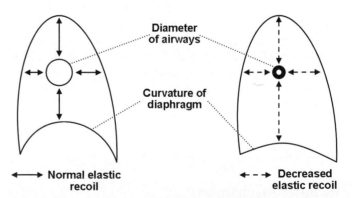

FIGURE 11-2. Aging-induced reduction of elastic recoil results in enlargement (barrel shaped) of the thorax and flattening of the diaphragm. The flatter diaphragm is less efficient in generating more muscle power which increases the work of breathing. The loss of elastic recoil results in a narrowing of small airways. Left panel: juvenile lung; right panel: aged lung. (Reprinted with permission from Zaugg and Lucchinetti.[1] Publisher: WB Saunders. Copyright © 2000 Elsevier.)

TABLE 11-1. Changes in respiratory function associated with aging and pathophysiologic mechanisms that explain perioperative complications.

Function alteration	Change	Pathophysiology	Potential complications
Upper airway patency	↓	Hypotonia of hypopharyngeal and genioglossal muscles, obesity (redundant tissues)	Upper airway obstruction and OSA
Swallowing reflexes and cough	↓ Clearance of secretions		Aspiration risk, inefficient expectoration, pneumonia, atelectasis, hypoxemia
Chest wall compliance	↓	Structural changes of the intercostal muscles and joints; and rib-vertebral articulations	↑ Work of breathing; delayed weaning from mechanical ventilation
Airway resistance	↑	↓ Diameter of small airways	Air trapping, propensity for developing intraoperative atelectasis; ↓ maximal expiratory flow (airflow limitation) during exercise
Lung compliance	↑	↓ Lung static elastic recoil pressure	Air trapping, potential for dynamic hyperinflation during mechanical ventilation
Closing volume	↑	Closing of small airways, sometimes within normal tidal volume breathing	Intraoperative hypoxemia, especially with ↓ FRC (mean lung volume) after induction of anesthesia; airflow limitation
Gas exchange	↓ Oxygenation	↑ Ventilation/perfusion heterogeneity and ↓ diffusing capacity	Hypoxemia
Gas exchange	↔ In CO_2	↑ In dead space ventilation counteracted by ↓ in CO_2 production because of ↓ in basal metabolic rate	
Exercise capacity	↓ Deconditioning	↓ $\dot{V}O_2$max because of ↓ in cardiac output	Associated with higher incidence of postoperative pulmonary complications
Regulation of breathing	↓	Dysfunction of central chemoreceptors and peripheral mechanoreceptors	↓ Ventilatory response to hypoxemia. Risk of hypercarbia and hypoxemia during use of opioids

$\dot{V}O_2$max = maximal oxygen uptake, CO_2 = carbon dioxide, OSA = obstructive sleep apnea, FRC = functional residual capacity, ↑ = increased, ↓ = decreased or reduced, ↔ = no change.

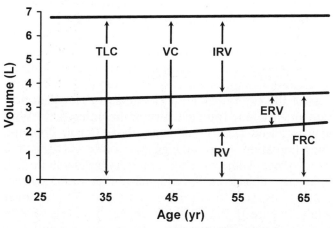

FIGURE 11-3. Evolution of lung volumes with aging. TLC = total lung volume, VC = vital capacity, IRV = inspiratory reserve volume, ERV = expiratory reserve volume, FRC = functional residual capacity, RV = residual volume. Aging produces an increase in RV with consequent reduction in ERV and VC, without changing TLC. (Reprinted with permission from Janssens et al.[7]; publisher: *European Respiratory Journal*; and adapted with permission from Crapo et al.[17]; publisher: *European Respiratory Journal*.)

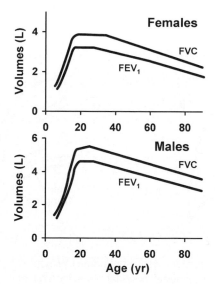

FIGURE 11-4. Effect of aging on FEV_1 (forced expiratory volume in 1 second) and FVC (forced vital capacity) in males and females. Both progressively decline after 20 years of age. (Reprinted with permission from Crapo[9]; and adapted with permission from Burrows et al.[21]; publisher: *Taylor & Francis Group*.)

65 years of age, this decline may be accelerated (38 mL per year).[22] Chronic smoking dramatically accelerates these age-related changes in FEV1 and FVC.[23] In healthy, elderly subjects from 65 to 85 years of age, the normal FEV_1/FVC ratio may be as low as 55%, compared with expected ≥70% in younger individuals.[24] Lung volume is a major determinant of airway resistance but, when adjusted for age-related change in mean lung volume, aging has no significant effect on airway resistance.[25] A decrease in small airway diameter with aging, associated with reduced mean lung volume (Figure 11-2, Table 11-1), contributes to a decrement in maximal expiratory flow with aging,[26] present even in lifetime nonsmokers.[27]

Airway Closure Concept (Closing Volume)

The loss of elastic recoil[7,17] also affects the caliber of intrathoracic airways (Figure 11-2).[26] These airways are normally distended by the transpulmonary pressure gradient (P_{tp}), i.e., the pressure gradient from inside the airway to the pleural space (Figure 11-5A).[28] In upright subjects, there is vertical gradient in pleural pressure, which results in gradient of P_{tp} from the top (high P_{tp}) to the bottom (low P_{tp}) of the lung. This P_{tp} gradient creates differences in the distending forces acting on small airways and causes airway diameter to be smaller in the dependent lung zones (Figure 11-5B).[28] When the patient exhales, the intrapleural pressure becomes less subatmospheric. At some point, the pressure at dependent parts of pleural space equals or exceeds atmospheric, and the airways in the dependent lung zones close (Figure 11-5B). Subsequent research has shown that this concept is an

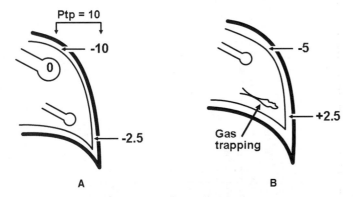

FIGURE 11-5. Effects of transpulmonary pressure (P_{tp}) on airway diameter at functional residual capacity (A) and at residual volume (B). Because of the vertical gradient of transpulmonary pressure, at residual volume the distending pressure across dependent airways becomes negative, and these dependent airways collapse. The lung volume at which this first occurs to a significant extend has been termed the "closing volume." (Reprinted with permission from Sykes et al.[28])

oversimplification of a complicated process. Nonetheless, this concept of "closing volume" is a useful means of conceptualizing lung behavior at low volumes. Because lung static recoil decreases with age, closing volume increases with age. In younger subjects, closing volume is less than FRC, and the airways remain open during resting tidal volume breathing. The increases in FRC with aging are less than increases in closing volume, such that in erect subjects without lung disease the closing volume starts to exceed FRC around the age of 65.[27] Because FRC decreases when a subject assumes the supine position, airway closure may be present during resting tidal volume breathing, and this typically occurs around the age of 45. When airways are closed during tidal breathing, it may lead to gas-exchange abnormalities (discussed below); indeed, changes in closing volume with age are correlated with hypoxemia.[1]

Just as the lung volume is determined by the P_{tp} gradient (as discussed above), the diameter of intrathoracic airways during breathing is determined in part by the transmural pressure gradient, i.e., the gradient of pressure from inside the airway to the intrapleural space.[29] For the larger intrathoracic airways, the pressure outside the airways is the same as intrapleural pressure (Figure 11-6A).[28] This transmural gradient is increased with increases in lung volume so that airway diameter increases with inspiration (Figure 11-6B).[28] During late nonforced expiration, the gradient of pressure between the pleural space and inside the airway is small, causing narrowing of the airway (Figure 11-6C). During forced expiration, active contraction of the expiratory muscles generates pleural pressure that is above atmospheric, and this creates a larger gradient of pressure down the airways (Figure 11-6D). The point in the small airway where intrapleural pressure equals the intra-airway pressure is called "equal pressure point." From that point downstream, the pleural pressure exceeds the intra-airway pressure causing it to close. Compression of airways limits the effectiveness of the expiratory muscles and sets a maximal flow rate for each lung volume ("airflow limitation").[29–31] With aging-induced loss of the lung elastic recoil pressure, "flow limitation" occurs at higher lung volumes compared with younger subjects. This expiratory airflow limitation in elderly subjects causes a significant alteration of ventilatory response to exercise compared with younger adults (Figure 11-7).[32,33] Older subjects have less ventilatory reserve to accommodate the increased ventilatory demand of exercise because of marked airflow limitation.[33] During similar levels of maximal exercise (minute ventilation of 114 L/min), 45% of the tidal volume of the 70-year-old subject is flow-limited because of airway compression, in comparison to less than 20% in the 30-year-old untrained adult (Figure 11-7).[32] Despite these limitations, arterial Pco_2 and Po_2 are well maintained, even during maximal exercise.

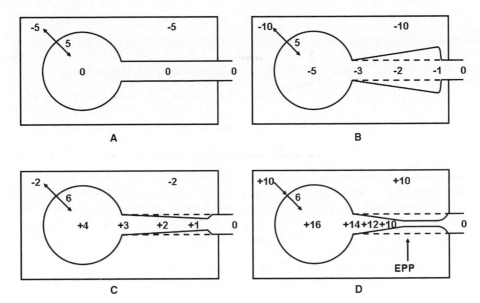

FIGURE 11-6. Factors affecting airway diameter. Schematic presentation of alveolus and intrathoracic airways. **(A)** At FRC: The intrapleural pressure (-5 cm H_2O) is generated by the elastic recoil pressure of the alveoli (-5 cm H_2O). The inside of the alveoli and airways are at atmospheric pressure (0 cm H_2O). A transairway pressure of 5 cm H_2O maintains airway patency. **(B)** Early inspiration: The gradient of pressure from alveolus (-5 cm H_2O) to pleural space (-10 cm H_2O) causes the alveolus to expand and draw air in through the airways. The resistance of the airways creates a gradient of pressure along the airways so that the transairway pressure gradient is greatest in the airways closer to the mouth. **(C)** Late expiration: The activity of the inspiratory muscles has ceased and the lung elastic recoil pressure is $+6$ cm H_2O. The resultant transairway gradient of $+4$ cm H_2O drives the remaining air out of the alveoli. The gradient of pressure between the pleural space and inside the airways is reversed and the airway is narrowed. **(D)** Forced expiration: Active contraction of the expiratory muscles generates above-atmospheric pleural pressure. Although the pressure in the alveolus still exceeds pleural pressure because of the lung elastic recoil pressure, there is a large gradient of pressure down the airways. The pleural pressure equals the intra-airway pressure at equal pressure point (EPP). Downstream from that point the pleural pressure exceeds the intraluminal pressure in the downstream portion of the airway which thus closes. This "dynamic compression" of the airway limits determines the maximal flow achievable at a given lung volume. (Reprinted with permission from Sykes et al.[28])

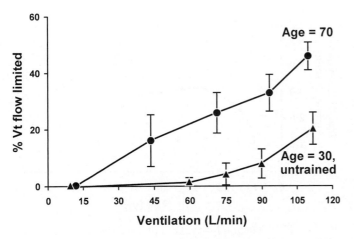

FIGURE 11-7. Flow limitation with progressive exercise in 30-year-old untrained adults and in 70-year-old adults. At a given minute ventilation, the incidence of flow limitation during tidal breathing is greater in the elderly than in the young. (Adapted with permission from Johnson et al.[32]; publisher: Elsevier.)

The Effects of Aging on Gas Exchange

The efficiency of alveolar gas exchange decreases with age. One explanation is an imbalance in the ventilation/perfusion ratio mainly caused by increase in physiologic dead space and shunting.[34,35] This imbalance leads to a gradual decrease in arterial P_{O_2} with aging (Figure 11-8).[19,36,37] At the same time, once arterial P_{CO_2} reaches 40 mm Hg in the newborn, it remains virtually constant for the remainder of life, and the CO_2 elimination remains unaffected despite an increase in dead space ventilation[38] and reduction in CO_2 sensitivity with aging. The latter is attributable at least in part to a decline in CO_2 production associated with a decrease in basal metabolic rate. Multiple factors contribute to the decline in arterial P_{O_2} related to age. In young, seated subjects breathing air at rest, the alveolar-arterial pressure difference for oxygen (A-aDO_2) is between 5 and 10 mm Hg. An increase in the A-aDO_2 with age occurs because of an increase in venti-

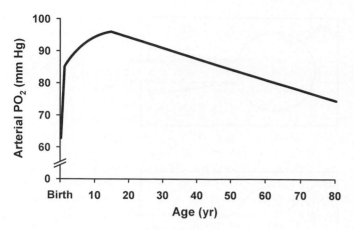

FIGURE 11-8. Arterial oxygenation (Po₂) as a function of age from birth to 80 years. Note the decline in arterial Po₂ after the age of 20. (Reprinted with permission from Murray.[19] Copyright © 1986 Elsevier.)

lation/perfusion heterogeneity, thought to be caused by a decrease in alveolar surface area and increase in closing volume.[39] Additionally, increased body mass index, as seen with obesity, that frequently accompanies aging, can contribute to the widening of A-aDO₂. After 75 years of age, arterial oxygen tension remains relatively stable at around 83 mm Hg.[40] The diffusing capacity of the lungs decreases with aging[41] at a rate between 0.2 and 0.3 mL/min/mm Hg/year,[19] with this decline being more pronounced after the age of 40. This deterioration is attributed to an increase in ventilation/perfusion mismatching, decline in pulmonary capillary blood volume,[41] and/or the loss of the alveolar surface area.[42]

Aging and Exercise Capacity

Age is a significant factor determining maximal O₂ uptake ($\dot{V}O_2max$). $\dot{V}O_2$ reaches a peak between 20 and 30 years of age and then decreases at a rate of 9% per decade (Figure 11-9).[19,43] The $\dot{V}O_2max$ decrease is more pronounced in sedentary elderly subjects than in the physically active.[44] In elderly individuals who maintain athletic exercise, the decline in $\dot{V}O_2max$ is slowed. Factors that limit the $\dot{V}O_2max$ in the elderly include a decrease in maximal minute ventilation, decrease in the maximum arterial-venous O₂ content difference, decrease in O₂ extraction by the tissues, and reduced peripheral muscle mass. The decrease in O₂ transport capacity during senescence is also linked to an age-related decrease in cardiac output. The O₂ cost of breathing (i.e., proportion of O₂ consumption by respiratory muscles) is higher than in younger subjects. Also, compared with younger individuals, the elderly are more responsive to CO₂ during exercise; for a given CO₂ production, the ventilatory response

increases with aging, unrelated to oxyhemoglobin desaturation or increase in metabolic acidosis.[45]

Regulation of Breathing

In humans, ventilation is adjusted by inputs from different chemoreceptors that respond to metabolic factors and by inputs from mechanoreceptors that provide feedback from the chest wall, lungs, and airways. Minute ventilation at rest is similar in young and elderly subjects, but tidal volumes are smaller and respiratory rates are higher in the elderly.[46] The mechanism is not fully understood, but it may represent an adaptation to decreases in chest wall compliance, as well as changes in the function of central chemoreceptors and peripheral mechanoreceptors in the chest wall and lung parenchyma.[47] Compared with younger subjects, elderly individuals have approximately 50% and 60% reduction in the ventilatory response to hypoxia and hypercapnia, respectively.[48] Moreover, studies have shown that the average increase in ventilation in response to an alveolar pressure of oxygen of 40 mm Hg in older men is 10 L/min, in contrast to 40 L/min for younger individuals.[49] Responses to normocapnic hypoxemia during sleep can be even more depressed. For example, elderly individuals may not arouse from the REM phase of sleep until their oxyhemoglobin saturation decreases below 70%. Although in elderly subjects the ventilatory response to hypercapnia is blunted compared with younger subjects, the ventilatory response to exercise is actually increased: for a given CO₂ production during exercise, the ventilatory response increases with aging compared with younger individuals.[45] This cannot be explained by either increased anaerobiosis or oxyhemoglobin desaturation, but it seems

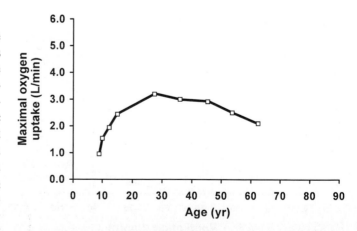

FIGURE 11-9. Maximal oxygen uptake ($\dot{V}O_2max$) measured during maximal exercise as a function of age. Note the decline in $\dot{V}O_2max$ starting near 30 years of age. (Reprinted with permission from Murray.[19] Copyright © 1986 Elsevier; and adapted from Grimby and Saltin[43] by permission from *Taylor & Francis Group*.)

that increased ventilation in the elderly compensates for increased inefficiency of gas exchange, allowing for the maintenance of normocapnia during exercise.[50]

Other respiratory control mechanisms may be altered in the elderly because of reduced efficiency in distinguishing respiratory stimuli and/or altered integration of perception of stimuli within the central nervous system.[51-53] The elderly also have a lesser ability to perceive methacholine-induced bronchoconstriction.[41] The loss of important protective and adaptive mechanisms, which may result in lesser awareness of disease and delayed diagnosis of pulmonary dysfunction in the elderly, are influenced by the blunted response to hypoxia and hypercapnia and a lower ability to perceive disease states such as bronchoconstriction.

Upper Airway Dysfunction

Hypotonia of the hypopharyngeal and genioglossal muscles predispose elderly subjects to upper airway obstruction, and the prevalence of sleep-disordered breathing increases with age.[54] Studies have found that up to 75% of subjects over 65 years old have obstructive sleep apnea (OSA).[55,56] Indeed, the prevalence of OSA in the elderly is so high that authorities are questioning whether OSA in the elderly is a different disease from OSA in middle age.[55] Some of the consequences of chronic hypoxemia associated with OSA may include cognitive impairment, personality changes, and hypertension.[56] OSA may be even more prevalent in elderly obese individuals, who may have increased postoperative risk of respiratory complications.[57]

The protective mechanisms of cough and swallowing are altered in elderly individuals, which may lead to ineffective clearance of secretions and increased susceptibility to aspiration. Mucociliary transport is also impaired in the elderly. Coughing is also less efficient in terms of volume, force, and flow rate. The loss of protective upper-airway reflexes is presumably attributable to an age-related alteration in peripheral signaling together with decreased central nervous system reflex activity.[58] In addition, elderly individuals have an increased prevalence of neurologic diseases that may be associated with dysphagia and an impaired cough reflex leading to the increased likelihood of pulmonary aspiration[58] and pneumonia,[59] which may have a significant impact on perioperative morbidity and mortality.

Perioperative Pulmonary Complications in the Elderly

With increased longevity, more elderly patients are potential candidates for major surgical procedures. For example, in 1997 in the United States, the Agency for Healthcare Policy and Research reported 1,350,000 major procedures in the 65- to 84-year-old age group and 233,000 procedures in the 85 and older age group.[60] Postoperative pulmonary complications, including atelectasis, pneumonia, respiratory failure, and exacerbation of underlying chronic lung disease, have a significant role in the risk for anesthesia and surgery.[61] These complications have been reported in 5%–10% of the general patient population[62] and usually prolong the hospital stay by an average of 1–2 weeks.[63] Pulmonary complications in nonthoracic surgery are as prevalent as cardiovascular complications and contribute in a similar manner to morbidity, mortality, and length of stay.[64,65]

Numerous factors may contribute to the development of postoperative pulmonary complications in the elderly (Figure 11-10). Advanced age is a significant independent predictor of pulmonary complications even after adjustment for various comorbid conditions.[61,64,66] Age increases the risk of pulmonary complications with an odds ratio of 2.1 for patients 60–69 years old, and 3.0 for those 70–79 years old compared with patients younger than 60 years.[61,64,67] Older age represents the second most common identified risk factor for pulmonary complications after the presence of chronic lung disease.[61,66,68] A multifactorial risk index for predicting postoperative respiratory failure in men after major noncardiac surgery[69] showed that age above 70 conferred a 2.6-fold increase in the risk of respiratory failure compared with subjects less than 60 years old.

Factors contributing to an increased risk of pulmonary complications in the elderly are: (a) decreases in chest wall compliance and muscle strength (increasing the work of breathing and the risk for respiratory failure); (b) changes in lung mechanics (including increased tendency for small airway closure which may impair gas exchange and promote atelectasis); (c) increased aspiration risk secondary to swallowing dysfunction; and (d) alterations in the control of breathing, including impaired responses to hypercapnia and hypoxia and increased sensitivity to drugs used during anesthesia (especially opioids) in the elderly.[70]

Intraoperative alterations in chest wall function lead to atelectasis, which forms within minutes after the induction of anesthesia and is an important cause of intraoperative gas-exchange abnormalities. Chest wall dysfunction persists into the postoperative period because of pain (which limits the voluntary actions of the chest wall muscles), reflex inhibition of the respiratory muscles, and mechanical disruption of respiratory muscles (surgery in the thoracic and abdominal cavities). Consequently, after thoracic or upper abdominal surgery, FRC and VC decrease and breathing becomes rapid and shallow, all of which may contribute to the development of pulmonary complications.[71] These effects apply to all ages but may be of special significance in the elderly patient with reduced respiratory reserve.

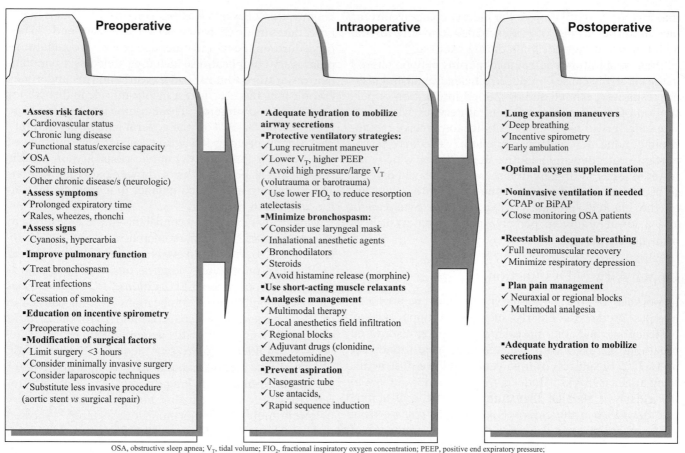

Preoperative	**Intraoperative**	**Postoperative**
■**Assess risk factors** ✓Cardiovascular status ✓Chronic lung disease ✓Functional status/exercise capacity ✓OSA ✓Smoking history ✓Other chronic disease/s (neurologic) ■**Assess symptoms** ✓Prolonged expiratory time ✓Rales, wheezes, rhonchi ■**Assess signs** ✓Cyanosis, hypercarbia ■**Improve pulmonary function** ✓Treat bronchospasm ✓Treat infections ✓Cessation of smoking ■**Education on incentive spirometry** ✓Preoperative coaching ■**Modification of surgical factors** ✓Limit surgery <3 hours ✓Consider minimally invasive surgery ✓Consider laparoscopic techniques ✓Substitute less invasive procedure (aortic stent *vs* surgical repair)	■**Adequate hydration to mobilize airway secretions** ■**Chronic ventilatory strategies:** ✓Lung recruitment maneuver ✓Lower V_T, higher PEEP ✓Avoid high pressure/large V_T (volutrauma or barotrauma) ✓Use lower FIO_2 to reduce resorption atelectasis ■**Minimize bronchospasm:** ✓Consider use laryngeal mask ✓Inhalational anesthetic agents ✓Bronchodilators ✓Steroids ✓Avoid histamine release (morphine) ■**Use short-acting muscle relaxants** ■**Analgesic management** ✓Multimodal therapy ✓Local anesthetics field infiltration ✓Regional blocks ✓Adjuvant drugs (clonidine, dexmedetomidine) ■**Prevent aspiration** ✓Nasogastric tube ✓Use antacids, ✓Rapid sequence induction	■**Lung expansion maneuvers** ✓Deep breathing ✓Incentive spirometry ✓Early ambulation ■**Optimal oxygen supplementation** ■**Noninvasive ventilation if needed** ✓CPAP or BiPAP ✓Close monitoring OSA patients ■**Reestablish adequate breathing** ✓Full neuromuscular recovery ✓Minimize respiratory depression ■ **Plan pain management** ✓ Neuraxial or regional blocks ✓ Multimodal analgesia ■**Adequate hydration to mobilize secretions**

OSA, obstructive sleep apnea; V_T, tidal volume; FIO_2, fractional inspiratory oxygen concentration; PEEP, positive end expiratory pressure; CPAP, continuous positive airway pressure; BiPAP, bi-level positive pressure pressure

FIGURE 11-10. Perioperative strategies used to minimize pulmonary complications.

Older, nonanesthetized individuals have less efficient gas exchange compared with younger subjects.[36] Upon assuming the supine position, there is a decrease in FRC and hence an increase in airway resistance, which is more marked in the elderly (especially those who are obese).[36] Alveolar gas exchange during anesthesia is less efficient in the elderly, and there is an inverse relationship between increased age and arterial Po_2 in spontaneously breathing anesthetized patients.[37,39] After the induction of anesthesia, atelectasis develops in dependent lung regions and may produce significant shunting. However, both the amount of atelectasis and pulmonary shunting do not increase significantly with age.[72,73] A similar phenomenon occurs in patients with chronic obstructive pulmonary disease (COPD); after the induction of anesthesia, there is less formation of atelectasis and less shunting compared with normal patients, which is explained by changes in the chest wall secondary to hyperinflation that prevents alveolar collapse.[74]

Decreased respiratory muscle strength, combined with diminished cough and swallowing reflexes (neurologic disorders, stroke, etc.), may diminish clearance of secre-tions and increase the risk of aspiration in the elderly.[75,76] This risk is even higher in the presence of gastroesopha-geal reflux, which is also more prevalent in the elderly. Selective, rather than routine, nasogastric tube decom-pression after abdominal surgery may improve the return of bowel function and reduce the risk of postoperative pulmonary complications, specifically a lower rate of atel-ectasis and pneumonia.[77,78] Interestingly a the aspiration rate was not lower in patients with selective nasogastric decompression.[78] Finally, age-related changes in control of breathing, increased sensitivity to anesthetic agents, and diminished response to gas-exchange abnormalities predispose elderly patients to postoperative respiratory failure. Elderly patients also have a higher incidence of postoperative sleep apnea episodes.[70,79]

General Health Status

Multiple measures of functional status and general health predict the risk of postoperative pulmonary complica-tions. An American Society of Anesthesiologists Physical Status Classification above II, poor exercise capacity, the presence of COPD, and congestive heart failure are all associated with increased risk of pulmonary complications in the elderly.[64,80,81] COPD is more prevalent in the elderly population and is the most important patient-related risk factor for the development of postoperative pulmonary complications, producing a three- to fourfold increase in relative risk.[66,81,82] Although obesity is prevalent in elderly patients and is associated with decreased perioperative arterial oxygenation, obesity is not a significant independent predictor of risk.[64,80,83]

Decreased functional status, which may accompany aging, is an independent risk factor for pulmonary complications.[64] Objective measurement of exercise capacity in geriatric patients demonstrated that inability to perform 2-minute supine bicycle exercise and an increase in the heart rate to above 99 beats/min was the best predictor of perioperative cardiopulmonary complications in patients older than 65 years undergoing elective abdominal or noncardiac thoracic surgery.[84] Patients with better exercise tolerance by self-report, better walking distance, or better cardiovascular classification had lower rates of postoperative pulmonary complications.[85]

Strategies Used to Minimize Pulmonary Risk in Elderly Patients: Preoperative Considerations

Preoperative Testing

The value of routine preoperative pulmonary function testing is controversial. For lung resection surgery, the results of pulmonary function testing, including measurement of arterial blood gases, have proven useful in predicting pulmonary complications and postoperative function; however, spirometry does not predict postoperative pulmonary complications after abdominal surgery.[85,86] Warner et al.[87] have demonstrated that the degree of airway obstruction assessed by spirometry does not represent an independent risk factor for postoperative respiratory failure, even in smokers with severe lung disease.[87] Spirometry, chest radiograms, and arterial blood gases should be obtained as indicated from the history and physical examination as a part of this evaluation, but should not be routinely ordered.[78]

Preoperative Therapies

To minimize postoperative pulmonary complications in elderly patients, it is important to optimize the respiratory status, beginning with a careful assessment of general physical status, with particular attention to the cardiopulmonary system. Specific therapy should be instituted preoperatively if such treatment is likely to result in improved functional status, so long as the therapeutic benefit outweighs any risk from surgical delay (Figure 11-10).

Preoperative spirometry should be used only to monitor the degree of therapeutic response to treatments such as bronchodilators used to treat reactive airway disease. Patients with a reversible component of airway obstruction must be treated with bronchodilators and/or corticosteroids. Antibiotics must be given if a pulmonary infection is suspected. Preoperative smoking cessation may decrease postoperative pulmonary complications, and all patients who smoke should be given help to quit.[88,89] Past studies have been interpreted as demonstrating that quitting within a few weeks of surgery actually increases pulmonary complications by stimulating mucous production.[90] However, careful review of these studies and more recent data show that, although it may take several weeks of abstinence before pulmonary outcomes are improved, brief abstinence does not worsen outcomes.[89,90] Thus, this consideration should not prevent practitioners from promoting preoperative abstinence from smoking, even for a brief period before surgery.

Strategies Used to Minimize Pulmonary Risk in Elderly Patients: Intraoperative Considerations

Surgical Considerations

The surgical site is the most important risk factor for the development of postoperative pulmonary complications and outweighs other patient-related risk factors.[67,69] There is a higher likelihood of pulmonary complications with incisions closer to the diaphragm because of diaphragmatic dysfunction, splinting, and decreased ability to take deep breaths. For example, pulmonary complications caused by upper abdominal surgeries range from 13% to 33% as compared with lower abdominal surgeries that range from 0% to 16%.[80] Duration of surgery also has a significant role in the development of pulmonary complications, and surgeries that last more than 3 hours have an increased risk of pulmonary complications.[91] When surgically feasible, laparoscopic techniques should be considered; however, significant respiratory dysfunction can occur even after laparoscopically performed operations,[78] and whether laparoscopic procedures may reduce the risk of clinically important pulmonary complications is not clear. Nonetheless, other considerations such as reduced postoperative pain and length of stay often favor the use of laparoscopic techniques. Placement of an aortic stent instead of an open aortic aneurysm repair may be desirable in patients with significant pulmonary comorbidity.

Induction of Anesthesia

Preoxygenation is recommended before the induction of general anesthesia. In contrast to younger patients, performing only four deep breaths before the induction may not be sufficient in elderly patients, who may require a full 3 minutes of 100% oxygen breathing to avoid oxyhemoglobin desaturation during rapid sequence induction.[92] In patients with intact oropharyngeal reflexes but significant reactive airway disease, avoidance of endotracheal intubation by using a laryngeal mask airway may be desirable.

Use of Muscle Relaxants During Anesthesia

In elderly patients, inadequate reversal of muscle paralysis may be an important factor for postoperative complications leading to hypoventilation and hypoxemia.[86] Pulmonary complications are three times higher among patients receiving a long-acting neuromuscular blocker than among those receiving shorter-acting relaxants.[93] Short-acting neuromuscular blocking agents should be used in the elderly to avoid prolonged muscle paralysis, and adequacy of reversal of neuromuscular block should be tested before extubation.[78]

Use of Regional Anesthetic Techniques for Surgery

Evidence is conflicting whether the use of regional techniques instead of general anesthesia will prevent postoperative pulmonary complications.[78] Regional anesthesia may be indicated for a variety of reasons in the elderly, but it has its own potential respiratory-related risks in these patients. Unintentional high anesthetic level during neuraxial anesthesia may be associated with paralysis of the chest wall (respiratory muscles) that may be poorly tolerated by the elderly, especially those with COPD. Regional techniques performed at the level of the neck (interscalene block, stellate ganglion block, axillary block) may be associated with paralysis of the phrenic nerve (diaphragm), and, if performed bilaterally, the patient may develop acute respiratory failure requiring urgent tracheal intubation.

Intraoperative Lung Expansion During General Anesthesia

As discussed before, in contrast to younger patients, atelectasis may be a less important cause of intraoperative hypoxemia during general anesthesia in the elderly[72]; however, in elderly obese patients, atelectasis may have a significant role in deterioration of intraoperative arterial oxygenation.[94] The isolated use of positive end-expiratory pressure (PEEP) does not predictably reverse atelectasis or increase arterial oxygenation.[95] Recently, there has been a considerable interest in maneuvers designated to recruit atelectatic lung regions. To reexpand the atelectatic lung, it is necessary to use a sustained lung insufflation (5–10 seconds long) with high inflation pressures (40 cm H_2O or above).[96–98] This technique is called a "recruitment maneuver" or "vital capacity maneuver" and should be followed by sufficient PEEP to maintain the alveolar units open.[99] It is crucial to closely monitor changes in blood pressure and heart rate while performing the recruitment maneuver because significant hypotension, especially in hypovolemic patients, may ensue.

Strategies Used to Minimize Pulmonary Risk in Elderly Patients: Postoperative Considerations

Neuraxial Blocks for Pain Management

Good postoperative pain control is necessary in all patients. There is a longstanding debate regarding whether neuraxial techniques such as epidural analgesia reduce the frequency of pulmonary complications. It is clear that these techniques provide excellent analgesia, but their benefits regarding pulmonary outcomes are less clear.[71] In one meta-analysis,[100] regional techniques reduced mortality by about a third with reductions of pulmonary embolism and pneumonia of 55% and 39%, respectively. However, many of the studies used in this and other meta-analyses have methodologic limitations. A recent unblinded, large clinical trial found few differences in outcome between those receiving and not receiving epidural analgesia, with the exceptions that: (1) respiratory failure was less frequent for some types of operations, and (2) postoperative pain control was improved by epidural analgesia.[101] A prospective, double-blind randomized trial performed by Jayr et al.[102] demonstrated that the use of epidural analgesia provided superior postoperative comfort without affecting the frequency of postoperative pulmonary complications. In addition, another blinded trial performed by Norris et al.[103] showed that in patients undergoing surgery of the abdominal aorta, thoracic epidural anesthesia combined with a light general anesthesia and followed by either intravenous or epidural patient-controlled analgesia offers no major advantage or disadvantage except for slightly shorter time to extubation. Postoperative pain management may include the use of a full range of adjunctive analgesia techniques, such as surgical field infiltration with local anesthetics, utilization of peripheral nerve blocks, nonsteroidal antiinflammatory agents, clonidine, and dexmedetomidine.[104] This "multimodal approach" of using the drugs that are associated with low potential for respiratory depression may be beneficial in elderly patients prone to developing postoperative respiratory depression.

Caution Regarding Perioperative Use of Opioids

Elderly patients may be especially sensitive to medications because of age-related altered pharmacokinetics and pharmacodynamics of the drugs.[70,105] Aging affects all pharmacokinetic processes, but the most important change is the reduction in the renal drug elimination. At the same time, pharmacodynamic changes also occur at the receptor or signal-transduction level or at the level of the homeostatic mechanisms.[105] This situation explains why the dosing of all anesthetic drugs should reflect the differences in pharmacokinetics and pharmacodynamics that accompany aging. Opioids are of particular concern in the elderly. Opioids reduce the respiratory response to chemical (hypoxemia, hypercapnia) load resulting in hypoventilation and hypoxemia. Given the fact that elderly patients may be particularly sensitive to opioids, they should be titrated carefully in order to avoid postoperative respiratory depression.[70]

Postoperative Respiratory Assistance to Maintain Lung Expansion

Decreased lung volumes and atelectasis attributable to surgery-related shallow breathing, bed rest, diaphragmatic dysfunction, pain, and impaired mucociliary clearance may be the first events in a cascade leading to postoperative pulmonary complications.[78] Postoperative use of lung expansion therapy such as incentive spirometry, chest physical therapy, effective cough, postural drainage, percussion-vibration, ambulation, continuous positive airway pressure (CPAP), and intermittent positive-pressure breathing is the mainstay of postoperative prevention of pulmonary complications in the elderly. Preoperative education in these maneuvers may reduce pulmonary complications more efficiently than when instruction is given after surgery.[106,107] Lung expansion maneuvers, when performed appropriately, lower the risk of atelectasis by 50%.[108] No modality seems superior, and combined modalities do not seem to provide additional risk reduction.[78] Incentive spirometry may be the least labor-intensive, whereas CPAP may be particularly beneficial for patients who cannot participate in incentive spirometry or deep-breathing exercises.[78] However, a most recent systematic review of randomized trials suggested that routine respiratory physiotherapy may not seem to be justified as a strategy for reducing postoperative pulmonary complications after abdominal surgery.[109] All patients with diagnosed OSA should have their status evaluated preoperatively, and, if they are CPAP-dependent, they should receive the CPAP treatment immediately after tracheal extubation. In addition, they may need close postoperative monitoring (i.e., oxygenation and ventilation). Depending on the severity of OSA, type of surgery, and anesthesia, they may require admission to a monitored bed overnight.

Noninvasive Positive Pressure Ventilation

Noninvasive positive pressure ventilation (NPPV) is the delivery of mechanically assisted breaths without placement of an artificial airway, such as an endotracheal or a tracheostomy tube. Bilevel positive airway pressure (BiPAP) is noninvasive ventilatory modality that seems to be more efficient than CPAP in supporting breathing. With BiPAP, continuous inspiratory positive airway pressure provides inspiratory assistance and expiratory positive airway pressure prevents alveolar closure.[104]

NPPV may be used in patients with COPD exacerbations, cardiogenic pulmonary edema, hypercapnic respiratory failure caused by neuromuscular disease, obesity-hypoventilation syndrome, and immunocompromised patients with respiratory failure. The role of nasal intermittent positive pressure ventilation (NIPPV) in hypoxemic respiratory failure attributable to other causes is still controversial and lacks adequate evidence support. The idea of utilizing NIPPV to manage patients with postextubation respiratory failure came from several trials demonstrating efficacy of NIPPV in postoperative respiratory failure, particularly when cardiogenic pulmonary edema was the etiology.[110–114] Immediately after extubation, elderly patients may need additional ventilatory support to maintain ventilation and oxygenation. CPAP has been successfully used to avoid tracheal reintubation in patients who developed hypoxemia after elective major abdominal surgery, and the use of CPAP was associated with lower incidence of other severe postoperative complications.[115] Outcomes of patients with postoperative postextubation hypoxemia treated by CPAP[115] may differ from that in the general intensive care population[116] or in patients with acute exacerbation of COPD.[117,118] Thus, Esteban et al.[116] demonstrated that NPPV does not prevent the need for reintubation and may be harmful in intensive care unit patients who develop respiratory failure after tracheal extubation. In contrast, in patients with acute exacerbation of COPD, comparing noninvasive ventilation with a standard intensive care unit approach in which endotracheal intubation was performed after failure of medical treatment, the use of noninvasive ventilation reduced complications, length of stay in the intensive care unit, and mortality.[117] The application of NIPPV has also been used successfully in the postoperative period with morbid obesity patients who were undergoing bariatric surgery.[119,120] Prophylactic BiPAP used during the first 12–24 hours after bariatric surgery resulted in significantly higher measures of pulmonary function, but did not translate into fewer hospital days or a lower complication rate.[119]

Mechanical Ventilation in the Elderly

An aging population is projected to substantially increase the demand for intensive care unit services during the next 25 years.[121,122] An increasing number of elderly patients will also require intensive care treatment after surgery. The risk of respiratory failure requiring mechanical ventilation in response to a variety of physiologic insults, including surgery, is increased in the elderly because of underlying pulmonary disease, loss of muscle mass, and other comorbid conditions.[123] In patients that develop adult respiratory distress syndrome, older age is clearly associated with higher mortality rates.[124,125] Ely et al.[126] prospectively studied whether age represents an independent effect on the outcomes in a cohort of patients requiring mechanical ventilation after admission to an intensive care unit. After adjustment for severity of illness, elderly patients, compared with younger patients, required a comparable length of mechanical ventilation. These effects could not be attributed to the differences in mortality; therefore, mechanical ventilation should not be withheld from elderly patients with respiratory failure on the basis of chronologic age.[126]

Patients aged 65 years or older account for 47% of intensive care unit admissions.[127] With aging, there are several factors known to affect weaning, such as decrease in lung elasticity, reduction in FVC, decreased respiratory muscle strength, and decreased chest wall compliance.[128] Kleinhenz and Lewis[129] reviewed the challenges of caring for elderly patients with chronic ventilator dependency. Long-term ventilator dependence, defined as need for mechanical ventilation for 6 hours per day for more than 21 days, is disproportionately higher in patients over 70 years of age.[129] Long-term ventilator dependence complicates 9% to 20% of the episodes of mechanical ventilation treated in the intensive care units of acute care hospitals, and it is associated with an average mortality rate of 40%.[129] This is an important socioeconomic issue, and more research is needed regarding the causes that may lead to respiratory failure in elderly patients. There is an ongoing investigation of the effects of "protective ventilatory strategies" (lower tidal volume, higher PEEP, recruitment lung strategies, as well as effects of intraoperatively administered fluids and blood products) on postoperative pulmonary outcomes. Literature evidence is slowly accumulating showing that the use of "protective ventilatory strategies" in high-risk patients may be beneficial in preventing postoperative ventilatory failure[130–133]; however, more studies are necessary before making definitive recommendations. Some specific areas that require further investigation are the relationship between the influence of age on weaning and the relationship between age and the work of breathing.

Conclusion

Aging causes significant changes in respiratory function, which leads to ventilation perfusion mismatching and diminished efficiency of gas exchange. The perioperative period represents a time of increased functional demand on the respiratory system, and elderly patients with reduced respiratory function may be prone to developing pulmonary complications. These complications are a significant source of morbidity, mortality, and prolonged hospitalization. These pulmonary complications may be attributed to diminished protective reflexes, increased sensitivity to respiratory depressants, and altered responses to hypoxemia and hypercapnia. After identifying patients at risk for postoperative pulmonary complications, anesthesiologists must consider strategies to try to reduce the risk throughout the perioperative period. Besides optimization of underlying comorbid conditions, anesthesiologists and other perioperative physicians may utilize strategies that facilitate lung expansion such as deep-breathing exercises, incentive spirometry, and adequate postoperative pain control. Select patients may benefit from postoperative application of NPPV.

References

1. Zaugg M, Lucchinetti E. Respiratory function in the elderly. Anesthesiol Clin North Am 2000;18(1):47–58, vi.
2. Pollock ML, Mengelkoch LJ, Graves JE, et al. Twenty-year follow-up of aerobic power and body composition of older track athletes. J Appl Physiol 1997;82(5):1508–1516.
3. McClaran SR, Babcock MA, Pegelow DF, Reddan WG, Dempsey JA. Longitudinal effects of aging on lung function at rest and exercise in healthy active fit elderly adults. J Appl Physiol 1995;78(5):1957–1968.
4. Kiyokawa H. Senescence and cell cycle control. Results Probl Cell Differ 2006;42:257–270.
5. Terman A, Gustafsson B, Brunk UT. Mitochondrial damage and intralysosomal degradation in cellular aging. Mol Aspects Med 2006;27(5–6):471–482.
6. Campbell EJ, Lefrak SS. How aging affects the structure and function of the respiratory system. Geriatrics 1978; 33(6):68–74.
7. Janssens JP, Pache JC, Nicod LP. Physiological changes in respiratory function associated with ageing. Eur Respir J 1999;13(1):197–205.
8. Turner JM, Mead J, Wohl ME. Elasticity of human lungs in relation to age. J Appl Physiol 1968;25(6):664–671.
9. Crapo RO. The aging lung. In: Mahler DA, ed. Pulmonary Disease in the Elderly Patient. New York: Marcel Dekker; 1993:1–21.
10. Larsson L. Histochemical characteristics of human skeletal muscle during aging. Acta Physiol Scand 1983;117(3):469–471.
11. Enright P, Kronmal R, Manolio T, Schenker M, Hyatt R. Respiratory muscle strength in the elderly. Correlates and reference values. Cardiovascular Health Study Research Group. Am J Respir Crit Care Med 1994;149(2):430–438.
12. Arora NS, Rochester DF. Respiratory muscle strength and maximal voluntary ventilation in undernourished patients. Am Rev Respir Dis 1982;126(1):5–8.
13. Tolep K, Higgins N, Muza S, Criner G, Kelsen SG. Comparison of diaphragm strength between healthy adult elderly and young men. Am J Respir Crit Care Med 1995; 152(2):677–682.

14. Niewohner D, Kleinerman J, Liotta L. Elastic behaviour of post-mortem human lungs: effects of aging and mild emphysema. J Appl Physiol 1975;25:664–671.

15. Verbeken E, Cauberghs M, Mertens I, Clement J, Lauweryns J, Van de Woestijne K. The senile lung. Comparison with normal and emphysematous lungs. 2. Functional aspects. Chest 1992;101(3):800–809.

16. Levitzky MG. Effects of aging on the respiratory system. Physiologist 1984;27(2):102–107.

17. Crapo RO, Morris AH, Clayton PD, Nixon CR. Lung volumes in healthy nonsmoking adults. Bull Eur Physiopathol Respir 1982;18(3):419–425.

18. Knudson RJ, Clark DF, Kennedy TC, Knudson DE. Effect of aging alone on mechanical properties of the normal adult human lung. J Appl Physiol 1977;43(6):1054–1062.

19. Murray JF. Aging. In: Murray JF, ed. The Normal Lung. Philadelphia: WB Saunders; 1986:339–360.

20. Knudson RJ, Slatin RC, Lebowitz MD, Burrows B. The maximal expiratory flow-volume curve. Normal standards, variability, and effects of age. Am Rev Respir Dis 1976; 113(5):587–600.

21. Burrows B, Cline MG, Knudson RJ, Taussig LM, Lebowitz MD. A descriptive analysis of the growth and decline of the FVC and FEV1. Chest 1983;83(5):717–724.

22. Brandstetter RD, Kazemi H. Aging and the respiratory system. Med Clin North Am 1983;67(2):419–431.

23. Griffith KA, Sherrill DL, Siegel EM, Manolio TA, Bonekat HW, Enright PL. Predictors of loss of lung function in the elderly: the Cardiovascular Health Study. Am J Respir Crit Care Med 2001;163(1):61–68.

24. Enright PL, Kronmal RA, Higgins M, Schenker M, Haponik EF. Spirometry reference values for women and men 65 to 85 years of age. Cardiovascular health study. Am Rev Respir Dis 1993;147(1):125–133.

25. Anthonisen N. Tests of mechanical function. In: Handbook of Physiology. Bethesda, MD: American Physiology Society; 1986:753–784.

26. Niewohner D, Kleinerman J. Morphologic basis of pulmonary resistance in human lung and effects of aging. J Appl Physiol 1974;36:412–418.

27. Fowler RW, Pluck RA, Hetzel MR. Maximal expiratory flow-volume curves in Londoners aged 60 years and over. Thorax 1987;42(3):173–182.

28. Sykes MK, McNicol MW, Campbell EJM. The mechanics of respiration. In: Sykes MK, McNicol MW, Campbell EJM, eds. Respiratory Failure. London: Blackwell Scientific Publications; 1976:3–30.

29. Hyatt RE, Flath RE. Influence of lung parenchyma on pressure-diameter behavior of dog bronchi. J Appl Physiol 1966;21(5):1448–1452.

30. Hyatt RE. Expiratory flow limitation. J Appl Physiol 1983; 55(1 Pt 1):1–7.

31. Babb TG, Rodarte JR. Mechanism of reduced maximal expiratory flow with aging. J Appl Physiol 2000;89(2):505–511.

32. Johnson BD, Badr MS, Dempsey JA. Impact of the aging pulmonary system on the response to exercise. Clin Chest Med 1994;15(2):229–246.

33. DeLorey DS, Babb TG. Progressive mechanical ventilatory constraints with aging. Am J Respir Crit Care Med 1999;160(1):169–177.

34. Wagner PD, Laravuso RB, Uhl RR, West JB. Continuous distributions of ventilation-perfusion ratios in normal subjects breathing air and 100 per cent O_2. J Clin Invest 1974; 54(1):54–68.

35. Wagner PD, Saltzman HA, West JB. Measurement of continuous distributions of ventilation-perfusion ratios: theory. J Appl Physiol 1974;36(5):588–599.

36. Craig DB, Wahba WM, Don HF, Couture JG, Becklake MR. "Closing volume" and its relationship to gas exchange in seated and supine positions. J Appl Physiol 1971;31(5): 717–721.

37. Sorbini CA, Grassi V, Solinas E, Muiesan G. Arterial oxygen tension in relation to age in healthy subjects. Respiration 1968;25(1):3–13.

38. Raine JM, Bishop JM. A-a difference in O_2 tension and physiological dead space in normal man. J Appl Physiol 1963;18:284–288.

39. Wahba WM. Influence of aging on lung function—clinical significance of changes from age twenty. Anesth Analg 1983; 62(8):764–776.

40. Cerveri I, Zoia MC, Fanfulla F, et al. Reference values of arterial oxygen tension in the middle-aged and elderly. Am J Respir Crit Care Med 1995;152(3):934–941.

41. Guenard H, Marthan R. Pulmonary gas exchange in elderly subjects. Eur Respir J 1996;9(12):2573–2577.

42. Thurlbeck WM, Angus GE. Growth and aging of the normal human lung. Chest 1975;67(2 Suppl):3S–6S.

43. Grimby G, Saltin B. Physiological effects of physical training. Scand J Rehabil Med 1971;3(1):6–14.

44. Mahler DA, Cunningham LN, Curfman GD. Aging and exercise performance. Clin Geriatr Med 1986;2(2):433–452.

45. Poulin MJ, Cunningham DA, Paterson DH, Rechnitzer PA, Ecclestone NA, Koval JJ. Ventilatory response to exercise in men and women 55 to 86 years of age. Am J Respir Crit Care Med 1994;149(2 Pt 1):408–415.

46. Krumpe PE, Knudson RJ, Parsons G, Reiser K. The aging respiratory system. Clin Geriatr Med 1985;1(1):143–175.

47. Mahler DA, Rosiello RA, Loke J. The aging lung. Part 1. Loss of elasticity. Clin Geriatr Med 1986;2(2):215–225.

48. Peterson DD, Pack AI, Silage DA, Fishman AP. Effects of aging on ventilatory and occlusion pressure responses to hypoxia and hypercapnia. Am Rev Respir Dis 1981; 124(4):387–391.

49. Kronenberg RS, Drage CW. Attenuation of the ventilatory and heart rate responses to hypoxia and hypercapnia with aging in normal men. J Clin Invest 1973;52(8):1812–1819.

50. Brischetto MJ, Millman RP, Peterson DD, Silage DA, Pack AI. Effect of aging on ventilatory response to exercise and CO_2. J Appl Physiol 1984;56(5):1143–1150.

51. Tack M, Altose MD, Cherniack NS. Effect of aging on respiratory sensations produced by elastic loads. J Appl Physiol 1981;50(4):844–850.

52. Tack M, Altose MD, Cherniack NS. Effect of aging on the perception of resistive ventilatory loads. Am Rev Respir Dis 1982;126(3):463–467.

53. Manning H, Mahler D, Harver A. Dyspnea in the elderly. In: Mahler D, ed. Pulmonary Disease in the Elderly Patient. New York: Marcel Dekker; 1993:81–111.

54. Hoch CC, Reynolds CF 3rd, Monk TH, et al. Comparison of sleep-disordered breathing among healthy elderly in the seventh, eighth, and ninth decades of life. Sleep 1990;13(6): 502–511.

55. Epstein CD, El-Mokadem N, Peerless JR. Weaning older patients from long-term mechanical ventilation: a pilot study. Am J Crit Care 2002;11(4):369–377.

56. Ancoli-Israel S, Coy T. Are breathing disturbances in elderly equivalent to sleep apnea syndrome? Sleep 1994; 17(1):77–83.

57. Krieger J, Sforza E, Boudewijns A, Zamagni M, Petiau C. Respiratory effort during obstructive sleep apnea: role of age and sleep state [see comment]. Chest 1997;112(4): 875–884.

58. Marik PE, Kaplan D. Aspiration pneumonia and dysphagia in the elderly. Chest 2003;124(1):328–336.

59. Rosenthal RA, Kavic SM. Assessment and management of the geriatric patient. Crit Care Med 2004;32(4 Suppl): S92–105.

60. McCormick KA, Cummings MA, Kovner C. The role of the Agency for Health Care Policy and Research (AHCPR) in improving outcomes of care. Nurs Clin North Am 1997;32(3):521–542.

61. Qaseem A, Snow V, Fitterman N, et al. Risk assessment for and strategies to reduce perioperative pulmonary complications for patients undergoing noncardiothoracic surgery: a guideline from the American College of Physicians. Ann Intern Med 2006;144(8):575–580.

62. Wightman JA. A prospective survey of the incidence of postoperative pulmonary complications. Br J Surg 1968; 55(2):85–91.

63. Lawrence VA, Dhanda R, Hilsenbeck SG, Page CP. Risk of pulmonary complications after elective abdominal surgery. Chest 1996;110(3):744–750.

64. Smetana GW, Lawrence VA, Cornell JE. Preoperative pulmonary risk stratification for noncardiothoracic surgery: systematic review for the American College of Physicians. Ann Intern Med 2006;144(8):581–595.

65. Lawrence VA, Hilsenbeck SG, Noveck H, Poses RM, Carson JL. Medical complications and outcomes after hip fracture repair. Arch Intern Med 2002;162(18):2053–2057.

66. Pedersen T, Eliasen K, Henriksen E. A prospective study of risk factors and cardiopulmonary complications associated with anaesthesia and surgery: risk indicators of cardiopulmonary morbidity. Acta Anaesthesiol Scand 1990; 34(2):144–155.

67. Smetana GW. Preoperative pulmonary assessment of the older adult. Clin Geriatr Med 2003;19(1):35–55.

68. McAlister FA, Khan NA, Straus SE, et al. Accuracy of the preoperative assessment in predicting pulmonary risk after nonthoracic surgery. Am J Respir Crit Care Med 2003;167(5):741–744.

69. Arozullah AM, Daley J, Henderson WG, Khuri SF. Multifactorial risk index for predicting postoperative respiratory failure in men after major noncardiac surgery. The National Veterans Administration Surgical Quality Improvement Program. Ann Surg 2000;232(2):242–253.

70. Freye E, Levy JV. Use of opioids in the elderly—pharmacokinetic and pharmacodynamic considerations [German].

Anasthesiol Intensivmed Notfallmed Schmerzther 2004; 39(9):527–537.

71. Warner DO. Preventing postoperative pulmonary complications: the role of the anesthesiologist. Anesthesiology 2000;92(5):1467–1472.

72. Gunnarsson L, Tokics L, Gustavsson H, Hedenstierna G. Influence of age on atelectasis formation and gas exchange impairment during general anaesthesia. Br J Anaesth 1991;66(4):423–432.

73. Holland J, Milic-Emili J, Macklem PT, Bates DV. Regional distribution of pulmonary ventilation and perfusion in elderly subjects. J Clin Invest 1968;47:81–92.

74. Gunnarsson L, Tokics L, Lundquist H, et al. Chronic obstructive pulmonary disease and anaesthesia: formation of atelectasis and gas exchange impairment. Eur Respir J 1991;4(9):1106–1116.

75. Sekizawa K, Ujiie Y, Itabashi S, Sasaki H, Takishima T. Lack of cough reflex in aspiration pneumonia. Lancet 1990;335(8699):1228–1229.

76. Smithard DG, O'Neill PA, Parks C, Morris J. Complications and outcome after acute stroke. Does dysphagia matter? Stroke 1996;27(7):1200–1204.

77. Nelson R, Tse B, Edwards S. Systematic review of prophylactic nasogastric decompression after abdominal operations. Br J Surg 2005;92(6):673–680.

78. Lawrence VA, Cornell JE, Smetana GW. Strategies to reduce postoperative pulmonary complications after noncardiothoracic surgery: systematic review for the American College of Physicians. Ann Intern Med 2006;144(8): 596–608.

79. Trayner E Jr, Celli BR. Postoperative pulmonary complications. Med Clin North Am 2001;85(5):1129–1139.

80. Smetana GW. Preoperative pulmonary evaluation [see comment]. N Engl J Med 1999;340(12):937–944.

81. Wong DH, Weber EC, Schell MJ, Wong AB, Anderson CT, Barker SJ. Factors associated with postoperative pulmonary complications in patients with severe chronic obstructive pulmonary disease. Anesth Analg 1995;80(2): 276–284.

82. Tarhan S, Moffitt EA, Sessler AD, Douglas WW, Taylor WF. Risk of anesthesia and surgery in patients with chronic bronchitis and chronic obstructive pulmonary disease. Surgery 1973;74(5):720–726.

83. Moulton MJ, Creswell LL, Mackey ME, Cox JL, Rosenbloom M. Obesity is not a risk factor for significant adverse outcomes after cardiac surgery. Circulation 1996;94 (9 Suppl):II87–92.

84. Gerson MC, Hurst JM, Hertzberg VS, Baughman R, Rouan GW, Ellis K. Prediction of cardiac and pulmonary complications related to elective abdominal and noncardiac thoracic surgery in geriatric patients. Am J Med 1990;88(2): 101–107.

85. Williams-Russo P, Charlson ME, MacKenzie CR, Gold JP, Shires GT. Predicting postoperative pulmonary complications. Is it a real problem? Arch Intern Med 1992;152(6): 1209–1213.

86. Beard K, Jick H, Walker AM. Adverse respiratory events occurring in the recovery room after general anesthesia. Anesthesiology 1986;64(2):269–272.

87. Warner DO, Warner MA, Offord KP, Schroeder DR, Maxson P, Scanlon PD. Airway obstruction and perioperative complications in smokers undergoing abdominal surgery. Anesthesiology 1999;90(2):372–379.
88. Warner DO. Helping surgical patients quit smoking: why, when, and how. Anesth Analg 2005;101(2):481–487.
89. Warner DO. Perioperative abstinence from cigarettes: physiologic and clinical consequences. Anesthesiology 2006;104(2):356–367.
90. Moller AM, Villebro N, Pedersen T, Tonnesen H. Effect of preoperative smoking intervention on postoperative complications: a randomised clinical trial. Lancet 2002; 359(9301):114–117.
91. Garibaldi RA, Britt MR, Coleman ML, Reading JC, Pace NL. Risk factors for postoperative pneumonia. Am J Med 1981;70(3):677–680.
92. Valentine SJ, Marjot R, Monk CR. Preoxygenation in the elderly: a comparison of the four-maximal-breath and three-minute techniques. Anesth Analg 1990;71(5): 516–519.
93. Berg H, Roed J, Viby-Mogensen J, et al. Residual neuromuscular block is a risk factor for postoperative pulmonary complications. A prospective, randomised, and blinded study of postoperative pulmonary complications after atracurium, vecuronium and pancuronium. Acta Anaesthesiol Scand 1997;41(9):1095–1103.
94. Eichenberger A, Proietti S, Wicky S, et al. Morbid obesity and postoperative pulmonary atelectasis: an underestimated problem. Anesth Analg 2002;95(6):1788–1792.
95. Bindslev L, Hedenstierna G, Santesson J, Norlander O, Gram I. Airway closure during anaesthesia, and its prevention by positive end expiratory pressure. Acta Anaesthesiol Scand 1980;24(3):199–205.
96. Rothen HU, Sporre B, Engberg G, Wegenius G, Hedenstierna G. Reexpansion of atelectasis during general anaesthesia may have a prolonged effect. Acta Anaesthesiol Scand 1995;39(1):118–125.
97. Rothen HU, Sporre B, Engberg G, Wegenius G, Hedenstierna G. Re-expansion of atelectasis during general anaesthesia: a computed tomography study. Br J Anaesth 1993; 71(6):788–795.
98. Whalen FX, Gajic O, Thompson GB, et al. The effects of the alveolar recruitment maneuver and positive end-expiratory pressure on arterial oxygenation during laparoscopic bariatric surgery. Anesth Analg 2006;102(1):298–305.
99. Lachmann B. Open up the lung and keep the lung open. Intensive Care Med 1992;18(6):319–321.
100. Rodgers A, Walker N, Schug S, et al. Reduction of postoperative mortality and morbidity with epidural or spinal anaesthesia: results from overview of randomised trials. BMJ 2000;321(7275):1493.
101. Myles PS, Power I, Jamrozik K. Epidural block and outcome after major surgery. Med J Aust 2002;177(10):536–537.
102. Jayr C, Thomas H, Rey A, Farhat F, Lasser P, Bourgain JL. Postoperative pulmonary complications. Epidural analgesia using bupivacaine and opioids versus parenteral opioids. Anesthesiology 1993;78(4):666–676; discussion 22A.
103. Norris EJ, Beattie C, Perler BA, et al. Double-masked randomized trial comparing alternate combinations of intraoperative anesthesia and postoperative analgesia in abdominal aortic surgery. Anesthesiology 2001;95(5): 1054–1067.
104. Sprung J, Gajic O, Warner DO. Review article: age related alterations in respiratory function—anesthetic considerations [Article de synthese : Les modifications de fonction respiratoire liees a l'age—considerations anesthesiques]. Can J Anaesth 2006;53(12):1244–1257.
105. Turnheim K. When drug therapy gets old: pharmacokinetics and pharmacodynamics in the elderly. Exp Gerontol 2003;38(8):843–853.
106. Celli BR, Rodriguez KS, Snider GL. A controlled trial of intermittent positive pressure breathing, incentive spirometry, and deep breathing exercises in preventing pulmonary complications after abdominal surgery. Am Rev Respir Dis 1984;130(1):12–15.
107. Castillo R, Haas A. Chest physical therapy: comparative efficacy of preoperative and postoperative in the elderly. Arch Phys Med Rehabil 1985;66(6):376–379.
108. Brooks-Brunn JA. Postoperative atelectasis and pneumonia. Heart Lung 1995;24(2):94–115.
109. Pasquina P, Tramer MR, Granier JM, Walder B. Respiratory physiotherapy to prevent pulmonary complications after abdominal surgery: a systematic review. Chest 2006; 130(6):1887–1899.
110. Pennock BE, Kaplan PD, Carlin BW, Sabangan JS, Magovern JA. Pressure support ventilation with a simplified ventilatory support system administered with a nasal mask in patients with respiratory failure. Chest 1991;100(5): 1371–1376.
111. Gust R, Gottschalk A, Schmidt H, Bottiger BW, Bohrer H, Martin E. Effects of continuous (CPAP) and bi-level positive airway pressure (BiPAP) on extravascular lung water after extubation of the trachea in patients following coronary artery bypass grafting. Intensive Care Med 1996; 22(12):1345–1350.
112. Matte P, Jacquet L, Van Dyck M, Goenen M. Effects of conventional physiotherapy, continuous positive airway pressure and non-invasive ventilatory support with bilevel positive airway pressure after coronary artery bypass grafting. Acta Anaesthesiol Scand 2000;44(1):75–81.
113. Aguilo R, Togores B, Pons S, Rubi M, Barbe F, Agusti AG. Noninvasive ventilatory support after lung resectional surgery. Chest 1997;112(1):117–121.
114. Kindgen-Milles D, Buhl R, Gabriel A, Bohner H, Muller E. Nasal continuous positive airway pressure: a method to avoid endotracheal reintubation in postoperative high-risk patients with severe nonhypercapnic oxygenation failure. Chest 2000;117(4):1106–1111.
115. Squadrone V, Coha M, Cerutti E, et al. Continuous positive airway pressure for treatment of postoperative hypoxemia: a randomized controlled trial. JAMA 2005;293(5):589–595.
116. Esteban A, Frutos-Vivar F, Ferguson ND, et al. Noninvasive positive-pressure ventilation for respiratory failure after extubation. N Engl J Med 2004;350(24):2452–2460.
117. Brochard L, Mancebo J, Wysocki M, et al. Noninvasive ventilation for acute exacerbations of chronic obstructive pulmonary disease. N Engl J Med 1995;333(13):817–822.
118. Brochard L. Non-invasive ventilation for acute exacerbations of COPD: a new standard of care. Thorax 2000;55(10): 817–818.

119. Ebeo CT, Benotti PN, Byrd RP Jr, Elmaghraby Z, Lui J. The effect of bi-level positive airway pressure on postoperative pulmonary function following gastric surgery for obesity. Respir Med 2002;96(9):672–676.

120. Joris JL, Sottiaux TM, Chiche JD, Desaive CJ, Lamy ML. Effect of bi-level positive airway pressure (BiPAP) nasal ventilation on the postoperative pulmonary restrictive syndrome in obese patients undergoing gastroplasty. Chest 1997;111(3):665–670.

121. Angus DC, Kelley MA, Schmitz RJ, White A, Popovich J Jr. Caring for the critically ill patient. Current and projected workforce requirements for care of the critically ill and patients with pulmonary disease: can we meet the requirements of an aging population? JAMA 2000; 284(21):2762–2770.

122. Rice DP, Fineman N. Economic implications of increased longevity in the United States. Annu Rev Public Health 2004;25:457–473.

123. Sevransky JE, Haponik EF. Respiratory failure in elderly patients. Clin Geriatr Med 2003;19(1):205–224.

124. Sloane PJ, Gee MH, Gottlieb JE, et al. A multicenter registry of patients with acute respiratory distress syndrome. Physiology and outcome. Am Rev Respir Dis 1992;146(2): 419–426.

125. Luhr OR, Karlsson M, Thorsteinsson A, Rylander C, Frostell CG. The impact of respiratory variables on mortality in non-ARDS and ARDS patients requiring mechanical ventilation. Intensive Care Med 2000;26(5):508–517.

126. Ely EW, Evans GW, Haponik EF. Mechanical ventilation in a cohort of elderly patients admitted to an intensive care unit. Ann Intern Med 1999;131(2):96–104.

127. Groeger JS, Guntupalli KK, Strosberg M, et al. Descriptive analysis of critical care units in the United States: patient characteristics and intensive care unit utilization. Crit Care Med 1993;21(2):279–291.

128. Thompson LF. Failure to wean: exploring the influence of age-related pulmonary changes. Crit Care Nurs Clin North Am 1996;8(1):7–16.

129. Kleinhenz ME, Lewis CY. Chronic ventilator dependence in elderly patients. Clin Geriatr Med 2000;16(4):735–756.

130. Gajic O, Dara SI, Mendez JL, et al. Ventilator-associated lung injury in patients without acute lung injury at the onset of mechanical ventilation. Crit Care Med 2004;32(9): 1817–1824.

131. Fernandez-Perez ER, Keegan MT, Brown DR, Hubmayr RD, Gajic O. Intraoperative tidal volume as a risk factor for respiratory failure after pneumonectomy. Anesthesiology 2006;105(1):14–18.

132. Choi G, Wolthuis EK, Bresser P, et al. Mechanical ventilation with lower tidal volumes and positive end-expiratory pressure prevents alveolar coagulation in patients without lung injury. Anesthesiology 2006;105(4):689–695.

133. Michelet P, D'Journo XB, Roch A, et al. Protective ventilation influences systemic inflammation after esophagectomy: a randomized controlled study. Anesthesiology 2006; 105(5):911–919.

12
Operative Debridements of Chronic Wounds

Andrew M. Hanflik, Michael S. Golinko, Melissa Doft, Charles Cain,
Anna Flattau, and Harold Brem

The term "chronic wound" does not refer to duration over time, but rather describes a wound that is physiologically impaired. All venous, pressure, and diabetic foot ulcers are defined as chronic wounds. Elderly patients are more likely to experience venous and pressure ulcers,[1–4] which lead to more than half of all lower extremity amputations in persons with diabetes.[5] Chronic wounds heal at the same frequency of closure in elderly populations as they do in younger populations, but may heal at a slower rate, primarily because of comorbidities associated with age.[6–9] The comorbidities that delay healing are prevalent among older populations and include venous insufficiency and diabetes. Although there are age-related changes to the skin, it has yet to be shown, clinically, that age alone decreases an elderly person's ability to heal.[7,10,11] A synergistic effect of advanced age and diabetes significantly slows healing.[12]

Chronic wounds in elderly patients heal successfully if the care regimen includes a coordinated effort to treat skin breakdown early and to prevent further ulceration. In the absence of ischemia and osteomyelitis, prompt medical treatment will heal most venous ulcers, diabetic foot ulcers, and stage I, II, and III pressure ulcers (defined below).[6] Delayed wound treatment, combined with multiple comorbidities affecting the elderly population, can lead to amputations, sepsis, and death. The established pathway from untreated chronic wound to death has been used as evidence for the manslaughter convictions of several care providers of the elderly.[13]

Pain is a complex and almost universal complication of this population, and appropriate pain management by an anesthesiologist is becoming increasingly recognized as essential in the optimal treatment of these patients.

The Operating Room

The only universally accepted treatment for chronic wounds is surgical debridement. This is the standard of care for nonviable and infected tissue and for the stimula-tion of healing.[14] Because these patients usually have multiple comorbidities and American Society of Anesthesiologists (ASA) scores of 3 or 4, we recommend operative debridement under local or regional anesthesia whenever possible. Regional blocks of the sciatic, popliteal, and femoral nerves are ideal. Many patients will require general anesthesia. It is essential that the patient and primary care physician understand this, as well as understand that the risks of not performing the debridement, i.e., leaving necrotic or infected tissue in an elderly person, is greater than the risks of anesthesia itself. For patients with peripheral arterial disease, treatment of underlying ischemia must be achieved before elective debridements unless infection is present.

Chronic Wounds in the Elderly Result in Significant Morbidity and Mortality

Diabetic Foot Ulcers

There are 20.8 million Americans diagnosed with diabetes.[15] The elderly are the largest constituent of this group because diabetes affects more than 18% of Americans greater than 60 years old.[16] In the United States between 1997 and 2004, the number of new cases of diabetes increased 54%.[17] By the year 2030, 366 million persons worldwide are estimated to have diabetes, with 130 million of them over the age of 64.[18] All of these patients are at risk for diabetic complications including retinopathy, nephropathy, neuropathy, and accelerated atherosclerosis. Neuropathy and atherosclerosis are associated with the development of diabetic foot ulcers and impaired healing.[19–21]

In the United States, the elderly account for 53.3% of diabetes-associated amputations per annum.[5] Diabetic foot ulcers are defined as any breakdown of skin on the foot of a diabetic person. Recent prevalence is as high as 12% of all people with diabetes.[22] These ulcers act

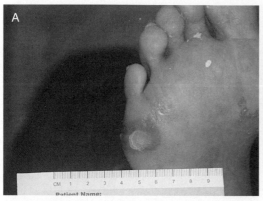
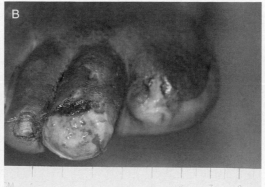
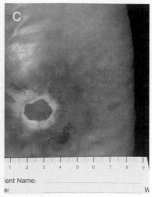

FIGURE 12-1. Examples of diabetic foot ulcers. Note: any break in the epidermis on the foot of a patient with diabetes is considered a diabetic foot ulcer. **A:** Typical-appearing ulcer under the fifth metatarsal head. **B:** A more advanced ulcer on the toe. **C:** A callous surrounded by central ulceration on the plantar aspect of the foot.

as portals for infectious organisms. A large multicenter study recently reported 58% of all patients with ulcers had concomitant foot infection.[23] Half of the patients who develop one foot lesion subsequently develop a contralateral wound.[24] Each wound is considered to be chronic from its inception and should be treated early. Individuals with diabetes have a 30- to 40-fold higher risk of lower limb amputation.[25] See Figure 12-1A–C for examples of the typical locations of diabetic foot ulcers.

Pressure Ulcers

The four stages of pressure ulcers are defined as[26,27]:

Stage I—Observable pressure-related alteration of intact skin whose indicators as compared with the adjacent or opposite area on the body may include changes in one or more of the following: skin temperature (warmth or coolness), tissue consistency (firm or boggy feel), and/or sensation (pain, itching). The ulcer appears as a defined area of persistent redness in lightly pigmented skin, whereas in darker skin tones the ulcer may appear with persistent red, blue, or purple hues. See Figure 12-2A.

Stage II—Partial-thickness skin loss involving epidermis, dermis, or both. The ulcer is superficial and presents clinically as an abrasion, blister, or shallow crater. See Figure 12-2B.

Stage III—Full-thickness skin loss involving damage to, or necrosis of, subcutaneous tissue that may extend down to, but not through, underlying fascia. The ulcer presents clinically as a deep crater with or without undermining of adjacent tissue. See Figure 12-2C.

Stage IV—Full-thickness skin loss with ulceration extending through the fascia, with extensive destruction, tissue necrosis, or damage to muscle, bone, or supporting structures (e.g., tendon, joint, capsule). Undermining and sinus tracts are frequently associated with stage IV pressure ulcers. See Figure 12-2D.

In 2003, 455,000 patients in the United States alone were hospitalized for pressure ulcers, representing a 63% increase from 1993: the most common reason for admission was septicemia.[28] The true incidence and prevalence of pressure ulcers is not known. A recent national study of acute care settings found that the prevalence of pressure ulcers ranged between 14% and 17%, whereas the incidence was between 7% and 9%.[29] At least 10% of hospitalized patients, more than 20% of nursing home patients, and 20%–30% of spinal cord injury patients are affected.[30] In a nursing home study, 6.5%–19.3% of patients developed a new pressure ulcer over a 3- to 21-month period. Patients at highest risk were those who had diabetes or fecal incontinence.[31] Recent studies have demonstrated that both age and immobility are strongly linked to development of pressure ulcers[32,33] as well as cognitive ability.[34]

The presence of a pressure ulcer doubles the risk of mortality in an elderly patient.[35,36] Elderly patients discharged with a hospital-acquired pressure ulcer have a much greater risk of death within a year than patients without a pressure ulcer, indicating that stage IV pressure ulcers should never be ignored.[37] A recent study of more than 100,000 patients revealed an overall age-adjusted mortality rate of 3.79%, for which pressure ulcers were listed as the cause of death in 18.7% of patients.[38] Stage IV pressure ulcers often lead to sepsis, a common cause of death in the elderly.[39,40]

Venous Ulcers

It is estimated that 1.7% of the elderly population is affected by venous ulcers, indicating that they are more prevalent in the elderly than in younger populations.[41–43]

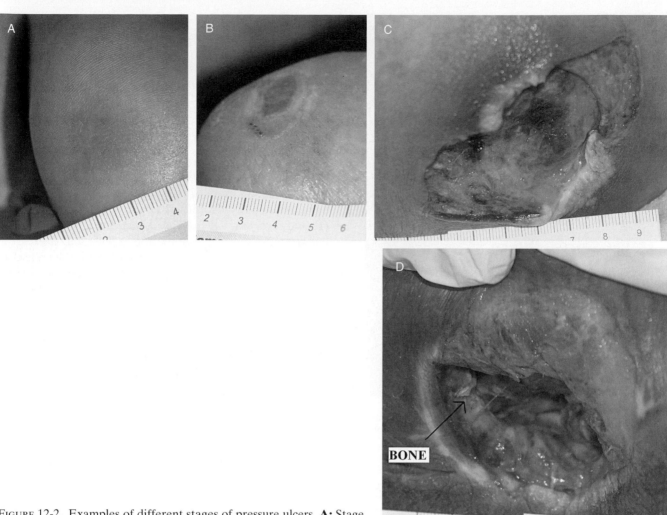

FIGURE 12-2. Examples of different stages of pressure ulcers. **A:** Stage I, heel. **B:** Stage II, ischium. **C:** Stage III, trochanter. **D:** Stage IV, ischium.

Venous ulcers are often misdiagnosed as traumatic injuries and are therefore undertreated.[44] Although these wounds are not frequently associated with osteomyelitis or amputation, when undertreated, they provide a gateway for infection that results in multiple hospitalizations, substantial suffering, and health care costs exceeding $1 billion annually.[45,46]

Venous ulcers are secondary to venous reflux disease, which correlates with increased age.[41,47,48] An example of a typical venous ulcer is shown in Figure 12-3. Venous reflux disease occurs when valvular incompetence prevents normal blood flow from superficial veins to deep veins. The most common etiologies for valvular dysfunction of the deep venous system are advanced age[41,49] and a history of deep vein thrombosis (DVT).[50] Valvular incompetence causes increased venous pressures, leading to venous distention and activation of apoptotic pathways, resulting in ulceration. Another hypothesis is that leukocytes and other large molecules become trapped in the dermis in response to endothelial damage and venous hypertension.[51] It is thought the extravasation of these large molecules, proteins, and leukocytes inhibits growth factors from reaching their targets.[52]

Ischemic Wounds

Peripheral arterial disease is often the primary etiology of an ischemic wound. It can also impair healing in venous, pressure, and diabetic foot ulcers because of a decreased blood flow to the affected area. Age, hypertension, smoking, and diabetes are each independent risk factors for developing peripheral arterial disease.[4,53] Although the incidence of peripheral arterial disease is only 4.3% in patients over 40 years old, the incidence sharply increases to 14.5% in patients over 70.[4] Additionally, a large study of Asian patients with diabetes over the age

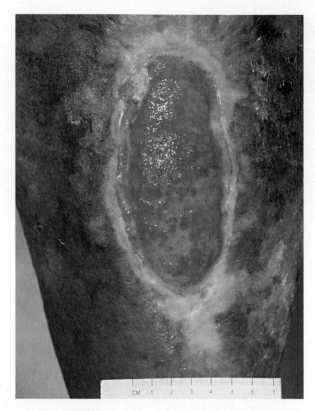

FIGURE 12-3. Example of a typical lower extremity venous ulcer.

of 50 showed the prevalence of peripheral arterial disease to be 17.7%.[54] Many if not most of these patients are asymptomatic.[55,56]

Experimental Evidence of Physiologic Impairments in the Elderly

Clinical and experimental studies have demonstrated that there is a greater frequency of physiologic impairments to wound healing in the elderly population.

Angiogenesis in Wound Healing

Laboratory research has identified more than 30 regulatory mechanisms of angiogenesis that occur during wound healing, including growth factors, growth factor receptors, chemotactic agents, and matrix metalloproteinases. In animal models, decreased angiogenesis significantly inhibits wound healing.[16,57–59] In these models, angiogenic cytokines such as vascular endothelial growth factor are present in smaller concentrations in the wounds of older animals compared with younger animals, resulting in smaller capillary densities within the wound bed.[60–62] It is theorized that the discrepancy is secondary to decreased macrophage function in the older animals.[63–65] The decrease in angiogenesis causes an initial delay in wound healing; yet, despite this, wounds contract with comparable frequency.[66] Therefore, a decreased angiogenic response in older animals contributes to an impaired wound-healing rate.

Decreased Immune Response

Review of experimental and clinical research has shown physiologic impairments in the immune response of the elderly, making them prone to infection.[67] Older animals have a markedly decreased adaptive immune response (B and T cells),[67] a bolstered but possibly dysfunctional regulatory T cell population (CD4+ CD25+),[68,69] a decrease in T cell receptor diversity,[70] and a decrease in toll-like receptors[65] and $\gamma\delta$-T cells.[71] The decreased immune response makes the elderly more susceptible to pathogenic invasion.

A Multidisciplinary Approach for Treating Venous, Pressure, and Diabetic Foot Ulcers

Many wounds that appear minor on initial physical examination signal extensive necrosis beneath the skin's surface and consequently may still be a significant source of sepsis (Figure 12-4). It is therefore critical to treat all wounds early and comprehensively. In the elderly population, patient care frequently focuses on the patient's comorbidities, whereas wounds are simply covered with a bandage and ignored. Too often, untreated wounds lead to preventable complications such as amputation, sepsis, and death. As part of an ongoing multidisciplinary collaboration among many specialists who care for elderly patients with chronic wounds, we have developed protocols to treat venous,[44] pressure, and diabetic foot ulcers.[6,44,72,73] Outlined below are the precepts of our treatment protocol (Table 12-1).

1. Contact the Primary Care Physician:
   A strong relationship with the primary care physician is essential to optimize the many comorbidities of the elderly patient. Common medical diseases that must be assessed include: coronary artery disease, diabetes, obesity, hypertension, dyslipidemia, chronic renal insufficiency, malnutrition, muscular atrophy, hepatic disease, chronic obstructive pulmonary disease, coagulopathy, and pain. In the diabetic population, seeking the counsel of a diabetologist may be necessary to maintain proper glucose control. The primary care physician, along with the assistance of a nutritionist, can also be helpful in evaluating the patient's nutritional status. A small number of prospective studies has found that nutritional

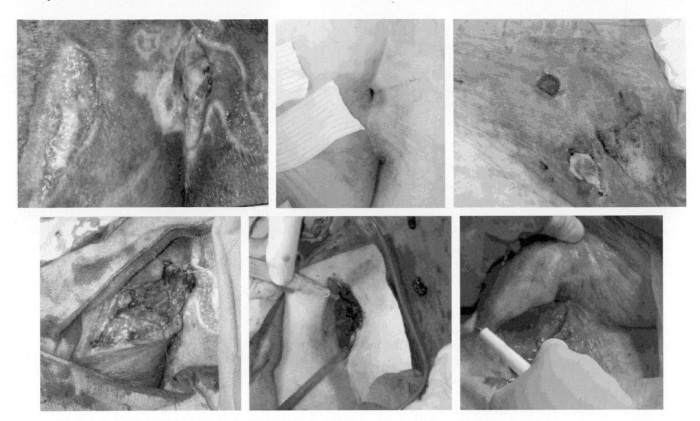

FIGURE 12-4. Pressure ulcers can be deceptively large. Pressure ulcers are often much larger than they appear to be. Wounds that may look quite small can contain extensive undermining and/or tunneling. This figure demonstrates three cases in which, upon debridement, the wound was shown to be substantially larger than it appeared at presentation.

supplements are beneficial in treating chronic wounds in malnourished patients.[74–76]

2. Comprehensive Physical Examination of At-Risk Patients:

TABLE 12-1. Summary of the current standard of care for the healing of venous ulcers, pressure ulcers, and diabetic foot ulcers.

1. Contact the primary care physician
2. Comprehensive physical examination of at-risk patients
3. Prevention of deep vein thrombosis
4. Laboratory and radiologic evaluations
5. Evaluation of blood flow in the lower extremities
6. Objective measurement of every wound weekly with digital photography, planimetry, and documentation of the wound-healing process
7. Elimination of cellulitis, drainage, and infection
8. Local wound care
9. Debridement of nonviable tissue and wound bed preparation
10. Offloading pressure from the wound and compression therapy
11. Growth factor therapies
12. Addressing comorbidities that may affect anesthesia
13. Physical therapy
14. Pain management

Diabetic and bed-bound patients are at high risk for developing diabetic foot and pressure ulcers, respectively. These patients often lack protective sensation. As a consequence, they do not sense skin breakdown and are unable to assess wound progression. All diabetics must have their feet examined daily for evidence of skin breakdown. All bed-bound patients should have their pressure points (heels, ischia, trochanters, and sacrum) examined daily for evidence of pressure ulcer development.

3. Prevention of Deep Vein Thrombosis:

The physical therapy team should ensure that every patient who is able to ambulate is doing so. In nonambulatory patients, we recommend moving from the bed to a chair at least twice a day. Standard deep vein prophylaxis is mandatory, including pneumatic compression boots and subcutaneous heparin or low-molecular-weight heparin.

4. Laboratory and Radiologic Evaluation:

Baseline laboratory tests should be obtained to evaluate the patient's overall health and to potentially detect underlying disease states. We recommend a complete blood count with differential, coagulation profile, creatinine and blood urea nitrogen levels, electrolyte panel, lipid panel, glycosylated hemoglobin, albumin and pre-albumin, erythrocyte sedimentation rate, hepatic panel, and thyroid-stimulating hormone level. Plain films of the affected area are recommended for all leg and foot wounds. Magnetic resonance imaging or bone scan is recommended to assess for osteomyelitis in stage IV pressure ulcers and in diabetic foot ulcers.

5. Evaluation of Blood Flow in the Lower Extremities:

Peripheral arterial disease and venous stasis disease are prevalent in the elderly population. All patients with limb ulcers should undergo arterial testing, regardless of what the primary etiology is thought to be, because the etiology may be multifactorial. Arterial testing is crucial because patients with ischemia should be revascularized before debridement and should not undergo compression therapy. Testing for venous stasis disease should be done in patients who clinically appear to have venous stasis ulcers.

Noninvasive flow studies, which include bilateral ankle brachial indices (comparison of pressures in ankles and arms) and pulse volume recordings (to determine the amount of blood flow when pressures are falsely elevated), are necessary to detect lower extremity ischemia. In particular, recent studies have suggested high sensitivity to detect peripheral arterial disease using the low ankle pressure test defined as the quotient of the lowest ankle artery pressure of two measurements and the highest of two brachial artery pressure measurements.[77,78] Depression of these values is associated with a greater risk of amputation.[79] An ankle brachial index less than 0.9 indicates significant arterial disease that requires referral to a vascular surgeon.[80] An elevated ankle brachial index greater than 1.30 has been found to be predictive of major amputation[81] and, particularly in the context of poor waveforms (i.e., monophasic),[82] may indicate atherosclerosis requiring vascular surgery referral.

When indicated, revascularization should proceed as soon as possible. Bypass grafting procedures are often avoided in elderly patients because their comorbidities make them poor surgical candidates. Alternatively, endovascular revascularization provides a minimally invasive and effective surgical option. Endovascular correction of arterial disease has proven safe and leads to 5-year limb salvage rates of more than 89% in diabetic and elderly populations.[83-87] If wound debridement is necessary, it should be done shortly after revascularization so as to utilize the improved blood supply.[88]

Duplex ultrasonography testing determines the presence and degree of venous insufficiency in patients with venous ulcers. Because venous incompetence is often attributable to a previous DVT, it is possible that the patient may concurrently have a DVT and a venous ulcer. In this scenario, the DVT will be identified by the venous flow studies.

Once venous ulcers have healed, venous insufficiency should be corrected. Minimally invasive techniques such as radiofrequency ablation of the greater saphenous vein, percutaneous vein valve bioprosthesis, and subfascial endoscopic perforator vein surgery are treatment options.[89-91] Correction of the underlying venous disease prevents recurrence of venous ulcers.[92-94]

6. Objective Assessment of Wound Healing:

Weekly wound-healing assessments should be objectively calculated by digital photography and planimetric measurements. Although a simple ruler has been shown to be reliable for predicting wound healing,[95] digital photography and computer-based wound measurements are more accurate for larger wounds and allow for easy transportation of data. Ideally, all data can be compiled into a wound electronic medical record (WEMR), if available, which plots a wound graph, demonstrating the healing curve of the wound based on planimetric measurements and allowing the team to objectively follow the progress of the wound. Serial objective measurements of the wound area allow the treatment team to accurately and rapidly detect a failure to heal and to adjust the treatment plan accordingly. A WEMR can also store the patient's medical history, wound history (wound graph, drainage, pain, associated pathology, surgery history, radiology, and microbiology), laboratory values, antibiotic history, vascular studies, medications, wound picture, and contact information for the patient's primary care doctor, pharmacist, and next of kin. The WEMR provides all of the patient's pertinent data needed for thorough treatment in an easy-to-read format.

7. Elimination of Infection:

Infection substantially impairs chronic wound healing. Drainage, cellulitis, and pain are indicators of infection. Deep tissue cultures reflect the pathogens populating the wound bed and surrounding tissue, and they allow the physician to tailor the patient's antibiotic regimen to cover only the pathogens grown from cultures, thereby helping to prevent drug-resistant organisms.[96-99] Deep tissue cultures are taken when the wound is debrided. If definitive debridement is not immediately planned, then an initial deep culture should be obtained at bedside, in the emergency room, or in the outpatient clinic, at the time when antibiotics are started.

8. Local Wound Care:

Homecare nursing is an integrated element in the wound-healing team. All wounds must be properly cleaned, treated with topical medications, and covered with the appropriate noncompressive or compressive dressing. Cleaning the wound includes washing with antimicrobial soap and water and scrubbing the wound with sterile saline and gauze. The topical therapy, such as cadexomer iodine (Iodosorb or Iodoflex; Smith & Nephew, Largo, FL), Acticoat (Smith & Nephew), and

Collagenase (Healthpoint, Fort Worth, TX), should provide a moist wound-healing environment and prevent bacterial colonization.

9. Debridement of Nonviable Tissue and Wound Bed Preparation:

Debridement of a chronic wound accelerates healing.[88] It is a recommended treatment for diabetic foot ulcers, pressure ulcers, and venous ulcers.[100–103] For ischemic ulcers, debridement should be deferred until after revascularization. Gene expression is altered in the nonhealing edge of a chronic wound, resulting in hyperkeratotic epidermis and up-regulation of the oncogene c-*myc*.[104] Debriding past this edge into healthy tissue stimulates the healthy epithelium to release growth factors and reduces local inflammation. It is thought that debridement encourages new fibroblasts to invade and replace the senescent cells of chronic wound beds, as well as

release of various growth factors that stimulate wound healing, although few rigorous studies demonstrate this.[88] Debridement also allows the surgeon to obtain microbiology and pathology samples that tailor antibiotic treatments and guide future debridements. For patients with active infection (such as cellulitis, fever, or elevated white blood cell count), debridement removes infected necrotic tissue that is the source of infection.

Venous ulcers should be debrided deeply enough to remove all underlying scar and infected tissue; only several millimeters of the surrounding epithelium need to be debrided. Pressure ulcers should be debrided to remove all infected, necrotic, and scarred tissue, as well as to allow deep packing during dressing changes. Diabetic foot ulcers often appear as a callus with a central ulceration. We consider the callus as part of the wound, and we recommend debridement of a diabetic foot ulcer 2–3 mm beyond the callus into healthy epithelium (Figure 12-5).

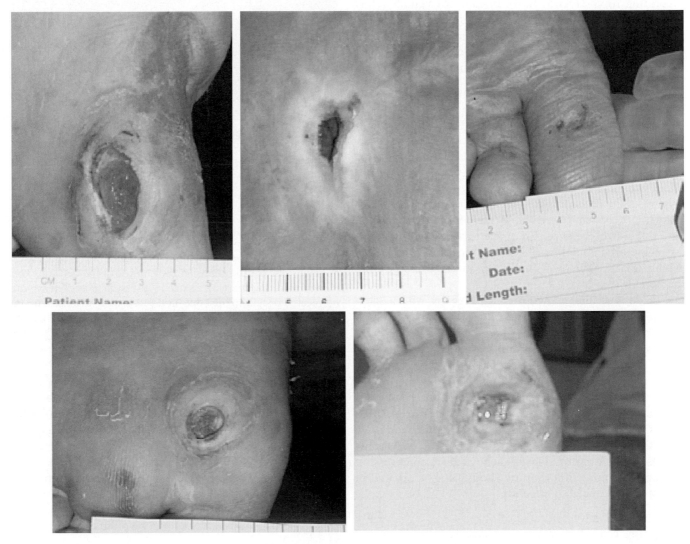

FIGURE 12-5. Proper debridement of diabetic foot ulcers. Diabetic foot ulcers are often associated with a thick hyperkeratotic callus. This callus impedes the healing process and needs to be removed. Debridement of diabetic foot ulcers must extend several millimeters past the nonmigratory edge into healthy epithelium. Debridement will aid in healing by removing nonviable tissue while stimulating reepithelialization with healthy tissue.

The surgeon should take pathology samples from the postoperative wound bed to confirm whether the remaining tissue is healthy. Almost all patients require multiple debridements, and the pathology results will guide the extent of future debridements.

Although it is possible to debride some ulcers at the bedside, many elderly patients are debrided in the operating room because of their significant cardiac and pulmonary comorbidities, the size of their wounds, dementia, pain control, and concerns regarding hemostasis. The personnel involved and close monitoring make the operating room the safest place for most elderly patients who require debridement.

Pressure ulcers often have a significant amount of tunneling and undermining that are revealed only after debridement has begun (Figure 12-4). Bone resection can cause significant bleeding, and most debridements of wounds extending to bone should be considered for the operating room (Figure 12-6). Because of venous reflux disease, venous ulcer debridement often causes significant blood loss from capillary bleeding, varicose veins, and venous perforators. Large venous ulcer debridements should be done in the operating room.

10. Offloading Pressure from the Wound and Compression Therapy:

Pressure is a significant contributor to the development and progression of pressure and diabetic foot ulcers. Pressure can be alleviated in pressure ulcer patients by using specialized air fluidized or alternating air mattresses. Heel pressure ulcer patients should be given a Multi-Podus splint (Restorative Care of America, St. Petersburg, FL) or a foam-based Heelift (DM Systems, Evanston, IL) to relieve pressure. Frequent turning and attentive skin care are mandatory for the treatment of all patients. Many devices have been created to offload pressure from diabetic foot ulcers.[105–109]

For venous ulcers, compression therapy with a measured multilayered bandage such as the Profore system (Smith & Nephew) should be used in conjunction with topical therapies.[110] These bandages decrease superficial vein distention and venous pressure, and they increase the efficacy of venous valves. This promotes the proper flow of blood from superficial to deep veins. High compression is more effective than low compression bandages, but their use is limited to nonischemic patients.[111] It is therefore imperative that all venous ulcer patients be evaluated for arterial insufficiency before compression therapy. Compression therapy should not be applied in the presence of active infection.

11. Growth Factor Therapies:

For the topical treatment of diabetic foot ulcers, the Food and Drug Administration has approved only Dermagraft[112] (Advanced Tissue Sciences, La Jolla, CA), Human Skin Equivalent (HSE), Apligraf,[113] a bilayered,

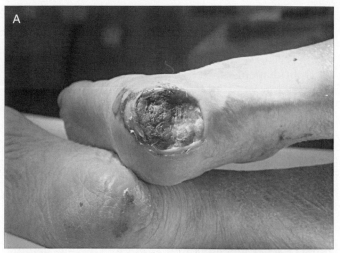

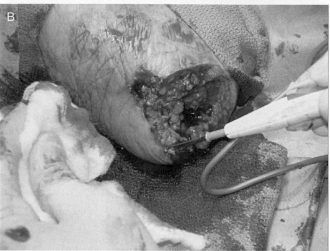

FIGURE 12-6. Proper hemostatic control often necessitates use of the operating room. **A:** Preoperative photo. **B:** Intraoperative debridement. The operating room provides a much higher level of hemostatic control than can be achieved at the bedside. This patient was admitted with a stage IV pressure ulcer. The wound permeated deep into the bone, and because of the large amount of bleeding that can be associated with the debridement of bone in these wounds, this case was safely completed in the operating room.

biologically active construct composed of a bovine collagen scaffold seeded with a layer of keratinocytes covering a layer of fibroblasts (Organogenesis Inc., Canton, MA), and Becaplermin (recombinant platelet-derived growth factor)[114,115] for safety and efficacy. Only Apligraf is approved for safety and efficacy in venous ulcers.[116] No treatment is approved for safety and efficacy in pressure ulcers. These agents should not be applied in the presence of active infection (cellulitis or wound drainage) and should be used only after surgical wound debridement.

12. Comorbidities Affecting Anesthesia:

Complicated cardiac conditions are common in the elderly and must be appropriately evaluated before surgery. If the patient has risk factors for coronary artery disease, an exercise stress test should be considered before surgery. If the patient has a history of coronary atherosclerosis, pacemaker placement, valvular disease, congestive heart failure, or cardiac arrhythmia, cardiac function should optimized.

Nephropathy is a common comorbidity in the elderly. The hypoproteinemia and acidemia seen in end-stage kidney disease patients can significantly affect the pharmacokinetics and pharmacodynamics of certain drugs used in anesthesia.[117] We recommend that end-stage kidney disease patients be dialyzed before surgery and that blood chemistries be closely monitored perioperatively. A venous blood gas is a safe, common approach to rapid evaluation of serum potassium and other electrolytes.

Neuropathy is also a common complication in people with diabetes and most notably in the vast majority of persons with diabetic foot ulcers: in a recent study, 78% of diabetic patients with ulcers also had neuropathy.[118] Because of the decrease in lower extremity sensation, it is rarely necessary to use a stronger anesthetic approach than a regional ankle block or Monitored Anesthesia Care with local anesthetic injections.

Pressure ulcers frequently affect spinal cord injury patients. The level of the spinal cord injury is particularly important. If the patient's injury is above thoracic vertebra 6, then the patient is at risk for autonomic dysreflexia.[119] Autonomic dysreflexia is an abrupt and exaggerated autonomic response to stimuli in patients with spinal cord injuries or dysfunction above the splanchnic sympathetic outflow (T5–6).[120] It is imperative that all patients with a T6 lesion or higher be debrided in the operating room under spinal or general anesthesia and with close blood pressure monitoring.

13. Physical Therapy:

Physical therapy is advised for patients with limited mobility and those with venous ulcers. For patients with limited mobility, physical therapy (1) decreases the incidence of DVT, (2) decreases respiratory complications, (3) increases mental acuity, and (4) decreases the development of contractures.[121] In patients with venous ulcers, musculoskeletal changes attributable to calf pain and venous hypertension dramatically affect the patient's gait. Physical therapy has been shown to improve underlying venous disease and patient ambulation.[122]

14. Pain Management:

Pain is common in patients with ulcers, and effective pain management regimens must be instituted. Pain should be quantified by the patient at each clinic visit. By using a Verbal Analogue Score in conjunction with the wound-healing graph from a wound data sheet, a physician can track the success of pain treatments as they relate to functional outcomes.[123] The end goal is to reduce

morbidity by eliminating pain. Pain control also facilitates appropriate cleaning and dressing of the wound, because patients may avoid these tasks if they are very painful. It may be necessary to incorporate a pain specialist into the treatment team.

Each category of chronic wounds presents with a unique type of pain. In venous ulcers, pain is believed to occur as a result of tissue damage, which stimulates the release of inflammatory mediators, sensitizing peripheral somatic pain receptors.[124] Because of intense pain in many venous ulcer patients, we recommend using a tiered system of pain medications based on the World Health Organization analgesic ladder,[125] in which patients are started on nonopioid drugs with or without adjuvant medications, to which increasing strengths of opioid medications are added depending on pain-control needs.[123,124] Patients with multiple comorbidities may have contraindications to common pain medications. In addition, in elderly patients, special attention must be given to the potential side effects of pain medications, such as constipation or mental status changes from narcotics.

Although often associated with neuropathy, diabetic foot ulcers and pressure ulcers can present with substantial pain management challenges. The pain associated with neuropathic diabetic foot ulcers can be treated with tricyclic antidepressants, anticonvulsants, capsaicin, mexiletine, lidocaine patches, N-methyl-D-aspartate (NMDA) inhibitors, clonidine, and tramadol.[124] All have been used with varying degrees of success. Spinal cord injury patients with pressure ulcers develop central pain that occurs when there is neuropathy in the area of the wound. Thus, spinal cord patients may also need pain control even though the wounded area is insensate.

Intraoperative Risk and Precautions for Development of Pressure Ulcers

Elderly patients with fragile skin and comorbid conditions are at highest risk for development of intraoperative pressure ulcers. Patients with a high ASA grade may be more likely to develop pressure ulcers.[126] The most comprehensive study was conducted in the United States in 1998 involving 104 hospitals and 1128 surgical patients, all undergoing procedures longer than 3 hours in duration. An overall prevalence of stage I and stage II pressure ulcers was 7.8% when examining patients up to 4 days postoperatively.[127]

Part of the intraoperative risk can be assessed by type of procedure. Vascular surgery, cardiac surgery, and orthopedic surgery are associated with higher risks, although rigorous studies have yet to emerge.[128] The risk may double for operations lasting more than 2.5 hours.[129] In a prospective Dutch study[130] of patients undergoing operations lasting more than 4 hours, 44 patients (21.2%)

developed 70 pressure ulcers in the first 2 days postoperatively. All but three were stage I and II.

Various locations may be at higher risk than others. The same Dutch study found that most heel ulcers were associated with cardiac procedures. They also found head and neck procedures most often associated with sacral ulcers and that use of a semi-Fowler position (elevating both head and lower extremities to 30 degrees) may be beneficial.[130]

Full examination of all areas at risk including the sacrum, heels, ischia, and trochanteric areas with documentation of any skin changes and existing ulcers can help identify postoperative changes. Because the heel has the smallest surface area, this area may be at greatest risk intraoperatively. An ordinary head-pillow placed underneath each heel during the operation and through the time the patient is immobile is likely the most effective pressure-reducing device, followed by a siliconized hollow-fiber–based heel protector.[131] Further studies into a variety of mattress (foam versus gel) and alternative positioning have yet to be evaluated by rigorous randomized controlled trials.

In most cases, if a wound is identified, extra care should be taken to relieve as much pressure from the surface as possible and to provide extra dressings either with 4 × 4 sterile gauze or circumferential roll gauze to account for extra drainage from the wound during prolonged procedures. After the procedure, the dressings on all chronic wounds should be examined and changed as necessary.

Conclusion

Elderly patients are frequently affected by chronic wounds including pressure, venous, and diabetic foot ulcers. The elderly have the ability to heal from chronic wounds, but they are prone to multiple comorbidities that may slow the rate of healing, and complications from infection pose significant risks to patients who are already fragile. Operative debridement is usually most important to remove the source of infection. Safety of the elderly patient can be optimized by focusing on glycemic control, hydration, and often beta-blockade. If all wounds are treated using the protocol described herein, we postulate that amputations will be decreased, stage IV pressure ulcers nearly eliminated, and morbidity from venous ulcers reduced.

References

1. Walker N, Rodgers A, Birchall N, Norton R, MacMahon S. The occurrence of leg ulcers in Auckland: results of a population-based study. NZ Med J 2002;115:159–162.
2. Livesley NJ, Chow AW. Infected pressure ulcers in elderly individuals. Clin Infect Dis 2002;35:1390–1396.
3. Margolis DJ, Bilker W, Santanna J, Baumgarten M. Venous leg ulcer: incidence and prevalence in the elderly. J Am Acad Dermatol 2002;46:381–386.
4. Selvin E, Erlinger TP. Prevalence of and risk factors for peripheral arterial disease in the United States: results from the National Health and Nutrition Examination Survey, 1999–2000. Circulation 2004;110:738–743.
5. Data & Trends. National Diabetes Surveillance System. Hospitalizations for nontraumatic lower extremity amputation, 1980–2003: Centers for Disease Control (CDC). Available at: http://www.cdc.gov/diabetes/statistics/lea/byAgetable1_2.htm. Accessed September 30, 2006.
6. Brem H, Tomic-Canic M, Tarnovskaya A, et al. Healing of elderly patients with diabetic foot ulcers, venous stasis ulcers, and pressure ulcers. Surg Technol Int 2003;11:161–167.
7. Gosain A, DiPietro LA. Aging and wound healing. World J Surg 2004;28:321–326.
8. Margolis DJ, Allen-Taylor L, Hoffstad O, Berlin JA. Diabetic neuropathic foot ulcers: predicting which ones will not heal. Am J Med 2003;115:627–631.
9. Margolis DJ, Allen-Taylor L, Hoffstad O, Berlin JA. The accuracy of venous leg ulcer prognostic models in a wound care system. Wound Repair Regen 2004;12:163–168.
10. Van de Kerkhof PC, Van Bergen B, Spruijt K, Kuiper JP. Age-related changes in wound healing. Clin Exp Dermatol 1994;19:369–374.
11. Thomas DR. Age-related changes in wound healing. Drugs Aging 2001;18:607–620.
12. Brem H, Tomic-Canic M, Entero H, et al. The synergism of age and db/db genotype impairs wound healing. Exp Gerontol 2007 Jan 31.
13. Di Maio VJ, Di Maio TG. Homicide by decubitus ulcers. Am J Forensic Med Pathol 2002;23:1–4.
14. Attinger CE, Janis JE, Steinberg J, Schwartz J, Al-Attar A, Couch K. Clinical approach to wounds: debridement and wound bed preparation including the use of dressings and wound-healing adjuvants. Plast Reconstr Surg 2006;117:72S–109S.
15. National Institute of Diabetes and Digestive and Kidney Diseases. National diabetes statistics fact sheet: general information and national estimates on diabetes in the United States, 2005. Bethesda, MD: U.S. Department of Health and Human Services, National Institute of Health. Available at: http://diabetes.niddk.nih.gov/. Accessed February 8, 2007.
16. Klein SA, Bond SJ, Gupta SC, Yacoub OA, Anderson GL. Angiogenesis inhibitor TNP-470 inhibits murine cutaneous wound healing. J Surg Res 1999;82:268–274.
17. Data & Trends. National Diabetes Surveillance System. Annual number (in thousands) of new cases of diagnosed diabetes among adults aged 18–79 years, United States, 1997–2004: Centers for Disease Control (CDC). Available at: http://www.cdc.gov/diabetes/statistics/incidence/fig1.htm. Accessed September 30, 2006.
18. Wild S, Roglic G, Green A, Sicree R, King H. Global prevalence of diabetes: estimates for the year 2000 and projections for 2030. Diabetes Care 2004;27:1047–1053.
19. Pecoraro RE, Reiber GE, Burgess EM. Pathways to diabetic limb amputation. Basis for prevention. Diabetes Care 1990;13:513–521.

20. Boyko EJ, Ahroni JH, Stensel V, Forsberg RC, Davignon DR, Smith DG. A prospective study of risk factors for diabetic foot ulcer. The Seattle Diabetic Foot Study. Diabetes Care 1999;22:1036–1042.

21. Abbott CA, Carrington AL, Ashe H, et al. The North-West Diabetes Foot Care Study: incidence of, and risk factors for, new diabetic foot ulceration in a community-based patient cohort. Diabet Med 2002;19:377–384.

22. Aguiar ME, Burrows NR, Wang J, Boyle JP, Geiss LS, Engelgau MM. History of foot ulcer among persons with diabetes—United States, 2000–2002. MMWR Morb Mortal Wkly Rep 2003;52:1098–1102.

23. Prompers L, Huijberts M, Apelqvist J, et al. High prevalence of ischaemia, infection and serious comorbidity in patients with diabetic foot disease in Europe. Baseline results from the Eurodiale study. Diabetologia 2007;50(1):18–25.

24. Klamer TW, Towne JB, Bandyk DF, Bonner MJ. The influence of sepsis and ischemia on the natural history of the diabetic foot. Am Surg 1987;53:490–494.

25. Cevera JJ, Bolton LL, Kerstein MD. Options for diabetic patients with chronic heel ulcers. J Diabetes Complications 1997;11:358–366.

26. Pressure ulcers prevalence, cost and risk assessment: consensus development conference statement—The National Pressure Ulcer Advisory Panel. Decubitus 1989;2:24–28.

27. Margolis DJ. Definition of a pressure ulcer. Adv Wound Care 1995;8:Suppl 8–10.

28. Russo CA, Elixhauser A. Hospitalizations Related to Pressure Sores, 2003 HCUP Statistical Brief #3. Rockville, MD: Agency for Healthcare Research and Quality; 2006.

29. Whittington KT, Briones R. National Prevalence and Incidence Study: 6-year sequential acute care data. Adv Skin Wound Care 2004;17:490–494.

30. Brem H, Nierman DM, Nelson JE. Pressure ulcers in the chronically critically ill patient. Crit Care Clin 2002;18:683–694.

31. Brandeis GH, Ooi WL, Hossain M, Morris JN, Lipsitz LA. A longitudinal study of risk factors associated with the formation of pressure ulcers in nursing homes. J Am Geriatr Soc 1994;42:388–393.

32. Allman RM, Goode PS, Patrick MM, Burst N, Bartolucci AA. Pressure ulcer risk factors among hospitalized patients with activity limitation. JAMA 1995;273:865–870.

33. Eachempati SR, Hydo LJ, Barie PS. Factors influencing the development of decubitus ulcers in critically ill surgical patients. Crit Care Med 2001;29:1678–1682.

34. Mecocci P, von Strauss E, Cherubini A, et al. Cognitive impairment is the major risk factor for development of geriatric syndromes during hospitalization: results from the GIFA study. Dement Geriatr Cogn Disord 2005;20:262–269.

35. Berlowitz DR, Brandeis GH, Anderson J, Du W, Brand H. Effect of pressure ulcers on the survival of long-term care residents. J Gerontol A Biol Sci Med Sci 1997;52:M106–110.

36. Dale MC, Burns A, Panter L, Morris J. Factors affecting survival of elderly nursing home residents. Int J Geriatr Psychiatry 2001;16:70–76.

37. Thomas DR, Goode PS, Tarquine PH, Allman RM. Hospital-acquired pressure ulcers and risk of death. J Am Geriatr Soc 1996;44:1435–1440.

38. Redelings MD, Lee NE, Sorvillo F. Pressure ulcers: more lethal than we thought? Adv Skin Wound Care 2005;18:367–372.

39. Anderson RN, Smith BL. Deaths: leading causes for 2002. Natl Vital Stat Rep 2005;53:1–89.

40. Angus DC, Linde-Zwirble WT, Lidicker J, Clermont G, Carcillo J, Pinsky MR. Epidemiology of severe sepsis in the United States: analysis of incidence, outcome, and associated costs of care. Crit Care Med 2001;29:1303–1310.

41. Baker SR, Stacey MC, Jopp-McKay AG, Hoskin SE, Thompson PJ. Epidemiology of chronic venous ulcers. Br J Surg 1991;78:864–867.

42. Abbade LPF, Lastoria S. Venous ulcer: epidemiology, physiopathology, diagnosis and treatment. Int J Dermatol 2005;44:449–456.

43. Margolis DJ, Bilker W, Santanna J, Baumgarten M. Venous leg ulcer: incidence and prevalence in the elderly. J Am Acad Dermatol 2002;46:381–386.

44. Brem H, Kirsner RS, Falanga V. Protocol for the successful treatment of venous ulcers. Am J Surg 2004;188:1–8.

45. Wissing U, Ek AC, Unosson M. Life situation and function in elderly people with and without leg ulcers. Scand J Caring Sci 2002;16:59–65.

46. Valencia IC, Falabella A, Kirsner RS, Eaglstein WH. Chronic venous insufficiency and venous leg ulceration. J Am Acad Dermatol 2001;44:401–421; quiz 422–424.

47. Capitao LM, Menezes JD, Gouveia-Oliveira A. A multivariate analysis of the factors associated with the severity of chronic venous insufficiency [in Portuguese]. Acta Med Port 1993;6:501–506.

48. Delis KT. Perforator vein incompetence in chronic venous disease: a multivariate regression analysis model. J Vasc Surg 2004;40:626–633.

49. Scott TE, LaMorte WW, Gorin DR, Menzoian JO. Risk factors for chronic venous insufficiency: a dual case-control study. J Vasc Surg 1995;22:622–628.

50. van Haarst EP, Liasis N, van Ramshorst B, Moll FL. The development of valvular incompetence after deep vein thrombosis: a 7 year follow-up study with duplex scanning. Eur J Vasc Endovasc Surg 1996;12:295–299.

51. Falanga V, Eaglstein WH. The "trap" hypothesis of venous ulceration. Lancet 1993;341:1006–1008.

52. Higley HR, Ksander GA, Gerhardt CO, Falanga V. Extravasation of macromolecules and possible trapping of transforming growth factor-beta in venous ulceration. Br J Dermatol 1995;132:79–85.

53. Kweon SS, Shin MH, Park KS, et al. Distribution of the ankle-brachial index and associated cardiovascular risk factors in a population of middle-aged and elderly Koreans. J Korean Med Sci 2005;20:373–378.

54. Rhee SY, Guan H, Liu ZM, et al. Multi-country study on the prevalence and clinical features of peripheral arterial disease in Asian type 2 diabetes patients at high risk of atherosclerosis. Diabetes Res Clin Pract 2007;76:82–92.

55. Cimminiello C. PAD: epidemiology and pathophysiology. Thromb Res 2002;106:V295–V301.

56. Doubeni CA, Yood RA, Emani S, Gurwitz JH. Identifying unrecognized peripheral arterial disease among asymptomatic patients in the primary care setting. Angiology 2006;57:171–180.

57. Brem H, Tsakayannis D, Folkman J. Time dependent suppression of wound healing with the angiogenesis inhibitor, AGM-1470. J Cell Biol 1991;115:403a.

58. O'Reilly MS, Brem H, Folkman J. Treatment of murine hemangioendotheliomas with the angiogenesis inhibitor AGM-1470. J Pediatr Surg 1995;30:325–330.

59. Bond SJ, Klein SA. TNP-470 reduces collagen and macrophage accumulation in expanded polytetrafluoroethylene tube implants. J Surg Res 2001;101:99–103.

60. Rivard A, Berthou-Soulie L, Principe N, et al. Age-dependent defect in vascular endothelial growth factor expression is associated with reduced hypoxia-inducible factor 1 activity. J Biol Chem 2000;275:29643–29647.

61. Rivard A, Fabre JE, Silver M, et al. Age-dependent impairment of angiogenesis. Circulation 1999;99:111–120.

62. Swift ME, Kleinman HK, DiPietro LA. Impaired wound repair and delayed angiogenesis in aged mice. Lab Invest 1999;79:1479–1487.

63. Nathan CF. Secretory products of macrophages. J Clin Invest 1987;79:319–326.

64. Cohen BJ, Danon D, Roth GS. Wound repair in mice as influenced by age and antimacrophage serum. J Gerontol 1987;42:295–301.

65. Plowden J, Renshaw-Hoelscher M, Engleman C, Katz J, Sambhara S. Innate immunity in aging: impact on macrophage function. Aging Cell 2004;3:161–167.

66. Ballas CB, Davidson JM. Delayed wound healing in aged rats is associated with increased collagen gel remodeling and contraction by skin fibroblasts, not with differences in apoptotic or myofibroblast cell populations. Wound Repair Regen 2001;9:223–237.

67. Yoshikawa TT. Perspective: aging and infectious diseases—past, present, and future. J Infect Dis 1997;176:1053–1057.

68. Gregg R, Smith CM, Clark FJ, et al. The number of human peripheral blood CD4 CD25 regulatory T cells increases with age. Clin Exp Immunol 2005;140:540–546.

69. Dejaco C, Duftner C, Schirmer M. Are regulatory T-cells linked with aging? Exp Gerontol 2006;41(4):339–345.

70. Naylor K, Li G, Vallejo AN, et al. The influence of age on T cell generation and TCR diversity. J Immunol 2005; 174:7446–7452.

71. Colonna-Romano G, Aquino A, Bulati M, et al. Impairment of gamma/delta T lymphocytes in elderly: implications for immunosenescence. Exp Gerontol 2004;39: 1439–1446.

72. Brem H, Lyder C. Protocol for the successful treatment of pressure ulcers. Am J Surg 2004;188:9–17.

73. Brem H, Sheehan P, Rosenberg HJ, Schneider JS, Boulton AJ. Evidence-based protocol for diabetic foot ulcers. Plast Reconstr Surg 2006;117:193S–209S; discussion 210S–211S.

74. Berlowitz DR, Wilking SV. Risk factors for pressure sores. A comparison of cross-sectional and cohort-derived data. J Am Geriatr Soc 1989;37:1043–1050.

75. Bergstrom N, Braden B. A prospective study of pressure sore risk among institutionalized elderly. J Am Geriatr Soc 1992;40:747–758.

76. Breslow RA, Hallfrisch J, Guy DG, Crawley B, Goldberg AP. The importance of dietary protein in healing pressure ulcers. J Am Geriatr Soc 1993;41:357–362.

77. Niazi K, Khan TH, Easley KA. Diagnostic utility of the two methods of ankle brachial index in the detection of peripheral arterial disease of lower extremities. Catheter Cardiovasc Interv 2006;68:788–792.

78. Schroder F, Diehm N, Kareem S, et al. A modified calculation of ankle-brachial pressure index is far more sensitive in the detection of peripheral arterial disease. J Vasc Surg 2006;44:531–536.

79. Carter SA, Tate RB. The relationship of the transcutaneous oxygen tension, pulse waves and systolic pressures to the risk for limb amputation in patients with peripheral arterial disease and skin ulcers or gangrene. Int Angiol 2006; 25:67–72.

80. ACC/AHA 2005 Practice Guidelines for the Management of Patients with Peripheral Arterial Disease (Lower Extremity, Renal, Mesenteric, and Abdominal Aortic): A Collaborative Report from the American Association for Vascular Surgery/Society for Vascular Surgery, Society for Cardiovascular Angiography and Interventions, Society for Vascular Medicine and Biology, Society of Interventional Radiology, and the ACC/AHA Task Force on Practice Guidelines (Writing Committee to Develop Guidelines for the Management of Patients with Peripheral Arterial Disease): Endorsed by the American Association of Cardiovascular and Pulmonary Rehabilitation; National Heart, Lung, and Blood Institute; Society for Vascular Nursing; TransAtlantic Inter-Society Consensus; and Vascular Disease Foundation. Circulation 2006;113:e463–654.

81. Silvestro A, Diehm N, Savolainen H, et al. Falsely high ankle-brachial index predicts major amputation in critical limb ischemia. Vasc Med 2006;11:69–74.

82. Williams DT, Harding KG, Price P. An evaluation of the efficacy of methods used in screening for lower-limb arterial disease in diabetes. Diabetes Care 2005;28:2206–2210.

83. Laird JR, Zeller T, Gray BH, et al. Limb salvage following laser-assisted angioplasty for critical limb ischemia: results of the LACI multicenter trial. J Endovasc Ther 2006; 13:1–11.

84. Costanza MJ, Queral LA, Lilly MP, Finn WR. Hemodynamic outcome of endovascular therapy for transatlantic intersociety consensus type B femoropopliteal arterial occlusive lesions. J Vasc Surg 2004;39:343–350.

85. Becquemin J-P, Favre J-P, Marzelle J, Nemoz C, Corsin C, Leizorovicz A. Systematic versus selective stent placement after superficial femoral artery balloon angioplasty: a multicenter prospective randomized study. J Vasc Surg 2003;37:487–494.

86. Faglia E, Mantero M, Caminiti M, et al. Extensive use of peripheral angioplasty, particularly infrapopliteal, in the treatment of ischaemic diabetic foot ulcers: clinical results of a multicentric study of 221 consecutive diabetic subjects. J Intern Med 2002;252:225–232.

87. Kudo T, Chandra FA, Ahn SS. The effectiveness of percutaneous transluminal angioplasty for the treatment of critical limb ischemia: a 10-year experience. J Vasc Surg 2005; 41:423–435.

88. Steed DL. Debridement. Am J Surg 2004;187:S71–S74.
89. Elias SM, Frasier KL. Minimally invasive vein surgery: its role in the treatment of venous stasis ulceration. Am J Surg 2004;188:26–30.
90. Puggioni A, Kalra M, Gloviczki P. Superficial vein surgery and SEPS for chronic venous insufficiency. Semin Vasc Surg 2005;18:41–48.
91. Ting AC, Cheng SW, Ho P, Poon JT, Wu LL, Cheung GC. Reduction in deep vein reflux after concomitant subfascial endoscopic perforating vein surgery and superficial vein ablation in advanced primary chronic venous insufficiency. J Vasc Surg 2006;43:546–550.
92. Barwell J, Davies CE, Deacon J, et al. Comparison of surgery and compression with compression alone in chronic venous ulceration (ESCHAR study): randomised controlled trial. Lancet 2004;363:1854–1859.
93. TenBrook J, John A, Iafrati MD, et al. Systematic review of outcomes after surgical management of venous disease incorporating subfascial endoscopic perforator surgery. J Vasc Surg 2004;39:583–589.
94. Roka F, Binder M, Bohler-Sommeregger K. Mid-term recurrence rate of incompetent perforating veins after combined superficial vein surgery and subfascial endoscopic perforating vein surgery. J Vasc Surg 2006;44: 359–363.
95. Kantor J, Margolis DJ. Efficacy and prognostic value of simple wound measurements. Arch Dermatol 1998;134: 1571–1574.
96. Edmonds M, Foster A. The use of antibiotics in the diabetic foot. Am J Surg 2004;187:25S–28S.
97. Weigelt J, Kaafarani HM, Itani KM, Swanson RN. Linezolid eradicates MRSA better than vancomycin from surgical-site infections. Am J Surg 2004;188:760–766.
98. Ruiz de Gopegui E, Oliver A, Ramirez A, Gutierrez O, Andreu C, Perez JL. Epidemiological relatedness of methicillin-resistant *Staphylococcus aureus* from a tertiary hospital and a geriatric institution in Spain. Clin Microbiol Infect 2004;10:339–342.
99. Fridkin SK, Hageman JC, Morrison M, et al. The Active Bacterial Core Surveillance Program of the Emerging Infections Program Network. Methicillin-resistant *Staphylococcus aureus* disease in three communities. N Engl J Med 2005;352:1436–1444.
100. Zacur H, Kirsner RS. Debridement: rationale and therapeutic options. Wounds Sep 2002;14:2S–6S.
101. Saap LJ, Falanga V. Debridement performance index and its correlation with complete closure of diabetic foot ulcers. Wound Repair Regen 2002;10:354–359.
102. Steed DL, Donohoe D, Webster MW, Lindsley L. Effect of extensive debridement and treatment on the healing of diabetic foot ulcers. Diabetic Ulcer Study Group. J Am Coll Surg 1996;183:61–64.
103. Williams D, Enoch S, Miller D, Harris K, Price P, Harding KG. Effect of sharp debridement using curette on recalcitrant nonhealing venous leg ulcers: a concurrently controlled, prospective cohort study. Wound Repair Regen 2005;13:131–137.
104. Stojadinovic O, Brem H, Vouthounis C, et al. The role of the beta-catenin and c-*myc* in pathogenesis of cutaneous wound healing. Am J Pathol 2005;167:59–69.
105. Steed DL. Foundations of good ulcer care. Am J Surg 1998;176:20S–25S.
106. Mueller MJ, Diamond JE, Sinacore DR, et al. Total contact casting in treatment of diabetic plantar ulcers. Controlled clinical trial. Diabetes Care 1989;12:384–388.
107. Armstrong DG, Nguyen HC, Lavery LA, van Schie CH, Boulton AJ, Harkless LB. Off-loading the diabetic foot wound: a randomized clinical trial. Diabetes Care 2001; 24:1019–1022.
108. Armstrong DG, Short B, Espensen EH, Abu-Rumman PL, Nixon BP, Boulton AJM. Technique for fabrication of an "instant total-contact cast" for treatment of neuropathic diabetic foot ulcers. J Am Podiatr Med Assoc 2002;92: 405–408.
109. Boulton AJ, Kirsner RS, Vileikyte L. Clinical practice. Neuropathic diabetic foot ulcers. N Engl J Med 2004; 351:48–55.
110. Nelson EA, Iglesias CP, Cullum N, Torgerson DJ. Randomized clinical trial of four-layer and short-stretch compression bandages for venous leg ulcers (VenUS I). Br J Surg 2004;91:1292–1299.
111. Fletcher A, Cullum N, Sheldon TA. A systematic review of compression treatment for venous leg ulcers. BMJ 1997; 315:576–580.
112. Marston WA, Hanft J, Norwood P, Pollak R. The efficacy and safety of Dermagraft in improving the healing of chronic diabetic foot ulcers: results of a prospective randomized trial. Diabetes Care 2003;26:1701–1705.
113. Veves A, Falanga V, Armstrong DG, Sabolinski ML. Graftskin, a human skin equivalent, is effective in the management of noninfected neuropathic diabetic foot ulcers: a prospective randomized multicenter clinical trial. Diabetes Care 2001;24:290–295.
114. Steed DL. Clinical evaluation of recombinant human platelet-derived growth factor for the treatment of lower extremity diabetic ulcers. Diabetic Ulcer Study Group. J Vasc Surg 1995;21:71–78; discussion 79–81.
115. Steed DL. Clinical evaluation of recombinant human platelet-derived growth factor for the treatment of lower extremity ulcers. Plast Reconstr Surg 2006;117:143S–149S; discussion 150S–151S.
116. Falanga V, Margolis D, Alvarez O, et al. Rapid healing of venous ulcers and lack of clinical rejection with an allogeneic cultured human skin equivalent. Human Skin Equivalent Investigators Group. Arch Dermatol 1998;134: 293–300.
117. Goyal P, Puri GD, Pandey CK, Srivastva S. Evaluation of induction doses of propofol: comparison between endstage renal disease and normal renal function patients. Anaesth Intensive Care 2002;30:584–587.
118. Reiber GE, Vileikyte L, Boyko EJ, et al. Causal pathways for incident lower-extremity ulcers in patients with diabetes from two settings. Diabetes Care 1999;22:157–162.
119. Curtin CM, Gater DR, Chung KC. Autonomic dysreflexia: a plastic surgery primer. Ann Plast Surg 2003;51:325–329.
120. Assadi F, Czech K, Palmisano JL. Autonomic dysreflexia manifested by severe hypertension. Med Sci Monit 2004;10: CS77–79.
121. Adam S, Forrest S. ABC of intensive care: other supportive care. BMJ 1999;319:175–178.

122. Padberg J, Frank T, Johnston MV, Sisto SA. Structured exercise improves calf muscle pump function in chronic venous insufficiency: a randomized trial. J Vasc Surg 2004; 39:79–87.

123. Freedman G, Cean C, Duron V, Tarnovskaya A, Brem H. Pathogenesis and treatment of pain in patients with chronic wounds. Surg Technol Int 2003;11:168–179.

124. Freedman G, Entero H, Brem H. Practical treatment of pain in patients with chronic wounds: pathogenesis-guided management. Am J Surg 2004;188:31–35.

125. World Health Organization. Cancer pain relief. Geneva: World Health Organization; 1996.

126. Scott EM, Leaper DJ, Clark M, Kelly PJ. Effects of warming therapy on pressure ulcers—a randomized trial. AORN J 2001;73:921–927, 929–933, 936–938.

127. Aronovitch S. Hospital acquired pressure ulcers: a comparison of costs in medical versus surgical patients, 1–18 First Annual OR-Acquired Pressure Ulcer Symposium. Atlanta, GA, 1998.

128. Scott EM, Buckland R. Pressure ulcer risk in the perioperative environment. Nurs Stand 2005;20:74, 76, 78 passim.

129. Hoshowsky VM, Schramm CA. Intraoperative pressure sore prevention: an analysis of bedding materials. Res Nurs Health 1994;17:333–339.

130. Schoonhoven L, Defloor T, Grypdonck MH. Incidence of pressure ulcers due to surgery. J Clin Nurs 2002;11:479–487.

131. De Keyser G, Dejaeger E, De Meyst H, Eders GC. Pressure-reducing effects of heel protectors. Adv Wound Care 1994;7:30–32, 34.

Part III
Anesthetic Management of the Aged Surgical Candidate

13
Preoperative Risk Stratification and Methods to Reduce Risk

Linda L. Liu and Jacqueline M. Leung

Aging increases the likelihood that a patient will have an operative procedure. Approximately 12% of those aged 45 to 60 years are operated on each year, and this number will increase to more than 21% by the year 2025.[1] Whereas operations performed on patients older than 50 years of age were contraindicated in the past, an increasingly larger number of elderly patients are undergoing surgery at present. Studies of perioperative outcomes in the elderly have shown a decline in perioperative mortality rate from 20% in the 1960s[2] to 10% in the 1970s[3] to 5%–8% in the 1980s.[4] These relatively low mortality rates have been attributed to improvement in anesthetic and surgical care.[5] As a result, many patients, including those who are elderly, do quite well after surgery and have improved quality of life as a result of their surgery.

In contrast to the immediate fatal postoperative complications, which are infrequent, more common occurrences are complications, which result in morbidity instead of mortality. As discussed in the previous chapters, age-related changes occur in most organ systems. Under normal conditions, the physiologic changes that occur with aging usually lead to minimal functional impairment. With an acute disease or a surgical procedure, however, the elderly may be more prone to complications given their diminished reserve capacity, their decreased ability to respond to stress, and pathologic changes resulting from their coexisting disease. Recent studies suggest that surgical risk increases as a result of this increased prevalence of comorbid disease and/or decreased physiologic reserve rather than simply as a result of increased age alone.[6,7]

The increasing number of elderly patients presenting for surgery will have a tremendous impact on anesthesia practice. As an example, in 1980, one million postoperative complications involving the cardiac system alone occurred, leading to an estimated $20 billion in annual costs from in-hospital and long-term care.[8] A critical component of the perioperative care of elderly patients is to identify and modify preoperative risk in order to decrease postoperative morbidity and mortality. This chapter will discuss how to perform risk stratification of elderly patients awaiting major surgery and to determine methods to reduce perioperative morbidity and mortality using an evidence-based approach.

The Importance of Coexisting Disease

Several previous studies have examined risk predictors of postoperative morbidity and mortality after major surgery and anesthesia. The majority of the studies agree that the most consistent risk predictor identified is the presence of coexisting disease. For example, Tiret et al.[9] determined that ASA PS classification (American Society of Anesthesiologists physical status), age, surgical procedure (major versus minor), and type (elective versus emergency) were significant predictors. Pedersen et al.[10] found similar predictors of risk, which included age, history of congestive heart failure, renal disease, emergency surgery, and the type of surgery to be performed. Rorbaek-Madsen et al.[11] studied 594 octogenarians undergoing surgery in Denmark. Mortality rates in this study ranged from 0% in those with no complicating coexisting disease undergoing elective surgery to 21% in those with coexisting disease who were undergoing emergency surgery. Bufalari et al.[12] found only the ASA PS, presence of two associated diseases, and laparotomy procedures to be predictors of risk in surgical octogenarians in Italy from 1989 to 1993. The combined results from our two previous studies in patients aged ≥80 years and those ≥70 years confirmed that the severity of preoperative comorbidities is a more important predictor of postoperative adverse outcomes than even intraoperative factors.[6,7]

Given the important impact of coexisting disease on anesthetic outcome, it should be noted that comorbid conditions are prevalent in elderly patients. Vaz and Seymour[13] prospectively studied 288 general surgical patients aged

65 years and older, and found a high prevalence of preexisting health problems in their cohort. Overall, 30% of the patients had three or more preoperative medical problems, involving pulmonary disease, a history of congestive heart failure, angina, and prior cerebrovascular accidents. In a consecutive cohort of patients ≥70 years of age undergoing noncardiac surgery, we similarly found that nearly 30% of patients had three or more comorbid conditions including a history of hypertension, cardiopulmonary disease, and neurologic disease.[6,7] In a study of a cohort of centenarians presenting for surgery, Warner et al.[14] found that nearly all of these very old patients had one or more pre-existing medical conditions.

Because mortality and morbidity rates are more affected by coexisting disease as opposed to age alone, efforts should be made to optimize any coexisting disease, if possible, before surgery. The remainder of this chapter will present evidence-based data addressing which of the coexisting diseases can be modified to reduce the likelihood of perioperative morbidity and mortality. However, for geriatric patients, postponing surgery to optimize any medical conditions must be weighed against the risk of delaying surgery because emergency surgical treatment is associated with higher morbidity and mortality. Certain surgical procedures, such as cancer surgery, may substantially alter the prognosis of the patients if delayed. As a result, good communication among the anesthesiologists, surgeons, and primary care physicians is critical to developing an optimal plan as to when a geriatric patient should be scheduled for the planned surgery.

Cognitive Dysfunction and Delirium after Noncardiac Surgery

One of the most common postoperative outcomes is an adverse event involving the neurologic system, with postoperative delirium and cognitive decline being the two most frequently occurring events in geriatric patients. Our previous retrospective cohort study in surgical octogenarians demonstrated that postoperative neurologic complications occurred in 15% of the patients, of which 91% were related to the occurrence of postoperative delirium.[6] Delirium is an acute disorder of attention and cognition and a serious problem for hospitalized geriatric patients. In contrast, cognitive dysfunction includes a wider range of neuropsychologic changes in several functional domains, and is often more subtle than delirium. It requires a different methodology for ascertainment and is frequently underestimated by health care professionals. A multinational study reported that postoperative cognitive dysfunction (POCD) was present in 26% of patients 1 week after surgery and in 10% of patients even 3 months after surgery.[15]

In the surgical setting, as demonstrated by our previous work[6,7] and work from others, postoperative delirium is common in elderly surgical patients.[16] In one study, 36% of elderly patients undergoing surgery for hip fracture under a variety of anesthetic agents were "confused" on the first postoperative day.[17] Patients who developed delirium required a hospital stay approximately four times longer than those who remained lucid.[18] More importantly, delirium resulted in increased rates of nursing home placement, and associated hospital mortality rates of 10%–65%.[19] Numerous risk factors for delirium in medical patients have been previously identified. They include the use of physical restraints, malnutrition, use of a bladder catheter, any iatrogenic event, and the use of more than three medications.[20–22]

In the perioperative setting, limited data exist as to whether specific intraoperative management precipitates POCD or delirium. The main areas that deserve consideration include:

1. Drugs: Although previous studies have demonstrated that certain drugs may be associated with postoperative delirium,[23] there has been no prospective randomized clinical trials to determine if the elimination of certain drugs used in the perioperative period will actually lead to a lowering of the incidence of delirium. As a result, no definitive guidelines can be provided at present regarding avoiding certain drugs in the perioperative period. However, a sensible guideline is that "polypharmacy" is best avoided in elderly patients because delirium has been shown to be related to the number of medications prescribed.[22,23]

2. Anesthetic techniques: Controversy persists as to whether any anesthetic technique (regional versus general) has an impact on postoperative neurologic dysfunction. Earlier studies suggested an association between a higher incidence of cognitive dysfunction and general anesthesia relative to epidural anesthesia.[18,24] More recent studies, in contrast, have concluded that there is no relationship between anesthetic technique and the magnitude or pattern of POCD.[25] In a study by Moller et al.,[15] only the duration of anesthesia was found to be one of the risk factors for early POCD. A retrospective cohort study of consecutive hip fracture patients, aged ≥60 years, undergoing surgical repair at 20 United States hospitals also found that the anesthesia technique (regional versus general) had no impact on postoperative mental status change.[26] More recently, a multicenter trial of patients ≥60 years of age, although not adequately powered, reported that the incidence of cognitive dysfunction at 3 months after surgery was not different after either general or regional anesthesia.[27]

3. Anesthetic management: Specifically, is the role of blood pressure or intraoperative hypotension associated with POCD? In a prospective, randomized study of older

adults (age >50 years) undergoing total hip replacement, Williams-Russo et al.[28] demonstrated that patients who underwent epidural anesthesia and were rendered markedly hypotensive had similar incidence of POCD as those who were maintained in the normotensive state. Moller et al.,[15] by a larger cohort study, also determined that neither hypotension nor hypoxemia were related to POCD.

4. Postoperative pain management: In one study of older patients undergoing major elective noncardiac operations,[29] after adjusting for known preoperative risk factors for delirium, higher pain scores at rest were associated with a slightly increased risk of delirium in the first three postoperative days. It remains to be proven whether better control of postoperative pain will reduce POCD.

Despite the importance and prevalence of postoperative neurologic decline, no single anesthetic technique has been identified to be superior for elderly surgical patients in minimizing POCD or delirium. Until more definitive clinical studies become available, minimizing the number of medications used, avoiding hypoxemia and hypercarbia, and providing adequate postoperative pain control seem to be the best approaches in minimizing the occurrence of postoperative delirium in geriatric surgical patients.

Cardiovascular Complications

The elderly are more likely to develop postoperative cardiovascular complications. Pedersen et al.[30] presented data on 7306 patients undergoing surgery in Denmark. The octogenarians had a 16.7% incidence of cardiovascular complications compared with a 2.6% incidence in patients younger than 50 years of age. The cardiovascular complications in this study were defined as systolic hypotension or hypertension (systolic blood pressures <60 mm Hg or >200 mm Hg, respectively), cardiac arrest, second- or third-degree heart block, chest pain, ventricular tachyarrhythmias, supraventricular tachycardia requiring treatment, myocardial infarction, or congestive heart failure. A high incidence of cardiovascular complications (40%) was found in patients with preoperative heart disease, especially in those with clinical signs of congestive heart failure, history of ischemic heart disease, or previous myocardial infarction. In two separate cohort studies of nearly 1000 patients older than 70 and 80 years of age undergoing noncardiac surgery, respectively, we found a similar cardiovascular complication rate of 10%–12%.[6,7] The most common postoperative cardiovascular events in these two separate cohorts were congestive heart failure, arrhythmias, and ischemic complications. In contrast to the Pedersen study, in which the severity of the operative case and elective versus emergent surgery

TABLE 13-1. Comparison between cardiac risk indexes developed by Goldman and Lee.

Goldman	Lee
• Preoperative S₃ or JVD	• High-risk type of surgery
• Myocardial infarction within 6 months	• Ischemic heart disease
• PVC >5 bpm	• History of congestive heart failure
• Rhythm other than sinus or presence of PACs	• History of cerebrovascular disease
• Age >70 years	• Insulin therapy for diabetes
• Intraperitoneal, intrathoracic, or aortic operations	• Preoperative serum creatinine >2 mg/dL
• Emergency surgery	
• Important valvular aortic stenosis	
• Poor general medical condition	

Source: Data from Goldman et al.[31] and Lee et al.[32]
JVD = jugular venous distention, PVC = premature ventricular contractions, PAC = premature atrial contractions.

were associated with the occurrence of cardiovascular complications, we found that intraoperative variables such as type of anesthesia and surgical procedure did not increase postoperative cardiovascular complications.

What are the characteristics of patients who develop postoperative complications? Many previous investigations have focused on clinical variables and diagnostic test procedures obtained preoperatively to identify patients at risk for postoperative complications. For example, a cardiac risk index was developed by Goldman et al. in 1977[31] and subsequently revised in 1999[32] to predict the occurrence of postoperative cardiac complications (Table 13-1). In this latter revised cardiac index,[32] variables that were associated with increased risk of postoperative cardiac complications included high-risk surgery, history of ischemic heart disease, congestive heart failure, or cerebrovascular disease, preoperative treatment of diabetes with insulin, and preoperative creatinine >2.0 mg/dL. Rates of major cardiac complication with 0, 1, 2, or ≥3 of the factors were 0.5%, 1.3%, 4%, and 9%, respectively.

The American College of Cardiology/American Heart Association (ACC/AHA) Task Force recently updated the guidelines for preoperative cardiac evaluation for patients presenting for noncardiac surgery[33] in an attempt to unify the risk stratification process. Although these guidelines are based on studies performed in the general surgical population and do not specifically target the geriatric population, some of the general principles are applicable. The main decision points of the guidelines are based on the patient's medical conditions, functional capacity, and the acuity and risk of the planned surgical procedure.

The first step is to stratify the patient by medical condition. Table 13-2 lists the minor, intermediate, and major clinical predictors as defined by the ACC/AHA guidelines. Advanced age, by itself, is considered only one of the minor clinical predictors. However, it should be noted that advanced age is associated with increased incidence of comorbid conditions, which may be intermediate predictors of postoperative cardiovascular complications. Diseases such as diabetes mellitus, renal insufficiency, and compensated congestive heart failure, are more likely to occur in the older population. Major predictors are unstable coronary syndromes, decompensated congestive heart failure, significant arrhythmias, and severe valvular disease.

The next area of focus in the guideline is the assessment of functional capacity. According to the ACC/AHA guidelines, the inability to perform activities beyond four metabolic equivalents (METs) requires further evaluation. A summary of how to evaluate METs is provided in Table 13-3. However, the accurate assessment of functional capacity may be difficult in the geriatric population because many elderly patients may have comorbid conditions or chronic pain, which limits their functional capacity. As a result, the functional limitation may be secondary to noncardiac causes, rather than attributable to a primary cardiac cause as the guideline would suggest. Therefore, direct adoption of the ACC/AHA algorithm without knowing the reason for the functional limitation may result in a great majority of elderly patients needing additional preoperative cardiac stress testing.

The ACC/AHA guidelines also take into account the operative procedure itself, which has an impact on the occurrence of cardiac morbidity and mortality. Emergency major operations, major vascular surgery, and any prolonged surgical procedures associated with large fluid shifts are stratified as procedures carrying higher cardiac

TABLE 13-2. Major, intermediate, and minor predictors of cardiovascular risk.

Predictors	
Major	Unstable coronary syndromes
	Decompensated heart failure
	Significant arrhythmias
	Significant valvular disease
Intermediate	Stable angina pectoris
	History of myocardial infarction
	Compensated heart failure
	Diabetes
	Renal insufficiency
Minor	Advanced age
	Abnormal electrocardiogram
	Rhythm other than sinus
	Poor exercise capacity
	History of cerebrovascular accident
	Uncontrolled hypertension

Source: Data adapted from Eagle et al.[33]

TABLE 13-3. Estimate of metabolic equivalent for different activities

MET estimate	Activity
1 MET	Activities of daily living
	Eating
	Dressing
	Walking indoors (2–3 mph)
	Dishwashing
4 MET	More strenuous activities
	Climbing stairs (1 flight)
	Walking (4 mph)
	Running short distance
	Scrubbing floors
	Playing golf, doubles tennis
10 MET	Playing sports
	Swimming
	Singles tennis
	Football

Source: Data adapted from Eagle et al.[33]
MET = metabolic equivalent.

risk. More minor surgeries such as cataract removal are deemed to be of low surgical risk. Taken together, the results of the medical history, current symptoms, and physical examination allow the physician to identify clinical predictors of increased perioperative cardiovascular risk. The clinical predictors, combined with an assessment of the patient's exercise tolerance and the risk of surgery, then provides additional guidance to the clinicians in determining the value of additional cardiac stress testing.

Strategies to Reduce Cardiac Risk

The basis of performing preoperative cardiac risk stratification assumes the possibility that some or all of these risk factors identified may be modifiable with the ultimate goal of improving patients' outcomes. However, this assumption has not been completely proven. Eagle et al.[34] determined that the risk of coronary artery bypass graft (CABG) surgery itself, when added to the risk of the noncardiac surgery, often exceeded the risk of the same surgery in patients who have not undergone CABG surgery. They showed that performance of CABG surgery before the planned noncardiac surgery may not be justified. In other words, it seems that for some of the patients, the risk of modifying their perioperative myocardial infarction risk by cardiac surgery may actually outweigh the benefits because of the risk of cardiac surgery itself.[34] In fact, a recent randomized multicenter trial in 510 male veterans scheduled for vascular operations demonstrates that coronary artery revascularization before elective vascular surgery does not significantly alter the long-term outcome.[35] As a result, a reexamination and further investigation of the appropriateness of the 2002 ACC/AHA guidelines for preoperative cardiac evaluation for elderly patients needs to be conducted.

Despite the varied nature of each study patient population, congestive heart failure (CHF) continues to be identified as a major predictor of surgical outcomes. In a prospective study of octogenarians, clinical signs of congestive heart failure increased the odds of an adverse cardiac event (odds ratio = 2.1, confidence interval = 1.1–5.1).[7] The strong association between clinical signs of CHF and postoperative complications emphasizes the importance of preoperative optimization of heart function in the elective surgical patient. The adequacy and accuracy of preoperative assessment of heart function seems to be a critical area deserving further investigation.

For the elderly patient, heart failure can often be caused by diastolic dysfunction associated with left ventricular hypertrophy. Older patients with CHF frequently present with normal left ventricular ejection fraction, suggesting the importance of diastolic dysfunction in this age group.[36] In fact, up to one third of patients with heart failure may have normal systolic function.[37] Other causes of diastolic dysfunction may include myocardial ischemia, accelerated hypertension, or intrinsic myocardial diseases such as fibrosis.[38] Unfortunately, this diagnosis may not be readily apparent preoperatively and the therapeutic approach is different.[39] The prognostic significance of diastolic function assessment, such as with preoperative Doppler echocardiography in patients with a history of heart failure remains to be determined. More studies are needed to better characterize diastolic function including defining normality in older patients before recommendations for preoperative care can be made.

The association between hypertension and end organ damage, such as ischemic heart disease, heart failure, cerebrovascular disease, and renal impairment, has been well established,[40,41] but in assessing perioperative risk, hypertension has not been recognized as a major predictor of perioperative cardiac risk.[31,32] Patients diagnosed with hypertension have increased systemic vascular resistance and cardiovascular lability during anesthesia.[42,43] Reich et al.[44] reported an association between intraoperative hypertension and tachycardia and adverse outcome in protracted surgery, but a direct causal relationship between hypertension and perioperative adverse cardiac outcomes is not as evident. In a meta-analysis of 30 studies, the risk of perioperative cardiovascular complications in hypertensive patients was only slightly increased (odds ratio = 1.35, confidence interval = 1.17–1.56) and the authors advised cautious interpretation of the data because of the heterogeneity of the observational studies.[45]

To date, there is no evidence to support the approach of deferring elective surgery to allow hypertension to be treated in order to reduce perioperative risk.[45] The ACC/AHA guidelines state that mild/moderate hypertension is not an independent risk factor for perioperative cardiovascular complications, but severe hypertension (systolic blood pressure ≥180 mm Hg and/or diastolic blood pressure ≥110 mm Hg) should be controlled before surgery.[33] Unfortunately, there are no data to suggest that this strategy reduces perioperative risk. In a meta-analysis report, Howell et al.[41] have suggested that surgery may proceed, but care should be taken to ensure perioperative cardiovascular stability, invasive arterial pressure monitoring should be started, and mean arterial blood pressure should be kept within 20% of baseline. In patients with severe hypertension and evidence of end organ damage, Howell et al. did suggest that it would be appropriate to defer surgery when possible, but this suggestion is based on evidence from medical patients, not from data in surgical patients.

In patients without contraindications, the use of perioperative beta-blockade may be of value in controlling blood pressure and also reducing perioperative myocardial ischemia. Several clinical trials have examined the potential beneficial effects of using beta-adrenergic blocking agents to improve perioperative surgical outcomes.[46,47] None, however, has directly focused on geriatric patients. The mechanism of beta-adrenergic blockade in prophylaxis of perioperative ischemia and postoperative cardiac events is probably multifactorial. Proposed mechanisms include decreased myocardial demand from a reduction in the inotropic and chronotropic state of the myocardium, and possible improved perfusion to ischemic regions from redistribution of myocardial blood flow. Because perioperative tachycardia increases myocardial oxygen demand and has been shown to be associated with myocardial ischemia,[48] the adequacy of the heart rate response to beta-blockers should be a critical guide to the dosing of the drug.

The hemodynamic effects of beta-blockers depend on the patient's cardiovascular status, underlying sympathetic tone, concurrent anesthesia, and vasoactive drug therapy. The decreased response to beta receptor stimulation with aging, together with interaction with anesthetic agents, may increase the risk for hypotension in the setting of prophylactic beta-blockade.[49] In a study of 63 elderly patients, Zaugg et al.[50] reported that perioperative beta-blockade actually resulted in better hemodynamic stability, decreased analgesic requirements, faster recovery from anesthesia, and decreased myocardial damage as diagnosed by increased levels of troponin I. This study is limited in size, but it is one of the first to suggest the relative safety and efficacy of beta-blockade in the elderly.

Current practice seems to suggest that beta-blockers are underutilized in all patients, especially the elderly. In a retrospective study, only 30% of patients who met

TABLE 13-4. Beta-blockers and suggested dosages used in the literature for perioperative myocardial protection.

Drug name	Dosage
Atenolol	50–100 mg PO daily
Metoprolol	25–50 mg PO twice daily
Bisoprolol	5–10 mg PO daily

criteria for perioperative beta-blockade after cholecystectomy received therapy.[51] This number is even lower for eligible elderly patients. Gottlieb et al.[52] performed a chart review of more than 200,000 cases after myocardial infarction. They determined that of the patients who should receive beta-blockade, only 27% of those 84 years old received beta-blockers versus 37% of those <75 years old. Some physicians are reluctant to prescribe beta-blockade to the elderly because of concerns of drug interactions, worsening of chronic obstructive pulmonary disease (COPD) symptoms, or exacerbation of hypotension, despite the fact that the underuse of beta-blockers in the elderly after myocardial infarction is associated with worse survival.[53]

It has been estimated that the implementation of a perioperative beta-blockade practice guideline would decrease mortality and hospital costs in all patients,[54] leading to the recommendation that beta-blockers be started in patients with known coronary artery disease or risk factors for coronary disease. Table 13-4 lists some beta-blockers and dosages that have been studied in the literature. Currently, there is no evidence to suggest the superiority of any one specific beta-blocker over another. Given the relative safety of perioperative beta-blockade, it seems that the benefits outweigh the risk of implementing perioperative beta-blockade in elderly surgical patients, although definitive randomized clinical trials in elderly patients are lacking.

Pulmonary Complications

Similar to the cardiac system, old age independently is not considered to be a risk factor for perioperative pulmonary dysfunction.[55] Intraoperative factors that have been shown to be associated with postoperative pulmonary complications include emergency surgery, the anatomic site of surgery (upper abdominal and thoracic procedures), duration of anesthesia, and general anesthesia.[56] A variety of preexisting factors prevalent in the elderly further predispose them to pulmonary complications. These factors include smoking, COPD, asthma, obesity, and preexisting pulmonary pathology.[57] Pulmonary complications have not been as well studied as cardiac complications, but recent evidence suggests that

postoperative pulmonary complications are more frequent and associated with longer hospital stays.[58]

Several previous investigators reported that postoperative pulmonary complications are prevalent in elderly patients. Pedersen et al.[30] reported a 10.2% rate of postoperative pulmonary complications, which were characterized as pulmonary aspiration, bronchospasm, hypoxemia, pneumothorax, respiratory failure requiring continuous positive airway pressure or reintubation, pneumonia, and atelectasis on chest radiograph. In our two cohort studies of consecutive elderly patients undergoing major noncardiac surgery, we found pulmonary complication rates of 5.5%–7%.[6,7] Postoperative signs of pneumonia requiring antibiotics were the most frequent adverse events followed by respiratory failure requiring reintubation, adult respiratory distress syndrome, and pulmonary embolus. In our study, patients with a history of congestive heart failure and a history of neurologic disorder were more likely to develop an adverse postoperative pulmonary event. Brooks-Brunn[59] similarly reported that age >60, impaired preoperative cognitive function, smoking history within the past 8 weeks, body mass index, history of cancer, and abdominal incision site were independent risk factors for postoperative pulmonary complications.

Of note, preoperative spirometry did not reliably predict the occurrence of postoperative complications in patients with obstructive lung disease.[60] In a study involving critically ill patients, the CO_2 levels on arterial blood gas and not spirometric testing predicted the need for postoperative intubation.[61] Taken together, the evidence to date suggests that pulmonary function tests should be selectively performed in patients undergoing nonthoracic surgery, because they can assess the presence and severity of the disease, but they do not have great predictive value for postoperative pulmonary complications.

Strategies to Reduce Pulmonary Risk

Preoperative optimization of respiratory function may improve patient outcomes. Several factors that deserve consideration include smoking cessation, optimization of asthma medications, and treatment of obstructive sleep apnea. Cigarette smoking is a known risk factor for COPD, coronary artery disease, and peripheral vascular disease. Current smokers are four times more likely to develop pulmonary complications than those who have never smoked.[62] Other trials have shown that smokers have a higher rate of wound infection than nonsmokers.[63] The institution of a smoking intervention program 6–8 weeks before joint replacement surgery reduced postoperative morbidity.[64] Warner et al.[65] showed that smoking cessation at least 2 months preoperatively maximized the reduction of postoperative respiratory complications.

From the above data, it seems that preoperative cessation of smoking will improve patient outcomes by decreasing adverse postoperative pulmonary outcomes and the incidence of wound infections. Smoking cessation should be encouraged even immediately before surgery, because smoking cessation has been associated with immediate decreases of carbon monoxide levels and reduced operative risk measured 6 weeks after surgery.[65]

Another condition common in geriatric patients is asthma. Asthma is often underdiagnosed in the elderly, and for those with the diagnosis, treatment may not be optimized. Asthma is often underdiagnosed in elderly for multiple reasons: (1) patient failure to report symptoms to the physician because of a lack of awareness of symptoms or misinterpreting the symptoms as deconditioning or normal process of aging; (2) presence of other conditions such as cardiac failure, ischemic cardiac failure, gastroesophageal reflux disease, respiratory tract tumors, laryngeal dysfunction, constrictive bronchiolitis, hypersensitive pneumonitis, or the use of medications (beta-blockers, angiotensin-converting enzyme inhibitors) that can mimic symptoms of asthma; (3) presence of other respiratory conditions such as COPD; or (4) general misperception that new-onset asthma is rare in the elderly.[66] With the appropriate diagnosis made, aggressive pulmonary rehabilitation, which includes exercise training, patient education, psychosocial, nutritional, and respiratory therapy counseling, smoking cessation, and optimization of medications, has been shown to be effective in the elderly population.[67] Unfortunately, some practitioners limit the use of beta agonists. They fear that systemic absorption of inhaled medications may result in tachycardia and hypertension, and precipitate cardiac ischemia in patients with coronary artery disease or result in drug interactions that may prolong the QT interval. The use of beta agonists is relatively safe in the elderly. Some earlier studies reported a decreased therapeutic response to inhaled beta receptor agonist with increasing age, but a recent study did not find any difference in the response to albuterol or ipratropium bromide with respect to age.[68]

Another comorbidity that is increasing in prevalence in the elderly is obesity and obstructive sleep apnea syndrome (OSAS). The prevalence of obesity is increasing at an alarming rate.[69] The number of obese adults aged 60 and older will increase from 32% in 2000 to 37.4% in 2010.[70] This increase has been attributed to a complex interaction between age-associated alterations in the metabolic rate, dietary changes, and sedentary lifestyles. Obesity causes diabetes, hypertension, hyperlipidemia, sleep apnea, and arthritis, resulting in reduced quality of life and life expectancy.[71] No specific studies addressed the impact of OSAS on postoperative complications in the elderly. However, in patients undergoing hip or knee replacement, procedures typically performed in older individuals, those with a preoperative diagnosis of OSAS were more than two times more likely to develop complications than those without OSAS. In fact, serious complications occurred in 24% of the OSAS group versus 9% in the control group, and hospital stay was significantly longer in the OSAS group.[72]

The data regarding the perioperative risk and best management techniques for patients with OSAS are scant and virtually nonexistent for elderly patients with OSAS. A Clinical Practice Review Committee of the American Academy of Sleep Medicine was unable to develop a standard of practice recommendation. They were only able to make a clinical practice statement based on a consensus of clinical experience and a few published peer-reviewed studies. They stated that important components of the perioperative management of OSAS patients include a high degree of clinical suspicion, control of the airway throughout the perioperative period, judicious use of medications, and appropriate monitoring.[73] At this point, this advice may be extrapolated to the elderly patient with OSAS. Other potentially prudent suggestions include having a lower threshold of admitting these patients to more intensive postoperative monitoring, use of supplemental oxygen, and use of nighttime continuous positive airway pressure.

Renal Dysfunction

The prevalence of renal insufficiency is quite common in the elderly because of a decrease in glomerular function with age. In populations ≥age 70, moderately or severely decreased glomerular filtration rate was observed in 75% of community-dwelling elderly, 78% of the patients from the geriatric ward, and 91% of nursing home patients. In populations ≥age 85, 99% had evidence of renal impairment necessitating dosing adjustments for drugs.[74] Kohli et al.[75] showed that surgery and nephrotoxic drugs are independent predictors of acute renal failure in elderly patients. They also found that mortality in patients with acute renal failure was significantly higher than similar patients without acute renal failure. In fact, it is estimated that acute renal failure contributes to at least one of every five perioperative deaths in elderly surgical patients.[76] A history of postoperative renal complications is a significant predictor of decreased long-term survival.[77] There are no clinical trials demonstrating that preoperative assessment for renal dysfunction will lead to better outcomes. However, recognizing that elderly patients are at risk of developing renal complications as a result of decreased renal function, effect of nephrotoxic drugs (aminoglycosides, nonsteroidal antiinflammatory drugs, angiotensin-converting enzyme inhibitors, and contrast dye), volume depletion, and hypotension seems prudent.

Diabetes Mellitus

Internationally, adults over age 60 will comprise two thirds of the diabetic population in developed countries by the year 2025.[78] In the United States, because of improvements in the identification of chronic diseases, declining death rates, and people living longer, diabetes is also increasing among persons aged 60 and older.[79] Currently, nearly one of every five adults in the United States over age 60 has diabetes, which puts them at increased risk for disability and morbidity.[80] Furthermore, the mortality risk is substantially higher in diabetics than nondiabetics. For example, McBean et al.[81] found that in individuals with diabetes, the overall risk of dying was 1.6 times greater than those without diabetes in a retrospective analysis of a 5% random sample of Medicare fee-for-service beneficiaries. The duration of diabetes also has a significant impact on the rate of developing complications as evidenced by a study demonstrating that patients with more than 10 years of diabetes have more significant compromise in one or more end-organ systems.[82] Diabetes is considered an intermediate clinical predictor for risk of perioperative myocardial ischemia[33] and is associated with increased risk of complications and death after myocardial infarction.

The recently published guidelines from the California Healthcare Foundation/American Geriatrics Society Panel on Improving Care for Elders with Diabetes provided recommendations on diabetes management for the elderly. These guidelines suggested that elderly persons in otherwise good health should have the same glycemic control goals as younger persons, which is a standard hemoglobin A1c target of <7%.[83] However, they acknowledged that there is not yet direct evidence that tight glycemic control is as beneficial in older populations as it has been shown to be in younger populations.[84]

There are no controlled trials demonstrating that preoperative assessment of glycemic control or duration of the disease will lead to better postoperative outcomes, but hyperglycemia has been shown to be associated with higher rates of postoperative complications. Hyperglycemia has been extensively associated with surgical-site infections. The National Veterans Administration Surgical Quality Improvement Program identified diabetes in a multiple logistic regression analysis as a significant preoperative risk factor for surgical-site infection.[85] Guvener et al.[86] demonstrated that high preoperative mean glucose levels were the main risk factor for development of postoperative deep sternal wound infection in diabetics undergoing coronary artery bypass grafting. Zerr et al.[87] demonstrated that implementation of a protocol to maintain postoperative blood glucose <200mg/dL decreased the incidence of deep sternal wound infection. Although not specifically studying elderly postoperative patients, Van den Berghe et al.[88] demonstrated that intensive

TABLE 13-5. Recommendations for insulin or oral hypoglycemic management for the day of surgery.

Type of insulin	Recommendations
Short-acting insulin	• Hold morning of surgery • Obtain a blood glucose and start an insulin infusion at 1–2U/h along with D5W at 75–100cc/h. • Check blood glucose every 1–2 hours and adjust infusion to keep glucose between 100–150mg/dL
Intermediate-acting insulin	• Give 1/2 to 2/3 of insulin morning of surgery • Check blood glucose every 1–2 hours and adjust infusion to keep glucose between 100–150mg/dL
Short-acting sulfonylureas	• Hold night before or morning of surgery
Long-acting sulfonylureas	• Hold 48–72 hours before surgery
Thiazolidinediones	• May be given morning of surgery or 1 dose may hold because of long half-life
Biguanides	• Hold 24 hours before surgery • Do not start until 48 hours after major surgery to ensure adequate renal function postoperatively

Source: Data adapted from Connery and Coursin.[89]

insulin therapy (blood glucose 80–110mg/dL) reduced morbidity and mortality in critically ill patients in the surgical intensive care unit when compared with regular insulin therapy (blood glucose 180–200mg/dL). The evidence to date would strongly argue for controlling blood glucose between 180–200mg/dL, but the evidence is weaker supporting the benefits of tighter control of blood glucose (80–100mg/dL) in the elderly surgical patient.

Below are some suggestions for management of diabetics in the perioperative period. These are mostly based on consensus opinion as opposed to randomized trials. Ideally, diabetic patients should have their operations scheduled early in the morning to reduce the time period of fasting and to minimize the disturbances in glycemic control.[89] Table 13-5 gives some examples of insulin and oral hypoglycemic management on the day of surgery. In the immediate postoperative period, blood glucose should be checked every 1–2 hours for several hours in Type 1 diabetics and every 4 hours in Type 2 diabetics.[89,90]

Nutritional Assessment

The prevalence of malnutrition in the elderly population varies from 2% to 10% in the community to 30% to 60% in the hospital or nursing home.[91] As early as the 1930s, it was noted that postoperative complications and deaths were more likely if patients had disease-related malnutrition.[92,93] A recent study from the Veterans Administration identified preoperative albumin level as a good predictor of postoperative mortality in the geriatric population.[94] The National Veterans Administration Surgical Risk Study examined 43 preoperative risk factors, 14 preoperative laboratory values, and 12 operative variables for predicting postoperative complications. The mean age in this study was 61 ± 13 years, and 97% of the subjects were men, but the results should apply to the general elderly surgical patient. The most important variable in predicting postoperative mortality was preoperative albumin level with ASA PS classification as the second best predictor. Albumin levels <2.1 g/dL was associated with 29% mortality and 65% morbidity.

Serum albumin is useful in gauging global nutritional status, but it is limited in its ability to assess acute changes because of its long half-life of 18–21 days.[95] It is also affected by changes in intravascular and extravascular fluid compartments and it is a negative acute-phase reactant, meaning there is a decline in levels during acute illness. Nevertheless, albumin has been extensively studied and testing is relatively inexpensive. Prealbumin and transferrin have increased sensitivity to changes in nutritional status because of much shorter half-lives.[96] However, their erratic responses to stress and illness[97,98] and the high cost of testing make them less useful as universal markers for nutritional status.

Despite the evidence linking albumin and possibly nutritional status to postoperative outcome, the use of preoperative total parenteral nutrition in surgical patients is somewhat controversial and has been studied only in selective populations with severe malnutrition.[99] An easier way to increase caloric intake is by providing a nutritional supplement.[100] Several trials have demonstrated that the use of a daily oral supplementation can maintain body weight and prevent malnutrition,[101] but trials specific to reducing perioperative risk are lacking. Although artificial enteral or parenteral nutrition is generally not indicated, the use of a multimodal intervention focused on aggressive postoperative pain control, and early return of gut function and mobility has been shown to be able to allow patients to commence oral intake quicker and be discharged from the hospital sooner.[102]

Exercise Capacity and Functional Status Assessment

Good exercise capacity may also affect perioperative outcome. Gerson et al.[103] used a supine bicycle exercise test before abdominal and noncardiac thoracic surgery in patients older than 65 years of age. In this study, perioperative cardiovascular complication rates were higher in patients who were unable to raise their heart rate more than 99 beats/minute or perform 2 minutes of supine bicycle exercise. For those unable to exercise, postoperative cardiopulmonary complication rate was 42% and mortality rate was 7.2% versus 9.3% and 0.9% respectively, for those who could exercise. In a study following patients referred for formal exercise treadmill testing, a 1 MET increase in treadmill performance was associated with a reduction in mortality in women and men, 17% and 12%, respectively. Exercise tolerance of less than 5 METs was associated with a twofold increase risk of death in men and a threefold increase risk of death in women.[104,105] A comparison between patients with good and poor exercise tolerance undergoing major noncardiac surgery demonstrated statistically significant increases in overall cardiovascular complications, myocardial ischemia, neurologic complications, unexpected transfer to intensive care unit or telemetry, and total serious complications in patients with poor exercise tolerance.[106] There are a number of possible explanations for these findings. Patients with poor exercise tolerance may be more likely to have significant medical problems such as diabetes, COPD, CHF, hypertension, and higher ASA scores, whereas patients with good exercise tolerance may better tolerate the physical rigors of surgery and mobilize more rapidly postoperatively.[106]

There are no studies to show that preoperative assessment and improvement of functional status in the elderly will result in improved postoperative outcomes. However, the preoperative assessment will allow for a baseline measurement, and physicians often fail to recognize mild-to-moderate impairments in functional status.[107] The activities of daily living (ADL), listed in Table 13-6, measures performance in bathing, dressing, toileting, transferring, continence, and feeding.[108] Lawton and Brody[109] then developed the instrumental activities of daily living scale (IADL) to describe a more complex set of behaviors reflecting the capacity of elders to adapt to their environment. The IADL (Table 13-7) includes use of the telephone, shopping, food preparation, doing housework and laundry, use of transportation, responsibility for own

TABLE 13-6. Activities of daily living.

Activity	Definition of independence
Bathing	Performs sponge bath, tub bath, or shower without assistance or with assistance in bathing only 1 body part
Dressing	Gets clothes from closet and gets dressed without assistance (except for tying shoes)
Toileting	Uses bathroom for bowel movements and urination; cleans self and redresses after using the bathroom
Transfers	Moves in and out of bed or chair without assistance or with use of mechanical device
Continence	Controls urination and bowel movement; may have an occasional accident
Feeding	Feeds self without assistance except for cutting meat or buttering bread

TABLE 13-7. Instrumental activities of daily living.

Instrumental activity	Definition of independence
Telephone	Able to use telephone; able to dial a few well-known numbers; able to answer the telephone
Shopping	Takes care of all shopping needs
Food preparation	Plans, prepares, serves adequate meals
Housekeeping	Performs light daily tasks, washes dishes, makes bed
Laundry	Does laundry
Mode of transportation	Travels by driving, or using public transportation alone or accompanied by another
Responsible for medications	Takes correct dosages at correct time
Handles finances	Manages day-to-day finances, can require assistance with banking or major purchases

medications, and ability to handle finances. Functional status before hospitalization has been found to be predictive of functional outcome, length of stay, mortality, and need for nursing home placement. Davis et al.[110] showed that ADL impairment was a powerful predictor of in-hospital mortality for the elderly and it was the single most important predictor of functional outcomes at 2 and 12 months after hospitalization.

A preoperative home-based physical therapy program, prehabilitation, has been described as a method of enhancing the functional capacity of a patient. It has been evaluated in frail, community-dwelling elders[111] and in preparation for the stress of an orthopedic surgical procedure[112] or an intensive care unit admission.[113] The goals of prehabilitation are to prevent deconditioning and improve the ability of the patient to withstand musculoskeletal and cardiovascular stressors of surgery. The efficacy of this type of approach remains to be validated by randomized controlled trials before prehabilitation can be recommended as a routine preoperative strategy in elderly patients.

Laboratory Values

Routine preoperative medical testing before elective surgery is estimated to cost $30 billion annually, but data show that laboratory abnormalities on routine screen often do not lead to changes in management. Schein et al.[114] studied nearly 20,000 patients undergoing cataract surgery who were randomized to either routine laboratory testing or no routine testing. They reported no difference in perioperative morbidity and mortality between those who did versus those who did not receive routine testing. In patients with few comorbidities, there is a low prevalence of abnormal laboratory tests. For example, in a population study of 7196 ambulatory patients, the pre-

valence of hemoglobin, glucose, and creatinine abnormalities was small (5.5%, 8.3%, and 2.7%, respectively).[115] In contrast, a substantially higher prevalence of abnormal results was demonstrated in a group of institutionalized elderly patients (11%–33% for hemoglobin, 25%–29% for glucose, and 11%–15% for creatinine).[116–118] Dzankic et al.[119] used a prospective cohort of patients ≥70 years of age undergoing elective noncardiac surgery to evaluate the prevalence and predictive value of abnormal preoperative laboratory tests. The prevalence of abnormal laboratory tests was quite high—electrolyte abnormalities (0.7%–5%), abnormal platelet counts (1.9%), glucose (7%), hemoglobin (10%), and abnormal creatinine (12%)—but in a separate analysis for patients classified as ASA 1–2, the incidence of laboratory abnormalities was as low as those in the general population (3.6%). In fact, in the entire elderly cohort, none of the abnormal laboratory values were significant independent predictors of adverse outcomes with multivariate regression. These results suggest that routine preoperative testing in geriatric surgical patients, particularly in those patients classified as ASA 1–2, generally produces few abnormal results.

Electrocardiogram (ECG) abnormalities also increase with age.[120] The most common abnormalities in a cohort of octogenarians[121] included arrhythmias, Q waves diagnosing previous myocardial infarction, left ventricular hypertrophy, bundle-branch block, and nonspecific segment changes. Although these abnormalities are common, they had limited value in predicting postoperative cardiac complications. There is no demonstrable evidence that measurement and investigation of preoperative ECGs reduce adverse outcomes, but current recommendations to obtain preoperative ECGs for men over age 40, women over age 50, and other patients with known coronary artery disease or cardiovascular risk factors such as diabetes or hypertension, are probably reasonable so that a baseline ECG is available before major surgery to determine whether subsequent abnormalities are new or preexistent.[122]

Preoperative chest X-rays (CXRs) have increased clinical relevance with increasing age and presence of cardiopulmonary disease.[123,124] In patients younger than age 50, the likelihood of an abnormal chest film ranges from 0% to 20%, whereas the likelihood increases to 20% to 60% in patients older than 50.[125] An evaluation of routine preoperative CXRs in vascular surgery patients demonstrated that no surgery cancellations occurred because of an abnormal X-ray, but the beneficial effects of a CXR increased in patients with known pulmonary disease. The study recommended that CXRs be ordered preoperatively only if there is clinical indication in the history and physical examination.[126]

There are no controlled clinical trials to show that routine laboratory tests, ECG or CXR, are associated with a decreased adverse event rate. However, information from preoperative ECG and/or CXR may be of value in the postoperative management because new abnormalities may be identified if preoperative baseline measurements are available. Although the actual rate of laboratory abnormalities is small in the elderly, it is still higher compared with the younger population.[127] Therefore, total abandonment of routine testing based on age must be weighed against the probability that unexpected disease may be detected by the testing and that the extent of surgery may be modified.[128]

Medications

Elderly patients frequently take multiple medications, both prescription and over-the-counter medications. The elderly constitute approximately 13% of the population but consume 32% of all prescription drugs in the United States.[129] Studies show that greater consumption of medications contributes to decreased medication adherence[130] and to greater risk of adverse drug events.[131] The impact of common herbal and alternative medicines is unclear, but is already becoming an important focus. In a survey of more than 2500 preoperative patients ≥age 18, almost 40% of the patients admitted to using some form of alternative medicine supplements.[132] Women ≥age 65 reported using an average of 2.6 herbal products.[133] Most important was the fact that more than 50% of the patients in the study indicated that they did not inform the anesthesiologists before surgery regarding their use of these products.[132] The Food and Drug Administration does not control these supplements and, therefore, quality is not rigorously regulated. Some reported side effects from herbal remedies include bleeding when warfarin is combined with ginkgo, garlic, or ginseng[134]; possible monoamine oxidase inhibition by St. John's wort[135]; coma when benzodiazepines are combined with kava[136]; and mania when antidepressants are combined with ginseng.[134] Other reported risks include contamination, inconsistencies and adulteration, and lead poisoning.[137] There are no randomized controlled trials to examine the effects of herbal medications in the perioperative period and to determine when the supplements should be stopped preoperatively. A few review articles made several suggestions (stopping ephedra, ginkgo, and kava 24–36 hours before surgery, and stopping garlic, ginseng, and St. John's wort 5–7 days before surgery) based on limited information on the pharmacokinetics of these agents[138,139] (Table 13-8).

In terms of prescription medications, the older patient is at risk for inappropriate drug use. Inappropriate medications may be defined as drugs that pose more risk than benefit.[140] In 1996, more than 20% of community-dwelling elderly received some inappropriate medication.[141]

TABLE 13-8. Recommendations for preoperative discontinuation of herbal medications.

Herbal medicine	Perioperative interactions	Discontinue before surgery
Echinacea	• Allergic reactions • Immunosuppression	No data
Ephedra	• Hypertension • Arrhythmias	24 hours
Garlic	• Inhibits platelet aggregation • Increases risk of bleeding	7 days
Ginkgo	• Inhibits platelet aggregation • Increases risk of bleeding	36 hours
Ginseng	• Hypoglycemia • Increases risk of bleeding	7 days
Kava	• Interactions with sedatives	24 hours
St. John's wort	• Induces cytochrome P-450 • Affects multiple drug levels	5 days

Source: Data adapted from Ang-Lee et al.[138] and Adusumilli et al.[139]

For example, specific medications such as antihistamines or benzodiazepines contribute to the risk of falls or confusion. Agostini et al.[142] showed that there is a linear relationship between the number of medications used and the risk of two frequently reported adverse drug effects—weight loss and impaired balance. This effect was apparent even when comorbidities and indications for many of the medications were adjusted for. In terms of risk reduction, a study showed that time taken to educate the patient on dosages and frequency of medicines, reasons for taking medicines, and information about adverse side effects improved patient compliance and outcomes.[143] The perioperative period has been proposed as an ideal time to critically review the medication list for polypharmacy, drug interactions, and adverse drug events.[144] Although these proposals make intuitive sense, no randomized trials have specifically addressed this issue.

Comprehensive Geriatric Assessment

The team approach to the elderly patient involves the geriatrician, nurse coordinator, physical therapist, and social worker. Randomized controlled trials have been variable in the benefits of a comprehensive geriatric assessment (CGA). The selective use of the CGA has been proven to be beneficial in the perioperative period. For instance, in community-dwelling elders who failed a screen for falls, urinary incontinence, depression, or functional impairment, CGA was found to be efficacious and cost-effective. Although not studied in the surgical population, a meta-analysis showed that CGA, along with long-term management, is effective for improving survival and function.[145] One recent randomized clinical trial that targeted patients aged ≥65 years after hip fracture surgery demonstrated that "proactive geriatric consultation" reduced delirium by more than one third and reduced severe delirium by more than half.[146] This important study demonstrates that certain adverse outcomes after surgery such as delirium may be modifiable, and suggests that similar strategies, which are multifactorial and targeted, may be possible to reduce the trajectory of decline after major surgery in the older population.

Conclusion

Although surgery in the geriatric population is not without risk, the mortality rate has decreased markedly. With more emphasis on preoperative medical optimization, along with early identification of surgical issues, most patients can expect to do well. Patients ≥80 years of age undergoing noncardiac surgery who did not have postoperative complications were found to survive just as well as the age- and gender-matched general population.[77] Chronologic age is less important as an independent risk predictor. A more important predictor is the presence of coexisting diseases. With the identification of the major risk factors associated with postoperative morbidity, opportunity to improve perioperative outcomes in elderly patients will be possible when risk factors for these adverse events can be modified through randomized prospective clinical trials. As more information becomes available on risk modification through future research, practitioners can then develop a comprehensive set of quality indicators for elderly surgical care and thereby improve the quality and safety of perioperative surgical care of geriatric patients.

References

1. Projections of the total resident population by 5-year age groups, and sex with special age categories: middle series, 2025–2045. Vol 2004. US Census Bureau; 2000.
2. Herron PW, Jesseph JE, Harkins HN. Analysis of 600 major operations in patients over 70 years of age. Ann Surg 1960;152:686–698.
3. Burnett W, McCaffrey J. Surgical procedures in the elderly. Surg Gynecol Obstet 1972;134:221–226.
4. Seymour DG, Vaz FG. A prospective study of elderly general surgical patients: II. Post-operative complications. Age Ageing 1989;18:316–326.
5. Milamed DR, Hedley-Whyte J. Contributions of the surgical sciences to a reduction of the mortality rate in the United States for the period 1968 to 1988. Ann Surg 1994;219:94–102.
6. Liu LL, Leung JM. Predicting adverse postoperative outcomes in patients aged 80 years or older. J Am Geriatr Soc 2000;48:405–412.
7. Leung JM, Dzankic S. Relative importance of preoperative health status versus intraoperative factors in predicting postoperative adverse outcomes in geriatric surgical patients. J Am Geriatr Soc 2001;49:1080–1085.
8. Mangano DT. Perioperative cardiac morbidity. Anesthesiology 1990;72:153–184.
9. Tiret L, Hatton F, Desmonts JM, et al. Prediction of outcome of anaesthesia in patients over 40 years: a multifactorial risk index. Stat Med 1988;7:947–954.
10. Pedersen T, Eliasen K, Henriksen E. A prospective study of mortality associated with anaesthesia and surgery: risk indicators of mortality in hospital. Acta Anaesthesiol Scand 1990;34:176–182.
11. Rorbaek-Madsen M, Dupont G, Kristensen K, et al. General surgery in patients aged 80 years and older. Br J Surg 1992;79:1216–1218.
12. Bufalari A, Ferri M, Cao P, et al. Surgical care in octogenarians. Br J Surg 1996;83:1783–1787.
13. Vaz FG, Seymour DG. A prospective study of elderly general surgical patients: I. Pre-operative medical problems. Age Ageing 1989;18:309–315.
14. Warner MA, Saletel RA, Schroeder DR, et al. Outcomes of anesthesia and surgery in people 100 years of age and older. J Am Geriatr Soc 1998;46:988–993.
15. Moller JT, Cluitmans P, Rasmussen LS, et al. Long-term postoperative cognitive dysfunction in the elderly ISPOCD1 study. ISPOCD investigators. International Study of Post-Operative Cognitive Dysfunction. Lancet 1998;351:857–861.
16. Marcantonio ER, Goldman L, Mangione CM, et al. A clinical prediction rule for delirium after elective noncardiac surgery. JAMA 1994;271:134–139.
17. Williams M, Holloway J, Winn M, et al. Nursing activities and acute confusional states in elderly hip-fractured patients. Nurs Res 1979;26:25–35.
18. Berggren D, Gustafson Y, Eriksson B, et al. Postoperative confusion after anesthesia in elderly patients with femoral neck fractures. Anesth Analg 1987;66:497–504.
19. Inouye S. The dilemma of delirium: clinical and research controversies regarding diagnosis and evaluation of delirium in hospitalized elderly medical patients. Am J Med 1994;97:278–288.
20. Gustafson Y, Berggren D, Brannstrom B, et al. Acute confusional states in elderly patients treated for femoral neck fracture. J Am Geriatr Soc 1988;36:525–530.
21. Francis J, Kapoor WN. Delirium in hospitalized elderly. J Gen Intern Med 1990;5:65–79.
22. Inouye SK, Charpentier PA. Precipitating factors for delirium in hospitalized elderly persons. Predictive model and interrelationship with baseline vulnerability. JAMA 1996;275:852–857.
23. Larson EB, Kukull WA, Buchner D, et al. Adverse drug reactions associated with global cognitive impairment in elderly persons. Ann Intern Med 1987;107:169–173.
24. Hole A, Terjesen T, Breivik H. Epidural versus general anaesthesia for total hip arthroplasty in elderly patients. Acta Anaesthesiol Scand 1980;24:279–287.
25. Williams-Russo P, Sharrock NE, Mattis S, et al. Cognitive effects after epidural vs general anesthesia in older adults. A randomized trial. JAMA 1995;274:44–50.

26. O'Hara DA, Duff A, Berlin JA, et al. The effect of anesthetic technique on postoperative outcomes in hip fracture repair. Anesthesiology 2000;92:947–957.

27. Rasmussen LS, Johnson T, Kuipers HM, et al. Does anaesthesia cause postoperative cognitive dysfunction? A randomised study of regional versus general anaesthesia in 438 elderly patients. Acta Anaesthesiol Scand 2003;47: 260–266.

28. Williams-Russo P, Sharrock NE, Mattis S, et al. Randomized trial of hypotensive epidural anesthesia in older adults. Anesthesiology 1999;91:926–935.

29. Lynch EP, Lazor MA, Gellis JE, et al. The impact of postoperative pain on the development of postoperative delirium. Anesth Analg 1998;86:781–785.

30. Pedersen T, Eliasen K, Henriksen E. A prospective study of risk factors and cardiopulmonary complications associated with anaesthesia and surgery: risk indicators of cardiopulmonary morbidity. Acta Anaesthesiol Scand 1990; 34:144–155.

31. Goldman L, Caldera DL, Nussbaum SR, et al. Multifactorial index of cardiac risk in noncardiac surgical procedures. N Engl J Med 1977;297:845–850.

32. Lee TH, Marcantonio ER, Mangione CM, et al. Derivation and prospective validation of a simple index for prediction of cardiac risk of major noncardiac surgery. Circulation 1999;100:1043–1049.

33. Eagle KA, Berger PB, Calkins H, et al. ACC/AHA guideline update for perioperative cardiovascular evaluation for noncardiac surgery—executive summary. A report of the American College of Cardiology/American Heart Association Task Force on Practice Guidelines (Committee to Update the 1996 Guidelines on Perioperative Cardiovascular Evaluation for Noncardiac Surgery). Circulation 2002;105:1257–1267.

34. Eagle KA, Rihal CS, Mickel MC, et al. Cardiac risk of noncardiac surgery: influence of coronary disease and type of surgery in 3368 operations. CASS Investigators and University of Michigan Heart Care Program. Coronary Artery Surgery Study. Circulation 1997;96:1882–1887.

35. McFalls EO, Ward HB, Moritz TE, et al. Coronary-artery revascularization before elective major vascular surgery. N Engl J Med 2004;351:2795–2804.

36. Aronow WS, Ahn C, Kronzon I. Normal left ventricular ejection fraction in older persons with congestive heart failure. Chest 1998;113:867–869.

37. Vasan RS, Benjamin EJ, Levy D. Prevalence, clinical features and prognosis of diastolic heart failure: an epidemiologic perspective. J Am Coll Cardiol 1995;26:1565–1574.

38. Tresch DD, McGough MF. Heart failure with normal systolic function: a common disorder in older people. J Am Geriatr Soc 1995;43:1035–1042.

39. Hamlin SK, Villars PS, Kanusky JT, et al. Role of diastole in left ventricular function. II: diagnosis and treatment. Am J Crit Care 2004;13:453–466; quiz 467–468.

40. Stamler J, Stamler R, Neaton JD. Blood pressure, systolic and diastolic, and cardiovascular risks. US population data. Arch Intern Med 1993;153:598–615.

41. Howell SJ, Sear JW, Foex P. Hypertension, hypertensive heart disease and perioperative cardiac risk. Br J Anaesth 2004;92:570–583.

42. Prys-Roberts C, Meloche R, Foex P. Studies of anaesthesia in relation to hypertension. I. Cardiovascular responses of treated and untreated patients. Br J Anaesth 1971;43: 122–137.

43. Prys-Roberts C, Greene LT, Meloche R, et al. Studies of anaesthesia in relation to hypertension. II. Haemodynamic consequences of induction and endotracheal intubation. Br J Anaesth 1971;43:531–547.

44. Reich DL, Bennett-Guerrero E, Bodian CA, et al. Intraoperative tachycardia and hypertension are independently associated with adverse outcome in noncardiac surgery of long duration. Anesth Analg 2002;95:273–277.

45. Stevens A, Abrams K. Consensus, reviews and metaanalysis. In: Stevens A, Abrams K, Brazier J, et al., eds. Methods in Evidence Based Healthcare. London: Sage; 2001:367–369.

46. Wallace A, Layug B, Tateo I, et al. Prophylactic atenolol reduces postoperative myocardial ischemia. McSPI Research Group. Anesthesiology 1998;88:7–17.

47. Poldermans D, Boersma E, Bax JJ, et al. The effect of bisoprolol on perioperative mortality and myocardial infarction in high-risk patients undergoing vascular surgery. Dutch Echocardiographic Cardiac Risk Evaluation Applying Stress Echocardiography Study Group. N Engl J Med 1999;341:1789–1794.

48. Mangano DT, Hollenberg M, Fegert G, et al. Perioperative myocardial ischemia in patients undergoing noncardiac surgery. I: incidence and severity during the 4 day perioperative period. The Study of Perioperative Ischemia (SPI) Research Group. J Am Coll Cardiol 1991;17:843–850.

49. Tuman KJ, McCarthy RJ. Individualizing beta adrenergic blocker therapy: patient-specific target-based heart rate control. Anesth Analg 1999;88:475–476.

50. Zaugg M, Tagliente T, Lucchinetti E, et al. Beneficial effects from beta-adrenergic blockade in elderly patients undergoing noncardiac surgery. Anesthesiology 1999;91: 1674–1686.

51. Lindenauer PK, Fitzgerald J, Hoople N, et al. The potential preventability of postoperative myocardial infarction: underuse of perioperative beta-adrenergic blockade. Arch Intern Med 2004;164:762–766.

52. Gottlieb SS, McCarter RJ, Vogel RA. Effect of betablockade on mortality among high-risk and low-risk patients after myocardial infarction. N Engl J Med 1998; 339:489–497.

53. Soumerai SB, McLaughlin TJ, Spiegelman D, et al. Adverse outcomes of underuse of beta-blockers in elderly survivors of acute myocardial infarction. JAMA 1997; 277:115–121.

54. Schmidt M, Lindenauer PK, Fitzgerald JL, et al. Forecasting the impact of a clinical practice guideline for perioperative beta-blockers to reduce cardiovascular morbidity and mortality. Arch Intern Med 2002;162:63–69.

55. Mohr DN. Estimation of surgical risk in the elderly: a correlative review. J Am Geriatr Soc 1983;31:99–102.

56. Dzankic S, Leung J. Anesthesia and aging. In: Lake C, Johnson J, McLoughlin T, eds. Advances in Anesthesia. Vol 21. Philadelphia: Mosby; 2003:1–42.

57. Zaugg M, Lucchinetti E. Respiratory function in the elderly. Anesthesiol Clin North Am 2000;18:47–58.

58. Lawrence VA, Hilsenbeck SG, Mulrow CD, et al. Incidence and hospital stay for cardiac and pulmonary complications after abdominal surgery. J Gen Intern Med 1995; 10:671–678.

59. Brooks-Brunn JA. Predictors of postoperative pulmonary complications following abdominal surgery. Chest 1997; 111:564–571.

60. Lawrence VA, Dhanda R, Hilsenbeck SG, et al. Risk of pulmonary complications after elective abdominal surgery. Chest 1996;110:744–750.

61. Jayr C, Matthay MA, Goldstone J, et al. Preoperative and intraoperative factors associated with prolonged mechanical ventilation. A study in patients following major abdominal vascular surgery. Chest 1993;103:1231–1236.

62. Bluman LG, Mosca L, Newman N, et al. Preoperative smoking habits and postoperative pulmonary complications. Chest 1998;113:883–889.

63. Sorensen LT, Karlsmark T, Gottrup F. Abstinence from smoking reduces incisional wound infection: a randomized controlled trial. Ann Surg 2003;238:1–5.

64. Moller AM, Villebro N, Pedersen T, et al. Effect of preoperative smoking intervention on postoperative complications: a randomised clinical trial. Lancet 2002;359: 114–117.

65. Warner MA, Offord KP, Warner ME, et al. Role of preoperative cessation of smoking and other factors in postoperative pulmonary complications: a blinded prospective study of coronary artery bypass patients. Mayo Clin Proc 1989;64:609–616.

66. Banerjee DK, Lee GS, Malik SK, et al. Underdiagnosis of asthma in the elderly. Br J Dis Chest 1987;81:23–29.

67. Couser JI Jr, Guthmann R, Hamadeh MA, et al. Pulmonary rehabilitation improves exercise capacity in older elderly patients with COPD. Chest 1995;107:730–734.

68. Kradjan WA, Driesner NK, Abuan TH, et al. Effect of age on bronchodilator response. Chest 1992;101:1545–1551.

69. Mokdad AH, Bowman BA, Ford ES, et al. The continuing epidemics of obesity and diabetes in the United States. JAMA 2001;286:1195–1200.

70. Arterburn DE, Crane PK, Sullivan SD. The coming epidemic of obesity in elderly Americans. J Am Geriatr Soc 2004;52:1907–1912.

71. Must A, Spadano J, Coakley EH, et al. The disease burden associated with overweight and obesity. JAMA 1999;282: 1523–1529.

72. Gupta RM, Parvizi J, Hanssen AD, et al. Postoperative complications in patients with obstructive sleep apnea syndrome undergoing hip or knee replacement: a case-control study. Mayo Clin Proc 2001;76:897–905.

73. Meoli AL, Rosen CL, Kristo D, et al. Upper airway management of the adult patient with obstructive sleep apnea in the perioperative period—avoiding complications. Sleep 2003;26:1060–1065.

74. Nygaard HA, Naik M, Ruths S, et al. Clinically important renal impairment in various groups of old persons. Scand J Prim Health Care 2004;22:152–156.

75. Kohli HS, Bhaskaran MC, Muthukumar T, et al. Treatment-related acute renal failure in the elderly: a hospital-based prospective study. Nephrol Dial Transplant 2000;15: 212–217.

76. John AD, Sieber FE. Age associated issues: geriatrics. Anesthesiol Clin North Am 2004;22:45–58.

77. Manku K, Bacchetti P, Leung JM. Prognostic significance of postoperative in-hospital complications in elderly patients. I. Long-term survival. Anesth Analg 2003;96: 583–589.

78. King H, Aubert RE, Herman WH. Global burden of diabetes, 1995–2025: prevalence, numerical estimates, and projections. Diabetes Care 1998;21:1414–1431.

79. Mokdad AH, Ford ES, Bowman BA, et al. Diabetes trends in the U.S.: 1990–1998. Diabetes Care 2000;23:1278–1283.

80. Jack L Jr, Boseman L, Vinicor F. Aging Americans and diabetes. A public health and clinical response. Geriatrics 2004;59:14–17.

81. McBean AM, Li S, Gilbertson DT, et al. Differences in diabetes prevalence, incidence, and mortality among the elderly of four racial/ethnic groups: whites, blacks, Hispanics, and Asians. Diabetes Care 2004;27:2317–2324.

82. Schiff RL, Welsh GA. Perioperative evaluation and management of the patient with endocrine dysfunction. Med Clin North Am 2003;87:175–192.

83. Brown AF, Mangione CM, Saliba D, et al. Guidelines for improving the care of the older person with diabetes mellitus. J Am Geriatr Soc 2003;51:S265–280.

84. American Diabetes Association. Implications of the diabetes control and complications trial. Diabetes Care 2003; 26(Suppl 1):S25–27.

85. Malone DL, Genuit T, Tracy JK, et al. Surgical site infections: reanalysis of risk factors. J Surg Res 2002;103:89–95.

86. Guvener M, Pasaoglu I, Demircin M, et al. Perioperative hyperglycemia is a strong correlate of postoperative infection in type II diabetic patients after coronary artery bypass grafting. Endocr J 2002;49:531–537.

87. Zerr KJ, Furnary AP, Grunkemeier GL, et al. Glucose control lowers the risk of wound infection in diabetics after open heart operations. Ann Thorac Surg 1997;63:356–361.

88. Van den Berghe G, Wouters P, Weekers F, et al. Intensive insulin therapy in the critically ill patients. N Engl J Med 2001;345:1359–1367.

89. Connery LE, Coursin DB. Assessment and therapy of selected endocrine disorders. Anesthesiol Clin North Am 2004;22:93–123.

90. Marks JB. Perioperative management of diabetes. Am Fam Physician 2003;67:93–100.

91. Guigoz Y, Lauque S, Vellas BJ. Identifying the elderly at risk for malnutrition. The Mini Nutritional Assessment. Clin Geriatr Med 2002;18:737–757.

92. Shils ME. Recalling a 63-year nutrition odyssey. Nutrition 2000;16:582–585.

93. Studley HO. Percentage of weight loss: a basic indicator of surgical risk in patients with chronic peptic ulcer. 1936. Nutr Hosp 2001;16:141–143.

94. Gibbs J, Cull W, Henderson W, et al. Preoperative serum albumin level as a predictor of operative mortality and morbidity: results from the National VA Surgical Risk Study. Arch Surg 1999;134:36–42.

95. Carney DE, Meguid MM. Current concepts in nutritional assessment. Arch Surg 2002;137:42–45.

96. Prealbumin in Nutritional Care Consensus Group. Measurement of visceral protein status in assessing protein and

energy malnutrition: standard of care. Nutrition 1995;11: 169–171.

97. Winkler MF, Gerrior SA, Pomp A, et al. Use of retinol-binding protein and prealbumin as indicators of the response to nutrition therapy. J Am Diet Assoc 1989; 89:684–687.

98. Hedlund JU, Hansson LO, Ortqvist AB. Hypoalbuminemia in hospitalized patients with community-acquired pneumonia. Arch Intern Med 1995;155:1438–1442.

99. Souba WW. Nutritional support. N Engl J Med 1997;336: 41–48.

100. Vellas B, Guigoz Y, Garry PJ, et al. The Mini Nutritional Assessment (MNA) and its use in grading the nutritional state of elderly patients. Nutrition 1999;15:116–122.

101. Gazzotti C, Arnaud-Battandier F, Parello M, et al. Prevention of malnutrition in older people during and after hospitalisation: results from a randomised controlled clinical trial. Age Ageing 2003;32:321–325.

102. Holte K, Kehlet H. Epidural anaesthesia and analgesia—effects on surgical stress responses and implications for postoperative nutrition. Clin Nutr 2002;21:199–206.

103. Gerson MC, Hurst JM, Hertzberg VS, et al. Prediction of cardiac and pulmonary complications related to elective abdominal and noncardiac thoracic surgery in geriatric patients. Am J Med 1990;88:101–107.

104. Gulati M, Pandey DK, Arnsdorf MF, et al. Exercise capacity and the risk of death in women: the St James Women Take Heart Project. Circulation 2003;108:1554–1559.

105. Myers J, Prakash M, Froelicher V, et al. Exercise capacity and mortality among men referred for exercise testing. N Engl J Med 2002;346:793–801.

106. Reilly DF, McNeely MJ, Doerner D, et al. Self-reported exercise tolerance and the risk of serious perioperative complications. Arch Intern Med 1999;159:2185–2192.

107. Pinholt EM, Kroenke K, Hanley JF, et al. Functional assessment of the elderly. A comparison of standard instruments with clinical judgment. Arch Intern Med 1987;147: 484–488.

108. Katz S, Ford AB, Moskowitz RW, et al. Studies of illness in the aged. The index of ADL: a standardized measure of biological and psychosocial function. JAMA 1963;185: 914–919.

109. Lawton MP, Brody EM. Assessment of older people: self-maintaining and instrumental activities of daily living. Gerontologist 1969;9:179–186.

110. Davis RB, Iezzoni LI, Phillips RS, et al. Predicting in-hospital mortality. The importance of functional status information. Med Care 1995;33:906–921.

111. Gill TM, Baker DI, Gottschalk M, et al. A prehabilitation program for the prevention of functional decline: effect on higher-level physical function. Arch Phys Med Rehabil 2004;85:1043–1049.

112. Ditmyer MM, Topp R, Pifer M. Prehabilitation in preparation for orthopaedic surgery. Orthop Nurs 2002;21:43–51; quiz 52–54.

113. Topp R, Ditmyer M, King K, et al. The effect of bed rest and potential of prehabilitation on patients in the intensive care unit. AACN Clin Issues 2002;13:263–276.

114. Schein OD, Katz J, Bass EB, et al. The value of routine preoperative medical testing before cataract surgery. Study

115. Collen MF, Feldman R, Siegelaub AB, et al. Dollar cost per positive test for automated multiphasic screening. N Engl J Med 1970;283:459–463.

116. Domoto K, Ben R, Wei JY, et al. Yield of routine annual laboratory screening in the institutionalized elderly. Am J Public Health 1985;75:243–245.

117. Levinstein MR, Ouslander JG, Rubenstein LZ, et al. Yield of routine annual laboratory tests in a skilled nursing home population. JAMA 1987;258:1909–1915.

118. Wolf-Klein GP, Holt T, Silverstone FA, et al. Efficacy of routine annual studies in the care of elderly patients. J Am Geriatr Soc 1985;33:325–329.

119. Dzankic S, Pastor D, Gonzalez C, et al. The prevalence and predictive value of abnormal preoperative laboratory tests in elderly surgical patients. Anesth Analg 2001;93: 301–308.

120. Gold BS, Young ML, Kinman JL, et al. The utility of preoperative electrocardiograms in the ambulatory surgical patient. Arch Intern Med 1992;152:301–305.

121. Liu LL, Dzankic S, Leung JM. Preoperative electrocardiogram abnormalities do not predict postoperative cardiac complications in geriatric surgical patients. J Am Geriatr Soc 2002;50:1186–1191.

122. Smetana GW, Macpherson DS. The case against routine preoperative laboratory testing. Med Clin North Am 2003;87:7–40.

123. Arozullah AM, Conde MV, Lawrence VA. Preoperative evaluation for postoperative pulmonary complications. Med Clin North Am 2003;87:153–173.

124. Seymour DG, Pringle R, Shaw JW. The role of the routine pre-operative chest X-ray in the elderly general surgical patient. Postgrad Med J 1982;58:741–745.

125. Marcello PW, Roberts PL. "Routine" preoperative studies. Which studies in which patients? Surg Clin North Am 1996;76:11–23.

126. Tape TG, Mushlin AI. How useful are routine chest X-rays of preoperative patients at risk for postoperative chest disease? J Gen Intern Med 1988;3:15–20.

127. Monro J, Booth A, Nicholl J. Routine preoperative testing: a systematic study of the evidence. Health Technol Assess 1997;1:1–62.

128. Fleisher LA. Routine laboratory testing in the elderly: is it indicated? Anesth Analg 2001;93:249–250.

129. Chrischilles EA, Foley DJ, Wallace RB, et al. Use of medications by persons 65 and over: data from the established populations for epidemiologic studies of the elderly. J Gerontol 1992;47:M137–144.

130. Gray SL, Mahoney JE, Blough DK. Medication adherence in elderly patients receiving home health services following hospital discharge. Ann Pharmacother 2001;35: 539–545.

131. Nolan L, O'Malley K. Prescribing for the elderly. Part I: sensitivity of the elderly to adverse drug reactions. J Am Geriatr Soc 1988;36:142–149.

132. Leung JM, Dzankic S, Manku K, et al. The prevalence and predictors of the use of alternative medicine in presurgical patients in five California hospitals. Anesth Analg 2001; 93:1062–1068.

133. Yoon SL, Horne CH. Perceived health promotion practice by older women: use of herbal products. J Gerontol Nurs 2004;30:9–15.

134. Fugh-Berman A. Herb-drug interactions. Lancet 2000;355: 134–138.

135. Bennett DA Jr, Phun L, Polk JF, et al. Neuropharmacology of St. John's wort (*Hypericum*). Ann Pharmacother 1998; 32:1201–1208.

136. Almeida JC, Grimsley EW. Coma from the health food store: interaction between kava and alprazolam. Ann Intern Med 1996;125:940–941.

137. Slifman NR, Obermeyer WR, Aloi BK, et al. Contamination of botanical dietary supplements by *Digitalis lanata*. N Engl J Med 1998;339:806–811.

138. Ang-Lee MK, Moss J, Yuan CS. Herbal medicines and perioperative care. JAMA 2001;286:208–216.

139. Adusumilli PS, Ben-Porat L, Pereira M, et al. The prevalence and predictors of herbal medicine use in surgical patients. J Am Coll Surg 2004;198:583–590.

140. Beers MH. Explicit criteria for determining potentially inappropriate medication use by the elderly. An update. Arch Intern Med 1997;157:1531–1536.

141. Zhan C, Sangl J, Bierman AS, et al. Potentially inappropriate medication use in the community-dwelling elderly: findings from the 1996 Medical Expenditure Panel Survey. JAMA 2001;286:2823–2829.

142. Agostini JV, Han L, Tinetti ME. The relationship between number of medications and weight loss or impaired balance in older adults. J Am Geriatr Soc 2004;52: 1719–1723.

143. Lowe CJ, Raynor DK, Courtney EA, et al. Effects of self medication programme on knowledge of drugs and compliance with treatment in elderly patients. BMJ 1995; 310:1229–1231.

144. Rich MW, Gray DB, Beckham V, et al. Effect of a multidisciplinary intervention on medication compliance in elderly patients with congestive heart failure. Am J Med 1996;101:270–276.

145. Stuck AE, Siu AL, Wieland GD, et al. Comprehensive geriatric assessment: a meta-analysis of controlled trials. Lancet 1993;342:1032–1036.

146. Marcantonio ER, Flacker JM, Wright RJ, et al. Reducing delirium after hip fracture: a randomized trial. J Am Geriatr Soc 2001;49:516–522.

14
Anesthetic Implications of Chronic Medications

Tamas A. Szabo and R. David Warters

The prevention and recognition of drug-related problems in older adults are of paramount importance. Medication-related problems are estimated to cause 106,000 deaths annually at a cost of $75–85 billion. Elderly patients presenting for surgery are often taking a large number and wide variety of chronic medications, greatly complicating their preoperative assessment and anesthesia management. The often daunting task of evaluating the potential interactions of these medications with one another as well as anesthetic medications is further complicated by the large number of inappropriate medications prescribed in this age group.

Inappropriate medications for elderly patients are defined as medications for which a better alternative drug exists and for which the potential risk outweighs the potential benefit. In 1997, Beers[1] devised a comprehensive set of explicit criteria for potentially inappropriate drug use in ambulatory older adults aged 65 years and older. Drugs were classified as inappropriate in three categories: (1) drugs that generally should be avoided in the elderly, (2) drugs that exceed a maximum recommended daily dose, and (3) drugs to be avoided in combination with specific comorbidities. Recently, the 1997 criteria were updated and presented as the 2002 Beers criteria.[2] In these updated criteria, the comorbidity list was modified, new medications were added, and several drugs were removed. The Beers criteria may not identify all causes of potentially inappropriate prescribing (e.g., drug–drug interactions are not included); however, they represent a widely used and standardized tool for pharmacologic research, despite the fact that nothing can substitute careful clinical judgment. A Dutch population-based cohort study revealed that 20% of ambulatory older adults receive at least one inappropriate drug prescription per year[3]; moreover, an epidemiologic study[4] from the United States reported that 23.5% of people aged >65 years receive >1 of the 20 medications on the Beers list. The prevalence of potentially inappropriate medications was found to be 21.3% among noninstitutionalized elderly patients.[5]

The safe administration of anesthesia to elderly patients requires a thorough evaluation and understanding of chronic medications and the potential for interactions. The aim of this chapter is to highlight (1) drugs that are common in elderly patients, and (2) drugs that have a potential interaction with medications used in the anesthetic practice.

Neuropsychiatric and Pain-Related Medications

Benzodiazepines

Benzodiazepines cause sedation, anterograde amnesia, anxiolysis, and muscle relaxation, as well as hypnotic and anticonvulsant effects. All effects and side effects of benzodiazepines are mediated through γ-aminobutyric acid $(GABA)_A$ receptors.

Long-acting benzodiazepines are considered potentially inappropriate in elderly patients[2,6] because of the risk of producing prolonged sedation and increasing the potential for falls and fractures. Patients most likely to be prescribed benzodiazepines are the elderly with a secondary complaint of insomnia. Although sleep fragmentation may be reduced by benzodiazepines, their long-term use may also elicit health problems, such as complete obstructive sleep apnea in heavy snorers.[7] Examples of long-acting benzodiazepines include halazepam (Paxipam), quazepam (Doral), flurazepam (Dalmane), chlordiazepoxide (Librium), chlordiazepoxide-amitriptyline (Limbitrol), clidinium-chlordiazepoxide (Librax), diazepam (Valium), and chlorazepate (Tranxene). Because of the increased sensitivity of long-acting benzodiazepines in elderly patients, smaller doses of short- or intermediate-acting benzodiazepines are considered preferable, safer, and more effective.

Midazolam (Versed), lorazepam (Ativan), and diazepam (Valium) are the primary benzodiazepines used in the anesthetic practice.[8] All three are highly protein bound, mainly by albumin. Patients with cirrhosis or chronic liver failure and subsequent hypoalbuminemia have a greater unbound fraction of benzodiazepines, which may increase their sensitivity to these agents.

Midazolam undergoes rapid hepatic metabolism to both active and inactive metabolites. Drugs that inhibit the cytochrome P-450 enzyme system [i.e., cimetidine, erythromycin, calcium channel blockers (CCBs), and antifungal agents] reduce the hepatic clearance of midazolam.[9]

Diazepam is metabolized in the liver through oxidative demethylation and glucuronidation to inactive metabolites that are excreted by the kidneys. An increased volume of distribution and reduced metabolic clearance may significantly increase the elimination half-life of diazepam in patients with cirrhosis. Elderly and/or obese patients are also susceptible to prolonged diazepam effects secondary to an increased volume of distribution. Lorazepam is hepatically conjugated to an inactive metabolite.

Respiratory depression secondary to the decrease in hypoxic drive is the most significant side effect of benzodiazepine administration. This effect is greater with midazolam than with lorazepam and diazepam in equipotent doses. Opioids may significantly enhance the respiratory depressant effects of benzodiazepines in patients with chronic obstructive pulmonary disease. Alpha$_2$ agonists, such as dexmedetomidine, have shown synergistic sedative effects,[10] while reversing the cardiovascular depressant effects of benzodiazepines. Moreover, the administration of even small doses of benzodiazepines in conjunction with opioids, propofol, or thiopental can also result in significant hypotension caused by the synergistic effects of these agents.[11]

Clinically significant hypotension may follow parenteral benzodiazepine administration in elderly patients. Parenteral benzodiazepines may be less effective in patients who take oral benzodiazepines on a chronic basis; moreover, the benzodiazepine antagonist flumazenil may precipitate withdrawal seizures in these patients.[12] Benzodiazepines reduce the anesthetic requirements for both intravenous and inhalational anesthetics, but may also decrease the analgesic effects of opiates.[13] Therefore, flumazenil may enhance the postoperative analgesic effects of morphine, reduce morphine requirements, and decrease the sedative, emetic, and cardiopulmonary depressant effects of morphine in patients who have received benzodiazepines after surgery.

Carbamazepine

Carbamazepine (Tegretol, Equetro, Carbatrol) is an anticonvulsant that blocks voltage- and frequency-dependent fast sodium currents. Sodium channels are kept in the inactivated state, inhibiting the spread of synchronized depolarization that is associated with the onset of seizures. Carbamazepine is structurally similar to tricyclic antidepressants.

The therapeutic index of carbamazepine for neurologic side effects is 8:1, making it a relatively nontoxic medication. Negative side effects include gastrointestinal (GI) irritation, diplopia, ataxia, vertigo, and sedation. Acute intoxication may lead to respiratory depression, unconsciousness, seizures, and cardiovascular collapse.[14]

The hepatic metabolism of carbamazepine may be inhibited by erythromycin, isoniazid, cimetidine, and propoxyphene,[15] leading to increased, possibly toxic, plasma levels. Carbamazepine can induce hepatic enzyme function and increase the metabolism of medications dependent on hepatic metabolism, including itself. Therefore, the half-life tends to decrease with regular use. Carbamazepine may reduce the plasma levels of primidone, valproic acid, phenytoin, and haloperidol.

Gabapentin

Gabapentin is a weak inhibitor of GABA transaminase which was originally developed for seizure disorder but is frequently used for postherpetic neuralgia and neuropathic pain. It has also been proposed as a component of perioperative pain control. It acts by increasing GABA synthesis. Nausea, vomiting, dizziness, somnolence, headache, ataxia, and fatigue are the most common side effects of the drug. Rarely, confusion, hallucinations, depression, and psychoses may occur.

Gabapentin is relatively free of drug interactions, its gastric absorption may be reduced by administration of antacids containing hydroxides of aluminum or magnesium, and its renal clearance can be reduced by cimetidine.

Monoamine Oxidase Inhibitors

Monoamine oxidase inhibitors (MAOIs) are used in the treatment of severe depression unresponsive to other antidepressants. Intraneuronal monoamine oxidase (MAO) is the primary enzyme involved in the oxidative deamination of amine neurotransmitters (epinephrine, norepinephrine, dopamine, and serotonin). MAOIs increase the level of intraneuronal transmitters, resulting in augmented postsynaptic depolarization and adrenergic stimulation. MAO exists in two isoforms: MAO-A preferentially metabolizes serotonin, dopamine, and norepinephrine, whereas MAO-B preferentially metabolizes phenylethylamine and tyramine.

Phenelzine (Nardil) is a nonselective MAOI that irreversibly inhibits the enzyme, and synthesis of new enzyme can take 10–14 days. It decreases pseudocholinesterase activity and subsequently prolongs depolarizing blockade. Tranylcypromine (Parnate) is a slightly shorter-acting MAOI derived from amphetamine. Selegiline (Deprenyl), a selective MAO-B inhibitor, is used as an adjunct in the treatment of Parkinson's disease.

The interactions of MAOIs with certain drugs (notably meperidine, which blocks neuronal uptake of serotonin) and foods containing tyramine (aged cheeses, chocolate, liver, fava beans, avocados, and Chianti wine) have limited their use.[16,17] Concurrent use of MAOI and meperidine may result in fatal excitatory reactions. Respiratory depression, hypotension, and coma are the signs of a depressive form that is secondary to the accumulation of free narcotic and has been described after the use of fentanyl, alfentanil, or sufentanil. If foods high in tyramine are ingested, there is the potential for massive displacement of norepinephrine into the cleft and for a life-threatening hypertensive crisis. Many patients taking MAOIs have symptoms of autonomic dysfunction such as orthostatic hypotension, because tyramine is not catabolized and remains at high levels in plasma. Tyramine is then taken up by sympathetic nerve terminals as a "false transmitter" and is converted to the biologically inactive octopamine.

MAOIs exaggerate the actions of indirect-acting and, to a lesser extent, direct-acting (phenylephrine, norepinephrine, epinephrine) sympathomimetics. A reduced dose of a direct-acting sympathomimetic is recommended[8] for the treatment of hypotension. Ketamine and pancuronium should not be used to avoid stimulation of the sympathetic nervous system. Morphine may be used for perioperative analgesia.

Selective Serotonin Reuptake Inhibitors

Selective serotonin reuptake inhibitors (SSRIs) inhibit the neuronal reuptake of serotonin. They are used primarily as antidepressants, but are also effective in the treatment of panic disorder, obsessive/compulsive disorder, posttraumatic stress disorder, and social phobia. SSRIs do not have anticholinergic effects, have little effect on norepinephrine reuptake, do not cause postural hypotension, do not cause delayed conduction of cardiac impulses, and do not affect the seizure threshold.

Fluoxetine is a potent inhibitor of certain hepatic cytochrome P-450 enzymes and may subsequently increase plasma concentrations of drugs that depend on hepatic metabolism. MAOIs, lithium, or carbamazepine combined with fluoxetine may cause the development of the potentially fatal (11% mortality) serotonin syndrome[18] characterized by hypo- or hypertension, anxiety, restlessness, confusion, chills, ataxia, insomnia, and seizures. This syndrome is most often reported in patients taking two or more medications that increase central nervous system (CNS) serotonin levels by different mechanisms.

Tricyclic Antidepressants

Amitriptyline and protriptyline are tricyclic antidepressants that exhibit the most prominent anticholinergic effects (tachycardia, blurred vision, dry mouth, delayed gastric emptying, urinary retention); therefore, they may be avoided in patients with glaucoma or prostatic hypertrophy. Cardiovascular abnormalities, including orthostatic hypotension and cardiac dysrhythmias (increased PR and QT intervals, widened QRS complexes), can be caused by these drugs.[19] Patients with coexisting heart block or prolonged QT intervals may be at increased risk for cardiac toxicity. Overdose may lead to cardiac conduction abnormalities, hypotension, mental status changes, seizures, coma, rhabdomyolysis, and renal failure. The sedation associated with tricyclic antidepressants may be beneficial for patients experiencing insomnia.

Patients taking tricyclic antidepressants may exhibit exaggerated systemic blood pressure responses after the administration of indirect-acting vasopressors because of the increased availability of norepinephrine at the postsynaptic receptors of the peripheral sympathetic nervous system. The combination of imipramine and pancuronium or ketamine may predispose anesthetized patients to tachydysrhythmias.[20] Postoperative delirium and confusion may result by the additive anticholinergic effects of the tricyclic antidepressants and centrally active anticholinergic drugs.

Antiparkinson Medications

The treatment of Parkinson's disease is directed toward increasing dopamine levels in the brain but preventing adverse peripheral effects of dopamine. Levodopa is the single most effective therapy for patients with Parkinson's disease. Side effects of levodopa administration include orthostatic hypotension, hypovolemia, depletion of myocardial norepinephrine stores, and peripheral vasoconstriction. The half-life of levodopa is short, and interruption of therapy for more than 6–12 hours can result in severe skeletal muscle rigidity that interferes with ventilation. Levodopa may alter some liver function tests, blood urea nitrogen, and positive Coombs test. Phenothiazines, butyrophenones (droperidol), and metoclopramide antagonize the effects of dopamine in the basal ganglia and should be avoided.[21]

Antidementia Drugs

Donepezil, rivastigmine, galantamine, and tacrine are reversible acetylcholinesterase inhibitors used in the treatment of mild to moderately severe dementia in Alzheimer's disease. Adverse effects include abdominal pain, nausea, vomiting, diarrhea, dizziness, headache, somnolence, muscle cramps, insomnia, sweating, tremor, and syncope. Angina, sinoatrial (SA), atrioventricular (AV), and bundle-branch blocks, bradycardia, cardiac arrest, peptic ulcers, GI hemorrhage, extrapyramidal symptoms, seizures, depression, hallucinations, agitation, confusion, and bladder outflow obstruction have been observed.[22] Rivastigmine, tacrine, and donepezil may prolong the action of succinylcholine. Cholinergic crisis may result from overdose.

Donepezil is selective for the CNS. It is highly protein bound, mainly by albumin. It undergoes partial metabolism via the cytochrome P-450 system. Ketoconazole, erythromycin, fluoxetine, and quinidine increase plasma donepezil concentrations by inhibiting the isoenzymes CYP 3A4 and CYP 2D6. Conversely, donepezil concentrations may be reduced by enzyme inducers such as phenytoin, carbamazepine, and rifampin.

Rivastigmine is selective for the CNS and has also been tried in the treatment of vascular dementia and in the treatment of psychosis in patients with Parkinson's disease. It is approximately 40% bound to plasma proteins and readily crosses the blood–brain barrier. The drug is metabolized by cholinesterase-mediated hydrolysis.[23]

Galantamine may also be effective in the treatment of vascular dementia. It is not recommended for treatment of mild cognitive impairment because of an association with increased mortality. Galantamine is partially metabolized by the cytochrome P-450 system. A reduced dose may be necessary in patients with hepatic or renal impairment or when galantamine is given with drugs that inhibit CYP 2D6 and CYP 3A4, such as quinidine, fluoxetine, fluvoxamine, paroxetine, and ketoconazole.

Tacrine may delay cognitive decline but many patients cannot tolerate the dosage required and have to stop treatment because of GI effects or signs of hepatotoxicity. It undergoes an extensive first-pass effect in the liver, and is metabolized by the cytochrome P-450 system. It may competitively inhibit the metabolism of other drugs that are also metabolized by the cytochrome P-450 isoenzyme CYP 1A2. Cimetidine has been shown to inhibit the metabolism of tacrine. Increased serum alanine aminotransferase concentrations, mostly within the first 12 weeks of therapy, are likely to occur in about 50% of patients.[24] Some patients may develop unpredictable life-threatening hepatotoxicity. There is no significant correlation between plasma-tacrine concentrations and hepatotoxicity. Abruptly stopping tacrine therapy may result in a decline in cognitive function.

The N-methyl-D-aspartate (NMDA) receptor antagonist memantine is used in the treatment of moderately severe to severe Alzheimer's disease and is thought to act through modulation of the effects of glutamate. It undergoes partial hepatic metabolism. The majority is excreted unchanged via the kidney. Use of other NMDA antagonists such as amantadine, ketamine, or dextromethorphan

may increase the incidence and severity of adverse effects and should be avoided. The effects of dopaminergics and antimuscarinics may also be enhanced, whereas memantine may reduce the actions of barbiturates and antipsychotics. Adverse effects include anxiety, hallucinations, confusion, constipation, dizziness, headache, somnolence, abnormal gait, hypertension, and seizures. Dosage adjustment may be required in patients with recent myocardial infarction, congestive heart failure, uncontrolled hypertension, and renal impairment.[25]

Cardiovascular Drugs

Alpha$_2$-Adrenergic Agonists

Three categories of alpha$_2$ agonists exist: phenylethylates (e.g., methyldopa), imidazolines (e.g., clonidine, dexmedetomidine), and oxaloazepines. The most prominent hemodynamic effects of alpha$_2$ agonists are hypotension and bradycardia. Hypotension can be reversed by standard vasoactive agents. The pressor response to ephedrine and phenylephrine are enhanced, but the response to norepinephrine is not.[26] The response to dopamine and to atropine is mildly attenuated. Rebound hypertension may occur after abrupt discontinuation of these drugs after chronic administration. The anesthetic-sparing and sedative effects of alpha$_2$ agonists result from inactivation of the locus ceruleus. The sedative effect is antagonized by alpha$_1$ agonists. Alpha$_2$ agonist or benzodiazepine premedication may attenuate the high incidence (up to 30%) of ketamine-induced disturbing emergence reactions. Alpha$_2$ agonists reduce GI motility and co-administration of opioids produces a synergistic inhibition of GI transit.

The potential for CNS adverse effects and orthostatic hypotension may contraindicate the use of clonidine in the elderly, whereas methyldopa (Aldomet) and methyldopa-hydrochlorothiazide (Aldoril) may cause bradycardia and exacerbate depression in elderly patients.[2]

Alpha$_1$-Adrenergic Antagonists

Doxazosin (Cardura) may cause orthostatic hypotension, edema, hepatitis, dry mouth, and urinary retention. Hypotension during epidural anesthesia may be exaggerated in the presence of alpha$_1$-blockers and the resulting decrease in systemic vascular resistance may not be responsive to alpha$_1$-adrenergic agonists (e.g., phenylephrine). The combination of alpha$_1$-blockers and a beta-blocker could result in refractory hypotension because of potentially blunted response to beta$_1$ as well as alpha$_1$ agonists.[26] Intoxication may result in nausea, vomiting, abdominal pain, hypotension, reflex tachycardia, and seizures.

Digoxin

Digoxin inhibits Na^+/K^+ adenosine triphosphatase, leads to an increase in the intracellular concentration of Na^+, and thus (by stimulation of Na^+–Ca^{2+} exchange) an increase in the intracellular concentration of Ca^{2+}. The beneficial effects of digoxin result from direct actions on cardiac muscle, as well as indirect actions on the cardiovascular system mediated by effects on the autonomic nervous system. The autonomic effects include: (1) a vagomimetic action, which is responsible for the effects of digoxin on the SA and AV nodes, and (2) baroreceptor sensitization, which results in increased afferent inhibitory activity and reduced activity of the sympathetic nervous system and renin-angiotensin system for any given increment in mean arterial pressure. The pharmacologic consequences of these direct and indirect effects are: (1) a positive inotropic effect, (2) a decrease in the degree of activation of the sympathetic nervous system and renin-angiotensin system (neurohormonal deactivating effect), and (3) negative dromotropic and negative chronotropic effects. The effects of digoxin in heart failure are mediated by its positive inotropic and neurohormonal deactivating effects, whereas the effects of the drug in atrial arrhythmias are related to its vagomimetic actions. The most frequent cause of toxicity is renal failure.[27] Digitalis toxicity is markedly increased in the presence of hypokalemia, and digitalis toxicity may be reversed to some degree by the administration of K^+. Other causes of digitalis toxicity include hypomagnesemia, hypercalcemia, and hypothyroidism. Administration of digitalis can lead to the development of a wide variety of arrhythmias including sinus bradycardia and arrest, AV conduction delays, and second- or third-degree heart blocks.[28] Sympathomimetics with beta-adrenergic agonist effects as well as pancuronium[29] and intravenous administration of Ca^{2+} may increase the likelihood of cardiac dysrhythmias. Oral antacids decrease the GI absorption of digitalis.[30,31]

Amiodarone

Amiodarone is a potent class III antidysrhythmic agent with a wide spectrum of activity against refractory supraventricular and ventricular tachydysrhythmias. The antiarrhythmic effect of amiodarone may be attributed to at least two major properties: (1) a prolongation of the myocardial cell-action potential duration and refractory period, and (2) noncompetitive alpha- and beta-adrenergic inhibition. Antiadrenergic and Ca^{2+} channel blocking effects contribute to peripheral vasodilation, bradycardia, conduction disturbances, negative inotropic effects, and hypotension. After oral dosing, however, amiodarone produces no significant change in left ventricular ejection fraction (LVEF), even in patients with depressed LVEF. After acute intravenous dosing, it may have a mild negative inotropic effect. Volatile anesthetics, beta-blockers, lidocaine, diltiazem, and verapamil can potentiate the cardiovascular and negative inotropic effects of amiodarone.[32] Proarrhythmic side effects of amiodarone are reported in less than 1%–2% of patients. Pulmonary toxicity is a severe complication that may occur in up to 17% of patients treated long term.[33] Pulmonary complications may progress to adult respiratory distress syndrome and pulmonary fibrosis. Both hypothyroidism and hyperthyroidism can occur with chronic amiodarone therapy.[34] Amiodarone treatment may also lead to increased liver function tests. Amiodarone inhibits CYP metabolisms resulting in increased levels of digoxin (by as much as 70%), procainamide, quinidine, warfarin, and cyclosporine. It may also directly depress vitamin K-dependent clotting factors. Cimetidine can reduce the metabolism of amiodarone, and phenytoin increases its metabolism.

Disopyramide

Disopyramide is a class IA antiarrhythmic indicated in the treatment of life-threatening ventricular arrhythmias and is also used to treat supraventricular arrhythmias caused by reentrant mechanisms. Of all antiarrhythmic drugs, this is the most potent negative inotrope and reversible heart failure has been reported after its use. As many as 50% of patients with a history of heart failure may have a recurrence of the disease with an incidence of less than 5% in other patients. Disopyramide should not be used in patients with cardiogenic shock, AV block, or long QT intervals. It can lead to the development of second- or third-degree AV block or torsade de pointes ventricular tachycardia.[35] Disopyramide has strong anticholinergic side effects including dry mouth, impotence, urinary retention, constipation, and exacerbation of glaucoma. Because of the large number and severity of side effects, disopyramide is contraindicated in elderly patients.

Beta Receptor Antagonists

Beta receptors are G protein–coupled receptors found throughout the myocardium and nodal conduction tissue. Beta receptor blockers are competitive antagonists at beta-adrenergic receptor sites and are used in the management of hypertension, stable and unstable angina pectoris, cardiac arrhythmias, myocardial infarction, and heart failure. These drugs have been shown to reduce mortality when administered prophylactically to patients undergoing major vascular surgery[36] who are at high risk for ischemia. Beta-blockers have also been found to reduce mortality and morbidity rates in patients with myocardial infarction[37] and congestive heart failure.[38] They are also given to control symptoms of sympathetic overactivity in alcohol withdrawal, anxiety states, hyperthyroidism, and tremor, and in the prophylaxis of migraine and of bleeding associated with portal hypertension. Beta receptor antagonism manifests in decreased heart rate and increased diastolic perfusion.

Beta-blockers belong to two general classifications, based on whether they are selective $beta_1$ antagonists or combined $beta_1$ and $beta_2$ antagonists. The $beta_1$ antagonists or those with intrinsic sympathomimetic activity at $beta_2$ receptors are "cardioselective" and are better suited for use in patients with asthma and bronchospastic disease and hypertension. With increasing doses of the cardioselective drugs, there is a decrease in receptor specificity. The beta-blockers with proven effects on prognosis include two selective $beta_1$ receptor blockers—metoprolol and bisoprolol—and three nonselective beta-blockers—timolol, propranolol, and carvedilol. Sotalol, a nonselective beta-blocker, which also has a pronounced class III antiarrhythmic effect, does not seem to have a significant effect on postinfarction mortality.

Beta-blockers are generally well tolerated and most adverse effects are mild. The most frequent and serious adverse effects are heart failure, heart block, and bronchospasm. For this reason, these drugs must be used judiciously in patients with severe obstructive pulmonary disease, bradycardia, heart block, or uncompensated congestive heart failure. Abrupt withdrawal of beta-blockers may exacerbate angina and may lead to sudden death. Reduced peripheral circulation may exacerbate peripheral vascular disease such as Raynaud's syndrome. CNS effects include headache, depression, dizziness, hallucinations, confusion, and sleep disturbances.

Beta-blockers are eliminated by several metabolic pathways. Propranolol and metoprolol undergo hepatic metabolism, esmolol is biotransformed in the blood by esterases, atenolol is renally excreted, and timolol is eliminated by the kidney and the liver. The metabolism and route of excretion is important when considering patients with renal or hepatic disease.

Coadministration of beta-blockers and propofol might result in cardiac events including severe bradycardia, sinus arrest, heart block, or even asystole. The myocardial depression seen with halothane is also exacerbated by beta-blockers.[39]

Calcium Channel Blockers

CCBs inhibit the cellular influx of calcium by binding to specific drug receptors on L-type calcium channels and maintaining the channels in an inactive state. The L-type channel is the predominant type in heart and vascular smooth muscle.

Three major classes of CCBs exist: the dihydropyridines, the phenylalkylamines, and the benzothiazepines. Each class binds to a unique site on the $alpha_1$-subunit of the L-type channel. Dihydropyridine CCBs (such as nife-

dipine, nimodipine, and amlodipine) have a greater selectivity for vascular smooth muscle than for myocardium and their main effect is vasodilatation. They have little or no action at the SA or AV nodes, and negative inotropic and chronotropic effects are minimal. They are used for their antihypertensive and antianginal properties. Nimodipine crosses the blood–brain barrier and is used in cerebral ischemia. Benzothiazepine CCBs (such as diltiazem) and phenylalkylamine CCBs (such as verapamil) have less selective vasodilator activity. They depress SA and AV nodal conduction and are used for their antiarrhythmic, antianginal, and antihypertensive properties. Verapamil has the most prominent negative inotropic effect and it may precipitate congestive heart failure in patients with preexisting left ventricular dysfunction. Diltiazem also reduces contractility, but the concurrent peripheral vasodilation may preserve cardiac output. Verapamil, nifedipine, and nicardipine are 90% protein-bound, and their clinical effects can be enhanced by drugs that increase the pharmacologically active unbound fraction (such as lidocaine or diazepam). Liver disease may necessitate reduced dosing of verapamil and diltiazem.[40]

CCBs may be responsible for several drug interactions and may have numerous adverse effects. The coadministration of diltiazem and beta-blockers may yield profound bradycardia. Diltiazem decreases the clearance of a single dose of propranolol, metoprolol, and possibly atenolol; therefore, elevated concentrations of beta-blockers may be responsible for the bradycardic effects. Cimetidine causes increases in plasma-diltiazem concentrations and in plasma-deacetyldiltiazem concentrations.

The combination of verapamil and beta-blockers may result in bradycardia, heart block, and left ventricular failure. The risks are especially increased when both drugs are given intravenously. Bradycardia has also been reported in a patient treated with oral verapamil and timolol eye drops.[41] Verapamil is extensively metabolized in the liver and interactions may occur with drugs that inhibit or enhance hepatic metabolism. Verapamil inhibits the cytochrome P-450 isoenzyme CYP 3A4 and therefore may increase plasma concentrations of carbamazepine, cyclosporine, digoxin (by up to 70%), midazolam, simvastatin, and theophylline. Verapamil and diltiazem have significant local anesthetic properties, because they block fast sodium channels, and therefore the risk of local anesthetic toxicity may be increased in patients taking these medications.

Enhanced antihypertensive effects may be seen with the combination of nifedipine and beta-blockers. Heart failure has also been reported in a few patients with angina who were given nifedipine and a beta-blocker. Nifedipine may modify insulin and glucose responses. Nifedipine is extensively metabolized in the liver by the cytochrome P-450 isoenzyme CYP 3A4, and interactions may occur with quinidine (resulting in increased serum nifedipine concentrations), which shares the same metabolic pathway, and with enzyme inducers, such as carbamazepine, phenytoin, and rifampicin. Inhibition of the cytochrome P-450 system by cimetidine and erythromycin may lead to potentiation of the hypotensive effect.

Decreased blood pressure from volatile anesthetics can be potentiated by concurrent administration of CCBs. Volatile anesthetics significantly decrease intracellular Ca^{2+} in the myocardium, and thus augment the negative inotropic, dromotropic, and vasodilatory effects of CCBs.[42] CCBs potentiate depolarizing and nondepolarizing neuromuscular blockade,[43] and the antagonism of a nondepolarizing neuromuscular blockade may be blunted, because calcium is essential for the release of acetylcholine at the neuromuscular junction. Edrophonium may be more effective than neostigmine in reversing neuromuscular blockade that has been enhanced by CCBs.[44]

Angiotensin-Converting Enzyme Inhibitors

Angiotensin-converting enzyme (ACE) inhibitors decrease angiotensin II and aldosterone levels. They have been shown to slow renal dysfunction in diabetic nephropathy and to improve long-term outcomes in heart failure trials.[45] Accumulation of captopril, lisinopril, and enalaprilat occurs in patients with renal impairment, and decreased glomerular filtration rate is seen in patients treated with ACE inhibitors. These drugs should be avoided in patients with renal artery stenosis. Hyperkalemia is possible[46] because of reduced production of aldosterone; therefore, potassium levels should be monitored. The adverse effects of ACE inhibitors on the kidneys may be potentiated by other drugs, such as nonsteroidal antiinflammatory drugs (NSAIDs). Several ACE inhibitors are designed as prodrugs, and they must undergo hepatic conversion. Enalapril is the prodrug of the active ACE inhibitor, enalaprilat, and conversion may be affected in patients with hepatic dysfunction. Captopril and lisinopril are not prodrugs.

The combination of NSAIDs and ACE inhibitors may have variable effects on renal function because they act at different parts of the glomerulus. When given to patients whose kidneys are underperfused (heart failure, hypovolemia, or cirrhosis), renal function may deteriorate. Indomethacin and possibly other NSAIDs, including aspirin, have been reported to reduce the hypotensive action of ACE inhibitors. Part of the hypotensive effect of ACE inhibitors may be prostaglandin-dependent, which might explain this interaction with drugs such as NSAIDs that block prostaglandin synthesis. Marked hypotension may occur during general anesthesia in patients receiving ACE inhibitors, therefore discontinuation of ACE inhibitor therapy before anesthesia should be considered. Excessive hypotension may occur when ACE inhibitors are used concurrently with diuretics or other antihypertensives. An additive hyperkalemic effect is possible in patients receiving ACE inhibitors with potassium-sparing diuretics, potassium supplements, or other drugs that can cause hyperkalemia (such as cyclosporine or indomethacin). Potassium-sparing diuretics and potassium supplements should generally be stopped before initiating ACE inhibitors in patients with heart failure.

Pulmonary Drugs

Beta Agonists

Inhaled beta receptor agonists are a mainstay in the treatment of asthma. The primary action of beta agonists is to stimulate adenylyl cyclase, and thus increase adenosine 3′,5′-cyclic monophosphate (cAMP). Increased levels of cAMP mediate smooth muscle relaxation and inhibit the inflammatory mediator release from mast cells. Metaproterenol was the first beta$_2$ selective agonist; however, albuterol is currently the most widely used agent. Adverse effects include tremor, tachycardia, hypertension, palpitations, nausea, and vomiting.[47] Direct-acting beta agonists should be administered with extreme caution to patients who are being treated with MAOIs (clorgyline, isocarboxazid, pargyline, phenelzine, selegiline), or within 2 weeks of the discontinuation of an MAOI, because the action of the beta agonist on the vascular system may be exaggerated. Acute metabolic responses include hyperglycemia, hypokalemia, and hypomagnesemia. Despite the relative beta$_2$ selectivity of these agents, higher doses can stimulate both beta$_1$ and beta$_2$ receptors. Prophylactic administration of beta agonists 1 hour before induction of general anesthesia results in reduced airway resistance after endotracheal intubation.[48]

Theophylline

Theophylline is a phosphodiesterase inhibitor, leading to increased cellular concentrations of cAMP and cGMP (cyclic guanosine 3′,5′-monophosphate). The combination of phosphodiesterase inhibition, inflammatory inhibition, and catecholamine release may all contribute to smooth muscle relaxation and bronchodilation. Theophylline is eliminated mainly by hepatic metabolism and usual doses can be given to patients with renal impairment. Its metabolism and clearance are greatly affected by concurrent disease states and altered physiology including liver disease, pulmonary edema, chronic obstructive pulmonary disease, and thyroid disease. Phenytoin markedly decreases the elimination half-life and increases the clearance of theophylline by up to 350%, probably as a result of hepatic enzyme induction. Carbamazepine and rifampin have been observed to increase theophylline elimination. However, cimetidine, erythromycin, amiodarone, mexiletine, and tacrine inhibit its hepatic metabolism. Theophylline may enhance lithium elimination with a consequent loss of effect.

Specific drug interactions with numerous anesthetic-related medications have been described. There is a risk of synergistic toxicity if theophylline is used in the presence of halothane[49] because of the sensitizing effects of halothane on the myocardium to increased catecholamines released by theophylline. Larger doses of benzodiazepines may be needed to achieve a desired effect, because benzodiazepines increase the CNS concentrations of adenosine, a potent CNS depressant, whereas theophylline blocks adenosine receptors. Ketamine may decrease the theophylline seizure threshold,[50] and theophylline can antagonize the effect of nondepolarizing neuromuscular blockers possibly because of phosphodiesterase inhibition. Theophylline can precipitate sinus tachycardia, multifocal atrial tachycardia, and supraventricular and ventricular premature contractions at therapeutic or supratherapeutic serum concentrations. It can also potentiate hypokalemia associated with the administration of beta$_2$ agonists, corticosteroids, and diuretics.

Gastrointestinal Drugs

Cimetidine

Cimetidine is a competitive antagonist for histamine at the H$_2$ receptor. Cimetidine is metabolized in the liver where it binds to cytochrome P-450 and interferes with the metabolism of several drugs including amiodarone, warfarin, theophylline, phenytoin, lidocaine, quinidine, tricyclic antidepressants, and propranolol.[51] The effects of cimetidine on carbamazepine plasma concentration may be temporary; however, carbamazepine toxicity, manifesting in ataxia, nystagmus, diplopia, headache, vomiting, apnea, seizures, and coma, may occur with cimetidine coadministration. Carvedilol is significantly metabolized by the cytochrome P-450 enzyme system. Increased adverse effects of carvedilol (dizziness, insomnia, GI symptoms, postural hypotension) may result when the drug is administered with cimetidine. Cimetidine also decreases the clearance of benzodiazepines that are metabolized by hydroxylation or dealkylation (e.g., diazepam, chlordiazepoxide, clorazepate, flurazepam, prazepam, halazepam, alprazolam, triazolam, midazolam, quazepam, bromazepam). Adverse effects such as pronounced sedation and impaired cognitive and psychomotor function have been reported. Benzodiazepines for which nitroreduction is a prominent metabolic pathway might also have their clearance decreased by cimetidine

(e.g., nitrazepam, clonazepam). Those benzodiazepines eliminated primarily by glucuronidation do not interact with cimetidine (e.g., lorazepam, oxazepam, temazepam). Hepatic metabolism of cimetidine may be enhanced if phenobarbital is administered concurrently. Cimetidine crosses the blood–brain barrier and interacts with cerebral H$_2$ receptors. Consequently, headaches, somnolence, confusion, and delirium may occur. Delayed awakening from anesthesia has been attributed to lingering CNS effects of cimetidine. Bradycardia, tachycardia, cardiac dysrhythmias, and hypotension may occur because of interaction with cardiac H$_2$ receptors. These events have generally been associated with rapid intravenous infusion. Cimetidine may cause impotence, loss of libido, and gynecomastia (by increasing the plasma concentration of prolactin) in male patients.

Metoclopramide

Metoclopramide is a dopamine antagonist and a selective peripheral cholinergic agonist useful for reducing gastric fluid volume by increasing lower esophageal sphincter tone, speeding gastric emptying time, and acting as an antiemetic. Side effects include hypotension, sedation, dysphoria, rash, and dry mouth. Anxiety, restlessness, and drowsiness may occur with rapid administration of undiluted metoclopramide. Bradycardia, supraventricular arrhythmias, complete heart block, and asystole have also been reported after administration of single doses of intravenous metoclopramide. The drug blocks dopaminergic receptors in the CNS, thereby inducing secretion of prolactin and creating the possibility of extrapyramidal symptoms.[51] Metoclopramide should be avoided in the presence of GI obstruction or after GI surgery and in patients taking MAOIs, tricyclic antidepressants, or other drugs that may cause extrapyramidal symptoms. By inhibiting pseudocholinesterase, metoclopramide may elicit prolonged responses to succinylcholine.[52]

Oral Anticoagulants

Warfarin

Warfarin is an anticoagulant that inhibits the hepatic conversion of four vitamin K-dependent coagulation factors (II, VII, IX, and X) and two anticoagulant proteins (protein C and S). It is indicated for the prophylaxis and/or treatment of venous thrombosis, pulmonary embolism, thromboembolic complications associated with atrial fibrillation, and/or cardiac valve replacement, and to reduce the risk of death, recurrent myocardial infarction, and stroke after myocardial infarction. An anticoagulation effect generally occurs within 24 hours after drug administration. However, peak anticoagulant effect may be delayed 72–96 hours when the vitamin K-dependent procoagulant proteins are reduced by 30%–50% of normal, which is consistent with international normalized ratio (INR) values in the range of 2–3. Warfarin is metabolized by hepatic cytochrome P-450 to inactive hydroxylated metabolites (predominant route) and by reductases to reduced metabolites. The metabolites are principally excreted into the urine and bile. No dosage adjustment is necessary for patients with renal failure. Hepatic dysfunction can potentiate the response to warfarin through impaired synthesis of clotting factors and decreased metabolism of warfarin. Discontinuation of warfarin will result in normalization of the prothrombin time (PT)/INR in 3 days unless the patient has substantial liver disease or vitamin K deficiency. Warfarin is >98% bound to albumin, meaning that only 1%–2% of the circulating drug accounts for the entire biologic effect.

Pyrazole NSAIDs (e.g., phenylbutazone) compete effectively for the same binding sites and may significantly increase bleeding risks when coadministered with warfarin. Amiodarone also inhibits the metabolic clearance of warfarin. Second- and third-generation cephalosporins augment the anticoagulant effect by inhibiting the cyclic interconversion of vitamin K. Aspirin and NSAIDs inhibit platelet function and have the potential to increase the risk of warfarin-associated bleeding.[53,54] Patients 60 years or older seem to exhibit greater than expected PT/INR response to the anticoagulant effects of warfarin. The cause of the increased sensitivity to warfarin in this age group is unknown. Therefore, as patient age increases, a lower dose of warfarin is usually required.

Ticlopidine

Ticlopidine is a platelet aggregation inhibitor. Its active metabolite blocks platelet surface adenosine 5′-diphosphate (ADP) receptors and, subsequently, ADP-induced binding of fibrinogen to the platelet GPIIb/IIIa receptor is inhibited. Ticlopidine may also block the binding of von Willebrand factor to platelets. The effect on platelet function is irreversible. Ticlopidine should be stopped 2 weeks before elective surgery. It may cause hepatic impairment, neutropenia, agranulocytosis, and thrombotic thrombocytopenic purpura. It should be avoided in patients with hepatic insufficiency. Intracranial and GI bleeding are also serious complications.[55–57] Ticlopidine potentiates the effect of aspirin or other NSAIDs on platelet aggregation. In clinical studies, ticlopidine was used concomitantly with beta-blockers, CCBs, and diuretics without evidence of clinically significant adverse interactions. The safety of concomitant use of ticlopidine and NSAIDs has not been established. Clearance of ticlopidine decreases with age. Steady-state trough values in elderly patients are approximately twice those in younger volunteer populations.

Nonsteroidal Antiinflammatory Drugs

NSAIDs are the most frequently prescribed drugs worldwide and are responsible for 21% of all adverse reactions reported each year to the spontaneous drug reporting system of the United States Food and Drug Administration.[58] NSAIDs are nonselective inhibitors of both cyclooxygenase (COX)-1 and COX-2. Absorption, peak plasma concentration, and metabolism can be significantly affected by GI pH, concomitant administration of other drugs, and the disease state of the patient. Antacids and mucoprotective agents can delay the absorption of NSAIDs. Elimination is largely dependent on hepatic biotransformation and renal excretion. Therefore, patients with hepatic and renal disease often demonstrate greater and more prolonged peak plasma concentrations. Acute renal impairment, papillary necrosis, acute interstitial nephritis, and nephrotic syndrome have all been attributed to NSAIDs.[59] In the presence of renal vasoconstriction, the vasodilator action of prostaglandins increases renal blood flow and thereby helps to maintain renal function. Patients whose renal function is being maintained by prostaglandins are therefore at risk from NSAIDs. Such patients include those with impaired circulation, the elderly, those taking diuretics, and those with heart failure or renal vascular disease. Serious hepatotoxicity is rare with typical therapeutic doses. The underlying mechanism seems to be immunologic; however, aspirin and phenylbutazone may have direct toxic effects. These drugs are frequently administered with opioid agents to enhance their analgesic potential. Naproxen (Naprosyn, Avaprox, Aleve), oxaprozin (Daypro), and piroxicam (Feldene) are considered potentially inappropriate for the elderly, because these medications all have the potential to produce hypertension, heart failure, renal failure, and GI adverse effects.

Ketorolac

Immediate and long-term use should be avoided in older patients, because a significant number have asymptomatic GI pathologic conditions. NSAID gastropathy (dyspepsia, nausea, epigastric pain) is one of the most frequent drug-related side effects in the United States.[60]

Indomethacin

All NSAIDs should be considered capable of causing confusion in the elderly. The more readily lipid-soluble agents would be expected to cross the blood–brain barrier easier and hence cause greater CNS adverse effects than less lipophilic NSAIDs. Of all available NSAIDs, indomethacin produces the most CNS adverse effects, including cognitive dysfunction, confusion, excessive somnolence, and behavioral disturbances.[61] Indomethacin may also accelerate the rate of cartilage destruction in patients with osteoarthritis.

H₁ Receptor Antagonists

These drugs are competitive, selective, and reversible antagonists of histamine on the H₁ receptor. First-generation antagonists may also activate muscarinic cholinergic, serotonin, or alpha-adrenergic receptors. Second-generation antagonists are unlikely to produce CNS side effects. Nonanticholinergic antihistamines are preferred in elderly patients when treating allergic reactions.

Diphenhydramine

Diphenhydramine is a first-generation H₁ receptor antagonist. It may cause confusion and sedation. Anticholinergic effects such as dry mouth, blurred vision, and urinary retention may be noted. Tachycardia, cardiac dysrhythmias, and prolongation of the QT interval may occur. The drug should not be used as a hypnotic, and when used to treat emergency allergic reactions, it should be used in the smallest possible dose.[62]

Hydroxyzine, Chlor-Trimeton

These are first-generation H₁ receptor antagonists with potent anticholinergic properties and as such are considered potentially inappropriate for older adults.

Opioids

Administration of narcotics (with the exception of meperidine) usually results in decreased heart rate. SA node depression and prolonged AV conduction can occur, as can sinus arrest and even asystole. Decreased sympathetic tone and histamine release (morphine and meperidine) can contribute to hypotension. Hypotensive effects are most prominent in patients with increased sympathetic tone, such as those with congestive heart failure or hypovolemia. Orthostatic hypotension may be seen in patients with autonomic neuropathy (e.g., diabetics). Meperidine, because of its structural similarity to atropine, may increase the heart rate. In large doses it has negative inotropic effects and can prolong the duration of action potential, potentiating class I antiarrhythmics. Meperidine has a bad reputation in the elderly for causing confusion and delirium.[63] Opioids may lessen total anesthetic requirements: a single dose of fentanyl may decrease the minimal anesthetic concentration (MAC) of isoflurane or desflurane by 50%. Likewise, alfentanil and remifentanil may also exhibit anesthetic-sparing effects.

Mixed agonist-antagonists are less effective than pure agonists in reducing MAC. The ceiling effect for MAC parallels the ceiling effect for respiratory depression. Nalbuphine decreases MAC by only 8%.

Pentazocine

Pentazocine is a benzomorphan derivative that possesses agonist (delta and kappa receptors) as well as weak antagonist actions. The most common side effect of pentazocine is sedation, followed by diaphoresis and dizziness. Pentazocine increases the plasma concentration of catecholamines, which may account for increases in heart rate, systemic blood pressure, and pulmonary artery pressure. Confusion and hallucinations limit its use in the elderly.[64] Pentazocine decreases MAC by 20%.

Propoxyphene

Propoxyphene offers few analgesic advantages over acetaminophen or aspirin, yet has the adverse effects of other narcotics. The only clinical use of propoxyphene is treatment of mild-to-moderate pain that is not adequately relieved by the above two drugs. It does not possess antipyretic or antiinflammatory effects, and its antitussive activity is not significant. The most common side effects of propoxyphene are vertigo, sedation, nausea, and vomiting. Overdose—especially in combination with alcohol—is complicated by seizures and depression of ventilation.[65,66] Propoxyphene may slow the metabolism of concomitantly administered antidepressants, anticonvulsants, or warfarin-like drugs. Severe neurologic signs, including coma, have occurred with concurrent use of carbamazepine.

Conclusions

The large number and variety of chronic medications prescribed to elderly patients presenting for surgery greatly complicate the preoperative assessment and anesthetic management of geriatric patients. The various interactions of medications on metabolism and end effects must be understood and considered when formulating an appropriate anesthetic plan.

References

1. Beers MH. Explicit criteria for determining potentially inappropriate medication use by the elderly. An update. Arch Intern Med 1997;157(14):1531–1536.
2. Fick DM, Cooper JW, Wade WE, et al. Updating the Beers criteria for potentially inappropriate medication use in older adults. Arch Intern Med 2003;163(22):2716–2724.
3. van der Hooft CS, Jong GW, Dieleman JP, et al. Inappropriate drug prescribing in older adults: the updated 2002 Beers

criteria—a population-based cohort study. Br J Clin Pharmacol 2005;60(2):137–144.

4. Willcox SM, Himmelstein DU, Woolhandler S. Inappropriate drug prescribing for the community-dwelling elderly. JAMA 1994;272(4):292–296.

5. Zhan C, Sangl J, Bierman AS, et al. Potentially inappropriate medication use in the community-dwelling elderly: findings from the 1996 Medical Expenditure Panel Survey. JAMA 2001;286(22):2823–2829.

6. Pitkala KH, Strandberg TE, Tilvis RS. Inappropriate drug prescribing in home-dwelling, elderly patients: a population-based survey. Arch Intern Med 2002;162(15):1707–1712.

7. Guilleminault C. Benzodiazepines, breathing, and sleep. Am J Med 1990;88(3A):25S–28S.

8. Faust RJ, Cucchiara RF, Rose SH, et al. Anesthesiology Review. 3rd ed. Philadelphia: Churchill Livingstone; 2002.

9. Sanders LD, Whitehead C, Gildersleve CD, et al. Interaction of H2-receptor antagonists and benzodiazepine sedation. A double-blind placebo-controlled investigation of the effects of cimetidine and ranitidine on recovery after intravenous midazolam. Anaesthesia 1993;48(4):286–292.

10. Salonen M, Reid K, Maze M. Synergistic interaction between alpha 2-adrenergic agonists and benzodiazepines in rats. Anesthesiology 1992;76(6):1004–1011.

11. Ruff R, Reves JG. Hemodynamic effects of a lorazepam-fentanyl anesthetic induction for coronary artery bypass surgery. J Cardiothorac Anesth 1990;4(3):314–317.

12. Spivey WH. Flumazenil and seizures: analysis of 43 cases. Clin Ther 1992;14(2):292–305.

13. Luger TJ, Hill HF, Schlager A. Can midazolam diminish sufentanil analgesia in patients with major trauma? A retrospective study of 43 patients. Drug Metabol Drug Interact 1992;10:177–184.

14. Megarbane B, Leprince P, Deye N, et al. Extracorporeal life support in a case of acute carbamazepine poisoning with life-threatening refractory myocardial failure. Intensive Care Med 2006;32(9):1409–1413.

15. Spina E, Pisani F, Perucca E. Clinically significant pharmacokinetic drug interactions with carbamazepine. An update. Clin Pharmacokinet 1996;31(3):198–214.

16. Sweet RA, Brown EJ, Heimberg RG, et al. Monoamine oxidase inhibitor dietary restrictions: what are we asking patients to give up? J Clin Psychiatry 1995;56(5):196–201.

17. Brown C, Taniguchi G, Yip K. The monoamine oxidase inhibitor-tyramine interaction. J Clin Pharmacol 1989;29(6):529–532.

18. Gillman PK. Monoamine oxidase inhibitors, opioid analgesics and serotonin toxicity. Br J Anaesth 2005;95(4):434–441.

19. Pacher P, Kecskemeti V. Cardiovascular side effects of new antidepressants and antipsychotics: new drugs, old concerns? Curr Pharm Des 2004;10(20):2463–2475.

20. Tung A, Chang JL, Garvey E, et al. Tricyclic antidepressants and cardiac arrhythmias during halothane-pancuronium anesthesia. Anesth Prog 1981;28(2):44, 48–49.

21. Young R. Update on Parkinson's disease. Am Fam Physician 1999;59(8):2155–2167.

22. Jackson S, Ham RJ, Wilkinson D. The safety and tolerability of donepezil in patients with Alzheimer's disease. Br J Clin Pharmacol 2004;58:1–8.

23. Hossain M, Jhee SS, Shiovitz T, et al. Estimation of the absolute bioavailability of rivastigmine in patients with mild to moderate dementia of the Alzheimer's type. Clin Pharmacokinet 2002;41:225–234.

24. Watkins PB, Zimmermann HJ, Knapp MJ, et al. Hepatotoxic effects of tacrine administration in patients with Alzheimer's disease. JAMA 1994;271:992–998.

25. Burns A, O'Brien J, BAP Dementia Consensus Group, et al. Clinical practice with anti-dementia drugs: a consensus statement from British Association for Psychopharmacology. J Psychopharmacol 2006;20:732–755.

26. Stoelting RK. Pharmacology and Physiology in Anesthetic Practice. 3rd ed. Philadelphia: Lippincott-Raven; 1999.

27. Van Deusen SK, Birkhahn RH, Gaeta TJ. Treatment of hyperkalemia in a patient with unrecognized digitalis toxicity. J Toxicol Clin Toxicol 2003;41(4):373–376.

28. Dec GW. Digoxin remains useful in the management of chronic heart failure. Med Clin North Am 2003;87(2):317–337.

29. Bartolone RS, Rao TL. Dysrhythmias following muscle relaxant administration in patients receiving digitalis. Anesthesiology 1983;58(6):567–569.

30. Crome P, Curl B, Holt D, et al. Digoxin and cimetidine: investigation of the potential for a drug interaction. Hum Toxicol 1985;4(4):391–399.

31. Mouser B, Nykamp D, Murphy JE, et al. Effect of cimetidine on oral digoxin absorption. DICP 1990;24(3):286–288.

32. Rooney RT, Marijic J, Stommel KA, et al. Additive cardiac depression by volatile anesthetics in isolated hearts after chronic amiodarone treatment. Anesth Analg 1995;85(5):917–924.

33. Camus P, Martin WJ 2nd, Rosenow EC 3rd. Amiodarone pulmonary toxicity. Clin Chest Med 2004;25(1):65–75.

34. Ursella S, Testa A, Mazzone M, et al. Amiodarone-induced thyroid dysfunction in clinical practice. Eur Rev Med Pharmacol Sci 2006;10(5):269–278.

35. Choudhury L, Grais IM, Passman RS. Torsades de pointes due to drug interaction between disopyramide and clarithromycin. Heart Dis 1999;1(4):206–207.

36. Feringa HH, Bax JJ, Bocrsma E, ct al. High-dose beta-blockers and tight heart rate control reduce myocardial ischemia and troponin T release in vascular surgery patients. Circulation 2006;114(1 Suppl):I344–349.

37. Kopecky SL. Effect of beta blockers, particularly carvedilol, on reducing the risk of events after acute myocardial infarction. Am J Cardiol 2006;98(8):1115–1119.

38. Pedersen ME, Cockcroft JR. The latest generation of beta-blockers: new pharmacologic properties. Curr Hypertens Rep 2006;8(4):279–286.

39. Hayashi Y, Sumikawa K, Kuro M, et al. Roles of beta 1- and beta 2-adrenoceptors in the mechanism of halothane myocardial sensitization in dogs. Anesth Analg 1991;72(4):435–439.

40. Grossman E, Messerli FH. Calcium antagonists. Prog Cardiovasc Dis 2004;47(1):34–57.

41. Pringle SD, MacEwen CJ. Severe bradycardia due to interaction of timolol eye drops and verapamil. BMJ 1987;294:155–156.

42. Wood M. Pharmacokinetic drug interactions in anaesthetic practice. Clin Pharmacokinet 1991;21(4):285–307.

43. Wali FA. Interaction of verapamil with gallamine and pancuronium and reversal of combined neuromuscular block ade with neostigmine and edrophonium. Eur J Anaesthesiol 1986;3(5):385–393.

44. Baciewicz AM, Baciewicz FA Jr. Effect of cimetidine and ranitidine on cardiovascular drugs. Am Heart J 1989;118(1):144–154.

45. Ray S, Dargie H. Infarct-related heart failure: the choice of ACE inhibitor does not matter. Cardiovasc Drugs Ther 1994;8(3):433–436.

46. Cruz CS, Cruz A, Marcilio de Souza CA. Hyperkalaemia in congestive heart failure patients using ACE inhibitors and spironolactone. Nephrol Dial Transplant 2003;18(9):1814–1819.

47. Huerta C, Lanes SF, Garcia Rodriguez LA. Respiratory medications and the risk of cardiac arrhythmias. Epidemiology 2005;16(3):360–366.

48. Wu RS, Wu KC, Wong TK, et al. Effects of fenoterol and ipratropium on respiratory resistance of asthmatics after tracheal intubation. Br J Anaesth 2000;84(3):358–362.

49. Koehntop DE, Liao JC, Van Bergen FH. Effects of pharmacologic alterations of adrenergic mechanisms by cocaine, tropolone, aminophylline, and ketamine on epinephrine-induced arrhythmias during halothane-nitrous oxide anesthesia. Anesthesiology 1977;46(2):83–93.

50. Hirshman CA, Krieger W, Littlejohn G, et al. Ketamine-aminophylline-induced decrease in seizure threshold. Anesthesiology 1982;56(6):464–467.

51. Flockhart DA, Desta Z, Mahal SK. Selection of drugs to treat gastro-oesophageal reflux disease: the role of drug interactions. Clin Pharmacokinet 2000;39(4):295–309.

52. Kao YJ, Tellez J, Turner DR. Dose-dependent effect of metoclopramide on cholinesterases and suxamethonium metabolism. Br J Anaesth 1990;65(2):220–224.

53. Gaga BF, Birman-Deych E, Kerzner R, et al. Incidence of intracranial hemorrhage in patients with atrial fibrillation who are prone to fall. Am J Med 2005;118(6):612–617.

54. Cappuzzo KA. Anticoagulation in elderly patients who fall frequently: a therapeutic dilemma. Consult Pharm 2005;20(7):601–605.

55. Sloane PD, Zimmerman S, Brown LC, et al. Inappropriate medication prescribing in residential care/assisted living facilities. J Am Geriatr Soc 2002;50(6):1001–1011.

56. Kubler PA, Pillans PI, Marrinan MC, et al. Concordance between clopidogrel use and prescribing guidelines. Intern Med J 2004;34(12):663–667.

57. Maio V, Yuen EJ, Novielli K, et al. Potentially inappropriate medication prescribing for elderly outpatients in Emilia Romagna, Italy: a population-based cohort study. Drugs Aging 2006;23(11):915–924.

58. Rossi AC, Hsu JP, Faich GA. Ulcerogenicity of piroxicam: an analysis of spontaneously reported data. Br Med J (Clin Res Ed) 1987;294(6565):147–150.

59. Johnson AG, Day RO. The problems and pitfalls of NSAID therapy in the elderly. Drugs Aging 1991;1(2):130–143.

60. Butt JH, Barthel JS, Moore RA. Clinical spectrum of the upper gastrointestinal effects of nonsteroidal anti-inflammatory drugs. Natural history, symptomatology, and significance. Am J Med 1988;84(2A):5–14.

61. Goodwin JS, Regan M. Cognitive dysfunction associated with naproxen and ibuprofen in the elderly. Arthritis Rheum 1982;25(8):1013–1015.

62. Caterino JM, Emond JA, Camargo CA Jr. Inappropriate medication administration to the acutely ill elderly: a nationwide emergency department study, 1992–2000. J Am Geriatr Soc 2004;52(11):1847–1855.

63. Fong HK, Sands LP, Leung JM. The role of postoperative analgesia in delirium and cognitive decline in elderly patients: a systematic review. Anesth Analg 2006;102:1255–1266.

64. Davis MP, Srivastava M. Demographics, assessment and management of pain in the elderly. Drugs Aging 2003;20(1):23–57.

65. Barkin RL, Barkin SJ, Barkin DS. Propoxyphene (dextropropoxyphene): a critical review of a weak opioid analgesic that should remain in antiquity. Am J Ther 2006;13(6):534–542.

66. Kamal-Bahl SJ, Stuart BC, Beers MH. Propoxyphene use and risk for hip fractures in older adults. Am J Geriatr Pharmacother 2006;4(3):219–226.

15
The Pharmacology of Opioids

Steven L. Shafer and Pamela Flood

There are a lot of old people. In the 1990 census, patients over the age of 65 comprised 12% of the United States population, or 30,000,000 people. That grew modestly, to 12.5%, by 2000. However, based on the United States population of 301,165,915 as of today,* that amounts to 38 million individuals. It should come as no surprise, therefore, that health care for the elderly consumes 5% of the United States gross domestic product.[1]

It is important that anesthesiologists understand the differences in pharmacology of opioids in elderly patients in order to be able to properly titrate these important analgesics. Below are the key points for this chapter:

1. Elderly patients need about half the dose as younger patients.

2. The reason is primarily pharmacodynamic (change in intrinsic sensitivity of the brain to the drug). The pharmacokinetic changes with age are modest.

3. Studies in elderly animals show reduced numbers of μ receptors with increased age. That does not explain the reduction in dose, as decreased receptor density should decrease sensitivity to opioids. The enhancement in drug effect seen in the clinic is more likely attributable to changes in cyclonucleotide coupling and other downstream changes that occur in aging.

4. Meperidine is a difficult drug to use in elderly patients. It should never be used in patient-controlled analgesia (PCA) and is best reserved for shivering.

General Observations

Opioids are among the most effective, and the most dangerous, of the drugs administered by anesthesiologists. This is why the World Health Organization proposed a three-step analgesic ladder for the treatment of chronic pain. They recommended starting with acetaminophen

and nonsteroidal analgesics, progressing to opioids of intermediate strength, such as codeine, and treating severe pain with strong opioids such as morphine.[2] The Agency for Health Care Policy and Research (now called the Agency for Healthcare Research and Quality) has issued similar guidelines.[3] Particular care must be taken when using opioids in elderly patients. It is nearly tautologic that elderly patients are more likely to suffer from chronic diseases than their younger counterparts. Some fortunate individuals remain physically vigorous until very late in life, whereas others seem to deteriorate physically at younger ages. Additionally, the cumulative effects of smoking, alcohol, and environmental toxins can accelerate the deterioration of aging in exposed individuals. Thus, it is not surprising that variability in physiology increases throughout life.[4] Increased physiologic variability results in increased pharmacokinetic and pharmacodynamic variability in elderly subjects. The clinical result of this increased variability is an increased incidence of adverse drug reactions in elderly patients.[5] Thus, elderly patients require more careful titration and, where possible and appropriate, therapeutic drug monitoring.[6]

In their secondary analysis of a retrospective cohort study, Cepeda and colleagues[7] noted that the risk of opioid-induced ventilatory depression increased with increasing age, with patients 61–70 years of age having 2.8 times the risk of ventilatory depression compared with patients 16–45 years old. Interestingly, in their analysis, they converted all of the opioids into morphine equivalents, and the conversion did not account for the increased potency of opioids in the elderly that will be described subsequently.

Although the risk of respiratory depression from opioids is greater in older people, the same is not true for all opioid side effects. Opioids are among the major causes of postoperative nausea and vomiting, increasing the risk nearly fourfold.[8] In the study by Cepeda et al., age was not a risk factor for nausea and vomiting.[7] In

---

*www.census.gov. Accessed February 17, 2007.

fact, age may actually decrease the risk of nausea and vomiting. Sinclair and colleagues[9] observed a 13% decrease in the risk of postoperative nausea and vomiting with each additional decade of life. This is consistent with the findings of Junger and colleagues.[8]

The Opioid Receptor

The existence of an opioid receptor was long suspected because of the high potency and stereoselectivity of pharmacologic antagonists. The biochemical discovery of opioid receptors was independently reported in 1973, by laboratories of Pert,[10] Simon,[11] and Terenius.[12] The finding of stereoselectivity led to an intense search for endogenous ligands, with identification of encephalin in 1975.[13] Other endogenous peptide ligands were isolated subsequently.[14,15] The fact that endogenous opioid ligands differed in their structure and binding sites suggested the existence of different opioid receptor types.[16] Three classes of opioid receptors were identified pharmacologically in the 1980s: μ (mu),[17] δ (delta),[18] and κ (kappa).[19]

Activation of the μ receptor is responsible for both the analgesic efficacy of the frequently used opioids and, unfortunately, for the majority of opioid toxicities. Shortly after characterization of the μ receptor, Pasternak and colleagues[20] demonstrated that there were two populations of opioid receptors: a high-affinity site, associated with analgesia and blocked by naloxazone, and a lower-affinity site, which was not blocked by naloxazone and seemed responsible for morphine lethality. It was subsequently demonstrated that morphine-induced analgesia was mediated by a population of receptors blocked by naloxonazine, which were termed μ1 receptors, whereas morphine-induced ventilatory depression was blocked by a population of receptors that were not affected by naloxonazine, which were termed the μ2 receptors.[21,22] To further complicate matters, a selective morphine-6-glucuronide antagonist was identified, 3-O-methylnaxtrexone, that had little effect on morphine analgesia.[23] This suggested that there was variability within the μ1 receptor itself. Although identification of a specific μ1 antagonist led to the hope that a μ1-specific agonist could be developed, no such agonist has ever been identified.

Additional evidence for μ receptor subtypes comes from the clinical observation of incomplete cross-tolerance among the opioids in patients,[24] so that if a patient is switched from an opioid to which the patient has become tolerant to an "equianalgesic" dosage of another opioid, the potential exists for serious overdose.[25] Additional evidence for multiple μ receptor subtypes comes from variance in the potency for analgesic efficacy and

toxicity among patients, such that there is no single opioid that has the best therapeutic window for all patients.[25] An extreme example of differential response to opioids is found in the CXBK mouse, which is insensitive to morphine but has normal sensitivity to fentanyl and morphine-6-glucuronide.[26]

The μ opioid subtypes have unique distributions within the body.[27] Specifically, μ1 is expressed in the brain, whereas μ2 is expressed in the brain, gastrointestinal tract, and the respiratory tract.[28] Activation of both μ receptor subtypes acts to decrease calcium and potassium conductance and intracellular adenosine 3',5'-cyclic monophosphate (cAMP). The recently discovered μ3 receptor is expressed on monocytes, granulocytes, and the vascular endothelium, where it acts to release nitric oxide.[29] Some of the vasodilatation that is associated with opioid administration that has been attributed to histamine release may be attributable to activation of the μ3 receptor.

The μ receptor is encoded by a single gene *Oprm*, located on chromosome 10 in the mouse[30,31] and on chromosome 6 in the human.[32] A variety of polymorphisms of *Oprm* have been identified in humans, as recently reviewed by Lötsch and Geisslinger.[32] The polymorphism that has generated the most interest has been the substitution of an aspartate for an asparagine in the 118 position, which is abbreviated the 118A > G SNP. This polymorphism has been associated with a decreased analgesic response to morphine. However, it does not reduce sensitivity to opioid-induced ventilatory depression.[33]

The *Oprm* gene gives rise to a family of μ receptors through selective splicing of the mRNA into μ opioid receptor subtypes.[34] In 1993, the first μ receptor was cloned, MOR-1.[35,36] Since then, at least 15 different splice variants of MOR-1 have been identified in mice, all derived from the same *Oprm* gene.[28] Several splice variants have been identified in humans as well.[37] Splice variants likely give rise to pharmacologically identified subtypes of μ receptors based on the exons that are translated. Unfortunately, mapping between individual splice variants and pharmacologically identified μ subtypes is incomplete. The currently identified splice variants are insufficient to explain the pharmacologic groupings, although this will likely become clearer as additional splice variants are discovered and characterized pharmacologically.

All opioid receptors so far identified are coupled to G proteins.[38] At the cellular level, the opioid receptors have an inhibitory effect. When the receptors are occupied by opioid agonists, intracellular cAMP content is reduced. Reduced levels of cAMP both increase the activation of K^+ channels and reduce the open probability of voltage-gated calcium channels. These changes cause hyperpolarization of the membrane potential and thus reduce neuronal excitability.[39]

Age and Opioid Receptors

End-organ sensitivity to various ligands changes with age. Part of this change is from differences at the level of the drug receptor-effector mechanism. For example, the number and structure of the β-adrenergic receptor is unchanged in the elderly myocardium. The decreased chronotropic and inotropic response of elderly patients to β-adrenergic drugs seems to result from downstream changes in the mechanism by which binding at the receptor is coupled to adrenergic response mechanism.[40] In the brain, there seems to be both decreased α- and β-adrenergic receptor density in elderly individuals.[41]

There is no decrease in the affinity or density of central nervous system benzodiazepine receptors with age.[42] Barnhill and colleagues[43] studied benzodiazepine binding in response to acute or chronic stress. In the absence of stress, there was no difference in the number or affinity of benzodiazepine receptors. In young rats, receptor binding was increased by acute stress, a response not observed in older animals. Chronic stress enhanced binding in both young and old rats, but the recovery following cessation of stress was delayed in older animals. Thus, there are age-associated changes in benzodiazepine binding, but only in the poststress condition.

Ueno and colleagues[44] examined opioid receptors in young, mature, and aged mice. Aged mice had reduced μ receptor density, but increased μ receptor affinity. Hess et al.[45] also observed decreased μ receptor density in rats with advancing age, associated with decreased sensitivity to pain. Similarly, Petkov and colleagues[46] observed decreased enkephalin receptors in aged rats, as well as decreased sensitivity to enkephalin. Aging may induce changes downstream of opioid receptor binding. In studies on opioid receptors in polymorphonuclear leucocytes, Fulop and colleagues[47] have shown that whereas cAMP was reduced on binding in cells from young adult animals, it was increased in cells from aged animals. Hoskins and Ho[48] have shown age-induced changes in the basal activities of adenylate cyclase, guanylate cyclase, cAMP phosphodiesterase, and cyclic guanosine monophosphate phosphodiesterase.

Smith and Gray[49] examined the analgesic response to opioids in young and aged rats. They applied noxious stimulus at two different stimulus intensities. At the low-intensity stimulus (immersing the tail in 50°C water), there was a trend toward increased sensitivity to opioids in the aged rats, but the difference was not statistically significant. However, when subjected to the high-intensity stimulus (immersing the tail in 55°C water), the aged rats were about twice as sensitive to opioids as the young rats, an effect that was statistically significant.

Other investigators have reached quite different conclusions using similar experimental paradigms (tail flick after immersion in hot water). Van Crugten and colleagues[50] looked at morphine antinociception in aged rats, and found no difference in antinociception between aged and adult animals. Hoskins and colleagues[51] found that aged mice were about half as sensitive to morphine as mature adult mice. Thus, the animal studies consistently show decreased numbers of opioid receptors in aged brains. However, the story about the antinociceptive response to morphine is less clear in animal models, with studies showing increased sensitivity, decreased sensitivity, or no change in sensitivity with advancing age.

Aging and Pain Perception

Pain is a part of daily life for many elderly patients, with about 50% of patients over the age of 70 reporting chronic pain.[52] Elderly patients are particularly more prone to chronic pain than younger people.[53,54] However, clinically it seems that pain in elderly subjects is indistinguishable from the experience of pain in younger subjects.[55]

There are some interesting differences between young and older subjects in their response to experimental pain. There is some evidence that older patients are more sensitive to experimental pain,[56] which may be explained, at least in part, by a reduction in the endogenous analgesic response to pain,[57,58] possibly mediated by reduced production of β-endorphin in response to noxious stimulation.[59] Older patients experience a more prolonged hyperalgesia after capsaicin injection compared with younger subjects.[60] However, older patients seem to also require a higher intensity of noxious stimulation before first reporting pain.[58]

Some of the differences between studies may also depend on exactly which pain pathways are activated during the assessment. Chakour and colleagues[61] demonstrated that pain transmission via C fibers was unchanged in young versus elderly subjects. However, there was a substantial reduction in pain transmission via Aδ fibers. Thus, the relative perceptions of pain in elderly subjects versus younger subjects were influenced by the extent of pain transmission via Aδ fibers.

The Onset and Offset of Opioid Drug Effect

Onset

The onset of opioid drug effect is determined by the route of delivery, the delivered dose, the pharmacokinetics of the opioid that determine the plasma concentrations over time, and the rate of blood–brain equilibration between the plasma and the site of drug effect. Table 15-1 shows adult pharmacokinetics of fentanyl,[62] alfentanil,[62]

TABLE 15-1. Pharmacokinetic parameters for frequently used opioids.

	Fentanyl	Alfentanil	Sufentanil	Remifentanil	Morphine	Methadone	Meperidine	Hydromorphone
Volumes (L)								
V_1	12.7	2.2	17.8	4.9	17.8	7.7	18.1	11.5
V_2	50	7	47	9	87	12	61	115
V_3	295	15	476	5	199	184	166	968
Clearances (L/min)								
Cl_1	0.62	0.20	1.16	2.44	1.26	0.13	0.76	1.33
Cl_2	4.82	1.43	4.84	1.75	2.27	2.19	5.44	3.45
Cl_3	2.27	0.25	1.29	0.06	0.33	0.38	1.79	0.92
Exponents (min^{-1})								
α	0.67	1.03	0.48	0.96	0.23	0.50	0.51	0.51
β	0.037	0.052	0.030	0.103	0.010	0.025	0.031	0.012
γ	0.0015	0.0062	0.0012	0.0116	0.0013	0.0005	0.0026	0.0005
Half-lives (min)								
$t_{1/2}\alpha$	1.03	0.67	1.43	0.73	2.98	1.38	1.37	1.35
$t_{1/2}\beta$	19	13	23	7	68	28	22	59
$t_{1/2}\gamma$	475	111	562	60	548	1377	271	1261
Blood–brain equilibration								
k_{e0} (min^{-1})	0.147	0.770	0.112	0.525	0.005	0.110	0.067	0.015
$t_{1/2}k_{e0}$ (min)	4.7	0.9	6.2	1.3	139	6.3	10.	46
T_{peak} (min)	3.7	1.4	5.8	1.6	93.8	11.3	8.5	19.6
VD peak effect (L)	76.9	6.0	94.9	17.0	590.2	30.9	143.3	383.3

Note: The references for the pharmacokinetic parameters are given in the text.
VD = volume of distribution.

sufentanil,[63] remifentanil,[64] morphine,[65] methadone,[66†] meperidine,[67‡] and hydromorphone.[68] Table 15-1 also shows k_{e0}, the rate constant for blood–effect-site equilibration, for fentanyl,[62] alfentanil,[62] sufentanil,[69] remifentanil,[64] morphine,[65] methadone,[70] meperidine,[71§] and hydromorphone.[72‖] Based on these data, it is possible to predict the time course of concentration change in the plasma following an intravenous bolus, as seen in Figure 15-1. The upper graph in Figure 15-1 shows the concentration during 24 hours following a bolus injection, whereas the lower graph just shows the first 30 minutes. In both cases, the curves have been normalized to start at 100%, which permits direct comparison of the pharmacokinetics despite differing potencies. As seen in the upper graph, the extremes of plasma elimination are remifentanil, which is ultra fast, and methadone, which has the longest half-life. Alfentanil has the second-shortest half-life among the eight opioids. Fentanyl, meperidine, sufentanil, hydromorphone, and morphine are all clustered in the middle. In particular, note how similar hydromorphone and morphine are when one examines the plasma pharmacokinetics. Approximately the same trend is observed in the first 30 minutes, although the initial distribution phase of hydromorphone takes it nearly as low as remi-

†Data extensively reanalyzed to obtain volume and clearance estimates.
‡Original data provided by S. Bjorkman and fit using population model to create estimates in Table 15-1.
§Based on a time to peak of 8.5 minutes in goats (!). It's not great, but it's the best onset data available.
‖Based on a time to peak effect of 15–20 minutes.

fentanil in the first 10 minutes. As will be seen shortly, this is significant in terms of recovery.

The plasma is not the site of drug effect, and thus the time course of concentration seen in Figure 15-1 will not reflect the time course of effect-site concentration or behavioral activity. By incorporating the plasma–effect-site equilibration delay into our calculations, we can examine the time course of the onset of drug effect, as shown in Figure 15-2. In this case, we have normalized the effect-site concentrations to peak-effect concentration[73] to again permit comparisons of the time course of drugs independent of the differences in potency. Alfentanil and remifentanil both reach a peak about 1.5 minutes after bolus injection, although the overall remifentanil drug effect is more evanescent. The peak fentanyl concentration occurs about 3.5 minutes after bolus injection, whereas the peak sufentanil effect is about 6 minutes after bolus injection. Methadone and meperidine are nearly indistinguishable following bolus injection, each reaching a peak about 12 minutes after a bolus. The peak for hydromorphone is 15–20 minutes after the bolus. Morphine is the outlier in terms of onset. Five minutes after a bolus injection, morphine is at 50% of the peak concentration. However, morphine reaches its peak concentration in the effect site about 90 minutes after the bolus injection. Table 15-1 shows the time to reach peak concentration for each of the opioids, as well as the volume of distribution at the time of peak effect, which is useful for calculating initial loading doses.[74–76]

One of the key benefits to knowing the time course of drug effect following bolus injection is logical programming of the lockout of PCA devices. A 10-minute lockout for hydromorphone and methadone is a logical choice, because patients are able to make a decision to redose themselves after reaching peak drug effect. The slower onset of morphine is somewhat problematic, because patients will administer another dose while the prior dose is still coming on, creating the possibility of stacking bolus doses.

Considerable attention is given to "equianalgesic dosing" of opioids. The calculation of the equianalgesic dose is complicated by both the relative intrinsic potency of the opioids, the different pharmacokinetic profiles, and the large differences in the rate of blood–brain equilibration. Table 15-2 shows equianalgesic doses of frequently used opioids, based on the "minimum effective analgesic concentrations" or "MEAC" (also called "MEC") of fentanyl,[77] alfentanil,[78] sufentanil,¶ remifentanil,# morphine,[79]** methadone,[80] meperidine,[81] and

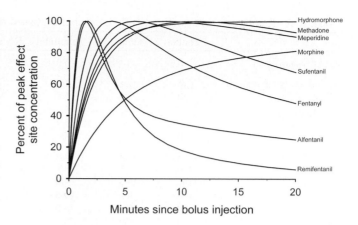

FIGURE 15-2. The time course of effect-site concentration following a bolus of fentanyl, alfentanil, sufentanil, remifentanil, morphine, methadone, meperidine, and hydromorphone, based on the pharmacokinetics and rate of plasma–effect-site equilibrium shown in Table 15-1. The curves have been normalized to the peak effect-site concentration, permitting comparison of the relative rate of increase independent of dose. The times to peak effect correspond to those shown in Table 15-1.

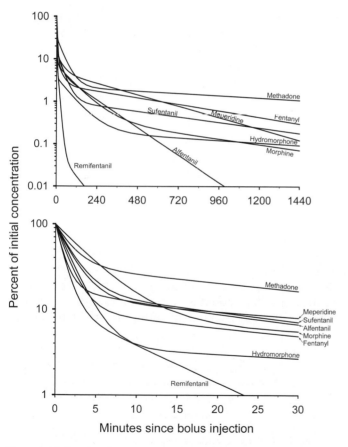

FIGURE 15-1. The time course of plasma concentration following a bolus of fentanyl, alfentanil, sufentanil, remifentanil, morphine, methadone, meperidine, and hydromorphone, based on the pharmacokinetics shown in Table 15-1. The y-axis is the percent of the initial concentration, which by definition is 100% at time 0, permitting display of the relative time courses of these opioids independent of the dose administered.

hydromorphone.[82,83]†† Reflecting anesthesiologists' familiarity with fentanyl, all of the calculations have been made using fentanyl as the reference opioid. The calculation of an equianalgesic bolus dose depends on when the observation of drug effect is made. For example, because fentanyl has a very rapid onset, and morphine has a very slow onset, 5 mg of morphine has the same effect at 10 minutes as 50 μg of fentanyl, whereas 60 minutes after the dose, 1 mg of morphine has the same effect as 50 μg of fentanyl. Similarly, because the drugs accumulate during infusions at different rates, the relative potencies of the opioids change depending on how long the infusion has been running, as shown in Table 15-2.

Figure 15-3 shows the increase in effect-site concentration during a continuous infusion for each of these opioids. As expected, remifentanil increases the fastest, whereas methadone increases the slowest. Note, however, that even after 10 hours of drug administration, most of these opioids are only at 60%–80% of the eventual

¶Scaled to fentanyl based on relative electroencephalogram (EEG) potency of fentanyl[62] and sufentanil.[69]
#Scaled to fentanyl based on the relative EEG potency of fentanyl and remifentanil.[64]
**The MEC range given by Dahlstrom was 6–31 ng/mL, with a mean of 16 ng/mL. We chose 8 ng/mL, at the lower end of the reported range, because the average value of 16 ng/mL predicted equianalgesic morphine that seemed excessive.
††This was the most difficult potency to determine from the literature. Hill and Zacny documented a tenfold bolus dose potency difference versus morphine, which was the final basis for calculating this number, and is similar to the value suggested by the Coda paper.

TABLE 15-2. Relative potency of frequently used opioids, based on the time of the observed effect.

	Fentanyl	Alfentanil	Sufentanil	Remifentanil	Morphine	Methadone	Meperidine	Hydromorphone
MEAC (ng/mL)	0.6	14.9	0.056	1.0	8	60	250	1.5
Equipotent bolus dose at:	(µg)	(µg)	(µg)	(µg)	(mg)	(mg)	(mg)	(mg)
Peak effect	50	92	5.5	17	4.9	1.9	37	0.6
10 minutes	50	197	4.4	72	5.3	1.4	28	0.4
30 minutes	50	174	3.9	282	2.0	0.9	17	0.2
60 minutes	50	175	4.8	1680	1.0	0.9	14	0.1
Equipotent infusion rate at:	(µg/h)	(µg/h)	(µg/h)	(µg/h)	(mg/h)	(mg/h)	(mg/h)	(mg/h)
1 hour	100	323	8.8	135	5.3	2.3	43	0.6
2 hours	100	332	9.6	182	3.3	2.3	38	0.4
4 hours	100	365	11.6	252	2.3	2.6	36	0.4
6 hours	100	409	13.0	310	2.1	2.9	37	0.4
12 hours	100	536	15.1	436	2.2	3.1	40	0.5
24 hours	100	675	16.3	554	2.4	2.9	45	0.6

Note: The references for the relative potency are given in the text.
MEAC = mean effective analgesic concentration.

steady-state concentration. This speaks to the problem of background infusions for PCA. Even after many hours, patients are not at steady state, and the increasing drug concentration from the background infusion may expose a patient to toxicity 12–24 hours after initiation of the infusion. Given the increased sensitivity of elderly patients to the effects of opioids, background infusions are likely a particularly poor choice in this population.

Offset

The offset of drug effect is a function of both the pharmacokinetic behavior and the rate of blood–brain equilibration. The "context sensitive half-time"[73,84] is a useful way to consider the plasma pharmacokinetic portion of the offset time, as shown in Figure 15-4. The *x*-axis on Figure 15-4 is the duration of an infusion that maintains

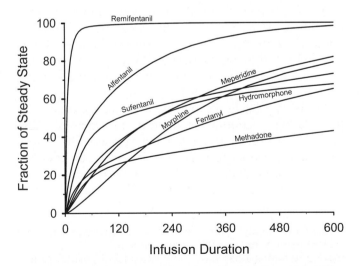

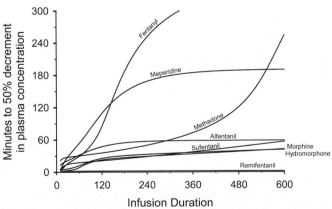

FIGURE 15-3. The increase to steady state during an infusion of fentanyl, alfentanil, sufentanil, remifentanil, morphine, methadone, meperidine, and hydromorphone, based on the pharmacokinetics and rate of plasma–effect-site equilibrium shown in Table 15-1. The curves have been normalized to the steady-state effect-site concentration, permitting comparison of the relative rate of increase independent of infusion rate. Only remifentanil and alfentanil are at steady state after 10 hours of continuous infusion.

FIGURE 15-4. The "context-sensitive half-time" (50% plasma decrement time) for fentanyl, alfentanil, sufentanil, remifentanil, morphine, methadone, meperidine, and hydromorphone, based on the pharmacokinetics shown in Table 15-1. Remifentanil shows virtually no accumulation over time with continuous infusions, whereas the offset of fentanyl changes considerably as it is administered to maintain a steady plasma concentration.

a steady concentration of drug in the plasma. The *y*-axis is the time required for the concentrations to decrease by 50% after the infusion is terminated. Remifentanil's pharmacokinetics are so fast that the context-sensitive half-time blurs right into the *x*-axis. Perhaps surprisingly, fentanyl is the outlier here. Fentanyl accumulates in fat, and so an infusion that maintains a steady concentration in the plasma winds up giving patients a whopping dose of fentanyl, resulting in slow recovery. Meperidine similarly shows long recovery. Note that for infusions of less than 10 hours, morphine, hydromorphone, and sufentanil are nearly indistinguishable based on the plasma pharmacokinetics.

Once again, we have to consider that the plasma is not the site of drug effect. Therefore, we must consider the 50% effect-site decrement time,[73,85] as shown in Figure 15-5. Because fentanyl and remifentanil have very rapid plasma–effect-site equilibration, they have changed little between Figures 15-4 and 15-6. Note, however, the huge change for morphine and hydromorphone. One might have thought from Figure 15-4 that these drugs would result in rapid offset of drug effect following a continuous infusion. This is clearly not the case, because the blood–brain equilibration delay results in these drugs having far slower offset than alfentanil or sufentanil. The "surprise" here is methadone. One would rarely think of methadone as a reasonable choice for infusion during anesthesia, but the pharmacokinetics of methadone

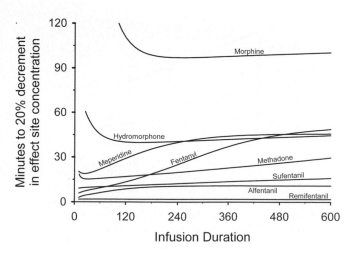

FIGURE 15-6. The 20% effect-site decrement curves for fentanyl, alfentanil, sufentanil, remifentanil, morphine, methadone, meperidine, and hydromorphone, based on the pharmacokinetics and rate of plasma–effect-site equilibrium shown in Table 15-1. The effect-site levels of all opioids, except morphine, will decrease by 20% quickly when an infusion is terminated. The slower decrease for morphine is because of its slow plasma–effect-site equilibration.

suggest that it might be a reasonable choice for anesthetics of 4 hours or less.

Figure 15-6 shows the 20% effect-site decrement curve for these eight opioids. Figure 15-6 speaks to how often one might expect to redose a patient with chronic pain who is titrating the analgesic level to a just-adequate concentration. Because of its slow blood–brain equilibration, morphine would need to be given approximately every 2 hours. Hydromorphone, fentanyl, and methadone would need to be given approximately every hour.

Specific Opioids

Morphine

Morphine has three unique aspects among the opioids frequently used in anesthesia practice: it is an endogenous ligand of the μ receptor, has an active metabolite, and has a very slow onset of effect. Morphine was initially identified in the brains of mice that had never been exposed to exogenous morphine.[86] It has subsequently been found in the brains of cows,[87] rats,[88] and humans.[89] Codeine has also been identified as an endogenously synthesized substance. However, because codeine is mostly an inactive prodrug of morphine, its presence in the brain does not diminish morphine's distinction as the only endogenous ligand of the μ receptor that is also a frequently administered drug.

Morphine is metabolized by glucuronidation into two metabolites, morphine-3-glucuronide, which is mostly

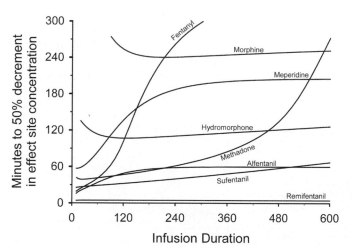

FIGURE 15-5. The 50% effect-site decrement curves for fentanyl, alfentanil, sufentanil, remifentanil, morphine, methadone, meperidine, and hydromorphone, based on the pharmacokinetics and rate of plasma–effect-site equilibrium shown in Table 15-1. For drugs with rapid plasma–effect-site equilibrium, the 50% effect-site decrement curve closely follows the context sensitive half-time curve. However, for drugs with slow plasma–effect-site equilibration, a 50% decrement in effect-site concentration is considerably slower than a 50% decrement in plasma concentration (e.g., morphine).

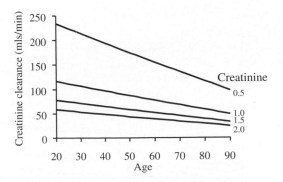

FIGURE 15-7. The relationship among age, serum creatinine, and creatinine clearance, based on the equation of Cockroft and Gault. (Adapted with permission from Cockcroft and Gault.[96])

inactive, and morphine-6-glucuronide, which is itself a potent analgesic.[90] Although the potency of intrathecal morphine-6-glucuronide is 650-fold higher than that of morphine,[91] morphine-6-glucuronide crosses the blood–brain barrier very slowly, so slowly that it is unlikely that it contributes to the acute analgesia provided by morphine.[92,93] However, with chronic administration, the levels of morphine-6-glucuronide will increase to pharmacologically active concentrations.[94]

Morphine-6-glucuronide is eliminated by the kidneys.[95] Creatinine clearance is reduced with advancing age, as shown in the often cited equation of Cockroft and Gault[96]:

Men: Creatinine clearance (mL/min)
  = {[140 − age (years)] × weight (kg)}/
    [72 × serum creatinine (mg%)]

Women: 85% of the above.

Figure 15-7 shows the relationship among creatinine, age, and creatinine clearance according to the above equation. The key observation from Figure 15-7 is that, *even in the presence of normal creatinine*, the creatinine clearance of an 80-year-old patient will be about half that in a 20-year-old patient. Thus, morphine-6-glucuronide will accumulate more in elderly patients, necessitating a reduction in dose of chronically administered morphine. Of course, if the patient has renal insufficiency, it might be better to select an opioid without an active metabolite.

The second unique aspect to morphine is the slow onset of effect. The peak effect following a bolus dose of morphine occurs approximately 90 minutes after the bolus. This has been demonstrated using pupillometry,[97–99] ventilatory depression,[98] and analgesia[99] as measures of morphine drug effect. The likely explanation for this is that morphine is a substrate for P-glycoprotein, which actively transports morphine out of the central nervous system.[100]

Figure 15-8 shows a simulation of the analgesic (y-axis > 1) and ventilatory (y-axis < 1) effects of three different morphine doses: a bolus of 0.2 mg/kg, a bolus of 0.2 mg/kg followed by an infusion of 1 mg/70 kg per hour, and repeated boluses of 0.1 mg/kg every 6 hours.[101] The solid line is the median prediction, whereas the shaded area represents the 95% confidence bounds. As seen in Figure 15-8, the time course of analgesia and ventilatory depression is similar, although the analgesia wanes somewhat faster than the ventilatory depression.

It is important to appreciate the slow onset of morphine when titrating to effect. Aubrun and colleagues[102,103] have advocated postoperative titration of morphine in elderly patients by administering 2- to 3-mg boluses every 5 minutes. This is not logical for a drug with a peak effect

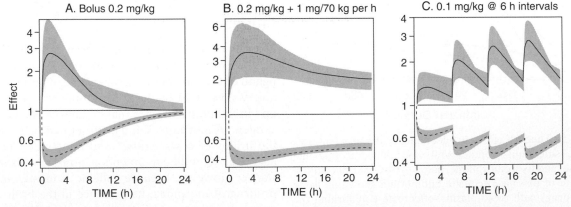

FIGURE 15-8. Simulated analgesic (y > 1) and ventilatory (y < 1) effects of three different doses of morphine: 0.2 mg/kg (**A**), 0.2 mg/kg plus an infusion of 1 mg/70 kg/h (**B**), and a bolus of 0.1 mg/kg every 6 hours (**C**). The analgesic and ventilatory effects peak concurrently, about 90 minutes after the morphine bolus. Because the concentration versus response relationship is steeper for analgesia than ventilatory depression, the analgesic effect dissipates before the ventilatory depression. (Reprinted with permission from Dahan et al.[101] Copyright © Lippincott Williams & Wilkins.)

about 1.5 hours after bolus injection. Aubrun and colleagues did not see any toxicity with this approach. That is surprising, given the potential for accumulation with repeated titration of small doses of morphine to effect. However, it does explain why their study is unique in finding that elderly patients require the same amount of opioid as younger patients.

Meperidine

The bottom line on meperidine is that it has little role in the management of pain. Meperidine is still a popular drug because of familiarity of its use, particularly among surgeons and obstetricians. Meperidine is unique among opioids in that it has significant local anesthetic activity.[104,105] Meperidine has been used as the sole analgesic intrathecally for obstetric anesthesia, but its benefit over a combination of local anesthetic with another opioid is unclear. One logical use of meperidine is in the treatment of postoperative shivering, in which doses of 10–20 mg are typically effective.

The problems with meperidine are its complex pharmacology and its toxic metabolite. Holmberg and colleagues[106] examined the pharmacokinetics of an intravenous meperidine bolus in young and elderly surgical subjects. They found that elderly patients had reduced meperidine clearance, resulting in a longer half-life for meperidine. There was minimal change in the initial volume of distribution. The clinical implication is that the initial dose of meperidine in elderly subjects should not be reduced based on pharmacokinetics, but meperidine will accumulate in elderly subjects with repeated administration. This makes meperidine a particularly poor choice for administration by PCA in elderly patients.[107]

A worrisome aspect of meperidine is the toxic metabolite, normeperidine. In a subsequent study, Holmberg and colleagues examined the renal excretion of both meperidine and normeperidine in elderly surgical patients.[108] Renal excretion was reduced in elderly patients, particularly for normeperidine. The result is that normeperidine will likely accumulate with repeated doses in elderly patients. Because normeperidine is highly epileptogenic, meperidine is probably a poor choice for PCA or other forms of continuous opioid delivery in elderly patients.

Meperidine has several other unique aspects to its pharmacology. It is the only negative inotrope among the opioids.[109] Meperidine also has intrinsic anticholinergic properties, which can result in tachycardia. Elderly patients with coronary artery disease are clearly at risk for adverse events if given drugs that have negative inotropic or positive chronotropic effects.

Last, meperidine is associated with several unusual reactions, including the potential for acute serotonergic syndrome when combined with a monoamine oxidase (MAO)-A inhibitor. Fortunately, the classic MAO-A inhibitors, phenelzine (Nardil), tranylcypromine (Parnate), and isocarboxazid (Marplan) are now rarely used. Selegiline, often used in Parkinson's disease, is a weak MAO-B inhibitor, and has been implicated in one nonfatal interaction with meperidine.[110] However, given the polypharmacy common in elderly patients, it would seem wise to avoid using meperidine when opioids with more selective pharmacology and inactive metabolites are available.

Hydromorphone

Hydromorphone in many aspects acts as a rapid-onset morphine. However, it lacks the histamine release associated with morphine and does not have active metabolites. There are no studies explicitly examining the role of age in hydromorphone pharmacokinetics or pharmacodynamics. In fact, there are surprisingly few studies examining perioperative use of hydromorphone. Keeri-Szanto[111] found intraoperative hydromorphone to be approximately 8 times more potent than morphine, with a half-life of 4 hours versus 5 hours for morphine. Kopp et al.[112] investigated whether 4 mg of hydromorphone provided any evidence of preemptive analgesia. It did not.

Rapp and colleagues[113] compared hydromorphone PCA to morphine PCA in postoperative patients following lower abdominal surgery. They found that hydromorphone PCA was associated with better mood scores, but with increased incidence of nausea and vomiting. They found that 1 mg of hydromorphone was approximately equianalgesic with 5 mg of morphine. This is about twice as potent as suggested by Hill and Zacny,[83] who determined that hydromorphone was tenfold more potent than morphine. Although Rapp and colleagues did not specifically study the effects of age, one would expect this ratio to be independent of age in the immediate postoperative period. Because morphine has an active metabolite that accumulates and hydromorphone does not, the apparent potency of morphine relative to hydromorphone may increase with chronic administration.

Lui and colleagues[114] compared epidural hydromorphone to intravenous hydromorphone, both administered by PCA in a double-blind/double-dummy protocol. They found more pruritus in patients receiving epidural hydromorphone, but no differences in postoperative analgesia, bowel function, or patient satisfaction. Overall, hydromorphone in the epidural group was half of that in the intravenous group, indicating that hydromorphone is acting spinally when administered via the epidural route. Hydromorphone and morphine both reach their peak concentrations in the cervical cerebrospinal fluid about 60 minutes after epidural administration,[115] suggesting they have similar potential for delayed ventilatory depression after epidural administration. In a study of obstetric patients, Halpern and colleagues[116] found 0.6 mg of hydromorphone to be clinically indistinguishable from 3 mg of morphine, consistent with the 1:5 relative potency reported for intravenous hydromorphone and morphine in the postoperative period.

Fentanyl

Fentanyl is among the "cleanest" opioids in terms of pharmacology. It has a rapid onset, predictable metabolism, and inactive metabolites. It is (obviously) the first of the "fentanyl" series of opioids, notable for their rapid metabolism and selective μ potency. It is the only one of the opioids that is available for transdermal and transmucosal delivery, although these methods of administration are being investigated for sufentanil as well.

Bentley et al.[117] studied aging and fentanyl pharmacokinetics in young and elderly groups of patients. They found that fentanyl clearance was decreased among the elderly, resulting in a prolonged half-life.

Scott and Stanski[62] used high-resolution arterial sampling during and after a brief fentanyl infusion to characterize the influence of age on the pharmacokinetics of fentanyl. These investigators did not find any effect of age on the pharmacokinetics of fentanyl or alfentanil, except for a small change in rapid intercompartmental clearance.

The minimal influence of age on the pharmacokinetics of fentanyl was subsequently confirmed by Singleton and colleagues.[118] These investigators found no change in the dose-adjusted concentration of fentanyl between young and elderly patients, except for a transient increase in concentration in elderly individuals at 2 and 4 minutes after the start of the infusion. These findings are consistent with the decreased rapid intercompartmental clearance reported by Scott and Stanski.

Scott and Stanski used the EEG as a measure of drug effect to estimate the potency of fentanyl.[62,119] They observed a decrease of approximately 50% in the dose required for 50% of maximal EEG suppression (C_{50}) from age 20 to age 85, as shown in Figure 15-9. Because the pharmacokinetics of fentanyl seem nearly unchanged by age, it is likely that elderly patients require less fentanyl because of intrinsic increased sensitivity to opioids. Put another way—the elderly brain is twice as sensitive to opioids as a younger brain. This predicts that elderly patients require half of the fentanyl that younger patients require. Because the pharmacodynamics of fentanyl (i.e., the C_{50}) is affected by age, and not the pharmacokinetics, the offset of fentanyl drug effect in elderly patients who receive an appropriately reduced dose of fentanyl should be as fast as it is in younger patients.

The 50% reduction in fentanyl suggested by Scott and Stanski's integrated pharmacokinetic/pharmacodynamic model is in reasonable agreement with an analysis by

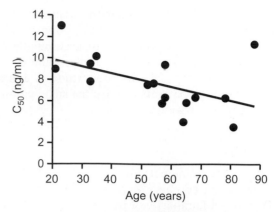

FIGURE 15-9. The influence of age on the 50% maximal effective dose (C_{50}) of fentanyl, as measured by electroencephalogram depression. Although there is considerable variability, overall there is about a 50% reduction in C_{50} from age 20 to age 80, reflecting increased brain sensitivity. This has been shown for alfentanil[62] and remifentanil,[64] and appears to be a class effect of opioids. (Adapted with permission from Scott JC, Stanski DR. Decreased fentanyl/alfentanil dose requirment with increasing age: A pharmacodynamic basis. J Pharmacol Exp Ther 240:159–166, 1987.)

Martin and colleagues[120] of intraoperative fentanyl utilization. Using the automated electronic record system in place at Duke University Hospital, they found that intraoperative doses of fentanyl decreased by about 10% per decade after age 30. Apparently, clinicians have integrated this information into their practice appropriately, at least at Duke University Hospital.

Other Fentanyl Delivery Systems

Fentanyl is also available in two unique dosage forms: oral transmucosal fentanyl citrate and transdermal fentanyl. Holdsworth and colleagues[121] studied pharmacokinetics and tolerability of a 20-cm^2 transdermal fentanyl patch in young and elderly subjects. Plasma fentanyl concentrations were nearly twofold higher in the elderly subjects compared with younger subjects, reflecting either increased absorption or decreased clearance. Given that fentanyl clearance seems unchanged in the elderly, the likely explanation is that transdermal fentanyl absorption is more rapid in elderly patients, possibly because the skin is thinner and poses less of a barrier to fentanyl absorption. The increased concentrations in elderly subjects were associated with increased adverse events—so much so that the patch was removed for the study in every elderly subject, whereas none of the patches were removed in younger subjects.

Davis and colleagues[122] also noted that the time course of absorption of fentanyl through the skin is delayed in the elderly, with subcutaneous fat acting as secondary reservoir leading to prolonged release even after the removal of the patch.

Kharasch and colleagues[123] examined the influence of age on the pharmacokinetics and pharmacodynamics of oral transmucosal fentanyl citrate (the fentanyl "lollipop"). They found no change in the pharmacokinetics of fentanyl with age, including the absorption characteristics of the buccal mucosa. Perhaps unexpectedly, they also found no increase in sensitivity to fentanyl, as measured by pupillary miosis. Thus, in their view, the data do not support reducing the dose of oral transmucosal fentanyl citrate in elderly patients.

Alfentanil

The relationship between opioids and age becomes more complex when we consider alfentanil. Scott and Stanski[62] reported similar findings for alfentanil as previously described for fentanyl. In particular, they did not find any effect of age on the pharmacokinetics of alfentanil, except for a small change in the terminal half-life. Shafer et al.[124] also reported no relationship between age and alfentanil pharmacokinetics. Sitar and colleagues[125] reported a modest decrease in alfentanil clearance and central compartment volume in elderly subjects. In a study that used historical control data, Kent and colleagues[126] also reported a modest decrease in alfentanil clearance with advancing age. Lemmens et al.[127] observed that the pharmacokinetics of alfentanil in men (as studied exclusively by Scott and Stanski) were unaffected by age, whereas the pharmacokinetics in women showed a clear negative correlation between age and clearance.

In an effort to sort out these modestly conflicting results, Maitre et al.[128] pooled alfentanil concentration data from multiple prior studies and performed a population pharmacokinetic analysis to estimate the influence of age and gender on the pharmacokinetics of alfentanil. Maitre et al. found that clearance decreased with age, and that the volume of distribution at steady state increased with age, the net effect being a longer terminal half-life with increasing age. That might sound like the end of the story, except that Raemer and colleagues[129] prospectively tested the Maitre et al. pharmacokinetics in two groups of patients, young women and elderly men, using computer-controlled drug administration. In this prospective test, the pharmacokinetics reported by Maitre et al. did *not* accurately predict the observed plasma alfentanil concentrations. However, pharmacokinetics reported by Scott and Stanski, which predict no influence of age or gender on alfentanil pharmacokinetics, accurately predicted the concentrations in both young women and elderly men. From these results, we can conclude that pharmacokinetics of alfentanil do not change in a clinically significant manner with age.

Although they found no change in pharmacokinetics with age, Scott and Stanski demonstrated that the C_{50} for EEG depression with alfentanil decreased by 50% in elderly subjects, nearly identical to the increased potency of fentanyl in elderly subjects.[62] This would suggest that, based on pharmacokinetic alterations with age, the dose of alfentanil in elderly patients should be about half of the dose that would be used in younger patients. Unfortunately, subsequent studies by Lemmens et al.,[130–132] based on clinical endpoints, found no influence of age on the pharmacodynamics of alfentanil. However, Lemmens et al.[133] observed that the alfentanil dose required to maintain adequate anesthesia, when administered by target-controlled infusion, was decreased by approximately 50% in elderly subjects. Thus, Lemmens et al. saw a similar change in dose-response relationship, in that the elderly required half as much opioid as younger subjects, but could not explain it as a pharmacodynamic difference. However, it is a bigger difference in concentration than any of the pharmacokinetic studies would have predicted, and there was no control group—the control group was a historical control group.

Where this leaves us is that there are many studies suggesting that the alfentanil dose in elderly subjects is about half of the dose in younger subjects. The available data suggest that the change is probably pharmacodynamic, but there may be a pharmacokinetic component to the increased sensitivity as well. If the change is mostly pharmacodynamic, perhaps, with a modest change in terminal half-life in elderly subjects, then the offset of alfentanil should be as fast in older subjects as it is in younger subjects, provided the dose has been appropriately reduced.

Sufentanil

Sufentanil is the most potent of the available opioids, with potency approximately tenfold greater than fentanyl.[134] Age has, at most, only a modest influence on sufentanil pharmacokinetics. Helmers and colleagues[135] found no change in sufentanil pharmacokinetics between young and elderly subjects. Similarly, Gepts and colleagues[136] found no effect of age on sufentanil pharmacokinetics in a complex population analysis. Matteo and colleagues[137] found that the central compartment volume of sufentanil was significantly decreased in elderly patients. This modest pharmacokinetic difference in elderly subjects would be expected to increase the effects of sufentanil in the first few minutes after a bolus dose and not subsequently. However, the elderly patients in Matteo's study were far more sensitive to sufentanil than the younger subjects. Six of seven elderly patients required naloxone at the end of this study, whereas only one of seven young patients required naloxone. Matteo et al. concluded that elderly patients had increased sensitivity to a given concentration of sufentanil, similar to the increased sensitivity to fentanyl and alfentanil in elderly patients described by Scott and Stanski.

Thus, based on the twofold increase in brain sensitivity to opioids demonstrated for fentanyl and alfentanil in elderly patients, one might expect similar increase in brain sensitivity to sufentanil in elderly patients. Thus, it is surprising that Hofbauer and colleagues[138] did not observe any influence of age on the sufentanil requirement of mechanically ventilated patients in the intensive care unit.

Remifentanil

Remifentanil has the fastest and most predictable metabolism of any of the available opioids. Remifentanil was introduced into clinical practice under Food and Drug Administration guidelines that mandated explicit pharmacokinetic and pharmacodynamic analysis for special populations, including elderly subjects. Thus, the influence of age on remifentanil pharmacokinetics and pharmacodynamics was established in high-resolution trials about 3 times larger than the trials for fentanyl, alfentanil, or sufentanil. The pharmacokinetic and pharmacodynamic models for remifentanil were reported by Minto and colleagues.[64] In a companion article, Minto et al.[139] used computer simulation to examine the implications of the complex age-related changes on remifentanil dosing. The pharmacokinetics of remifentanil change with age, as shown in Figure 15-10. With advancing age, V_1, the volume of the central compartment, decreases about 20% from

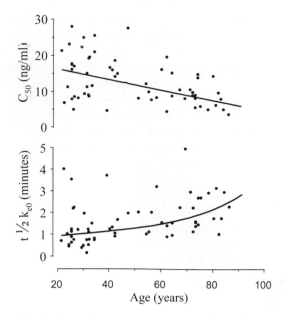

FIGURE 15-11. The influence of age on remifentanil pharmacodynamics. With advancing age, the 50% effective concentration (EC_{50}) declines, reflecting a nearly identical increase in intrinsic potency as seen with fentanyl and alfentanil. Additionally, half-time of blood–brain equilibration ($t_{1/2} k_{e0}$) increases. (Adapted with permission from Minto et al.[64])

age 20 to 80. Concurrently, clearance decreases about 30% from age 20 to age 80. Figure 15-11 shows the age-related changes in remifentanil pharmacodynamics. As also observed for fentanyl and alfentanil, the C_{50} for EEG depression is reduced by 50% in elderly subjects, suggesting that remifentanil has about twice the intrinsic potency in elderly subjects as in younger subjects. The $t_{1/2} k_{e0}$, half-time of plasma–effect-site equilibration, is also increased in elderly subjects. In the absence of other changes, this would mean that the onset and offset of remifentanil drug effect will be slower in elderly patients.

Figure 15-12 uses computer simulations to examine the time course of blood concentration (solid lines) and effect-site concentration (dashed lines) after a unit bolus of remifentanil. The blood concentrations are higher in elderly subjects because of the smaller central compartment concentration. However, the slower $t_{1/2} k_{e0}$ in elderly subjects results in less-rapid equilibration. As a result, the effect-site concentrations in elderly individuals do not increase higher than the effect-site concentrations in young individuals. However, the onset and offset are slower in elderly individuals. For example, in a young individual, the peak drug effect is expected about 90 seconds after a bolus injection. In an elderly individual, the peak effect is expected about 2–3 minutes after bolus injection.

Figure 15-13 shows the influence of age and weight on remifentanil dosing. As seen in the top graph of Figure

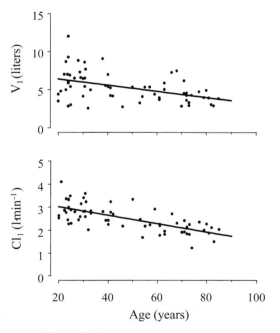

FIGURE 15-10. The influence of age on remifentanil pharmacokinetics. With advancing age, the volume of the central compartment decreases by 50% from age 20 to age 80, and the clearance decreases by 66%. (Adapted with permission from Minto et al.[64])

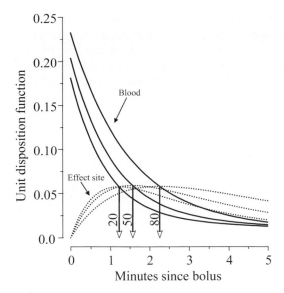

FIGURE 15-12. Simulations showing the effect-site concentration from identical bolus doses in a 20-, 50-, and 80-year-old subject. The concentrations are highest in the 80-year-old subject because of the reduced size of the central compartment. However, because of the slower blood–brain equilibrium in the 80-year-old subject, the peak effect-site concentration is almost identical in the three simulations. Thus, the smaller V_1 is offset by the slower plasma–effect-site equilibration. However, a bolus of remifentanil takes about a minute longer to reach peak effect-site concentrations in elderly subjects. (Adapted with permission from Minto et al.[139])

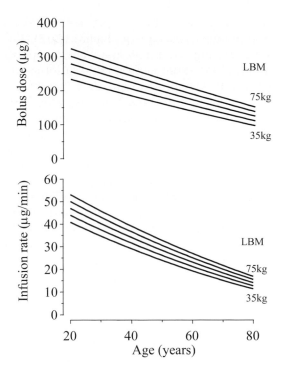

FIGURE 15-13. The influence of age and weight on remifentanil bolus dose and infusion rates. Bolus doses should be reduced by 50% in elderly subjects, reflecting the increased brain sensitivity. Infusion rates should be reduced by 66%, reflecting the combined effects of increased brain sensitivity and decreased clearance. LBM = lean body mass. (Adapted with permission from Minto et al.[139])

15-13, elderly subjects need about half of the bolus dose as younger subjects to achieve the same level of drug effect. This is not because of the change in pharmacokinetics. As shown in Figure 15-12, the peak effect-site levels after a bolus of remifentanil are nearly identical in young and elderly subjects. Rather, the remifentanil bolus is reduced in elderly subjects because of the increased sensitivity of the elderly brain to opioid drug effect, exactly as reported for fentanyl and alfentanil. The bottom graph in Figure 15-13 shows that elderly subjects require about one third as rapid an infusion as younger subjects. This reflects the combined influences of the increased sensitivity and the decreased clearance in elderly individuals.

As seen in Figure 15-13, the influence of weight on remifentanil dosing is considerably less than the influence of age. We point this out because anesthesiologists reflexively adjust remifentanil infusions to body weight, but seem reluctant to make an adequate reduction in infusion rate for elderly individuals.

Figure 15-14 shows the time required for decreases in effect-site concentration of 20%, 50%, and 80% as a function of remifentanil infusion duration. These would be the "20% effect-site decrement time," the "50% effect-site decrement time," and the "80% effect-site decrement

time," respectively. For each decrement time, the expected relationship is shown for a 20-year-old patient and an 80-year-old patient. Figure 15-14 suggests that elderly patients can be expected to recover from remifentanil

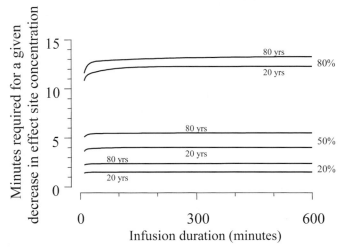

FIGURE 15-14. The 20%, 50%, and 80% effect-site decrement curves for 20- and 80-year-old subjects. Provided remifentanil dose is adequately reduced, as shown in Figure 15-13, there should be little difference in the awakening time as a function of age.

about as fast as younger subjects, provided the dose has been appropriately reduced (e.g., Figure 15-13).

The unique features of remifentanil are its rapid clearance and rapid k_{e0}, resulting in a rapid onset and offset of drug effect. It is tempting to speculate that these characteristics will make remifentanil an easy drug to titrate and that clinicians will not need to consider patient covariates such as advanced age when choosing a dosing regimen. However, the rapid onset of drug effect may be accompanied by rapid onset of adverse events such as apnea and muscle rigidity. The rapid offset of drug effect can result in patients who are in severe pain at a time when the anesthesiologist is ill-equipped to deal with the problem, for example, when the patient is in transit to the recovery room. It is thus important that anesthesiologists understand the proper dose adjustment required for the elderly. By adjusting the bolus and infusion doses, the anesthesiologist can hope to avoid the peaks and valleys in remifentanil concentration that might expose elderly patients to risk. When the proper adjustment is made, the variability in remifentanil pharmacokinetics is considerably less than for any other intravenous opioid. This makes remifentanil the most predictable opioid for treatment of the elderly.

Methadone

Methadone has several distinguishing characteristics, including having the longest terminal half-life and being supplied as a racemic mixture with surprising stereospecific pharmacology. As shown in Table 15-1 and as evident in Figure 15-1, the terminal half-life of methadone is approximately 1 day.[66] As a result, it will take nearly a week of methadone dosing to reach steady state. When methadone is used as a chronic analgesic, particularly in elderly patients, the patient and physician must be made aware that steady state will not be reached for several days, requiring vigilance for accumulation to toxicity during the "run-in" titration of methadone for analgesia. Also, adequate arrangements for rescue analgesia must be available during the period before steady-state levels.

Methadone's other unique feature is that it is supplied as a racemate with two enantiomers. L-Methadone is an opioid agonist, whereas D-methadone is an N-methyl-D-aspartate (NMDA) antagonist.[140] The potency of the D-methadone in blocking NMDA is such that, at clinically used doses, it may be effective in attenuating opioid tolerance and preventing central sensitization (hyperalgesia).[141,142] There are no specific studies examining the pharmacokinetics and pharmacodynamics of methadone in elderly subjects. However, as the increased brain sensitivity to opioid drug effect seems to be a class effect for opioids, it seems prudent to reduce methadone doses by about 50% in elderly patients compared with younger

patients. Additionally, the NMDA blocking activity of D-methadone may provide some analgesic synergy between the enantiomers. Provided methadone is titrated in a manner that is mindful of the long half-life and the potential for accumulation, methadone's rapid onset and sustained effect make it a rational choice for postoperative analgesia.

Patient-Controlled Anesthesia

PCA devices are very effective means to provide postoperative analgesia in elderly patients. Lavand'Homme and De Kock[143] have reviewed the use of PCA in the elderly. They observed that poor pain management places elderly patients at risk of confusion and outright delirium, and this may be associated with poorer clinical outcomes. They emphasized that increased monitoring and individualization of dosage are essentials in PCA management of elderly patients. They also observed that elderly patients may need additional time to become familiar with PCA devices and that the devices will become ineffective if elderly patients become confused or agitated.

Macintyre and Jarvis[144] examined morphine PCA in elderly patients and observed that age is the best predictor of postoperative morphine requirements. They found that the average PCA morphine use in the first 24 hours after surgery was approximately 100 – age. However, they also emphasized that the dose needed to be individualized, because there was tenfold variation in the dose in each age category.

This is similar to the results of Woodhouse and Mather.[145] They found that elderly patients required significantly less fentanyl and morphine administered by PCA following surgery. They also identified a similar trend for meperidine, but it was less steep and characterized by higher variability. As seen in Figure 15-15, elderly patients required about half as much morphine and fentanyl as younger subjects, consistent with the "50% reduction" suggestion at the beginning of the chapter.

Gagliese and colleagues[146] also found an approximately 50% reduction in PCA opioid use in elderly patients. In their study, patients in the younger group (average age = 39) expected more severe pain than those in the older group (average age = 67). However, both groups obtained similar efficacy from their PCA devices and expressed similar levels of satisfaction with PCA as a means of managing postoperative analgesia. The average 24 hour dose of morphine (or morphine equivalents) in the younger patients was 67 mg at the end of day one and 44 mg at the end of day two. In the older patients, the average dose was 39 mg at the end of day one and 28 mg at the end of day two. In an accompanying editorial, Ready[147] emphasized that patients must be able to understand and participate in their care, emphasizing the need to individualize therapy

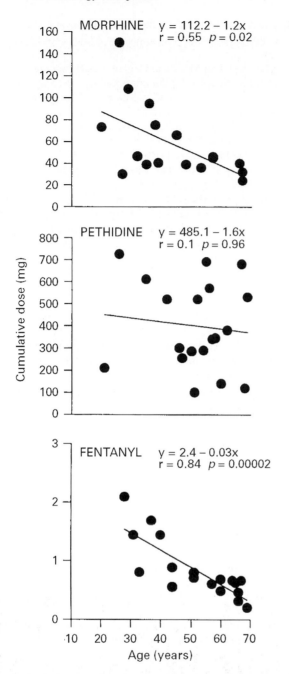

FIGURE 15-15. Twenty-four-hour cumulative patient-controlled analgesia opioid administration as a function of age. Morphine and fentanyl both show the expected reduction in dose of about 50%, as predicted by the pharmacokinetic/pharmacodynamic modeling. Meperidine (pethidine) is more variable, perhaps reflecting its more complex pharmacology, or the stimulating effects of normeperidine. (Reprinted with permission from Woodhouse and Mather.[145] Copyright © Blackwell Publishing.)

for elderly patients in whom a cognitive assessment might be appropriate before using PCA.

It is reasonable that other interventions, such as nerve blocks, infusions of local anesthetic, and adjuvant analge-

sic therapy, be combined with PCA to provide adequate analgesia at the lowest possible opioid dose in elderly patients. Beattie et al.[148] have reported that ketorolac effectively reduces morphine doses in elderly subjects. In this case, the reduced opioid requirement must be balanced against the risk of gastric bleeding and fluid retention induced by ketorolac. However, in appropriate patients, one or two doses of ketorolac are associated with only modest risk and would be expected to provide significant synergy with morphine.[149,150]

Suggested Guidelines for Chronic Opioids in the Elderly

The subject of opioids in the management of chronic pain in the elderly has been extensively reviewed.[151–153] A few basic principles will be emphasized here:

1. In general, opioids should be reserved for those elderly patients in whom less-toxic alternatives, such as acetaminophen and nonsteroidal antiinflammatory drugs, have proven ineffective.

2. It is best to start with the weaker opioids, such as codeine, and titrate to effect. The stronger opioids should be reserved for patients whose symptoms are inadequately treated by weaker opioids.

3. Careful monitoring during the initial dose titration is absolutely essential, particularly with opioids or delivery systems associated with long half-lives and time to steady state, such as methadone, oral sustained-release preparations, and transdermal fentanyl.

4. Opioid-induced constipation may be reduced by the use of a peripheral opioid antagonist, such as alvimopan[154] and methylnaltrexone.[155] Elderly patients are at increased risk of drug interactions. The risk of drug interactions particularly precludes the use of chronic meperidine in elderly patients. However, opioids should be used with great caution if combined with any drugs that decrease consciousness (e.g., benzodiazepines). Figure 15-16 shows the interaction between remifentanil and propofol on ventilation in healthy volunteers as reported by Nieuwenhuijs and colleagues.[156] Whereas propofol and remifentanil individually have modest effects on ventilation, when combined (solid triangles), they demonstrate profound depression of ventilation. This effect will be exaggerated in elderly patients because of the increased sensitivity to opioid drug effects.

5. Elderly patients are at increased risk of confusion in response to opioids.

6. Rotation of opioids may permit lower doses to be used, because of the incomplete cross-tolerance and individual differences in analgesic versus toxicity profiles among individuals.

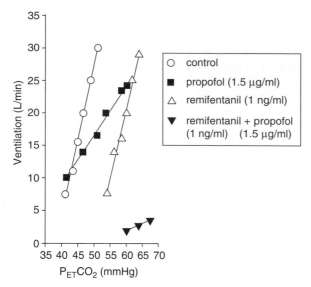

FIGURE 15-16. The interaction between remifentanil and propofol on ventilation demonstrates a class effect for opioid/hypnotic synergy. In this figure, propofol very slightly changes the slope of the CO_2 versus ventilation curve, and remifentanil very slightly changes the apnea threshold without changing the slope. However, the combination of propofol and remifentanil (triangles, lower right) profoundly displaces both the slope and the apneic threshold. (Reprinted with permission from Nieuwenhuijs et al.[156] Copyright © Lippincott Williams & Wilkins.)

Conclusion

Opioids are appropriate for both acute and chronic pain in elderly patients, particularly when nonopioid analgesics have failed to provide adequate pain relief. Elderly patients, on average, need about half the dose of opioids as younger patients to achieve the same level of analgesic effect. The biologic basis for the increased brain sensitivity (pharmacodynamic increased potency) to opioids in elderly patients is not completely understood. Elderly patients have factors that place them at increased risk of opioid toxicity, including increased pharmacologic variability, frequent polypharmacy, noncompliance with dosage regimens, and impaired renal and hepatic function.

References

1. Anderson GF, Hussey PS. Population aging: a comparison among industrialized countries. Health Aff 2000;19:191–203.
2. Ventafridda V, Tamburini M, Caraceni A, De Conno F, Naldi F. A validation study of the WHO method for cancer pain relief. Cancer 1987;59:850–856.
3. Jacox A, Carr DB, Payne R. New clinical-practice guidelines for the management of pain in patients with cancer. N Engl J Med 1994;330:651–655.
4. Bafitis H, Sargent F 2nd. Human physiological adaptability through the life sequence. J Gerontol 1977;32:402–410.
5. Klein U, Klein M, Sturm H, et al. The frequency of adverse drug reactions as dependent upon age, sex and duration of hospitalization. Int J Clin Pharmacol Biopharm 1976;13:187–195.
6. Crooks J. Aging and drug disposition—pharmacodynamics. J Chronic Dis 1983;36:85–90.
7. Cepeda MS, Farrar JT, Baumgarten M, Boston R, Carr DB, Strom BL. Side effects of opioids during short-term administration: effect of age, gender, and race. Clin Pharmacol Ther 2003;74:102–112.
8. Junger A, Hartmann B, Benson M, et al. The use of an anesthesia information management system for prediction of antiemetic rescue treatment at the postanesthesia care unit. Anesth Analg 2001;92(5):1203–1209.
9. Sinclair DR, Chung F, Mezei G. Can postoperative nausea and vomiting be predicted? Anesthesiology 1999;91:109–118.
10. Pert CB, Snyder SH. Opiate receptor: demonstration in nervous tissue. Science 1973;179:1011–1014.
11. Simon EJ, Hiller JM, Edelman I. Stereospecific binding of the potent narcotic analgesic (3H) Etorphine to rat-brain homogenate. Proc Natl Acad Sci USA 1973;70:1947–1949.
12. Terenius L. Characteristics of the "receptor" for narcotic analgesics in synaptic plasma membrane fraction from rat brain. Acta Pharmacol Toxicol (Copenh) 1973;33:377–384.
13. Hughes J, Smith TW, Kosterlitz HW, Fothergill LA, Morgan BA, Morris HR. Identification of two related pentapeptides from the brain with potent opiate agonist activity. Nature 1975;258:577–580.
14. Li CH, Chung D. Isolation and structure of an untriakontapeptide with opiate activity from camel pituitary glands. Proc Natl Acad Sci USA 1976;73:1145–1148.
15. Goldstein A, Tachibana S, Lowney LI, Hunkapiller M, Hood L. Dynorphin-(1-13), an extraordinarily potent opioid peptide. Proc Natl Acad Sci USA 1979;76:6666–6670.
16. Martin WR, Eades CG, Thompson JA, Huppler RE, Gilbert PE. The effects of morphine- and nalorphine-like drugs in the nondependent and morphine-dependent chronic spinal dog. J Pharmacol Exp Ther 1976;197:517–532.
17. Chang KJ, Cooper BR, Hazum E, Cuatrecasas P. Multiple opiate receptors: different regional distribution in the brain and differential binding of opiates and opioid peptides. Mol Pharmacol 1979;16:91–104.
18. Robson LE, Kosterlitz HW. Specific protection of the binding sites of D-Ala2-D-Leu5-enkephalin (delta-receptors) and dihydromorphine (mu-receptors). Proc R Soc Lond B Biol Sci 1979;205:425–432.
19. Schulz R, Wuster M, Krenss H, Herz A. Selective development of tolerance without dependence in multiple opiate receptors of mouse vas deferens. Nature 1980;285:242–243.
20. Pasternak GW, Childers SR, Snyder SH. Opiate analgesia: evidence for mediation by a subpopulation of opiate receptors. Science 1980;208:514–516.

21. Ling GS, Spiegel K, Nishimura SL, Pasternak GW. Dissociation of morphine's analgesic and respiratory depressant actions. Eur J Pharmacol 1983;86:487–488.
22. Ling GS, Spiegel K, Lockhart SH, Pasternak GW. Separation of opioid analgesia from respiratory depression: evidence for different receptor mechanisms. J Pharmacol Exp Ther 1985;232:149–155.
23. Brown GP, Yang K, King MA, et al. 3-Methoxynaltrexone, a selective heroin/morphine-6beta-glucuronide antagonist. FEBS Lett 1997;412:35–38.
24. Crews JC, Sweeney NJ, Denson DD. Clinical efficacy of methadone in patients refractory to other mu-opioid receptor agonist analgesics for management of terminal cancer pain. Case presentations and discussion of incomplete cross-tolerance among opioid agonist analgesics. Cancer 1993;72:2266–2272.
25. Mercadante S. Opioid rotation for cancer pain: rationale and clinical aspects. Cancer 1999;86:1856–1866.
26. Chang A, Emmel DW, Rossi GC, Pasternak GW. Methadone analgesia in morphine-insensitive CXBK mice. Eur J Pharmacol 1998;351:189–191.
27. Abbadie C, Rossi GC, Orciuolo A, Zadina JE, Pasternak GW. Anatomical and functional correlation of the endomorphins with mu opioid receptor splice variants. Eur J Neurosci 2002;16:1075–1082.
28. Cadet P. Mu opiate receptor subtypes. Med Sci Monit 2004;10:MS28–32.
29. Stefano GB, Hartman A, Bilfinger TV, et al. Presence of the mu3 opiate receptor in endothelial cells. Coupling to nitric oxide production and vasodilation. J Biol Chem 1995;270:30290–30293.
30. Kozak CA, Filie J, Adamson MC, Chen Y, Yu L. Murine chromosomal location of the mu and kappa opioid receptor genes. Genomics 1994;21:659–661.
31. Belknap JK, Mogil JS, Helms ML, et al. Localization to chromosome 10 of a locus influencing morphine analgesia in crosses derived from C57BL/6 and DBA/2 strains. Life Sci 1995;57:PL117–124.
32. Lötsch J, Geisslinger G. Are mu-opioid receptor polymorphisms important for clinical opioid therapy? Trends Mol Med. 11:82–89, 2005.
33. Romberg RR, Olofsen E, Bijl H, et al. Polymorphism of mu-opioid receptor gene (OPRM1:c.118A > G) does not protect against opioid-induced respiratory depression despite reduced analgesic response. Anesthesiology 2005;102:522–530.
34. Pasternak GW. Multiple opiate receptors: deja vu all over again. Neuropharmacology 2004;47(Suppl 1):312–323.
35. Chen Y, Mestek A, Liu J, Hurley JA, Yu L. Molecular cloning and functional expression of a mu-opioid receptor from rat brain. Mol Pharmacol 1993;44:8–12.
36. Wang JB, Imai Y, Eppler CM, Gregor P, Spivak CE, Uhl GR. Mu opiate receptor: cDNA cloning and expression. Proc Natl Acad Sci USA 1993;90:10230–10234.
37. Pan YX, Xu J, Mahurter L, Xu M, Gilbert AK, Pasternak GW. Identification and characterization of two new human mu opioid receptor splice variants, hMOR-1O and hMOR-1X. Biochem Biophys Res Commun 2003;301:1057–1061.
38. Connor M, Christie MD. Opioid receptor signalling mechanisms. Clin Exp Pharmacol Physiol 1999;26:493–499.
39. North RA. Opioid actions on membrane ion channels. In: Herz A, ed. Opioids. Handbook of Experimental Pharmacology. Vol 104. Berlin: Springer-Verlag; 1993:773–797.
40. Scarpace PJ, Tumer N, Mader SL. Beta-adrenergic function in aging. Basic mechanisms and clinical implications. Drugs Aging 1991;1:116–129.
41. Scarpace PJ, Abrass IB. Alpha- and beta-adrenergic receptor function in the brain during senescence. Neurobiol Aging 1988;9:53–58.
42. Barnhill JG, Greenblatt DJ, Miller LG, Gaver A, Harmatz JS, Shader RI. Kinetic and dynamic components of increased benzodiazepine sensitivity in aging animals. J Pharmacol Exp Ther 1990;253:1153–1161.
43. Barnhill JG, Miller LG, Greenblatt DJ, Thompson ML, Ciraulo DA, Shader RI. Benzodiazepine receptor binding response to acute and chronic stress is increased in aging animals. Pharmacology 1991;42:181–187.
44. Ueno E, Liu DD, Ho IK, Hoskins B. Opiate receptor characteristics in brains from young, mature and aged mice. Neurobiol Aging 1988;9:279–283.
45. Hess GD, Joseph JA, Roth GS. Effect of age on sensitivity to pain and brain opiate receptors. Neurobiol Aging 1981;2:49–55.
46. Petkov VV, Petkov VD, Grahovska T, Konstantinova E. Enkephalin receptor changes in rat brain during aging. Gen Pharmacol 1984;15:491–495.
47. Fulop T Jr, Kekessy D, Foris G. Impaired coupling of naloxone sensitive opiate receptors to adenylate cyclase in PMNLs of aged male subjects. Int J Immunopharmacol 1987;9(6):651–657.
48. Hoskins B, Ho IK. Age-induced differentiation of morphine's effect on cyclic nucleotide metabolism. Neurobiol Aging 1987;8:473–476.
49. Smith MA, Gray JD. Age-related differences in sensitivity to the antinociceptive effects of opioids in male rats. Influence of nociceptive intensity and intrinsic efficacy at the mu receptor. Psychopharmacology (Berl) 2001;156:445–453.
50. Van Crugten JT, Somogyi AA, Nation RL, Reynolds G. The effect of old age on the disposition and antinociceptive response of morphine and morphine-6 beta-glucuronide in the rat. Pain 1997;71:199–205.
51. Hoskins B, Burton CK, Ho IK. Differences in morphine-induced antinociception and locomotor activity in mature adult and aged mice. Pharmacol Biochem Behav 1986;25:599–605.
52. Helme RD, Gibson SJ. Pain in older people. In: Crombie IK, Croft PR, Linton SJ, Le Resche L, Von Korff M, eds. The Epidemiology of Pain. 2nd ed. Seattle: IASP Press; 1999:103–112.
53. Helme RD, Gibson SJ. The epidemiology of pain in elderly people. Clin Geriatr Med 2001;17:417–431.
54. Verhaak PF, Kerssens JJ, Dekker J, Sorbi MJ, Bensing JM. Prevalence of chronic benign pain disorder among adults: a review of the literature. Pain 1998;77:231–239.
55. Sorkin BA, Rudy TE, Hanlon RB, Turk DC, Stieg RL. Chronic pain in old and young patients: differences appear less important than similarities. J Gerontol 1990;45:P64–P68.
56. Edwards RR, Fillingim RB. Age-associated differences in responses to noxious stimuli. J Gerontol A Biol Sci Med Sci 2001;56:M180–M185.

57. Edwards RR, Fillingim RB, Ness TJ. Age-related differences in endogenous pain modulation: a comparison of diffuse noxious inhibitory controls in healthy older and younger adults. Pain 2003;101:155–165.

58. Washington LL, Gibson SJ, Helme RD. Age-related differences in the endogenous analgesic response to repeated cold water immersion in human volunteers. Pain 2000; 89:89–96.

59. Casale G, Pecorini M, Cuzzoni G, de Nicola P. Beta-endorphin and cold pressor test in the aged. Gerontology 1985;31:101–105.

60. Zheng Z, Gibson SJ, Khalil Z, Helme RD, McMeeken JM. Age-related differences in the time course of capsaicin-induced hyperalgesia. Pain 2000;85:51–58.

61. Chakour MC, Gibson SJ, Bradbeer M, Helme RD. The effect of age on A delta- and C-fibre thermal pain perception. Pain 1996;64:143–152.

62. Scott JC, Stanski DR. Decreased fentanyl/alfentanil dose requirement with increasing age: a pharmacodynamic basis. J Pharmacol Exp Ther 1987;240:159–166.

63. Hudson RJ, Bergstrom RG, Thomson IR, Sabourin MA, Rosenbloom M, Strunin L. Pharmacokinetics of sufentanil in patients undergoing abdominal aortic surgery. Anesthesiology 1989;70:426–431.

64. Minto CF, Schnider TW, Egan T, et al. The influence of age and gender on the pharmacokinetics and pharmacodynamics of remifentanil. I. Model development. Anesthesiology 1997;86:10–23.

65. Lotsch J, Skarke C, Schmidt H, Liefhold J, Geisslinger G. Pharmacokinetic modeling to predict morphine and morphine-6-glucuronide plasma concentrations in healthy young volunteers. Clin Pharmacol Ther 2002;72:151–162.

66. Inturrisi CE, Colburn WA, Kaiko RF, Houde RW, Foley KM. Pharmacokinetics and pharmacodynamics of methadone in patients with chronic pain. Clin Pharmacol Ther 1987;41:392–401.

67. Bjorkman S. Reduction and lumping of physiologically based pharmacokinetic models: prediction of the disposition of fentanyl and pethidine in humans by successively simplified models. J Pharmacokinet Pharmacodyn 2003; 30:285–307.

68. Drover DR, Angst MS, Valle M, et al. Input characteristics and bioavailability after administration of immediate and a new extended-release formulation of hydromorphone in healthy volunteers. Anesthesiology 2002;97: 827–836.

69. Scott JC, Cooke JE, Stanski DR. Electroencephalographic quantitation of opioid effect: comparative pharmacodynamics of fentanyl and sufentanil. Anesthesiology 1991; 74:34–42.

70. Inturrisi CE, Portenoy RK, Max MB, Colburn WA, Foley KM. Pharmacokinetic-pharmacodynamic relationships of methadone infusions in patients with cancer pain. Clin Pharmacol Ther 1990;47:565–577.

71. Qiao GL, Fung KF. Pharmacokinetic-pharmacodynamic modelling of meperidine in goats (II): modelling. J Vet Pharmacol Ther 1994;17:127–134.

72. Hill JL, Zacny JP. Comparing the subjective, psychomotor, and physiological effects of intravenous hydromorphone and morphine in healthy volunteers. Psychopharmacology (Berl) 2000;152:31–39.

73. Shafer SL, Varvel JR. Pharmacokinetics, pharmacodynamics, and rational opioid selection. Anesthesiology 1991;74: 53–63.

74. Shafer SL, Gregg KM. Algorithms to rapidly achieve and maintain stable drug concentrations at the site of drug effect with a computer-controlled infusion pump. J Pharmacokinet Biopharm 1992;20:147–169.

75. Henthorn TK, Krejcie TC, Shanks CA, Avram MJ. Time-dependent distribution volume and kinetics of the pharmacodynamic effector site. J Pharm Sci 1992;81: 1136–1138.

76. Wada DR, Drover DR, Lemmens HJ. Determination of the distribution volume that can be used to calculate the intravenous loading dose. Clin Pharmacokinet 1998;35:1–7.

77. Gourlay GK, Kowalski SR, Plummer JL, Cousins MJ, Armstrong PJ. Fentanyl blood concentration-analgesic response relationship in the treatment of postoperative pain. Anesth Analg 1988;67:329–337.

78. Lehmann KA, Ribbert N, Horrichs-Haermeyer G. Postoperative patient-controlled analgesia with alfentanil: analgesic efficacy and minimum effective concentrations. J Pain Symptom Manage 1990;5:249–258.

79. Dahlstrom B, Tamsen A, Paalzow L, Hartvig P. Patient-controlled analgesic therapy. Part IV. Pharmacokinetics and analgesic plasma concentrations of morphine. Clin Pharmacokinet 1982;7:266–279.

80. Gourlay GK, Willis RJ, Wilson PR. Postoperative pain control with methadone: influence of supplementary methadone doses and blood concentration-response relationships. Anesthesiology 1984;61:19–26.

81. Mather LE, Glynn CJ. The minimum effective analgetic blood concentration of pethidine in patients with intractable pain. Br J Clin Pharmacol 1982;14:385–390.

82. Coda B, Tanaka A, Jacobson RC, Donaldson G, Chapman CR. Hydromorphone analgesia after intravenous bolus administration. Pain 1997;71:41–48.

83. Hill JL, Zacny JP. Comparing the subjective, psychomotor, and physiological effects of intravenous hydromorphone and morphine in healthy volunteers. Psychopharmacology (Berl) 2000;152:31–39.

84. Hughes MA, Glass PS, Jacobs JR. Context-sensitive half-time in multicompartment pharmacokinetic models for intravenous anesthetic drugs. Anesthesiology 1992;76: 334–341.

85. Youngs EJ, Shafer SL. Pharmacokinetic parameters relevant to recovery from opioids. Anesthesiology 1994;81: 833–842.

86. Gintzler AR, Gershon MD, Spector S. A nonpeptide morphine-like compound: immunocytochemical localization in the mouse brain. Science 1978;199:447–448.

87. Goldstein A, Barrett RW, James IF, et al. Morphine and other opiates from beef brain and adrenal. Proc Natl Acad Sci USA 1985;82:5203–5207.

88. Donnerer J, Oka K, Brossi A, Rice KC, Spector S. Presence and formation of codeine and morphine in the rat. Proc Natl Acad Sci USA 1986;83:4566–4567.

89. Cardinale GJ, Donnerer J, Finck AD, Kantrowitz JD, Oka K, Spector S. Morphine and codeine are endogenous com-

ponents of human cerebrospinal fluid. Life Sci 1987;40: 301–306.

90. Lotsch J, Geisslinger G. Morphine-6-glucuronide: an analgesic of the future? Clin Pharmacokinet 2001;40:485–499.

91. Paul D, Standifer KM, Inturrisi CE, Pasternak GW. Pharmacological characterization of morphine-6 beta-glucuronide, a very potent morphine metabolite. J Pharmacol Exp Ther 1989;251:477–483.

92. Lotsch J, Kobal G, Stockmann A, Brune K, Geisslinger G. Lack of analgesic activity of morphine-6-glucuronide after short-term intravenous administration in healthy volunteers. Anesthesiology 1997;87(6):1348–1358.

93. Lotsch J, Kobal G, Geisslinger G. No contribution of morphine-6-glucuronide to clinical morphine effects after short-term administration. Clin Neuropharmacol 1998;21: 351–354.

94. Wolff T, Samuelsson H, Hedner T. Morphine and morphine metabolite concentrations in cerebrospinal fluid and plasma in cancer pain patients after slow-release oral morphine administration. Pain 1995;62:147–154.

95. Portenoy RK, Foley KM, Stulman J, et al. Plasma morphine and morphine-6-glucuronide during chronic morphine therapy for cancer pain: plasma profiles, steady-state concentrations and the consequences of renal failure. Pain 1991;47:13–19.

96. Cockcroft DW, Gault MH. Prediction of creatinine clearance from serum creatinine. Nephron 1976;16:31–41.

97. Lotsch J, Skarke C, Schmidt H, Grosch S, Geisslinger G. The transfer half-life of morphine-6-glucuronide from plasma to effect site assessed by pupil size measurement in healthy volunteers. Anesthesiology 2001;95:1329–1338.

98. Skarke C, Jarrar M, Erb K, Schmidt H, Geisslinger G, Lotsch J. Respiratory and miotic effects of morphine in healthy volunteers when P-glycoprotein is blocked by quinidine. Clin Pharmacol Ther 2003;74:303–311.

99. Skarke C, Darimont J, Schmidt H, Geisslinger G, Lotsch J. Analgesic effects of morphine and morphine-6-glucuronide in a transcutaneous electrical pain model in healthy volunteers. Clin Pharmacol Ther 2003;73:107–121.

100. Letrent SP, Polli JW, Humphreys JE, Pollack GM, Brouwer KR, Brouwer KL. P-glycoprotein-mediated transport of morphine in brain capillary endothelial cells. Biochem Pharmacol 1999;58:951–957.

101. Dahan A, Romberg R, Teppema L, Sarton E, Bijl H, Olofsen E. Simultaneous measurement and integrated analysis of analgesia and respiration after an intravenous morphine infusion. Anesthesiology 2004;101:1201–1209.

102. Aubrun F, Monsel S, Langeron O, Coriat P, Riou B. Postoperative titration of intravenous morphine in the elderly patient. Anesthesiology 2002;96:17–23.

103. Aubrun F, Bunge D, Langeron O, Saillant G, Coriat P, Riou B. Postoperative morphine consumption in the elderly patient. Anesthesiology 2003;99:160–165.

104. Wagner LE 2nd, Eaton M, Sabnis SS, Gingrich KJ. Meperidine and lidocaine block of recombinant voltage-dependent Na+ channels: evidence that meperidine is a local anesthetic. Anesthesiology 1999;91:1481–1490.

105. Wolff M, Olschewski A, Vogel W, Hempelmann G. Meperidine suppresses the excitability of spinal dorsal horn neurons. Anesthesiology 2004;100:947–955.

106. Holmberg L, Odar-Cederlof I, Boreus LO, Heyner L, Ehrnebo M. Comparative disposition of pethidine and norpethidine in old and young patients. Eur J Clin Pharmacol 1982;22:175–179.

107. Seifert CF, Kennedy S. Meperidine is alive and well in the new millennium: evaluation of meperidine usage patterns and frequency of adverse drug reactions. Pharmacotherapy 2004;24:776–783.

108. Odar-Cederlof I, Boreus LO, Bondesson U, Holmberg L, Heyner L. Comparison of renal excretion of pethidine (meperidine) and its metabolites in old and young patients. Eur J Clin Pharmacol 1985;28:171–175.

109. Huang YF, Upton RN, Rutten AJ, Mather LE. The hemodynamic effects of intravenous bolus doses of meperidine in conscious sheep. Anesth Analg 1994;78:442–449.

110. Zornberg GL, Bodkin JA, Cohen BM. Severe adverse interaction between pethidine and selegiline. Lancet 1991; 337:246.

111. Keeri-Szanto M. Anaesthesia time/dose curves IX: the use of hydromorphone in surgical anaesthesia and postoperative pain relief in comparison to morphine. Can Anaesth Soc J 1976;23:587–595.

112. Kopp A, Wachauer D, Hoerauf KH, Zulus E, Reiter WJ, Steltzer H. Effect of preemptive hydromorphone administration on postoperative pain relief—a randomized controlled trial. Wien Klin Wochenschr 2000;112:1002–1006.

113. Rapp SE, Egan KJ, Ross BK, Wild LM, Terman GW, Ching JM. A multidimensional comparison of morphine and hydromorphone patient-controlled analgesia. Anesth Analg 1996;82:1043–1048.

114. Liu S, Carpenter RL, Mulroy MF, et al. Intravenous versus epidural administration of hydromorphone. Effects on analgesia and recovery after radical retropubic prostatectomy. Anesthesiology 1995;82:682–688.

115. Brose WG, Tanelian DL, Brodsky JB, Mark JB, Cousins MJ. CSF and blood pharmacokinetics of hydromorphone and morphine following lumbar epidural administration. Pain 1991;45:11–15.

116. Halpern SH, Arellano R, Preston R, et al. Epidural morphine vs hydromorphone in post-caesarean section patients. Can J Anaesth 1996;43:595–598.

117. Bentley JB, Borel JD, Nenad RE Jr, Gillespie TJ. Age and fentanyl pharmacokinetics. Anesth Analg 1982;61:968–971.

118. Singleton MA, Rosen JI, Fisher DM. Pharmacokinetics of fentanyl in the elderly. Br J Anaesth 1988;60:619–622.

119. Scott JC, Ponganis KV, Stanski DR. EEG quantitation of narcotic effect: the comparative pharmacodynamics of fentanyl and alfentanil. Anesthesiology 1985;62:234–241.

120. Martin G, Glass PS, Breslin DS, et al. A study of anesthetic drug utilization in different age groups. J Clin Anesth 2003;15:194–200.

121. Holdsworth MT, Forman WB, Killilea TA, et al. Transdermal fentanyl disposition in elderly subjects. Gerontology 1994;40:32–37.

122. Davis MP, Srivastava M. Demographics, assessment and management of pain in the elderly. Drugs Aging 2003;20: 23–57.

123. Kharasch ED, Hoffer C, Whittington D. Influence of age on the pharmacokinetics and pharmacodynamics of oral

transmucosal fentanyl citrate. Anesthesiology 2004;101: 738–743.

124. Shafer A, Sung ML, White PF. Pharmacokinetics and pharmacodynamics of alfentanil infusions during general anesthesia. Anesth Analg 1986;65:1021–1028.

125. Sitar DS, Duke PC, Benthuysen JL, Sanford TJ, Smith NT. Aging and alfentanil disposition in healthy volunteers and surgical patients. Can J Anaesth 1989;36:149–154.

126. Kent AP, Dodson ME, Bower S. The pharmacokinetics and clinical effects of a low dose of alfentanil in elderly patients. Acta Anaesthesiol Belg 1988;39:25–33.

127. Lemmens HJ, Burm AG, Hennis PJ, Gladines MP, Bovill JG. Influence of age on the pharmacokinetics of alfentanil. Gender dependence. Clin Pharmacokinet 1990;19:416–422.

128. Maitre PO, Vozeh S, Heykants J, Thomson DA, Stanski DR. Population pharmacokinetics of alfentanil: the average dose-plasma concentration relationship and interindividual variability in patients. Anesthesiology 1987;68:59–67.

129. Raemer DB, Buschman A, Varvel JR, et al. The prospective use of population pharmacokinetics in a computer-driven system for alfentanil. Anesthesiology 1990;73: 66–72.

130. Lemmens HJ, Burm AG, Bovill JG, Hennis PJ. Pharmacodynamics of alfentanil as a supplement to nitrous oxide anaesthesia in the elderly patient. Br J Anaesth 1988; 61:173–179.

131. Lemmens HJ, Bovill JG, Hennis PJ, Burm AG. Age has no effect on the pharmacodynamics of alfentanil. Anesth Analg 1988;67:956–960.

132. Lemmens HJ, Burm AG, Bovill JG, Hennis PJ, Gladines MP. Pharmacodynamics of alfentanil. The role of plasma protein binding. Anesthesiology 1992;76:65–70.

133. Lemmens HJ, Bovill JG, Burm AG, Hennis PJ. Alfentanil infusion in the elderly. Prolonged computer-assisted infusion of alfentanil in the elderly surgical patient. Anaesthesia 1988;43:850–856.

134. Scott JC, Cooke JE, Stanski DR. Electroencephalographic quantitation of opioid effect: comparative pharmacodynamics of fentanyl and sufentanil. Anesthesiology 1991; 74:34–42.

135. Helmers JH, van Leeuwen L, Zuurmond WW. Sufentanil pharmacokinetics in young adult and elderly surgical patients. Eur J Anaesthesiol 1994;11:181–185.

136. Gepts E, Shafer SL, Camu F, et al. Linearity of pharmacokinetics and model estimation of sufentanil. Anesthesiology 1995;83:1194–1204.

137. Matteo RS, Schwartz AE, Ornstein E, Young WL, Chang WJ. Pharmacokinetics of sufentanil in the elderly surgical patient. Can J Anaesth 1990;37:852–856.

138. Hofbauer R, Tesinsky P, Hammerschmidt V, et al. No reduction in the sufentanil requirement of elderly patients undergoing ventilatory support in the medical intensive care unit. Eur J Anaesthesiol 1999;16:702–707.

139. Minto CF, Schnider TW, Shafer SL. The influence of age and gender on the pharmacokinetics and pharmacodynamics of remifentanil. II. Model application. Anesthesiology 1997;86:24–33.

140. Shimoyama N, Shimoyama M, Elliott KJ, Inturrisi CE. d-Methadone is antinociceptive in the rat formalin test. J Pharmacol Exp Ther 1997;283:648–652.

141. Davis AM, Inturrisi CE. d-Methadone blocks morphine tolerance and N-methyl-D-aspartate-induced hyperalgesia. J Pharmacol Exp Ther 1999;289:1048–1053.

142. Callahan RJ, Au JD, Paul M, Liu C, Yost CS. Functional inhibition by methadone of N-methyl-D-aspartate receptors expressed in Xenopus oocytes: stereospecific and subunit effects. Anesth Analg 2004;98:653–659.

143. Lavand'Homme P, De Kock M. Practical guidelines on the postoperative use of patient-controlled analgesia in the elderly. Drugs Aging 1998;13:9–16.

144. Macintyre PE, Jarvis DA. Age is the best predictor of postoperative morphine requirements. Pain 1996;64: 357–364.

145. Woodhouse A, Mather LE. The influence of age upon opioid analgesic use in the patient-controlled analgesia environment. Anaesthesia 1997;52:949–955.

146. Gagliese L, Jackson M, Ritvo P, Wowk A, Katz J. Age is not an impediment to effective use of patient-controlled analgesia by surgical patients. Anesthesiology 2000;93: 601–610.

147. Ready LB. PCA is effective for older patients, but are there limits? Anesthesiology 2000;93:597–598.

148. Beattie WS, Warriner CB, Etches R, et al. The addition of continuous intravenous infusion of ketorolac to a patient-controlled analgetic morphine regime reduced postoperative myocardial ischemia in patients undergoing elective total hip or knee arthroplasty. Anesth Analg 1997;84: 715–722.

149. Malmberg AB, Yaksh TL. Pharmacology of the spinal action of ketorolac, morphine, ST-91, U50488H, and L-PIA on the formalin test and an isobolographic analysis of the NSAID interaction. Anesthesiology 1993;79:270–281.

150. Lashbrook JM, Ossipov MH, Hunter JC, Raffa RB, Tallarida RJ, Porreca F. Synergistic antiallodynic effects of spinal morphine with ketorolac and selective COX1- and COX2-inhibitors in nerve-injured rats. Pain 1999;82: 65–72.

151. Gloth FM 3rd. Pain management in older adults: prevention and treatment. J Am Geriatr Soc 2001;49:188–199.

152. Wilder-Smith OH. Opioid use in the elderly. Eur J Pain 2005;9:137–140.

153. Nikolaus T, Zeyfang A. Pharmacological treatments for persistent non-malignant pain in older persons. Drugs Aging 2004;21:19–41.

154. Taguchi A, Sharma N, Saleem RM, et al. Selective postoperative inhibition of gastrointestinal opioid receptors. N Engl J Med 2001;345:935–940.

155. Kurz A, Sessler DI. Opioid-induced bowel dysfunction: pathophysiology and potential new therapies. Drugs 2003; 63:649–671.

156. Nieuwenhuijs DJ, Olofsen E, Romberg RR, et al. Response surface modeling of remifentanil-propofol interaction on cardiorespiratory control and bispectral index. Anesthesiology 2003;98:312–322.

16
Intravenous Hypnotic Anesthetics

Matthew D. McEvoy and J.G. Reves

This chapter discusses the pharmacology of frequently used intravenous hypnotic agents in the geriatric patient. The focus of this chapter is the changes in pharmacokinetics and pharmacodynamics in the geriatric patient specific to propofol, thiopental, midazolam, and etomidate, the four most popular intravenous agents for sedation, induction, and maintenance of general anesthesia.

Propofol

Propofol was first investigated in Europe in the 1980s. Initially the drug was suspended in a solvent that caused anaphylactoid reactions in some patients. It was reformulated in a different preparation and it has gained widespread use ever since. Because of its quick onset of action, fairly predictable dose-response, and quick termination of action, propofol is only second to thiopental in use for the intravenous induction of general anesthesia.[1] Propofol is also the focus of a tremendous amount of research in target-controlled infusion techniques, both in the operating room (OR) and in non-OR anesthesia.

Pharmacology: Structure/Action

Propofol (2,6-diisopropylphenol) is a hypnotic drug in the class of the alkylphenols that principally works at the gamma-aminobutyric acid-A (GABA$_A$) receptor site in the central nervous system (CNS).[2] However, it has also been postulated in recent years that propofol might have additional action at excitatory amino acid receptors.[2,3] Propofol is composed of a phenol ring with two isopropyl groups attached to it. It is not water soluble and is thus prepared in an oil-water emulsion consisting of soybean oil, egg lecithin, and glycerol.[4] This is important because this preparation can support the growth of bacteria, even though it contains disodium edetate to retard bacterial growth. Because of this unique preparation, propofol is not considered to be antimicrobially preserved under

United States Pharmacopeia specifications. Thus, the current recommendations are that sterile technique should be used when handling and administering this drug, as with all intravenous anesthetics, and that any propofol withdrawn from a vial should be used within 6 hours and any vial that is spiked and used as an intravenous infusion should be completely used within 12 hours. Any amount remaining after those times should be discarded.[5,6]

Pharmacodynamics

Central Nervous System Effects

Propofol has numerous effects on various organ systems throughout the body. Like thiopental, it has favorable effects on CNS parameters, as it lowers cerebral metabolic rate (CMRO$_2$), cerebral blood flow (CBF), and intracranial pressure (ICP) (Table 16-1).[7] If a large bolus is given, propofol does have the ability to lower the mean arterial pressure (MAP) considerably, possibly lowering cerebral perfusion pressure (CPP) below a critical level (<50 mm Hg). This latter consideration is of prime importance in the elderly patient population because they are more apt to have critical carotid or aortic valvular stenosis. Particularly in candidates for carotid endarterectomy and/or aortic valve replacement, even moderate afterload reduction can threaten cerebral perfusion because the cerebral autoregulation curve is shifted to the right such that the baseline hypertension in these patients is required in order to perfuse past the fixed stenotic lesions.[8]

Propofol induces a biphasic pattern of electroencephalogram (EEG) activation and then slowing with increasing doses. After the initial activation, EEG slowing is dose-related and proceeds to burst-suppression and then to complete electrical silence.[9] During induction, patients older than 70 years reach significantly deeper EEG stages than younger patients, need a longer time to reach the deepest EEG stage, and need more time until a light

TABLE 16-1. Cardiovascular, respiratory, and cerebral effects of several intravenous hypnotic agents.

Agent	Cardiovascular*		Respiratory*		Cerebral*		
	HR	MAP	Vent	B'dil	CBF	CMRO$_2$	ICP
Propofol	0/↓↓	↓↓↓	↓↓/↓↓↓	?	↓↓↓	↓↓↓	↓↓↓
Thiopental	↑↑/↑	↓↓/↓↓↓	↓↓/↓↓↓	↓	↓↓↓	↓↓↓	↓↓↓
Etomidate	0	0/↓	↓/↓↓	0	↓↓↓	↓↓↓	↓↓↓
Midazolam	↑	↓↓	↓↓/↓↓↓	0	↓↓	↓↓	↓↓

Source: Modified with permission from Morgan GE Jr, Mikhail MS, Murray MJ. Clinical Anesthesiology. 3rd ed. New York/Stamford, CT: McGraw-Hill/Appleton & Lange; 2002.

0 = no change, ↑/↓ = minimal change in corresponding direction, ↑↑/↓↓ = moderate change in corresponding direction, ↑↑↑/↓↓↓ = marked change in corresponding direction, HR = heart rate, MAP = mean arterial pressure, Vent = ventilation, B'dil = bronchodilation, CBF = cerebral blood flow, CMRO$_2$ = cerebral metabolic rate, ICP = intracranial pressure.

*Where there is a difference between the young adult and the geriatric patient, the first set of arrows indicates the response in the young adult and the second set of arrows indicates the response in the geriatric patient.

EEG stage is regained.[10] The EEG changes described above cause a shorter duration of seizure in the electroconvulsive therapy (ECT) patient, but they also allow for a blunted hypertensive and hyperdynamic response that is often seen in these patients.[11] Methohexital will allow for longer seizure duration, but it does not block the hypertensive response to ECT as much and thus it is not as ideal in the geriatric patient who is likely to have cardiac disease. Although propofol often allows for seizures of a clinically acceptable duration,[11] many psychiatrists prefer methohexital for ECT.

The brain becomes more sensitive to propofol with increasing age. Schnider et al.[12] reported that geriatric patients were approximately 30% more sensitive to the pharmacodynamic effects of propofol than younger subjects, as measured by EEG changes. This was found to be true for both induction doses and infusions. Thus, it seems that increasing age causes changes in the brain that increase the effective potency of propofol for the geriatric patient.

Respiratory Effects

Propofol causes dose-related depression of ventilation and it is thought to produce some bronchodilation, although this is controversial (Table 16-1).[13,14] In standard induction doses, propofol causes apnea.[15] However, when compared with thiopental, respirations are lost later and recovered earlier.[16] With intravenous infusions for sedation, propofol causes increasing levels of respiratory depression, mainly by affecting the tidal volume. Furthermore, airway reflexes are depressed more so with propofol than with equivalent doses of thiopental or etomidate, and this effect is greatly enhanced by the addition of opioids.[17] Also, although propofol does not inhibit hypoxic pulmonary vasoconstriction, it does seem to blunt both the hypoxic and hypercapnic ventilatory responses.[16,18–20]

All of these changes described above have particular relevance for the elderly patient. Because of increases in closing capacity with increasing age, which will exceed functional residual capacity (FRC) even in the upright position in a 65-year-old individual, desaturation can occur at a faster rate. In the elderly, this occurs as a result of an increase in shunt fraction rather than a reduced FRC, as is seen with the obese or in patients with restrictive lung disorders.[21] The elderly also have a decreased cough reflex and thus a decreased ability to clear secretions.[22] This inherently decreased cough reflex in the elderly patient combined with the suppression of this reflex from propofol puts the elderly person at higher risk for aspiration during its use. Furthermore, the elderly patient already has a blunted hypoxic and hypercapnic ventilatory response compared with the average adult patient.[22] These changes call for great vigilance when administering propofol to an elderly patient for minimal alveolar concentration (MAC) anesthesia or even light sedation. Ventilation should be closely monitored, particularly if supplemental oxygen is used, because the hypercapnic ventilatory response will become the primary regulator of respiration. This is important because supplemental oxygen could prevent hypoxemia, but allow for a progressive hypercapnia that could be dangerous to the patient. Finally, all of these effects are increased with the concurrent use of opioids, thus requiring even greater attention in operative and procedural situations when the elderly patient is maintaining oxygenation and ventilation through spontaneous respirations without a secure airway or end-tidal carbon dioxide monitoring. However, all of the evidence cited thus far would suggest that increased pharmacodynamic sensitivity in the elderly patient moves in a parallel manner for respiratory depression and sedation/hypnosis; that is, the patient is not fully awake and merely experiencing decreased respiratory drive. Thus, in the spontaneously ventilating patient, the gradual titration of propofol matched with a vigilance attentive to signs of adequate respiration and level of sedation should provide for a safe and effective anesthetic.

Cardiovascular Effects

Propofol causes little change in heart rate but can cause profound changes in MAP when given in induction bolus doses (Table 16-1).[23] These changes are caused by a reduction in systemic vascular resistance (via inhibition of sympathetic vasoconstriction) and preload, as well as through direct effects on myocardial contractility. This hypotension is more pronounced than that which is seen with the administration of thiopental, etomidate, or midazolam. In the normal adult patient, this hypotension is well tolerated and it is readily reversed during the stimulation of laryngoscopy and intubation. However, studies have shown that the degree of hypotension is increased and an adequate hemodynamic response to a bolus induction is decreased in the geriatric patient. This occurs by several mechanisms. First, propofol impairs the arterial baroreceptor reflex to hypotension, which is already decreased in the geriatric patient.[24] Second, the geriatric patient is more likely to have ventricular dysfunction. A decrease in preload in these patients may result in a significant decrease in cardiac output. Third, these patients are often taking beta-blockers and diuretics or other therapies that cause hypovolemia in the perioperative period. The former will reduce the magnitude of any baroreceptor-mediated reflex tachycardia to a decrease in blood pressure, whereas the latter will tend to make the patient more sensitive to changes in systemic vascular resistance and preload secondary to being relatively intravascularly hypovolemic.[24] Finally, it is possible for a profound decrease in preload to result in a vagally mediated reflex bradycardia.[25] Practically speaking, these concerns can be applied clinically in two general categories. First, for the geriatric patient with significant cardiac disease, it is best to avoid a rapid bolus induction with propofol. Second, many of the untoward effects noted above can be greatly minimized if a slower infusion induction is performed with laryngoscopy being performed after reaching a pharmacodynamic endpoint, such as a bispectral index (BIS) value of less than 60 (see discussion below).[26]

Other Effects

Two unique beneficial effects of propofol are noteworthy. Propofol has both antiemetic and antipruritic properties.[27,28] Thus, its intraoperative and perioperative use has the potential to reduce the need for traditional antiemetic and possibly antipruritic medications in the postoperative period. This is particularly important in the geriatric patient who may be more susceptible to the untoward effects of drugs that work at cholinergic and dopaminergic sites in the normal treatment of nausea and pruritus.

Metabolism and Disposition (Pharmacokinetics)

The pharmacokinetics of propofol involve a very large volume of distribution, rapid redistribution, and rapid elimination via hepatic and extrahepatic routes. Because of high lipid solubility, it has an onset of action of one arm-to-brain circulation time (almost as fast as thiopental). Rapid awakening from a single bolus is the result of extensive redistribution to non-CNS sites throughout the body. Its initial distribution half-life in a healthy adult patient is approximately 2 minutes.[29,30]

There are various changes in the pharmacokinetics of propofol in the elderly patient. The central volume of distribution is less, systemic clearance is reduced, and intercompartmental clearance is reduced. During a propofol infusion, the plasma concentration of the drug is about 20% higher in the elderly patient as compared with the average adult.[31] Furthermore, the context-sensitive half-time changes with increasing age. Studies have shown that the time required for a 50% reduction in effect-site concentration (50% effect-site decrement time) is significantly prolonged with advancing age in an exponential manner. For propofol infusions less than 1 hour, there is little difference between the young adult patient and the elderly patient in recovery time. However, after a 4-hour infusion, there is a doubling of the 50% effect-site decrement time in an 80-year-old versus a 20-year-old patient, and this difference becomes even greater with infusions of 10 hours and longer.[31] This fact is of particular importance because this assumes that there have already been dosage adjustments for other pharmacokinetic parameters such that the plasma concentration is the same in both patients. Thus, even at reduced infusion rates, the elderly patient will take longer to emerge than the young patient.

Indications

Propofol, as noted above, is routinely used for induction and maintenance phases of general anesthesia, as well as for various levels of sedation in OR, and non-OR anesthesia,[1] as well as in the intensive care unit.

Dosing in the Elderly

When the pharmacokinetic and pharmacodynamic changes are considered together, the current literature suggests a 20% reduction in the induction dose of propofol, if given as a bolus. Practically, this has been reported as a reduction of the bolus dose from 2.0–2.5 to 1.5–1.8 mg/kg.[32] Of note, it is the authors' clinical experience that if the induction dose is titrated to a neurologic endpoint (such as BIS or PSA4000) or given slowly in order to account for the effect-site hysteresis time (k_{e0}), this

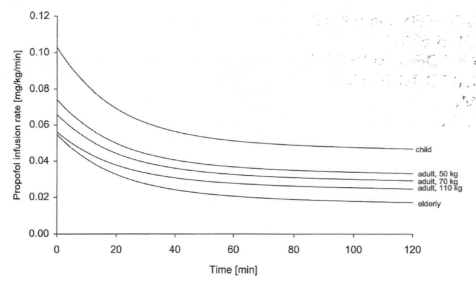

FIGURE 16-1. Propofol infusion rate required to maintain 1 μg/mL plasma level of propofol in patients of various ages. These dosing guidelines take into account the pharmacokinetic changes with aging. This correlates with a mild level of sedation. (Reprinted with permission from Schüttler and Ihmsen.[29])

dose is reduced to as low as 0.8–1.2 mg/kg in the elderly, which corresponds with the findings of Kazama et al.[26] Furthermore, numerous reports have shown that there is less hemodynamic instability if this bolus is given over a longer period of time in the elderly patient than as one fast bolus.[26,29,31]

Dosing requirements during an infusion are even less for the elderly patient. Schüttler and Ihmsen[29] have shown that for continuous low plasma level infusions, such as those used during the maintenance phase of an anesthetic for sedation (plasma concentration 1 μg/mL), a 75-year-old patient will require approximately 30% less drug than

a 25-year-old patient to maintain the same level of drug concentration. However, this only takes into account the pharmacokinetic changes with age (Figure 16-1).[29] The age-related decline in the amount of propofol required for the same level of anesthesia becomes even more profound when one considers the pharmacodynamic data along with the pharmacokinetic data. For a surgical level of anesthesia, Shafer proposes an age-adjusted dosing guideline based on the compilation of several pharmacokinetic and pharmacodynamic studies (Figure 16-2).[12,32] This pharmacodynamic change is also illustrated in Figure 16-3, which shows that a 75-year-old patient will require

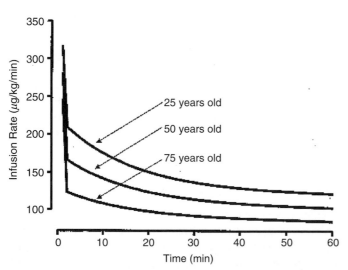

FIGURE 16-2. Propofol infusion rate required to maintain adequate surgical anesthesia in patients of various ages. These dosing guidelines account for the changes with age in propofol pharmacokinetics and pharmacodynamics. (Reprinted with permission from Shafer.[32])

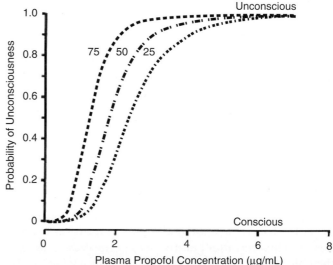

FIGURE 16-3. Effect of age on propofol pharmacodynamics. This logistic regression shows the age-related probability of being asleep after a 1-hour infusion of propofol. A 75-year-old patient is 30%–50% more sensitive to propofol than is a 25-year-old patient. (Reprinted with permission from Schnider et al.[12])

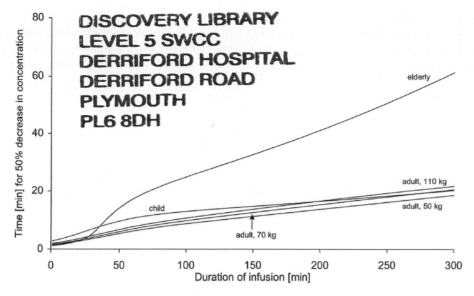

FIGURE 16-4. Context-sensitive half-time of propofol in patients of various ages. Altered pharmacokinetics in the elderly become clinically significant after a 1-hour infusion. (Reprinted with permission from Schüttler and Ihmsen.[29])

a 50% lower propofol plasma concentration than a 25-year-old patient in order to have the same likelihood of being asleep after a 1-hour infusion.[12] Additionally, as aforementioned, it must be noted that a prolonged propofol infusion should be stopped earlier in the elderly patient in order to have recovery at the same time as the younger patient (Figure 16-4).[29]

Adverse Effects and Contraindications

The major adverse effect of propofol, a significant decrease in blood pressure, has been mentioned already. If proper dosage adjustments are made, propofol is a well-tolerated induction and infusion medication in the elderly. However, in the patient with significant ventricular dysfunction or hemodynamic instability, it may be best to use etomidate or thiopental for bolus induction. It is also of note that propofol routinely causes pain on intravenous injection. However, this is normally brief and well tolerated if it is injected into a briskly running intravenous line.

Future Considerations

The dosing adjustments mentioned above are well supported in the pharmacokinetic and pharmacodynamic literature.[12,29–32] Clinical application of some of the mathematical models that have been simulated has proven successful for the authors without the use of target-controlled infusion pumps. The authors have confirmed a less profound hemodynamic change when several models

have been tested. In our experience, many geriatric patients can be induced (as measured by a BIS of less than 60) with 0.8–1.2 mg/kg propofol over a 180- to 240-second time frame with a less than 10% change from baseline heart rate and blood pressure. This is done through the application of several pharmacokinetic and pharmacodynamic models mentioned above. For instance, slightly modifying models proposed by Schüttler, Schnider, and Kazama, we induce many geriatric patients at an initial rate of 400 μg/kg/min propofol with 1–2 μg/kg fentanyl given 2–3 minutes before the start of the infusion. When the BIS reaches 70 (usually within 90–150 seconds), the neuromuscular blocker (NMBD) of choice (normally cisatracurium or rocuronium) is given while the propofol infusion is continued. When sufficient time has passed for the NMBD to have taken effect and the BIS is <60, laryngoscopy is performed and the patient is intubated. The infusion of propofol is then reduced and titrated to a BIS level of 50–60, which tends to conform to the curve in Figure 16-2. Of note, for cases in the 4- to 6-hour range, the infusion rate of propofol (with opioid supplementation) in our elderly patients is often as low as 30–35 μg/kg/min near the end of the case, with this rate of infusion providing a BIS level of 55–60. The benefit of this is that, because we are using less propofol but still maintaining a level of general anesthesia, we are able to give a more individualized anesthetic which results in a lessened need for vasopressors and an increased use of beta-blockers and opioids. We find that with this technique our geriatric patients wake up smooth and quick with good analgesia and well-controlled hemodynamics.

Of further consideration with the use of propofol in the geriatric patient is the possible benefit of its antiinflammatory and antioxidant properties.[33,34] New research is being conducted which *may* show that a propofol infusion for the maintenance of anesthesia decreases the magnitude of the rise of inflammatory markers in the elderly patient compared with volatile agents. This is of profound importance when it is viewed in light of the research showing that increases in inflammatory markers, such as interleukin-6, tumor necrosis factor-alpha, C-reactive protein, and myeloperoxidase, are associated with increased rates of cardiovascular mortality and morbidity.[35,36]

Thiopental

Barbituric acid, a combination of urea and malonic acid that is lacking in sedative properties, was first synthesized in 1864 by J.F.W. Adolph von Baeyer, a Nobel prize-winning organic chemist.[37] The thiobarbiturates were first described in 1903. However, because of fatal experiments in dogs, their use was not further explored until the 1930s.[38–40] In 1935, Tabern and Volwiler synthesized a series of sulfur-containing barbiturates, of which thiopental became the most widely used. Thiopental was introduced clinically by Ralph Waters and John Lundy, and became preferred clinically because of its rapid onset of action and short duration, without the excitatory effects of hexobarbital.[41]

Pharmacology: Structure/Action

Thiopental is a hypnotically active drug that works at $GABA_A$ receptor sites in the CNS.[42] Thiopental is in the class of thiobarbiturates, which is defined by having a sulfur substituted at the position C2. Substitutions at the 5, 2, and 1 positions of the barbiturate ring confer different pharmacologic activities to the barbiturate nucleus. Substitutions at position 5 with either aryl or alkyl groups produce hypnotic and sedative effects. A phenyl group substitution at C5 produces anticonvulsant activity. An increase in length of one or both side-chains of an alkyl group at C5 increases hypnotic potency. Substitution of a sulfur at position 2 produces a more rapid onset of action, as seen with thiopental.[43]

Pharmacodynamics

Thiopental produces sedation and sleep. Sufficient doses produce a CNS depression that is attended by loss of consciousness, amnesia, and respiratory and cardiovascular depression. The response to pain and other noxious stimulation during general anesthesia seems to be obtunded. However, the results of pain studies reveal that barbiturates may actually decrease the pain threshold in low doses, such as with small induction doses of thiopental or after emergence from thiopental when the blood levels are low.[44] The amnesic effect of barbiturates has not been well studied, but it is decidedly less pronounced than that produced by benzodiazepines or propofol.[45]

Central Nervous System Effects

Barbiturates, similar to other CNS depressants, have potent effects on cerebral metabolism. Several studies in the 1970s demonstrated the effect of barbiturates as a dose-related depression of the $CMRO_2$, which produces a progressive slowing of the EEG, a reduction in the rate of adenosine triphosphate consumption, and protection from incomplete or focal cerebral ischemia.[46,47] When the results of the EEG became isoelectric, a point at which cerebral metabolic activity is approximately 50% of baseline, no further decrements in $CMRO_2$ occurred.[48] These findings support the hypothesis that metabolism and function are coupled. However, it must be noted that it is the portion of metabolic activity concerned with neuronal signaling and impulse traffic that is reduced by barbiturates, not that portion corresponding to basal metabolic function. The only way to suppress baseline metabolic activity concerned with cellular activity is through hypothermia. Thus, the effect of barbiturates on cerebral metabolism is maximized at a 50% depression of cerebral function in which less oxygen is required as $CMRO_2$ is diminished, leaving all metabolic energy to be used for the maintenance of cellular integrity.[48] This may be of importance to the elderly patient undergoing neurosurgery for aneurysm clipping or carotid endarterectomy in which focal ischemia may occur.

With the reduction in $CMRO_2$, there is a parallel reduction in cerebral perfusion, which is seen in decreased CBF and ICP (Table 16-1). With reduced $CMRO_2$, cerebral vascular resistance increases and CBF decreases.[49] However, for thiopental, the ratio of CBF to $CMRO_2$ is unchanged. Thus, the reduction in CBF after the administration of barbiturates causes a concurrent decrease in ICP. Furthermore, even though the MAP decreases, barbiturates do not compromise the overall CPP, because the CPP = MBP − ICP. In this relationship, ICP decreases more relative to the decrease in MAP after barbiturate use, thus preserving CPP. This is in contrast to propofol, which has a greater likelihood in the elderly patient of decreasing MAP to an extent that may compromise CPP, as noted above.[50]

Onset of Central Nervous System Effects

Barbiturates produce CNS effects when they cross the blood–brain barrier. There are several well-known factors that help to determine the rapidity with which a drug enters the cerebral spinal fluid (CSF) and brain tissue. These factors include the degree of lipid solubility, degree of ionization, level of protein binding, and the plasma drug concentration. Drugs with high lipid solubility and low degree of ionization cross the blood–brain barrier rapidly, producing a fast onset of action. Approximately 50% of thiopental is nonionized at physiologic pH, which accounts in part for the rapid accumulation of thiopental in the CSF after intravenous administration. Protein binding also affects the onset of action in the CNS. Barbiturates are highly bound to albumin and other plasma proteins. Because only unbound drug (free drug) can cross the blood–brain barrier, an inverse relationship exists between the degree of plasma protein binding and the rapidity of drug passage across the blood–brain barrier.

The final factor governing the rapidity of drug penetration of the blood–brain barrier is the plasma drug concentration. Simply because of concentration gradient, higher levels of drug concentrations in the plasma produce greater amounts of drug that diffuses into the CSF and brain. The two primary determinants of the plasma concentration are the dose administered and the rate (speed) of administration. The higher the dose and the more rapid its administration, the more rapid is the effect. This is of particular importance in the elderly patient who may have a reduced central volume of distribution and thus require a reduced dose of thiopental in order to reach the same plasma concentration as a younger adult.[51]

Cardiovascular System

Cardiovascular depression from barbiturates is a result of both central and peripheral (direct vascular and cardiac) effects.[52] The hemodynamic changes produced by barbiturates have been studied in healthy subjects and in patients with heart disease. The primary cardiovascular effect of barbiturate induction is peripheral vasodilation that results in a pooling of blood in the venous system. A decrease in contractility is another effect, which is related to reduced availability of calcium to the myofibrils. There is also an increase in heart rate. Mechanisms for the decrease in cardiac output include (1) direct negative inotropic action, (2) decreased ventricular filling because of increased capacitance, and (3) transiently decreased sympathetic outflow from the CNS. The increase in heart rate (10%–36%) that accompanies thiopental administration probably results from the baroreceptor-mediated sympathetic reflex stimulation of the heart in response to the decrease in output and pressure. Thiopental produces dose-related negative inotropic effects, which seem to result from a decrease in calcium influx into the cells with a resultant diminished amount of calcium at sarcolemma sites. The cardiac index is unchanged or is reduced, and the MAP is maintained or is slightly reduced.[52] Thiopental infusions and lower doses tend to be accompanied by smaller hemodynamic changes than those noted with rapid bolus injections.[26]

The increase in heart rate encountered in patients with coronary artery disease anesthetized with thiopental (1–4 mg/kg) is potentially deleterious because of the obligatory increase in myocardial oxygen consumption (MVO_2) that accompanies the increased heart rate. Patients who have normal coronary arteries have no difficulty in maintaining adequate coronary blood flow to meet the increased MVO_2.[53] When thiopental is given to hypovolemic patients, there is a significant reduction in cardiac output (69%) as well as a substantial decrease in blood pressure.[38–41] Patients without adequate compensatory mechanisms, therefore, may have serious hemodynamic depression with thiopental induction. All of these concerns are of particular importance in geriatric patients, because they are more likely to have clinically significant coronary artery disease, they are more likely to be intravascularly hypovolemic, and their compensatory mechanisms to maintain heart rate and blood pressure may be reduced because of age-related alterations and pharmacologic treatments such as beta-blockers or calcium channel blockers. Thus, it is of prime importance in the elderly patient to understand proper dose reduction (discussed below) and the effects of the rate of administration of an induction bolus. If these are not heeded, it becomes common to have significant hypotension in the geriatric patient with the need to administer vasopressors after induction, a practice that can be avoided if a proper understanding of the above principle is gained.

Respiratory System

Barbiturates produce dose-related central respiratory depression. There is also a significant incidence of transient apnea after their administration for induction of anesthesia.[16] The evidence for central depression is a correlation between EEG suppression and minute ventilation.[54] With increased anesthetic effect, there is diminished minute ventilation. The time course of respiratory depression has not been fully studied, but it seems that peak respiratory depression (as measured by the slope of CO_2 concentration in the blood) and minute ventilation after delivery of thiopental 3.5 mg/kg occurs 1–1.5 minutes after administration. These parameters return to predrug levels rapidly, and within 15 minutes the drug effects are barely detectable.[55] Of note, respirations are lost sooner and return later than that seen with propofol. Patients with chronic lung disease are slightly more susceptible to the respiratory depression of thiopental. The usual ventilatory pattern with thiopental induction has been described as "double apnea." The initial apnea that occurs during drug administration lasts a few seconds and is succeeded by a few breaths of reasonably adequate tidal volume, which is followed by a longer apneic period. During the induction of anesthesia with thiopental, ventilation must be assisted or controlled to provide adequate respiratory exchange. This is of particular concern in the elderly patient who will have an increased closing capacity, which will produce a shorter time to becoming hypoxemic, as compared with the young adult patient.[22]

Metabolism and Disposition (Pharmacokinetics)

Thiopental pharmacokinetics have been described in both physiologic and compartmental models. These models basically describe a rapid mixing of the drug with the central blood volume followed by a quick distribution of the drug to the highly perfused, low-volume tissues (i.e., brain) with a slower redistribution of the drug to lean tissue (muscle). In these models, adipose tissue uptake and metabolic clearance (elimination) have only a minor role in the termination of the effects of the induction dose because of the minimal perfusion ratio compared with other tissues and the slow rate of removal, respectively. Both of these pharmacokinetic models describe rapid redistribution as the primary mechanism that terminates the action of a single induction dose.[32,56]

Awakening may be delayed in older patients mainly because of a decreased central volume of distribution relative to younger adults.[57] The initial volume of distribution is less in elderly patients when compared with that in young patients (80-year-old versus 35-year-old), which explains a 50%–75% lower dose requirement for the onset of EEG and hypnotic effects.[51,57] However, except in disease states, the clearance of thiopental is not reduced in the elderly, and thus, awakening should only be prolonged in the elderly with a bolus administration and not with a constant infusion.

Indications

Thiopental is an excellent hypnotic for use as an intravenous induction agent.[1] The prompt onset (15–30 seconds) of action and smooth induction noted with its use make thiopental superior to most other available drugs. The relatively rapid emergence, particularly after single use for induction, has also been a reason for the widespread use of thiopental in this setting. Thiopental does not possess analgesic properties and therefore it must be supplemented with analgesic drugs in order to obtund reflex responses to noxious stimuli during anesthesia induction and surgical procedures. Thiopental can be used to maintain general anesthesia, because repeated doses reliably sustain unconsciousness and contribute to amnesia. However, the ease of use of propofol for light sedation and total intravenous anesthesia has sup-

planted the use of thiopental for this purpose and relegated it mainly for use in the induction portion of an anesthetic.

Dosing in the Elderly

Numerous studies have shown that the brain of the elderly patient is not intrinsically more sensitive to the effects of thiopental than that of the younger patient.[51] Further studies concluded that the need for a reduction in the induction dose of thiopental in the elderly is attributable to a reduction in the central volume of distribution.[58] Shafer[32] collated the results of several studies to suggest that the optimal dose in an 80-year-old patient is 2.1 mg/kg, which is approximately 80% of the dose needed for a young adult. However, it should again be noted that slower bolusing of the induction dose will generally result in less-acute hemodynamic alterations. Furthermore, monitoring of an EEG-related endpoint during a slow induction can guide the amount of drug given and may allow for a more individualized dosing regimen.[59]

Adverse Effects and Contraindications

The effects of barbiturates on various organ systems have been studied extensively. There are several side effects that occur in unpredictable, varying proportions of patients, whereas the cardiovascular and pulmonary are dose-related.[60] The complications of injecting barbiturates include a garlic or onion taste (40% of patients), allergic reactions, local tissue irritation, and rarely, tissue necrosis. An urticarial rash may develop on the head, neck, and trunk that lasts a few minutes. More severe reactions such as facial edema, hives, bronchospasm, and anaphylaxis can occur. Treatment of anaphylaxis is to stop any further administration of the drug, administer 1-mL increments of 1:10,000 epinephrine with boluses of intravenous fluids, give inhaled bronchodilators, such as albuterol, for bronchospasm, and then administer histamine antagonists, such as Benadryl and Pepcid.

Studies have shown pain on injection to be 9% and phlebitis to be approximately 1% with thiopental use.[61] Tissue and venous irritation are more common if a 5% solution is used rather than the standard 2.5% solution. Rarely, intraarterial injection can occur. The consequences of accidental arterial injection may be severe. The degree of injury is related to the concentration of the drug. Treatment consists of (1) dilution of the drug by the administration of saline into the artery, (2) heparinization to prevent thrombosis, and (3) brachial plexus block. Overall, the proper administration of thiopental intravenously into a briskly running IV is remarkably free of local toxicity.[60] However, it should be noted that thiopental can precipitate if the alkalinity of the solution is decreased, which is why it cannot be reconstituted with lactated Ringer's solution or mixed with other acidic solutions. Examples of drugs that are not to be coadministered or mixed in solution with the barbiturates are pancuronium, vecuronium, atracurium, alfentanil, sufentanil, and midazolam. Studies have shown that in rapid-sequence induction, the mixing of thiopental with vecuronium or pancuronium results in the formation of precipitate that may occlude the intravenous line.[62]

Midazolam

The first benzodiazepine found to have sedative-hypnotic effects was chlordiazepam (Librium) in 1955.[63] Diazepam (Valium) was synthesized in 1959 and became the first benzodiazepine used for sedation and anesthesia induction. Subsequently, a number of benzodiazepines have been produced including lorazepam and the antagonist flumazenil. The benzodiazepines produce many of the elements important in anesthesia. They produce their actions by occupying the benzodiazepine receptor, which was first presented in 1971.[62] In 1977, specific benzodiazepine receptors were described when ligands were found to interact with a central receptor.[64] The most frequently used benzodiazepine in the elderly is midazolam. Fryer and Walser's 1976 synthesis of midazolam (Versed) produced the first clinically used water-soluble benzodiazepine[65] and it also was the first benzodiazepine that was produced primarily for use in anesthesia.[66]

Pharmacology: Structure/Action

Midazolam is water soluble in its formulation, but highly lipid soluble at physiologic pH.[67] Midazolam solution contains 1 or 5 mg/mL midazolam with 0.8% sodium chloride and 0.01% disodium edetate, with 1% benzyl alcohol as a preservative. The pH is adjusted to 3 with hydrochloric acid and sodium hydroxide. The imidazole ring of midazolam accounts for its stability in solution and rapid metabolism. The high lipophilicity accounts for the rapid CNS effect, as well as for the relatively large volume of distribution.[68]

Pharmacodynamics

Central Nervous System Effects

All benzodiazepines have hypnotic, sedative, anxiolytic, amnesic, anticonvulsant, and centrally produced muscle-relaxant properties. The drugs differ in their potency and efficacy with regard to each of these pharmacodynamic actions. The binding of benzodiazepines to their respective receptors is of high affinity, is stereospecific, and is able to fully saturate the receptors; the order of receptor affinity (thus potency) of the three agonists is lorazepam > midazolam > diazepam. Midazolam is approximately three to six times as potent as diazepam.[69]

The mechanism of action of benzodiazepines is reasonably well understood.[70–72] The interaction of ligands with the benzodiazepine receptor represents an example in which the complex systems of biochemistry, molecular pharmacology, genetic mutations, and clinical behavioral patterns are seen to interact. Through recent genetic studies, the $GABA_A$ subtypes have been found to mediate the different effects (amnesic, anticonvulsant, anxiolytic, and sleep).[73] Sedation, anterograde amnesia, and anticonvulsant properties are mediated via $a1$ receptors,[73] and anxiolysis and muscle relaxation are mediated by the $a2$ $GABA_A$ receptor.[73] The degree of effect exerted at these receptors is a function of plasma level. By using plasma concentration data and pharmacokinetic simulations, it has been estimated that a benzodiazepine receptor occupancy of less than 20% may be sufficient to produce the anxiolytic effect, whereas sedation is observed with 30%–50% receptor occupancy and unconsciousness requires 60% or higher occupation of benzodiazepine agonist receptors.[73]

Agonists and antagonists bind to a common (or at least overlapping) area of the benzodiazepine portion of the $GABA_A$ receptor by forming differing reversible bonds with it.[74] The effects of midazolam can be reversed by use of flumazenil, a benzodiazepine antagonist that occupies the benzodiazepine receptor, but produces no activity and therefore blocks the actions of midazolam. The duration of reversal is dependent on the dose of flumazenil and the residual concentration of midazolam.

The onset and duration of action of a bolus intravenous administration of midazolam depends largely on the dose given and time at which the dose is administered; the higher the dose given over a shorter time (bolus), the faster the onset. Midazolam has a rapid onset (usually within 30–60 seconds) of action. The time to establish equilibrium between plasma concentration and EEG effect of midazolam is approximately 2–3 minutes and is not affected by age.[75] Like onset, the duration of effect is related to lipid solubility and blood level.[76] Thus, termination of effect is relatively rapid after midazolam administration. But some physicians have a general sense that midazolam is associated with the production of confusion even after the termination of sedation. This has been reported in prior studies and case reports.[77,78] However, a more recent study suggests that this might not be the case, particularly at lower doses.[79] Taken together, these data seem to suggest that single, lower doses of midazolam (0.03 mg/kg) will not cause confusion, whereas higher doses (0.05–0.07 mg/kg) plus an infusion of midazolam will have a greater association with confusion in the geriatric patient, as opposed to that seen with the use of a low-dose propofol infusion.

Respiratory Effects

Midazolam, like most intravenous anesthetics and other benzodiazepines, produces dose-related central respiratory system depression. The peak decrease in minute ventilation after midazolam administration (0.15 mg/kg) is almost identical to that produced in healthy patients given diazepam (0.3 mg/kg).[80] Respiratory depression is potentiated with opioids and must be carefully monitored in elderly patients getting both. The peak onset of ventilatory depression with midazolam (0.13–0.2 mg/kg) is rapid (about 3 minutes), and significant depression remains for about 60–120 minutes.[56,81] The depression is dose-related. The respiratory depression of midazolam is more pronounced and of longer duration in patients with chronic obstructive pulmonary disease, and the duration of ventilatory depression is longer with midazolam (0.19 mg/kg) than with thiopental (3.3 mg/kg).[56]

At sufficient doses, apnea occurs with midazolam as with other hypnotics. The incidence of apnea after thiopental or midazolam when these drugs are given for induction of anesthesia is similar. In clinical trials, apnea occurred in 20% of 1130 patients given midazolam for induction and 27% of 580 patients given thiopental.[67] Apnea is related to dose and is more likely to occur in the presence of opioids. Old age, debilitating disease, and other respiratory depressant drugs probably also increase the incidence and degree of respiratory depression and apnea with midazolam.

Cardiovascular Effects

Midazolam alone has modest hemodynamic effects. The predominant hemodynamic change is a slight reduction in arterial blood pressure, resulting from a decrease in systemic vascular resistance. The hypotensive effect is minimal and about the same as seen with thiopental.[82] Despite the hypotension, midazolam, in doses as high as 0.2 mg/kg, is safe and effective for induction of anesthesia even in patients with severe aortic stenosis. The hemodynamic effects of midazolam are dose-related: the higher the plasma level, the greater the decrease in systemic blood pressure[83]; however, there is a plateau plasma drug effect above which little change in arterial blood pressure occurs. The plateau plasma level for midazolam is 100 ng/mL.[83] Heart rate, ventricular filling pressures, and cardiac output are maintained after induction of anesthesia with midazolam.

The stresses of endotracheal intubation and surgery are not blocked by midazolam.[84] Thus, adjuvant anesthetics, usually opioids, are often combined with benzodiazepines. The combination of benzodiazepines with opioids and nitrous oxide has been investigated in patients with ischemic and valvular heart diseases.[85–88] Whereas the addition of nitrous oxide to midazolam (0.2 mg/kg) has trivial hemodynamic consequences, the combination of benzodiazepines with opioids does have a synergistic effect.[89] The combination of midazolam with fentanyl[86] or sufentanil[88] produces greater decreases in systemic blood pressure than does each drug alone.

Metabolism and Disposition (Pharmacokinetics)

Biotransformation of all benzodiazepines occurs in the liver. The two principal pathways involve either hepatic microsomal oxidation (N-dealkylation or aliphatic hydroxylation) or glucuronide conjugation.[90,91] The difference in the two pathways is significant, because oxidation is susceptible to outside influences and can be impaired by certain population characteristics (specifically old age), disease states (e.g., hepatic cirrhosis), or the coadministration of other drugs that can impair oxidizing capacity (e.g., cimetidine). Of the two, conjugation is less susceptible to these factors.[90] Midazolam undergoes oxidation reduction, or phase I reactions, in the liver.[92] The cytochrome P450 3A4 is primarily responsible for metabolism.[93] The fused imidazole ring of midazolam is oxidized rapidly by the liver, which accounts for the high rate of hepatic clearance. Neither age nor smoking decreases midazolam biotransformation.[94] Chronic alcohol consumption increases the clearance of midazolam.[95]

The metabolites of the benzodiazepines can be important. Midazolam is biotransformed to hydroxymidazolams, which have activity, and when midazolam is given in prolonged infusions these metabolites can accumulate.[96] These metabolites are rapidly conjugated and excreted in the urine. The 1-hydroxymidazolam has an estimated clinical potency 20%–30% of midazolam.[97] It is primarily excreted by the kidneys and can cause profound sedation in patients with renal impairment.[98] Overall, the metabolites of midazolam are less potent and normally more rapidly cleared than the parent drug, making them of little concern in patients with normal hepatic and renal function. However, they may be a consideration in elderly patients with impaired renal function.

Midazolam is classified as a short-lasting benzodiazepine. The plasma disappearance curves of midazolam can be fitted to a two- or three-compartment model. The clearance rate of midazolam ranges from 6 to 11 mL/kg/min.[94] Although the termination of action of these drugs is primarily a result of redistribution of the drug from the CNS to other tissues after bolus or maintenance use for surgical anesthesia, after daily (long-term) repeated administration or after prolonged continuous infusion, midazolam blood levels will decrease more slowly.

Factors known to influence the pharmacokinetics of benzodiazepines are age, gender, race, enzyme induction, and hepatic and renal disease. Age reduces the clearance of midazolam to a modest degree.[99] Among the pharmacokinetic parameters of midazolam that vary significantly with age, it is clearance which does so most consistently.[100] In healthy adults, midazolam clearance is high, approximating 50% of hepatic blood flow.[101] However, with advanced age, there is a loss of functional hepatic tissue and a decrease in hepatic perfusion such that clearance is reduced in the elderly by as much as 30% from that of a young adult.[39] As a result of the normal decline in lean tissue mass and concomitant increase in percent body fat in the aged, a slight increase is also observed in volume of distribution.[102] Moreover, according to one study, advanced age is in itself enough to cause the mean elimination half-life of midazolam to double.[38] Neither oral bioavailability nor midazolam protein binding are affected by age, despite reduced hepatic albumin synthesis and lower serum albumin concentrations in the elderly.[39,100]

Midazolam pharmacokinetics are affected by obesity. The volume of distribution is increased as drug goes from the plasma into the adipose tissue. Although clearance is not altered, elimination half-lives are prolonged, because of the delayed return of the drug to the plasma in obese persons.[99] This can be of concern in elderly obese patients. Although the pharmacokinetics of midazolam are clearly affected by age, they are, with the exception of total clearance, not consistently altered to statistical significance.[39,98] These pharmacokinetic changes with age do not explain the increased sensitivity of the elderly to midazolam discussed above. There are pharmacodynamic factors that are yet to be fully understood that make midazolam more potent in the elderly than the young.

Indications

Intravenous Sedation

Midazolam is used for sedation as preoperative premedication, intraoperatively during regional or local anesthesia, and postoperatively for sedation. The anxiolysis, amnesia, and elevation of the local anesthetic seizure threshold are desirable benzodiazepine actions for regional anesthesia. It should be given by titration for this use; endpoints of titration are adequate sedation or dysarthria and maintained ventilation. The onset of action is relatively rapid with midazolam, usually with peak effect reached within 2–3 minutes of administration. The duration of action depends primarily on the dose used. There is often a disparity in the level of sedation compared with the presence of amnesia (patients can be seemingly conscious and coherent, yet they are amnesic for events and instructions). The degree of sedation and the reliable amnesia, as well as preservation of respiratory and hemodynamic function, are better overall with midazolam than with other sedative-hypnotic drugs used for conscious sedation. When midazolam is compared with propofol for

sedation, the two are generally similar except that emergence or wake-up is more rapid with propofol and amnesia is more reliable with midazolam. Propofol requires closer medical supervision because of its respiratory depression and hypotension.[103,104] Despite the wide safety margin with midazolam, respiratory function must be monitored when it is used for sedation to prevent undesirable degrees of respiratory depression. This is especially true in the geriatric patient. There may be a slight synergistic action between midazolam and spinal anesthesia with respect to ventilation.[103] Thus, the use of midazolam for sedation during regional and epidural anesthesia requires vigilance with regard to respiratory function, as when these drugs are given with opioids. Sedation for longer periods, for example, in the intensive care unit, is accomplished with benzodiazepines. Prolonged infusion will result in accumulation of drug and, in the case of midazolam, significant concentration of the active metabolite. The chief advantages are the amnesia and hemodynamic stability and the disadvantage, compared with propofol, is the longer dissipation of effects when infusion is terminated.

Induction and Maintenance of Anesthesia

With midazolam, induction of anesthesia is defined as unresponsiveness to command and loss of the eyelash reflex. When midazolam is used in appropriate doses, induction occurs less rapidly than with thiopental or propofol,[67] but the amnesia is more reliable. Numerous factors influence the rapidity of action of midazolam. These factors are dose, speed of injection, degree of premedication, age, American Society of Anesthesiologists (ASA) physical status, and concurrent anesthetic drugs.[67,105] In a well-premedicated, healthy patient, midazolam (0.2 mg/kg given in 5–15 seconds) will induce anesthesia in 28 seconds. Emergence time is related to the dose of midazolam as well as to the dose of adjuvant anesthetic drugs.[67] Emergence is more prolonged with midazolam than with propofol.[106,107] This difference accounts for some anesthesiologists' preference for propofol induction for short operations. The best method of monitoring depth with midazolam is use of the EEG-BIS.[108]

The amnesic period after an anesthetic dose is about 1–2 hours. Infusions of midazolam have been used to ensure a constant and appropriate depth of anesthesia.[109] Experience indicates that a plasma level of more than 50 ng/mL when used with adjuvant opioids (e.g., fentanyl) and/or inhalation anesthetics (e.g., nitrous oxide, volatile anesthetics) is achieved with a bolus loading dose of 0.05–0.15 mg/kg and a continuous infusion of 0.25–1 μg/kg/min.[110] This is sufficient to keep the patient asleep and amnesic but arousable at the end of surgery. Lower infusion doses almost certainly are required in elderly patients and with certain opioids.

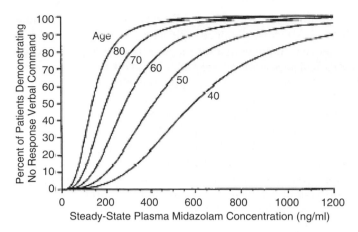

FIGURE 16-5. Response curves to verbal commands in patients of various ages at varying plasma levels of midazolam. This demonstrates a pharmacodynamic change associated with aging in response to midazolam. (Reprinted with permission from Jacobs et al.[112])

Effects of Age on Pharmacology

Elderly patients require lower doses of midazolam than younger patients to reach various standard clinical endpoints of sedation, such as response to verbal command (Figure 16-5).[111,112] The usual induction dose of midazolam in elderly premedicated patients is between 0.05 and 0.15 mg/kg. Some studies show that patients older than 55 years and those with ASA physical status higher than 3 require a 20% or more reduction in the induction dose of midazolam.[67] However, Shafer, who collated the results of numerous pharmacokinetic and pharmacodynamic studies, recommends a 75% reduction in dose from the 20-year-old to the 90-year-old. Thus, there is definitely a graded decrease in the amount of drug needed as a result of aging.[32] Furthermore, when midazolam is used with other anesthetic drugs (coinduction), there is a synergistic interaction,[110,113,114] and the induction dose is less than 0.1 mg/kg. The synergy is seen when midazolam is used with opioids and/or other hypnotics such as thiopental, propofol, and etomidate.

Awakening after midazolam anesthesia is the result of the redistribution of drug from the brain to other, less well-perfused tissues. The emergence (defined as orientation to time and place) of young, healthy volunteers who received 10 mg of intravenous midazolam occurred in about 15 minutes,[113] and, after an induction dose of 0.15 mg/kg, it occurred in about 17 minutes.[78] The effect of age on emergence has not been studied, but it likely is prolonged compared with younger patients because of greater potency in the elderly.

Adverse Effects and Contraindications

Midazolam is a remarkably safe drug. It has a relatively high margin of safety, especially compared with barbitu-

rates and propofol. It is also free of allergenic effects and does not suppress the adrenal gland.[114] The most significant problem with midazolam is respiratory depression. It is free of venous irritation and thrombophlebitis, problems related to aqueous insolubility and requisite solvents in other drug formulations.[67] When used as a sedative or for induction and maintenance of anesthesia, midazolam can produce an undesirable degree or prolonged interval of postoperative amnesia, sedation, and, rarely, respiratory depression. These residual effects can be reversed with flumazenil.

Etomidate

Pharmacology: Structure/Action

Etomidate is a hypnotic drug that is structurally unrelated to all other induction medications. It contains a carboxylated imidazole ring that provides water solubility in an acidic milieu and lipid solubility at physiologic pH. It is dissolved in propylene glycol, which often causes pain on injection. Etomidate works by depressing the reticular activating system and it enhances the inhibitory effects of GABA by binding to a subunit of the $GABA_A$ receptor and thereby increasing its affinity for GABA. However, unlike the barbiturates, which have global depressant effects on the reticular activating system, etomidate has some disinhibitory effects, which accounts for the 30%–60% rate of myoclonus with administration. Interestingly, one study has shown that this unwanted side effect can be reduced with pretreatment, similar to a defasciculating dose of NMBDs.[115]

Pharmacodynamics

Central Nervous System Effects

Etomidate induces changes in CBF, metabolic rate, and ICP to the same extent as thiopental and propofol. However, because this is not the result of a large reduction in arterial blood pressure, CPP is well maintained.[115] This is of particular importance in the elderly person who is at risk for ischemic stroke secondary to carotid occlusion. Etomidate has EEG changes similar to thiopental with a biphasic pattern of activation followed by depression. However, etomidate has been shown to activate somatosensory evoked potentials.[50] Of note, etomidate does have a higher rate of postoperative nausea and vomiting associated with it than with the other intravenous induction drugs.[116] Finally, there are no pharmacodynamic changes with age with respect to etomidate as measured by EEG.[115]

Cardiovascular Effects

Unlike propofol, etomidate has minimal effects on the cardiovascular system. There is a slight decline in the arterial blood pressure secondary to a mild reduction in the systemic vascular resistance. Etomidate does not seem to have direct myocardial depressant effects, because myocardial contractility, heart rate, and cardiac output are usually unchanged.[117] Etomidate does not cause histamine release. These aspects of the pharmacodynamics of etomidate make it very useful in the patient with compromised intravascular volume, coronary artery disease, or reduced ventricular function, as is often encountered in the elderly patient.

Respiratory Effects

Etomidate causes less respiratory depression than benzodiazepines, barbiturates, or propofol in induction doses. In fact, even an induction dose of etomidate often does not cause apnea.[118] This fact, combined with its minimal cardiovascular effects, makes etomidate a very useful drug in the setting of a hemodynamically brittle elderly patient with a possible difficult airway and little respiratory reserve.

Endocrine Effects

Induction doses of etomidate temporarily inhibit the synthesis of cortisol and aldosterone.[119] However, with a single bolus dose there is little clinical significance. Alternatively, long-term infusions or closely repeated exposures can lead to adrenocortical suppression, which may be associated with an increased susceptibility to infection and an increased mortality rate in the critically ill patient.[120]

Metabolism and Disposition (Pharmacokinetics)

Etomidate is used only in intravenous formulations and is generally used for the induction of general anesthesia. Etomidate is similar to thiopental in its distribution and onset of action. Although it is highly protein bound, etomidate has a very rapid onset of action because of its high lipid solubility and its large nonionized fraction. Redistribution to noncentral compartments is responsible for its rapid offset of action. Hepatic microsomal enzymes as well as plasma esterases rapidly hydrolyze etomidate to its nonactive metabolites. This rate of biotransformation is five times greater than that of thiopental, but less than that of propofol.

The volume of distribution is slightly larger than that of the barbiturates and the elimination clearance is greater. However, the elimination clearance is still less than propofol. Thus, the elimination half-life of etomidate is faster than thiopental, but longer than propofol. Both of these parameters are decreased in the elderly, which causes a higher plasma concentration of etomidate for any given dose. Furthermore, to our knowledge, no study has ever shown an increased brain sensitivity to etomidate with increasing age. Therefore, like thiopental, any dose reduction in the elderly is attributable to pharmacokinetic, not pharmacodynamic, changes.[121]

Indications

Etomidate is used for the intravenous induction of anesthesia.[1] It can be used with an intermittent bolus technique for short procedures. Typically, 25% of the induction dose is given every 15–30 minutes to maintain surgical anesthesia. Etomidate is not approved in the United States for maintenance infusions.

Dosing in the Elderly

The standard induction dose of etomidate is intravenous 0.3–0.4 mg/kg. However, the elderly may only require 0.2 mg/kg. This change in dosage is attributable only to pharmacokinetic parameters, not pharmacodynamic.[121]

Adverse Effects and Contraindications

Etomidate has a high incidence of side effects, most of which are minor. As mentioned above, etomidate has a higher rate of postoperative nausea and vomiting than either propofol or thiopental. The incidence of myoclonic movements on induction is reported to be as high as 60%. This effect as well as pain on injection can be reduced with a slow injection into a rapidly running intravenous carrier line, preferably in a large vein. When etomidate is injected into veins in the hand, the incidence of pain is reported to exceed 40%. Furthermore, because of the propylene glycol solvent, studies have shown that 10%–20% of patients experience venous sequelae after its use.[122]

Summary

This chapter has surveyed the pharmacology of frequently used intravenous hypnotic agents in the geriatric patient. There is substantial evidence of significant changes in the pharmacokinetic and pharmacodynamic behavior of propofol, thiopental, midazolam, and etomidate in this population. A few final points remain when considering the general changes for each of these hypnotic agents. First, practitioners should perform a thorough review of the cardiopulmonary status of all geriatric patients, because an absence of complaints in a review of systems may merely be a function of a sedentary lifestyle. A more extensive history may elicit findings that would alter the method of induction or the combination/doses of drugs used for anesthesia. Second, a full review of the current medical management of systemic disease should be performed, because the elderly population often presents for surgery with outpatient polypharmacy. Particular attention should be given to current use of antihypertensive, diuretic, antidepressant, anti-Parkinsonian, and erectile dysfunction agents, with vigilance given to careful blood pressure monitoring when using the induction agents reviewed in this chapter in patients who are taking one or several of these medications. Third, a thorough understanding of the changes in the pharmacokinetics and pharmacodynamics of opioids in the geriatric patient is critical when combining them for sedation or general anesthesia in this population. Finally, unless a rapid sequence induction is indicated, a slow and careful titration of the induction of anesthesia using smaller doses of hypnotic agents and some form of an EEG monitor will prevent overdosing, subsequent hypotension, and delayed awakening in this population.

References

1. Martin G, Glass PS, Breslin DS, et al. A study of anesthetic drug utilization in different age groups. J Clin Anesth 2003; 15(3):194–200.
2. Trifune M, Takarada T, Shimizu Y, et al. Propofol-induced anesthesia in mice is mediated by gamma-aminobutyric acid-A and excitatory amino acid receptors. Anesth Analg 2003;97(2):424–429.
3. Dong XP, Xu TL. The actions of propofol on gamma-aminobutyric acid-A and glycine receptors in acutely dissociated spinal dorsal horn neurons of the rat. Anesth Analg 2002;95(4):907–914.
4. Glen JB, Hunter SC. Pharmacology of an emulsion formulation of ICI 35 868. Br J Anaesth 1984;56:617–626.
5. Carr S, Waterman S, Rutherford G, et al. Postsurgical infections associated with an extrinsically contaminated intravenous anesthetic agent: California, Illinois, Maine, and Michigan, 1990. MMWR Morb Mortal Wkly Rep 1990;39: 426–427.
6. Bennett SN, McNeil MM, Bland LA, et al. Postoperative infections traced to contamination of an intravenous anesthetic, propofol. N Engl J Med 1995;333:147–154.
7. Ludbrook GL, Visco E, Lam AM. Propofol: relation between brain concentrations, electro-encephalogram, middle cerebral artery blood flow velocity, and cerebral oxygen extraction during induction of anesthesia. Anesthesiology 2002;97(6):1363–1370.
8. van der Starre PJA, Guta C. Choice of anesthetics. Anesthesiol Clin North Am 2004;22(2):251–264.
9. Kuizenga K, Wierda JM, Kalkman CJ. Biphasic EEG changes in relation to loss of consciousness during induction with thiopental, propofol, etomidate, midazolam or sevoflurane. Br J Anaesth 2001;86(3):354–360.
10. Schultz A, Grouven U, Zander I, Beger FA, Siedenberg M, Schultz B. Age-related effects in the EEG during propofol anaesthesia. Acta Anaesthesiol Scand 2004;48(1):27–34.
11. Ding Z, White PF. Anesthesia for electroconvulsive therapy. Anesth Analg 2002;94(5):1351–1364.
12. Schnider TW, Minto CF, Shafer SL, et al. The influence of age on propofol pharmacodynamics. Anesthesiology 1999;90(6):1502–1516.
13. Brown RH, Greenberg RS, Wagner EM. Efficacy of propofol to prevent bronchoconstriction: effects of preservative. Anesthesiology 2001;94:851–855; discussion 6A.
14. Conti G, Dell'Utri D, Vilardi V, et al. Propofol induces bronchodilation in mechanically ventilated chronic obstructive pulmonary disease (COPD) patients. Acta Anaesthesiol Scand 1993;37:105–109.
15. Streisand JB, Nelson P, Bubbers S, et al. The respiratory effects of propofol with and without fentanyl. Anest Analg 1987;66:S171.
16. Bluoin RT, Conrad PF, Gross JB. Time course of ventilatory depression following induction doses of propofol and thiopental. Anesthesiology 1991;75:940–944.
17. Tagaito Y, Isono S, Nishino T. Upper airway reflexes during a combination of propofol and fentanyl anesthesia. Anesthesiology 1998;88(6):1459–1466.
18. Van Keer L, Van Aken H, et al. Propofol does not inhibit hypoxic pulmonary vasoconstriction in humans. J Clin Anesth 1989;1:284–288.
19. Abe K, Shimizu T, Takashina M, Shiozaki H, Yoshiya I, et al. The effects of propofol, isoflurane, and sevoflurane on oxygenation and shunt fraction during one-lung ventilation. Anesth Analg 1998;87(5):1164–1169.
20. Blouin RT, Seifert HA, Babenco HD, Conard PF, Gross JB. Propofol depresses the hypoxic ventilatory response during conscious sedation and isohypercapnia. Anesthesiology 1993;79:1177–1182.
21. Chan ED, Welsh CH. Geriatric respiratory medicine. Chest 1998;114(6):1704–1733.
22. Zaugg M, Lucchinetti E. Respiratory function in the elderly. Anesthesiol Clin North Am 2000;18(1):47–58, vi.
23. Kirkbride DA, Parker JL, Williams GD, Buggy DJ. Induction of anesthesia in the elderly ambulatory patient: a double-blinded comparison of propofol and sevoflurane. Anesth Analg 2001;93(5):1185–1187.
24. John AD, Sieber FE. Age associated issues: geriatrics. Anesthesiol Clin North Am 2004;22(1):45–58.
25. Rooke GA. Autonomic and cardiovascular function in the geriatric patient. Anesthesiol Clin North Am 2000;18(1): 31–46, v–vi.
26. Kazama T, Ikeda K, Morita K, et al. Comparison of the effect-site k(eO)s of propofol for blood pressure and EEG bispectral index in elderly and younger patients. Anesthesiology 1999;90(6):1517–1527.
27. Tramèr M, Moore A, McQuay H. Propofol anaesthesia and postoperative nausea and vomiting: quantitative systematic review of randomized controlled studies. Br J Anaesth 1997;78(3):247–255.
28. Borgeat A, Wilder-Smith OH, Saiah M, Rifat K. Sub-hypnotic doses of propofol relieve pruritus induced by epidural and intrathecal morphine. Anesthesiology 1992;76(4):510–512.
29. Schüttler J, Ihmsen H. Population pharmacokinetics of propofol: a multicenter study. Anesthesiology 2000;92: 727–738.
30. Shafer A, Doze VA, Shafer SL, White PF. Pharmacokinetics and pharmacodynamics of propofol infusions

during general anesthesia. Anesthesiology 1988;69: 348–356.

31. Schnider TW, Minto CF, Gumbus PL, et al. The influence of method of administration and covariates on the pharmacokinetics of propofol in adult volunteers. Anesthesiology 1998;88(5):1170–1182.

32. Shafer SL. The pharmacology of anesthetic drugs in elderly patients. Anesthesiol Clin North Am 2000;18(1):1–29, v.

33. Takaono M, Yogosawa T, Okawa-Takatsuji M, Aotsuka S. Effects of intravenous anesthetics on interleukin (IL)-6 and IL-10 production by lipopolysaccharide-stimulated mononuclear cells from healthy volunteers. Acta Anaesthesiol Scand 2002;46(2):176–179.

34. Alvarez-Ayuso L, Calero P, Granado F, et al. Antioxidant effect of gamma-tocopherol supplied by propofol preparations (Diprivan) during ischemia-reperfusion in experimental lung transplantation. Transpl Int 2004;17(2):71–77.

35. Lombardo A. Inflammation as a possible link between coronary and carotid plaque instability. Circulation 2004; 109(25):3158–3163.

36. Willerson JT. Inflammation as a cardiovascular risk factor. Circulation 2004;109(21 Suppl 1):II2–10.

37. Dundee JW, Hassard TH, McGowan WAW, et al. The "induction" dose of thiopentone: a method of study and preliminary illustrative results. Anaesthesia 1982;37:1176.

38. Ball C, Westhorpe R. The history of intravenous anaesthesia: the barbiturates. Part 1. Anaesth Intensive Care 2001; 29(2):97.

39. Ball C, Westhorpe R. The history of intravenous anaesthesia: the barbiturates. Part 2. Anaesth Intensive Care 2001; 29(3):219.

40. Ball C, Westhorpe R. The history of intravenous anaesthesia: the barbiturates. Part 3. Anaesth Intensive Care 2001; 29(4):323.

41. Dundee JW. Fifty years of thiopentone. Br J Anaesth 1984;56:211.

42. Tanelian DL, Kosek P, Mody I, et al. The role of the GABAA receptor/chloride channel complex in anesthesia. Anesthesiology 1993;78:757.

43. Dundee JW. Molecular structure-activity relationships of barbiturates. In: Halsey MJ, Millar RA, Sutton JA, eds. Molecular Mechanisms in General Anesthesia. New York: Churchill Livingstone; 1974:16.

44. Archer DP, Ewen A, Froelich J, Roth SH, Samanani N. Thiopentone induced enhancement of somatic motor responses to noxious stimulation: influence of GABAA receptor modulation. Can J Anaesth 1996;43(5 Pt 1):503–510.

45. Veselis RA, Reinsel RA, Feshchenko VA, Wroński M. The comparative amnestic effects of midazolam, propofol, thiopental, and fentanyl at equisedative concentrations. Anesthesiology 1997;87(4):749–764.

46. Stulken EH Jr, Milde JH, Michenfelder JD, et al. The nonlinear response of cerebral metabolism to low concentrations of halothane, enflurane, isoflurane and thiopental. Anesthesiology 1977;46:28.

47. Smith AL. Barbiturate protection in cerebral hypoxia. Anesthesiology 1977;47:285.

48. Baughman VL. Brain protection during neurosurgery. Anesthesiol Clin North Am 2002;20(2):315–327, vi.

49. Albrecht RF, Miletich DJ, Rosenberg R, et al. Cerebral blood flow and metabolic changes from induction to onset of anesthesia with halothane or pentobarbital. Anesthesiology 1977;47:252.

50. Cheng MA, Theard MA, Tempelhoff R. Intravenous agents and intraoperative neuroprotection. Beyond barbiturates. Crit Care Clin 1997;13(1):185–199.

51. Stanski DR, Maitre PO. Population pharmacokinetics and pharmacodynamics of thiopental: the effect of age revisited. Anesthesiology 1990;72:412–422.

52. Russo H, Bressolle E. Pharmacodynamics and pharmacokinetics of thiopental. Clin Pharmacokinet 1998;35:95–134.

53. Sonntag H, Hellberg K, Schenk HD, et al. Effects of thiopental (Trapanal) on coronary blood flow and myocardial metabolism in man. Acta Anaesthesiol Scand 1975;19(1): 69–78.

54. Choi SD, Spaulding BC, Gross JB, Apfelbaum JL. Comparison of the ventilatory effects of etomidate and methohexital. Anesthesiology 1985;62(4):442–447.

55. Hung OR, Varvel JR, Shafer SL, Stanski DR. Thiopental pharmacodynamics. II. Quantitation of clinical and electroencephalographic depth of anesthesia. Anesthesiology 1992;77(2):237–244.

56. Gross JB, Zebrowski ME, Carel WD, Gardner S, Smith TC. Time course of ventilatory depression after thiopental and midazolam in normal subjects and in patients with chronic obstructive pulmonary disease. Anesthesiology 1983;58(6):540–544.

57. Wada DR, Bjorkman S, Ebling WF, et al. Computer simulation of the effects of alterations in blood flows and body composition on thiopental pharmacokinetics in humans. Anesthesiology 1997;87:884.

58. Homer TD, Stanski DR. The effect of increasing age on thiopental disposition and anesthetic requirement. Anesthesiology 1985;62:714–724.

59. Avram MJ, Krejcie TC, Henthorn TK. The relationship of age to the pharmacokinetics of early drug distribution: the concurrent disposition of thiopental and indocyanine green. Anesthesiology 1990;72:403–411.

60. Mortier E, Struys M, De Smet T, Versichelen L, Rolly G. Closed-loop controlled administration of propofol using bispectral analysis. Anaesthesia 1998;53(8):749–754.

61. Dundee JW, Wyant GM. Intravenous Anaesthesia. 2nd ed. Edinburgh: Churchill Livingstone; 1988.

62. Reves JG, Glass PSA, Lubarsky DA. Nonbarbiturate intravenous anesthetics. In: Miller RD, ed. Anesthesia. 5th ed. New York: Churchill Livingstone; 2000:228–272.

63. Kawar P, Dundee JW. Frequency of pain on injection and venous sequelae following the I.V. administration of certain anaesthetics and sedatives. Br J Anaesth 1982; 54(9):935–939.

64. Haefely W, Hunkeler W. The story of flumazenil. Eur J Anaesthesiol 1988;2:3.

65. Squires RF, Braestrup C. Benzodiazepine receptors in rat brain. Nature 1977;266:732.

66. Walser A, Benjamin LES, Flynn T, et al. Quinazolines and 1,4-benzodiazepines. 84. Synthesis and reactions of imidazo (1,5)(1,4)-benzodiazepines. J Org Chem 1978;43:936.

67. Reves JG, Fragen RJ, Vinik HR, et al. Midazolam: pharmacology and uses. Anesthesiology 1985;62:310.

68. Greenblatt DJ, Shader RI, Abernethy DR. Medical intelligence drug therapy: current status of benzodiazepines. N Engl J Med 1983;309:354.

69. Arendt RM, Greenblatt DJ, DeJong RH, et al. In vitro correlates of benzodiazepine cerebrospinal fluid uptake, pharmacodynamic action and peripheral distribution. J Pharmacol Exp Ther 1983;227:98.

70. Mould DR, DeFeo TM, Reele S, et al. Simultaneous modeling of the pharmacokinetics and pharmacodynamics of midazolam and diazepam. Clin Pharmacol Ther 1995; 58:35.

71. Mohler H, Richards JG. The benzodiazepine receptor: a pharmacological control element of brain function. Eur J Anaesthesiol 1988;2:15.

72. Amrein R, Hetzel W. Pharmacology of Dormicum (midazolam) and Anexate (flumazenil). Acta Anaesthsiol Scand 1990;92:6.

73. Mohler H, Fritschy JM, Rudolph U. A new benzodiazepine pharmacology. J Pharmacol Exp Ther 2002;300:2.

74. Amrein R, Hetzel W, Harmann D, et al. Clinical pharmacology of flumazenil. Eur J Anaesthesiol 1988;2:65.

75. Haefely W. The preclinical pharmacology of flumazenil. Eur J Anaesthesiol 1988;2:25.

76. Breimer LTM, Burm AGL, Danhof M, et al. Pharmacokinetic-pharmacodynamic modelling on the interaction between flumazenil and midazolam in volunteers by aperiodic EEG analysis. Clin Pharmacokinet 1991;20:497.

77. White PF, Negus JB. Sedative infusions during local and regional anesthesia: a comparison of midazolam and propofol. J Clin Anesth 1991;3(1):32–39.

78. Burnakis TG, Berman DE. Hostility and hallucinations as a consequence of midazolam administration. DICP 1989; 23(9):671–672.

79. Christe C, Janssens JP, Armenian B, Herrmann F, Vogt N. Midazolam sedation for upper gastrointestinal endoscopy in older persons: a randomized, double-blind, placebo-controlled study. J Am Geriatr Soc 2000;48(11):1398–1403.

80. Forster A, Gardaz JP, Suter PM, et al. Respiratory depression by midazolam and diazepam. Anesthesiology 1980; 53:494.

81. Brodgen RN, Goa KL. Flumazenil. Drugs 1991;42:1061.

82. Lebowitz PW, Core ME, Daniels AL, et al. Comparative cardiovascular effects of midazolam and thiopental in healthy patients. Anesth Analg 1982;61:771.

83. Sunzel M, Paalzow L, Berggren L, et al. Respiratory and cardiovascular effects in relations to plasma levels of midazolam and diazepam. Br J Clin Pharmacol 1988;25: 561.

84. Samuelson PN, Reves JG, Kouchoukos NT, et al. Hemodynamic responses to anesthetic induction with midazolam or diazepam in patients with ischemic heart disease. Anesth Analg 1981;60:802.

85. Ruff R, Reves JG. Hemodynamic effects of a lorazepam-fentanyl anesthetic induction for coronary artery bypass surgery. J Cardiothorac Anesth 1990;4:314.

86. Heikkila H, Jalonen J, Arola M, et al. Midazolam as adjunct to high-dose fentanyl anaesthesia for coronary artery bypass grafting operation. Acta Anaesthesiol Scand 1984; 28:683.

87. Benson KT, Tomlinson DL, Goto H, et al. Cardiovascular effects of lorazepam during sufentanil anesthesia. Anesth Analg 1988;67:966.

88. Windsor JW, Sherry K, Feneck RO, et al. Sufentanil and nitrous oxide anaesthesia for cardiac surgery. Br J Anaesth 1988;61:662.

89. Reves JG, Croughwell N. Valium-fentanyl interaction. In: Reves JG, Hall K, eds. Common Problems in Cardiac Anaesthesia. Chicago: Year Book; 1987:356.

90. Greenblatt DL, Shader RI. Benzodiazepines in Clinical Practice. New York: Raven Press; 1974.

91. Elliott HW. Metabolism of lorazepam. Br J Anaesth 1976; 48:1017.

92. Blitt CD. Clinical pharmacology of lorazepam. In: Brown BRJ, ed. New Pharmacologic Vistas in Anesthesia. Philadelphia: FA Davis; 1983:135.

93. Kronbach T, Mathys D, Umeno M, Gonzalez FJ, Meyer UA. Oxidation of midazolam and triazolam by human liver cytochrome P450IIIA4. Mol Pharmacol 1989;36:89–96.

94. Reves JG. Benzodiazepines. In: Prys-Roberts C, Hugg CC, eds. Pharmacokinetics of Anesthesia. Boston: Blackwell Scientific Publications; 1984:157.

95. Kassai A, Eichelbaum M, Klotz U. No evidence of a genetic polymorphism in the oxidative metabolism of midazolam. Clin Pharmacokinet 1988;15:319.

96. Barr J, Donner A. Optimal intravenous dosing strategies for sedatives and analgesics in the intensive care unit. Crit Care Clin 1995;11:827.

97. Mandema JW, Tuk B, van Steveninck AL, et al. Pharmacokinetic-pharmacodynamic modeling of the central nervous system effects of midazolam and its main metabolite α-hydroxymidazolam in healthy volunteers. Clin Pharmacol Ther 1992;51:715.

98. Bauer TM, Ritz R, Haberthur C, et al. Prolonged sedation due to accumulation of conjugated metabolites of midazolam. Lancet 1995;346:145.

99. Greenblatt DJ, Abernethy DR, Loeniskar A, et al. Effect of age, gender, and obesity on midazolam kinetics. Anesthesiology 1984;61:27.

100. Weese H, Scharpf W. Evipan ein neuartiges Einschlafmittel. Dtsch Med Wochenschr 1932;58:1205.

101. Tabern TW, Volwiler EH. Sulfur-containing barbiturate hypnotics. J Am Chem Soc 1935;57:1961.

102. Halford FJ. A critique of intravenous anaesthesia in war surgery. Anaesthesiology 1943;4:67–69.

103. Sanchez-Izquierdo-Riera JA, Caballero-Cubedo RE, Perez-Vela JL, Ambros-Checa A, Cantalapiedra-Santiago JA, Alted-Lopez E. Propofol versus midazolam: safety and efficacy for sedating the severe trauma patient. Anesth Analg 1998;86:1219.

104. Vargo JJ, Zuccaro G Jr, Dumot JA, et al. Gastroenterologist-administered propofol versus meperidine and midazolam for advanced upper endoscopy: a prospective, randomized trial. Gastroenterology 2002;123:8.

105. Gauthier RA, Dyck B, Chung R, et al. Respiratory interaction after spinal anesthesia sedation with midazolam. Anesthesiology 1992;77:909.

106. Kanto J, Sjoval S, Vuori A. Effect of different kinds of premedication on the induction properties of midazolam. Br J Anaesth 1982;54:507.

107. Norton AC, Dundas CR. Induction agents for day-case anaesthesia. Anaesthesia 1990;45:198.
108. Liu J, Singh H, White PF. Electroencephalogram bispectral analysis predicts the depth of midazolam-induced sedation. Anesthesiology 1996;84:64–69.
109. Melvin MA, Johnson BH, Quasha AL, et al. Induction of anesthesia with midazolam decreases halothane MAC in humans. Anesthesiology 1982;57:238.
110. Theil DR, Stanley TE, White WD, et al. Continuous intravenous anesthesia for cardiac surgery: a comparison of two infusion systems. J Thorac Cardiovasc Anesth 1993; 7:300.
111. Gamble JAS, Kawar P, Dundee JW, et al. Evaluation of midazolam as an intravenous induction agent. Anaesthesia 1981;36:868.
112. Jacobs JR, Reves JG, Marty J, et al. Aging increases pharmacodynamic sensitivity to the hypnotic effects of midazolam. Anesth Analg 1995;80:143.
113. Brown CR, Sarnquist FH, Canup CA, et al. Clinical electroencephalographic and pharmacokinetic studies of water-soluble benzodiazepine, midazolam maleate. Anesthesiology 1979;50:467.
114. Nilsson A, Persson MP, Hartvig P, et al. Effect of total intravenous anaesthesia with midazolam/alfentanil on the adrenocortical and hyperglycaemic response to abdominal surgery. Acta Anaesthesiol Scand 1988;32: 379.
115. Doenicke AW, Roizen MF, Kugler J, Kroll H, Foss J, Ostwald P. Reducing myoclonus after etomidate. Anesthesiology 1999;90(1):113–119.
116. Watcha MF, White PF. Postoperative nausea and vomiting. Its etiology, treatment, and prevention. Anesthesiology 1992;77:162–184.
117. Kettler D, Sonntag H, Donath U, Regensburger D. Schenk HD. Haemodynamics, myocardial mechanics, oxygen requirement and oxygenation of the human heart during induction of anaesthesia with etomidate. Anaesthesist 1974;23:116.
118. Choi SD, Spaulding BC, et al. Comparison of the ventilatory effects of etomidate and methohexital. Anesthesiology 1985;62:442.
119. Allolio B, Dörr H, Stuttmann R, Knorr D, Engelhardt D, Winkelmann W. Effect of a single bolus dose of etomidate upon eight major corticosteroid hormones and plasma ACTH. Clin Endocrinol (Oxf) 1985;22:281.
120. Wagner RL, White PF. Etomidate inhibits adrenocortical function in surgical patients. Anesthesiology 1984;61: 647–651.
121. Arden JR, Holley OF, Stanski DR. Increased sensitivity to etomidate in the elderly: initial distribution versus altered brain response. Anesthesiology 1986;65:19–27.
122. Korttila K, Aromaa U. Venous complications after intravenous injection of diazepam, flunitrazepam, thiopentone and etomidate. Acta Anaesthesiol Scand 1980;24:227.

17
Inhalational Anesthetics

Gary R. Haynes

General anesthesia with inhalational anesthetic agents is the most common method of surgical anesthesia. Although regional and neuroaxial anesthetics are preferred in some circumstances, the use of general anesthesia with inhalational agents remains widespread. Total intravenous anesthesia has greater acceptance in Europe where it accounts for approximately 40% of general anesthesia cases. However, only a small portion of general anesthesia cases in the United States use this technique.

General anesthesia in older adults with inhalational agents compares favorably to intravenous anesthesia.[1] However, there are many gaps in our knowledge of volatile anesthetic drug effects in the elderly. Many of the most comprehensive studies on inhalational anesthetics were done in young adults. Clinical drug trials demonstrating their safety, dosing, and efficacy frequently involve younger patients. When clinical trials enroll subjects over a range of ages, they frequently do not stratify patients into age groups. Consequently, it is often impossible to make statements describing any differences between younger and older patients.

The focus of past clinical studies investigating inhalational anesthetic agents was their immediate effects and short-term outcomes. The control of cardiovascular responses and time for emergence from general anesthesia are typical examples. There is only limited information on the immediate perioperative outcome of elderly patients and even fewer reports regarding their long-term outcomes. When the concern is the elderly patient, there are often more questions than answers.

The Pharmacokinetics of Inhalational Agents in the Elderly

The pharmacokinetic aspects of inhalational anesthetic agents include the absorption, distribution, and metabolism of these drugs. Profound age-related changes occur in the pharmacokinetics of intravenous drugs, so it is anticipated that age will also change inhalational anesthetic behavior. However, there are few studies describing how their pharmacokinetics change with age.

Advancing age modifies every aspect of systems controlling the movement of these drugs. Consequently, the assumptions based on the behavior of inhaled anesthetics in younger patients may not hold when administered to older individuals. Some insight comes from the results of studies in middle-aged adults or from studies in the elderly conducted for some purpose other than examining pharmacokinetics.

The pharmacokinetics of volatile anesthetics can be studied in one of two ways. Under laboratory conditions, subanesthetic doses of several agents can be administered in combination to a single subject. This approach has the advantage of limiting the variability between individuals while measuring the kinetics of each drug. The drawback of this method is the inability to measure the pharmacologic effect specific to each drug.[2,3] The other method is to administer a single agent and track it in an individual subject. These studies require validation in many subjects. Frequently, the design of such studies does not address the issue of age.

Influence of the Aging Pulmonary System

Uptake of anesthetics begins when the fresh gas inflow from the anesthesia machines carries a volatile agent into the patient. The uptake of an inhalational agent is simply the difference between the inspired and expired concentrations multiplied by the alveolar ventilation.

The total gas flow passing through the vaporizer determines the rate of inhalational agent consumption.[4] In young subjects, saturation is most rapid with desflurane. Saturation is next most rapid with sevoflurane. High fresh gas flow (>3 L/min) will consume volatile agents more rapidly than when using low flows, and anesthetic drug cost can be reduced by using a low-flow technique.

With the low-flow technique, fresh gas flow rate is reduced to less than half the patient's minute ventilation, usually to less than 3.0 L/min. Monitoring of inspired and expired gas concentrations is mandatory. At a low flow rate, consumption of an insoluble agent, such as desflurane, depends on fresh gas flow whereas halothane does not. Consumption of isoflurane and enflurane vary with minimal and low fresh gas flow rates.[5]

Do anesthetic agents control the response to surgical stimulation in the same manner at low flows? The partial pressure of agents in pulmonary arterial blood that have a low blood/gas solubility should change rapidly with changes in vaporizer settings. Desflurane provides faster control of hemodynamic responses at 1 and 3 L/min flows, and its use requires fewer incremental increases to control acute responses to surgical stimulation. At fresh gas flow rates of 1 L/min, more interventions are necessary to control blood pressure in older patients receiving isoflurane compared with desflurane.[6]

The respiratory changes characterizing advanced age have been thoroughly reviewed by others.[7–11] The principal anatomic changes include lung atrophy and a loss of pulmonary elasticity. There is a loss of alveolar walls, a depletion of the connective tissue elastin, and an increase in interstitial fibrous tissue. The histopathologic change in the senescent lung is sometimes termed "senile emphysema," and it refers to the atrophic changes and dilatation of the alveoli that mimic mild emphysema (Figure 17-1).

The destruction of alveolar walls results in small alveoli coalescing to form larger sacs. Consequently, the lungs have less elasticity and less natural recoil to hold small airways open as lung volumes change with respiration.[12,13] Airways from the level of bronchioles to the alveolar ducts lack a cartilaginous support. Without a semirigid structure to keep them open during passive exhalation, these airways depend on the elastic recoil of the lung parenchyma to prevent collapse at low lung volumes (Figure 17-2). There is an age-related decrease in the diameter of small bronchioles from the fourth decade that is consistent with decreased compliance.[14] In the older patient, these dependent airways close at a higher lung volume than in younger subjects. The physiologic consequence of these changes is increasing ventilation-perfusion (V/Q) mismatching with advancing age. A progressive hypoxemia develops as the number of alveoli gradually decreases and anatomic dead space increases.[15]

The increased closing volume makes it more likely an older patient will experience hypoxia at some time in the perioperative period. Older patients experience hemoglobin desaturation at a faster rate because of greater V/Q mismatching. In the operating room, the transfer of oxygen is not as efficient when using positive pressure ventilation in the supine position as it is when breathing spontaneously. The combination of altered ventilatory response to hypoxia, sedation from residual inhalational agents, and analgesics increases the risk of hypoxia after general anesthesia. The likelihood of hypoxia is further compounded if pulmonary disease is superimposed on age-related changes.

An age-related mismatching of pulmonary ventilation and perfusion may influence the uptake of volatile anesthetic agents. Areas of the lung that are well ventilated but with less perfusion will contribute more anesthetic gas and can be expected to cause a more rapid increase in the ratio of alveolar (F_A) to inspired (F_I) agent concentrations. However, there is little evidence to confirm this.

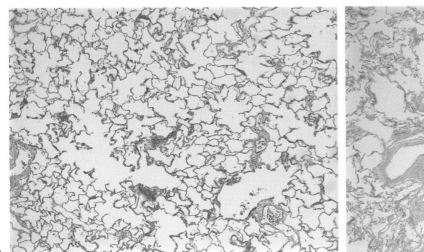 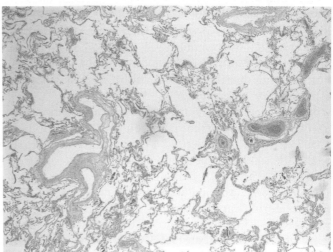

A

B

FIGURE 17-1. Histologic sections of normal lung from a nonsmoking (A) 22-year-old homicide victim, and (B) a 75-year-old individual (hematoxylin and eosin stain, 2×).

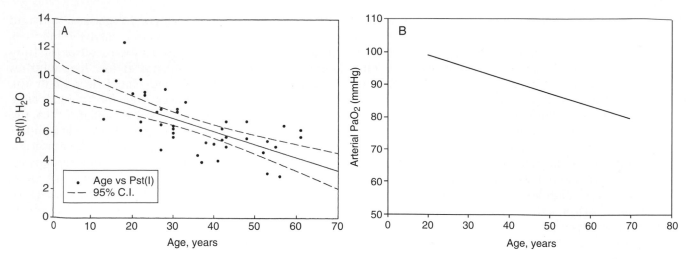

FIGURE 17-2. **(A)** The change in static recoil of the lung measured at 60% of total lung capacity. The decrease in recoil with age is apparent. Atrophy of pulmonary parenchyma results in less elastic recoil to hold open small airways at low tidal volumes. (Data from Turner et al.[13]) **(B)** Increasing ventilation-perfusion mismatching occurring with age leads to lower resting PaO_2. The resting arterial tension was determined by the equation PaO_2 (mm Hg) $= 143.6 - (0.39 \times age) - (0.56 \times BMI) - (0.57 \times Paco_2)$, assuming a BMI of 25 and $Paco_2$ of 40 mm Hg. (Data from Cerveri et al.[15])

In the absence of grossly abnormal pulmonary function, the small increase in the F_A/F_I ratio caused by a progressive V/Q mismatch is probably offset by a lower metabolic rate, and hence lower ventilation and perfusion per kilogram body weight in the elderly. It is difficult to demonstrate any difference in anesthetic uptake attributable to age alone in normal patients (Edmond Eger, personal communication, 2005). However, patients with chronic pulmonary obstructive disease from emphysema, chronic bronchitis, or asthma will have a slower increase in the alveolar concentration (F_A) of volatile anesthetic agents (Figure 17-3).

There is no evidence that an obstruction to diffusion of anesthetic agents develops with age. Alveolar thickening from unusual disorders such as idiopathic pulmonary fibrosis or common problems such as lung congestion from cardiac failure should slow diffusion of anesthetic gases, but it is not likely that this results in a slower increase in the partial pressure of the inhalational agent in pulmonary venous blood.

Any change in V/Q mismatching has a more pronounced effect on inhalational agents with low blood/gas partition (B/G) coefficients.[16] This includes sevoflurane, desflurane, and the inorganic compound nitrous oxide (Table 17-1). Lu et al.[17] measured sevoflurane concentration in arterial and jugular venous blood samples in patients during cardiac surgery. Their study population consisted of 10 patients between the ages of 51 and 73 years who received a constant 3.5% inspired sevoflurane concentration for 1 hour. It took 40 minutes before the concentration of sevoflurane in venous blood became equal to the arterial blood. The arterial sevoflurane concentration was also approximately 40% less than the end-tidal expired sevoflurane. Thus, the end-tidal sevoflurane concentration did not reliably reflect the parallel concentration of sevoflurane in the brain. The equilibration between arterial blood and brain tissues takes four times longer than predicted and sevoflurane uptake in the brain takes approximately 1 hour.[17] As a result of the changes showing slower uptake, it should also be anticipated there

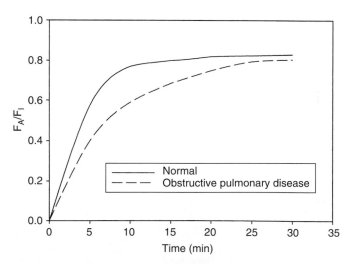

FIGURE 17-3. The effect of pulmonary disease on the increase of alveolar concentration (F_A) compared with inspired concentration (F_I) versus time. The increase in F_A/F_I is slower in subjects with pulmonary disease. (Adapted with permission from Gloyna DF. Effects of inhalation agents. In: McLeskey CH, ed. Geriatric Anesthesiology. Baltimore: Williams & Wilkins; 1997.)

TABLE 17-1. Physical properties of inhalational agents including nitrous oxide.

Agent	Molecular weight*† (g)	Boiling* point (°C)	Vapor pressure*‡	Partition coefficient Oil/gas*	Blood/gas*	Fat/blood§	Recovered as metabolites‖ (%)
Halothane	197.4	50	243	224	2.3	51	11–25
Enflurane	184.5	57	172	98.5	1.91	36	2.4
Isoflurane	184.5	49	238	90.8	1.4	45	0.2
Desflurane	168	24	669	19	0.45	27	0.02
Sevoflurane	200	59	157	53.4	0.60	48	5.0
Nitrous oxide¶	44	−88	38,770	1.4	0.47	2.3	0

Note: Values are based on measurement at 37°C unless otherwise noted.
*Data from Stevens WC, Kingston HGG. Inhalational Anesthesia. In: Barash PG, ed. Clinical Anesthesia. Philadelphia: JB Lippincott; 1989:295.
†Data from Eger EI, Weiskopf RB, Eisenkraft JB. The Pharmacology of Inhaled Anesthetics. The Dannemiller Memorial Educational Foundation; 2002.
‡At 20°C, in mm Hg.
§Data from Eger EI. Uptate and Distribution. In: Miller RD, ed. Anesthesia. Philadelphia: Elsevier Churchill Livingstone; 2005:132.
‖Data from Carpenter et al.[73]
¶For individuals aged 30–60 years.

will be slower elimination of inhalational anesthetics from altered pulmonary function.[18]

Alveolar ventilation does not change with age. However, there are changes that lead to degrees of V/Q mismatching and changes in the control of minute ventilation in response to hypoxia and hypercarbia. The normal partial pressure of carbon dioxide in arterial blood is 4.6–5.3 kPa (34.5–39.8 mm Hg) in older patients.[19,20] With advancing age, the control of ventilation is less sensitive. The normal response to hypercarbia is an increase in the minute ventilation. In young individuals, there is a profound response, about 2–5 L/min per torr carbon dioxide.[21,22] Where the response to rebreathing carbon dioxide is 3.4 L/min in men whose average age is 26 years, the response is only 1.8 L/min in men who are about 70 years of age.[23] The likelihood of respiratory acidosis from impaired ventilation after general anesthesia is therefore greater but it is not documented.

The ventilatory response to hypoxia greatly diminishes with advanced age.[23] When combined with the sedative effect of inhalational anesthetics, the profoundly impaired drive to increase minute ventilation in response to hypoxia leaves the elderly patient at risk for hypoxia. This may contribute to the numerous instances of respiratory complications in the recovery period including hypoxia hypoventilation, and atelectasis.[24] Therefore, less-soluble inhalational anesthetic drugs for elderly patients are reasonable choices. Transporting elderly patients with supplemental oxygen from the operating room to the postanesthesia care unit (PACU) is prudent. Generous use of supplemental oxygen and close monitoring while in the PACU are imperative.

Aside from being the frequent target of disease, the cardiovascular system experiences a decline in function with age. One general measure of cardiac function, the maximum oxygen transport or VO_{2-max}, decreases at the rate of approximately 1% per year after age 30.[28-30] It is tempting to rely on cardiac output as a way of assessing the effect of age. However, changes in cardiovascular function are variable and not easily attributed to a single cause. Cardiac output has several determinants, and, as a single index, it is not an adequate measure to understand anesthetic effects in the elderly.

In healthy older subjects, the peripheral flow of blood decreases and peripheral vascular resistance increases in comparison to younger counterparts. Physical conditioning does not alter these changes[31] (Figure 17-4). Increasing vascular resistance may explain some decrease in

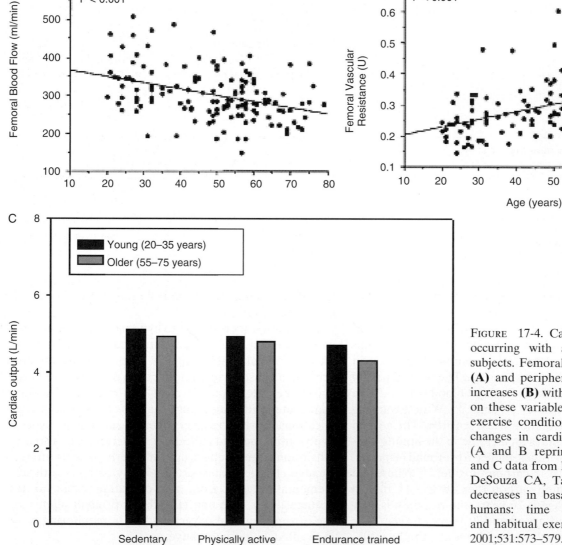

FIGURE 17-4. Cardiovascular changes occurring with age in healthy male subjects. Femoral blood flow decreases (A) and peripheral vascular resistance increases (B) with age. The effect of age on these variables is not influenced by exercise conditioning. (C) Age-related changes in cardiac output are minor. (A and B reprinted with permission, and C data from Dienno FA, Seals DR, DeSouza CA, Tanaka H. Age-related decreases in basal limb blood flow in humans: time course, determinants and habitual exercise effects. J Physiol 2001;531:573–579.)

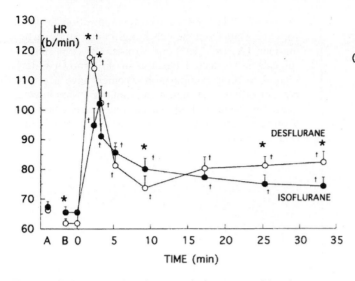

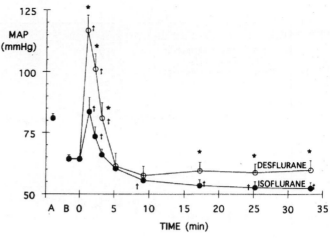

FIGURE 17-8. A transient increase in heart rate, blood pressure, and sympathetic activity occurs with isoflurane and desflurane when the concentrations are increased rapidly to more than 1 minimal alveolar concentration. Several interventions have been described to effectively counter this occurrence, including avoiding the "over pressuring" technique. HR = heart rate, MAP = mean arterial pressure. (Reprinted with permission from Weiskopf et al.[33])

Fat tissue has a great capacity to retain lipid-soluble drugs. For those inhalational agents with greater lipid solubility, the volume of distribution increases (Tables 17-1 and 17-3). Fat acts as a reservoir for volatile agents, resulting in the accumulation of inhalational agents during maintenance and delaying emergence. Depending on many variables, including the lipid solubility of the agent, less blood flow to fat tissue than other tissues, and the duration of anesthesia, an increase in the proportion of body fat may prolong emergence. Although the changes in body fat composition are greater in men, and women have a greater percent body fat at all ages, there is no indication of a gender difference with the pharmacokinetics of inhalational anesthetic agents.

The lipid-soluble drugs redistribute slowly from fat tissue so their effect may be prolonged. The loss of skeletal muscle mass has a significant impact on drug pharmacokinetics because this tissue receives a large portion of the blood supply. As the body fat content increases, a smaller part of each circulating blood volume perfuses this tissue and it diminishes the volume of distribution for the agents that are not very lipid soluble.

Most body fat resides in subcutaneous and abdominal areas. However, body fat may be heterogeneous and various anatomic fat stores may differ in their capacity to act as a reservoir for lipid-soluble drugs.[36] Subcutaneous fat that develops from excessive eating may function differently from the epicardial or mesenteric fat that is present even in very lean individuals. How this might affect the uptake and retention of lipid-soluble inhalational agents is yet to be determined.

The steady-state volume of distribution, V_{dss}, is greatest for isoflurane and least with desflurane[37] (Table 17-3). The movement of volatile agent from the central to peripheral compartments is fastest for desflurane and intermediate for sevoflurane, whereas isoflurane is the slowest.

TABLE 17-2. The influence of halothane or enflurane on myocardial contractility, E_{ES}, in a canine model and during coronary artery bypass surgery.

| | Canine model | | |
	Halothane (n = 7)	Enflurane (n = 7)	CABG surgery	
Control	10.1 ± 0.6	15.2 ± 0.4	Control	11.5 ± 2.0
1%	6.7 ± 0.4	12.3 ± 0.6	60% N_2O	9.0 ± 2.2
2%	4.2 ± 0.5	9.3 ± 0.5	0.5% halothane	8.1 ± 2.4

Source: Data from Van Trigt P, Christian CC, Fagraeus L, et al. Myocardial depression by anesthetic agents (halothane, enflurane, and nitrous oxide): quantitation based on end-systolic pressure-dimension relations. Am J Cardiol 1984;53:243–247.

E_{ES} (mm Hg/mm) = slope of the end-systolic pressure-diameter relation, a sensitive index of contractility unaffected by volume loading; CABG = coronary artery bypass graft.

A

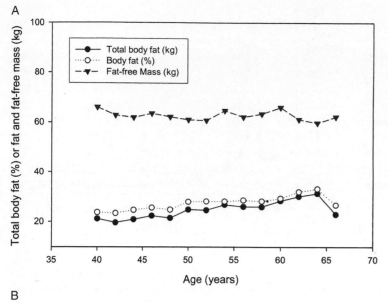

B

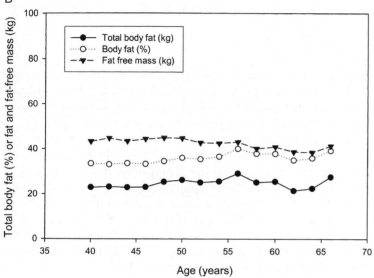

FIGURE 17-9. The change in body composition occurring with age. Data from the Fels Longitudinal Study including men **(A)** (n = 102) and women **(B)** (n = 108) for subjects not selected because of any known criteria related to body composition. Women have a greater percent of body fat than men at all ages. Men have an increasing trend in body weight and percent body fat. Women tend to lose fat-free mass as they become older. (Data from Guo et al.[34])

It is not just the greater solubility of isoflurane that accounts for its V_d being six times that of desflurane. Isoflurane increases blood flow to tissues such as skeletal muscle, a tissue with large storage capacity.[37,38]

The partial pressure of anesthetic permitting wakefulness, the MAC-awake value, determines the emergence from general anesthesia. The MAC-awake value for all volatile anesthetics is about one third the MAC value. A slow, continued release of volatile agent from fat tissue can maintain a partial pressure of agent in the blood causing excessive sedation, respiratory depression, and contribute to postanesthesia delirium. This action may

TABLE 17-3. Pharmacokinetics of newer volatile anesthetic agents.

Agent	MAC	B/G*	FGF†	k_{12}^3 (min^{-1})	Cl_{12}‡ (mL$_{vapor}$ kg^{-1} min^{-1})	V_{dss}‡ (mL$_{vap}$/kg$_{bw}$)
Sevoflurane	2.1	0.69	2	0.117 (0.070–0.344)	13.0 (9.8–22.4)	1748 (819–8997)
Isoflurane	1.2	1.4	<1	0.158 (0.065–0.583)	30.7 (15.9–38.7)	4285 (1509–9640)
Desflurane	6	0.42	<1	0.078 (0.029–0.186)	7.0 (4.4–11.1)	698 (408–1917)

MAC = minimal alveolar concentration, B/G = blood gas partition, k_{12} = microconstant for transport from central to peripheral compartment, Cl_{12} = transport clearance from central to peripheral compartment, V_{dss} = total volume of distribution during steady state.
*Data from Eger EI. In: Miller RD, ed. Uptake and Distribution. Philadelphia: Elsevier Churchill Livingstone; 2005:132.
†Data from FDA Product Prescribing Information: Desflurane and Sevoflurane.
‡Data from Wissing et al.[37]

contribute to a greater incidence of postoperative complications and prolonged stays in the PACU.

The increasing proportion of body fat suggests an advantage with the less-soluble volatile anesthetic drugs. Emergence from general anesthesia has been studied by comparing desflurane and isoflurane anesthesia in elderly patients. Compared with isoflurane anesthesia, signs of early recovery and endotracheal tube removal occurred in approximately half the time with desflurane. Emergence was also faster than with intravenous anesthesia.[39] For short procedures (less than 2 hours), patients reached signs of early recovery and experienced endotracheal tube removal sooner with desflurane compared with sevoflurane.[40]

Influence of Renal Changes

Renal atrophy occurs with age, mainly through the loss of cortical nephrons. The kidney loses about 20% of its mass by age 80, and functional changes accompany renal atrophy. The majority of subjects experience a decrease in renal blood flow, glomerular filtration rate (GFR), and creatinine clearance. The reduction in renal blood flow probably results from cardiovascular changes in addition to renal changes.[41] However, the Baltimore Longitudinal Study of Aging showed that a decline in the GFR is not inevitable because 30% of healthy individuals have no decrease in GFR with age.[42] The plasma creatinine level varies with the muscle mass and with age-related changes in body composition accompanying the aging process. Thus, it is better to evaluate renal function in the elderly using the Cockroft-Gault formula [(140 − age) × weight

(kg)/Cr × 72] than simply using the plasma creatinine value[43] (Figure 17-10).

All volatile anesthetic agents in clinical use are fluorinated ether compounds. The constellation of renal changes may place the older patient at greater risk for fluoride toxicity[44] (Table 17-1). Inorganic free fluoride ions form during metabolism of these agents by the hepatic cytochrome P-450 enzyme system. Toxic levels of free fluoride produce a high output, vasopressin-resistant form of acute renal failure.[45] This disorder was first reported with methoxyflurane in 1966.

The only inhalation agents used today that can produce enough fluoride to be of concern are enflurane, isoflurane, and sevoflurane.[46-48] The threshold fluoride level for causing mild defects in renal concentrating ability is 50 μmol/L.[49] Experiments with cultured collecting duct cells indicate mitochondria may be the target of the free fluoride ion.[50]

Whether fluoride toxicity results from the use of modern inhalational anesthetics is in doubt. Concern surrounded the use of sevoflurane because about 5% of it is metabolized by the cytochrome P-450 2E1 isoform.[51] Of that, 3.5% appears in the urine as free fluoride ion.[52] This is less than the fluoride production from methoxyflurane metabolism but more than that seen with either enflurane or isoflurane.

The likelihood of fluoride toxicity has been questioned because fluoride levels in excess of 50 μg/L were reached in studies comparing sevoflurane and enflurane administration in humans, yet they did not demonstrate nephrotoxicity.[53] The mean fluoride level in patients receiving sevoflurane was 47 μmol/L, twice the 23 μmol/L level in

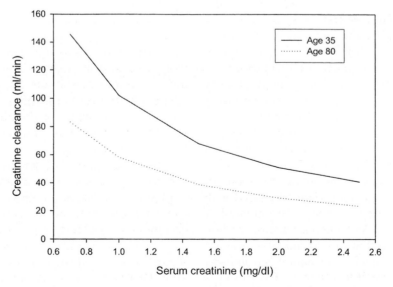

FIGURE 17-10. The relationship between serum creatinine and creatinine clearance by age. The glomerular filtration rate (GFR) decreases in the majority of individuals after age 30 but a decline in GFR is not inevitable. The graphs are standardized for a 70-kg male with values calculated using the Cockroft-Gault formula. (Data from Hughes et al.[35])

patients that received prolonged enflurane anesthesia. More than 40% of subjects having prolonged sevoflurane anesthesia had plasma fluoride levels greater than 50 μmol/L, with no impairment of renal concentrating ability. The results of this study should be cautiously extrapolated to the elderly because it included only young volunteers in their mid-twenties.[54] Neither enflurane nor halothane produced a further decrease of renal function in patients with moderate renal insufficiency.[55] At this time, enflurane is infrequently used for general anesthesia. There are no clinical reports that actively assert that enflurane should be avoided in elderly patients with renal insufficiency.

A toxic fluoride threshold more likely will be met with prolonged exposure to isoflurane than halothane. The peak plasma level of fluoride occurs 24 hours after an average 10-hour administration of isoflurane. This is equivalent to 19.2 MAC hours of isoflurane exposure. With this level of exposure, 40% of patients studied had fluoride levels slightly greater than 50 μmol/L. In contrast, similar exposure to halothane produced lower fluoride levels with the highest plasma levels occurring at the end of the surgical cases. Among elderly patients with renal insufficiency, no further deterioration of renal function resulted with the use of isoflurane, enflurane, or sevoflurane anesthesia.[56] Desflurane poses very little risk to patients with renal insufficiency because so very little of it is metabolized.[57]

Sevoflurane breaks down in the alkaline environment of the carbon dioxide absorber to form fluoromethyl-2,2-difluoro-1-(trifluoromethyl)vinyl ether, or Compound A. This happens particularly at low total gas flows. Similar to free fluoride ion, compound A is also nephrotoxic. The production of Compound A is increased with greater production and absorption of carbon dioxide because the degradation of sevoflurane increases with absorber temperature.[58–60] The combination favoring production of Compound A includes not only increased CO_2 absorption but also absorber temperature, decreased CO_2 washout, and high levels of sevoflurane.[23,61,62] Compound A is clearly nephrotoxic in the laboratory, but it is not certain whether any instances of renal failure occurred from using sevoflurane. In patients with normal renal function and ranging in age from 30 to 69 years, Compound A accumulated during anesthesia with 1 LPM gas flows. Yet, there was no difference detected in clinical or biochemical markers of renal function when those patients were compared with subjects receiving isoflurane anesthesia.[63] Compound A does not accumulate in breathing circuits or carbon dioxide absorbers when gas flows are 5 L/min, but because of the potential for Compound A formation, sevoflurane is not recommended for use at less than 2 LPM fresh gas flow.[64] Nevertheless, no differences in biochemical markers were noted among patients receiving sevoflurane at low-flow (1 L/min), high-flow (5–6 L/min), or low-flow isoflu-

rane anesthesia, and no evidence of renal toxicity exists.[65] Furthermore, in older patients with moderately impaired renal function, sevoflurane anesthesia does not cause apparent injury to the renal tubules,[66] and low-flow anesthesia with sevoflurane does not result in any greater change in blood urea nitrogen, creatinine, or creatinine clearance than isoflurane.[67]

Influence of Hepatic Changes

There is a similar atrophy of the liver that is accompanied by a reduction in hepatic blood flow.[68–70] Decreased hepatic blood flow results in diminished metabolism of drugs that rely on hepatic clearance. The decrease in hepatic blood flow seems responsible for the decreased hepatic metabolism of drugs and not changes in hepatic enzyme activity.[71]

The newer inhalational agents are not extensively metabolized. Of all the volatile agents, halothane is the most extensively transformed with approximately 20% of it metabolized in the liver.[72] The other agents in common use are metabolized to a much lesser extent. Approximately 5% of sevoflurane, 2.4% of enflurane, 0.2% of isoflurane, and 0.02% of desflurane are metabolized[16,73–75] (Table 17-1). Metabolism of halothane, isoflurane, and desflurane produces trifluoroacetic acid. The amount of this metabolite produced is lowest with desflurane.[72,76–79]

The hepatic-function changes associated with aging are probably important only for halothane and sevoflurane because the other agents undergo only minimal transformation. The loss of hepatic tissue with age may be associated with decreased metabolism of the volatile agents, but this is not documented. If decreased metabolism of these drugs occurs, it is probably not clinically significant.

Volatile anesthetic agents have a variable effect on liver function. Sevoflurane decreases production of fibrinogen, transferrin, and albumin in cultured hepatocytes more than exposure to halothane, isoflurane, or enflurane does.[80] However, enflurane causes greater depression of albumin synthesis than sevoflurane. The effects of desflurane on hepatic synthesis are not known. It is not anticipated that it would have much effect because so little of it is metabolized.[81]

Many drugs bind to plasma proteins, and several intravenous anesthetic drugs are carried in the blood bound to plasma proteins. Albumin is a carrier for many drugs, and low blood concentrations of albumin are frequently encountered in elderly patients. This probably contributes to the exaggerated effects of many drugs in older subjects because of the greater fraction of unbound free drug. There is no evidence suggesting that volatile agents rely on protein binding for transport or that the increased sensitivity to volatile anesthetics works through this mechanism.

The Pharmacodynamics of Inhalational Agents in the Elderly

The introduction of halogenated ethers with progressively lower solubility characterizes the era of modern agents. As the solubility of newer agents approaches that of nitrous oxide, the result is a more rapid uptake and faster elimination of the drug. Theoretically, low solubility and faster uptake also allow greater control of anesthetic blood levels during the maintenance phase of anesthesia. Faster elimination with low-solubility agents should provide for a rapid emergence from anesthesia. Inhalational agents used for general anesthesia include isoflurane, sevoflurane, desflurane, halothane, and enflurane. For practical purposes, the first three warrant most consideration because they represent the majority of volatile agents used. The properties of the inhalational agents are found in Table 17-1.

Aging and the Minimal Alveolar Concentration

The classic expression of pharmacodynamic effect for volatile anesthetic agents is the MAC. MAC is the minimal alveolar concentration of a volatile drug at 1 atm that prevents movement in 50% of subjects following surgical incision.[82] The concentrations of volatile agents defined by MAC values are usually not enough for adequate anesthesia during surgical cases. Frequently, about 1.3 times MAC, or essentially an ED_{95} dose of anesthetic, is needed.[83]

For adult subjects, the MAC is 1.15% for isoflurane, 6% for desflurane, and 1.85% for sevoflurane. As patients age, MAC decreases for all the volatile drugs, generally occurring at approximately 6% per decade.[84] The decrease in drug requirement does not follow a linear relationship but accelerates after 40–50 years of age. This phenomenon also applies to intravenous anesthetic drugs in which the pharmacokinetics of injected drugs changes substantially with age.[85] Guedel[86] was the first to note that inhalational anesthetic requirements decrease with age. This has subsequently been documented for halothane,[87] isoflurane,[88] enflurane, desflurane,[89,90] and sevoflurane.[91] The mathematic relationship of MAC, age, end-expired concentration of anesthetic agent, and the contribution by nitrous oxide has been determined.[92] A nomogram for estimating age-related changes in MAC is available (Figure 17-11).

Martin et al.[93] reviewed the use of the most common anesthetic drug combinations for general anesthesia.

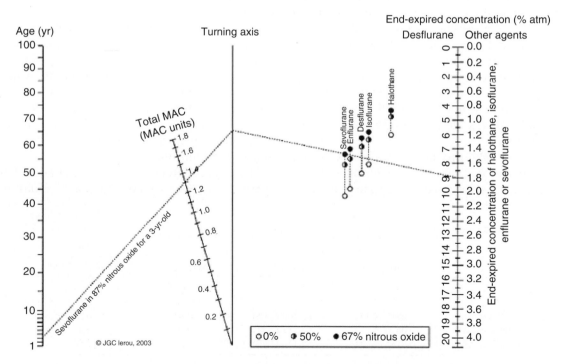

FIGURE 17-11. Nomogram relating age, total minimal alveolar concentration (MAC) expressed in MAC units, and end-expiratory concentrations of volatile agent and nitrous oxide. A result is found by drawing two straight lines. Example (dotted lines): if the measured end-expired concentrations of sevoflurane and nitrous oxide are 1.8% and 67% (at 1 atm), respectively, then the total age-related MAC is 1.3 in a 3-year-old. Reverse example: a total MAC of 1.3 in a 3-year-old, when using sevoflurane and nitrous oxide 67% in oxygen, requires an end-expired sevoflurane concentration of 1.8%. (Reprinted with permission from Lerou.[92])

258   G.R. Haynes

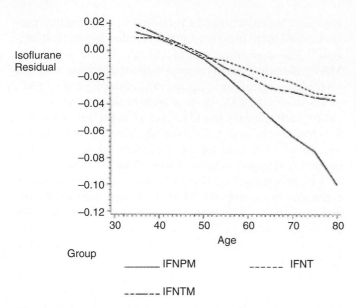

Group

————— IFNPM   –––––– IFNT

––––– IFNTM

FIGURE 17-12. The trend in reduction of isoflurane concentration with age. Compared with maximum values at age 30, there is an 11%–16% reduction in isoflurane requirement by age 80. IFNTM, isoflurane, fentanyl, nitrous oxide, thiopental, midazolam; IFNPM, isoflurane, fentanyl, nitrous oxide, propofol, midazolam; IFNT, isoflurane, fentanyl, nitrous oxide, thiopental. (Reprinted with permission from Martin et al.[93])

When controlling for the synergistic interaction of intravenous and inhalational agents, the authors demonstrated a decrease in drug requirements for 80-year-old patients. The decrease was not the same for drugs of different classes. The utilization of intravenous drugs decreased 30%–50%, whereas the requirement for isoflurane decreased only 11%–26% (Figure 17-12). Although older patients do not require as much anesthetic drug, there is little known that explains the decreased requirement of inhalational anesthetics.

MAC is a value that provides a way to compare the potency of inhalational anesthetic agents on a specific endpoint. Depth of anesthesia is one endpoint of interest.

Other endpoints have received less attention in the aged patient. This is generally one third the MAC value except in the case of halothane, for which MAC_{awake} is 0.55 MAC. MAC_{awake} decreases with age.[94] The MAC-BAR is the MAC of agent that inhibits a sympathetic nervous system response such as tachycardia or hypertension when subjects are stimulated. It is expressed as a multiple of the MAC (Table 17-4). However, there is no information on the concentration of volatile agent needed to attenuate autonomic reflexes (MAC-BAR) with increasing age.

There are several possible explanations of how age decreases the inhalational anesthetic requirements. Several changes contribute to this change: an increase in body fat; reductions in metabolism, reduced cardiac output, decreased drug clearance; and atrophy of organ systems, particularly the central nervous system.[95] A combination of factors probably accounts for the decreased dose of hypnotic drugs needed for loss of consciousness and shifting the electroencephalogram pattern.[96-98] Several factors associated with increasing and decreasing MAC are listed in Tables 17-5 and 17-6. Factors not associated with a change in MAC are listed in Table 17-7.

Drugs frequently used in the elderly influence the effective dose of volatile agents. These include calcium channel blockers[99] and clonidine.[100] Some drugs may affect MAC by depletion of neurotransmitters.[101,102] Benzodiazepines and opioids have an additive effect with volatile anesthetic agents.[43]

Slow emergence and prolonged sedation in the recovery room are usually regarded as detrimental for elderly patients. Postoperative sedation occurs in approximately 10% of elderly general surgery patients. Among elderly patients, the incidence of postoperative sedation after general anesthesia can be as high as 61% for those having emergency surgery. Intraoperative hypotension and anesthetic drugs contribute to postoperative sedation and longer hospitalization.[103]

The physical properties of the inhalational anesthetics contribute to the speed of action and resolution of these

TABLE 17-4. Clinical properties of volatile anesthetic agents in routine use.

	MAC [atm, (%)] at various ages*			MAC‡§		
	2–5 years†	36–49 years†	65 years†	MAC_{awake}	MAC_{awake}/MAC	MAC-BAR
N₂O		1.04		0.68	0.64	—
Halothane				0.0041	0.55	1.3
Isoflurane	0.0160 (1.6)	0.0115 (1.15)	0.0105 (1.05)	0.0049	0.38	1.3
Desflurane	0.0854 (8.54)	0.0600 (6)	0.0517 (5.17)	0.025	0.34	1.45
Sevoflurane	0.0250 (2.5)	0.0185 (1.85)	0.0177 (1.77)	0.0062	0.34	2.24

MAC = minimal alveolar concentration.
*Data from Eger EI II, Eisenkraft JB, Weiskopf RB. The Pharmacology of Inhaled Anesthetics. Dannemiller Memorial Educational Foundation; 2002:7–19.
†Volatile agent delivered in oxygen without nitrous oxide.
‡Values for subjects aged 20–60 years.
§Data from Stevens WC, Kingston HCG. Inhalation anesthesia. In: Barash PG, et al. Clinical Anesthesia. 3rd ed. Philadelphia: Lippincott-Raven; 1997:359–383.

TABLE 17-5. Factors that increase minimal alveolar concentration.

Increased central neurotransmitters
• Monoamine oxidase inhibitors
• Acute dextroamphetamine use
• Cocaine ingestion
• Ephedrine
• Levodopa
Hyperthermia
Chronic ethanol abuse
Hypernatremia

Source: Modified with permission from Ebert TJ, Schmid PG. Inhalation anesthesia. In: Barash PG, Cullen BF, Stoelting RK, eds. Clinical Anesthesia. 4th ed. Philadelphia: Lippincott Williams & Wilkins; 1997:389.

drugs. The blood level of agents with low blood/gas and blood/lipid solubility changes rapidly in response to varying the administered dose. At the conclusion of general anesthesia, the resolution of the hypnotic effect resolves faster with these agents. Faster emergence from general anesthesia is an important way to minimize postoperative complications in the elderly. Reports indicate faster emergence from anesthesia and shorter time spent in the PACU with desflurane.[29]

TABLE 17-6. Factors that decrease minimal alveolar concentration.

Metabolic acidosis
Hypoxia (PaO$_2$ < 38 mm Hg)
Hypotension (mean arterial pressure < 50 mm Hg)
Decreased central neurotransmitters (alpha methyldopa, reserpine, chronic dextroamphetamine use, levodopa)
Clonidine
Hypothermia
Hyponatremia
Lithium
Hypoosmolality
Pregnancy
Acute ethanol use
Ketamine
Pancuronium
Physostigmine (10 times clinical doses)
Neostigmine (10 times clinical doses)
Lidocaine
Opioids
Opioid agonist-antagonist analgesics
Barbiturates
Chlorpromazine
Diazepam
Hydroxyzine
Δ-9-Tetrahydrocannabinol
Verapamil

Source: Modified with permission from Ebert TJ, Schmid PG. Inhalation anesthesia. In: Barash PG, Cullen BF, Stoelting RK, eds. Clinical Anesthesia. 4th ed. Philadelphia: Lippincott Williams & Wilkins; 1997:389.

TABLE 17-7. Factors that do not reduce minimal alveolar concentration.

Duration of anesthesia
Type of stimulation
Gender
Hypocarbia (Paco$_2$ to 21 mm Hg)
Hypercarbia (Paco$_2$ to 95 mm Hg)
Metabolic alkalosis
Hyperoxia
Isovolemic anemia (hematocrit to 10%)
Arterial hypertension
Thyroid function
Magnesium
Hyperkalemia
Hyperosmolality
Propranolol
Isoproterenol
Promethazine
Naloxone
Aminophylline

Source: Modified with permission from Stevens WC, Kingston HG. Inhalational anesthesia. In: Barash PG, ed. Clinical Anesthesia. Philadelphia: JB Lippincott; 1992:443.)

Cardiovascular Actions of Inhalational Agents in the Elderly

The elderly patient's heart and vascular system are anatomically and functionally different from younger patients. The most striking are a decrease in the maximum heart rate response to exercise, decreased sensitivity to catecholamines, increased pulmonary artery, and left ventricular diastolic filling pressures.[104–107] Determining whether these changes are a direct result of aging and if they can be modified are current issues. Both mechanisms of aging in the cardiovascular system and lifestyle undoubtedly have a role in these changes.[108]

The physiologic response of elderly patients during anesthesia must be evaluated carefully because impressions about how elderly patients will respond may be incorrect. For example, Joris et al.[109] found that cardiac index decreases significantly in young patients when abdominal insufflation impairs venous return to the right side of the heart. Because cardiovascular changes inevitably occur with age, it is reasonable to expect greater hemodynamic changes in elderly patients. However, the response of elderly patients may be better than expected. In patients over age 75 years, the cardiac function decreased with induction of general anesthesia with isoflurane and nitrous oxide. But during laparoscopic cholecystectomy, the cardiac performance increased and blood pressure returned to preanesthetic levels with the onset of surgery. Surprisingly, elderly patients tolerated the decreased preload and increased afterload from abdominal insufflation rather well.[110]

Hemodynamic changes during general anesthesia in sicker American Society of Anesthesiologists (ASA) physical status 3 and 4 patients are similar to changes in healthier ASA 1 and 2 patients.[111–117] Inhalation anesthesia produces a dose-dependent decrease in blood pressure and depression of the cardiovascular system.[118–121] Volatile anesthetics reduce blood pressure by reducing cardiac output and vasodilatation.

Inhalation anesthetics affect cardiac systolic function. Depression of myocardial contractility in the elderly varies with the inhalational agent. Isoflurane does not maintain the cardiac output in older patients as it does in younger individuals during anesthesia.[120] The addition of nitrous oxide to isoflurane helps maintain the cardiac index; however, its ability to maintain myocardial contractility is inconsistent. There are reports suggesting nitrous oxide both helps maintain[122] and depresses[123] myocardial contractility when combined with halothane.

Inhalational anesthetics also affect diastolic function. Myocardial relaxation has two components: an energy-dependent active component and a passive component, influenced by myocardial stiffness. In patients over the age of 60, halothane and isoflurane decrease the early, energy-dependent component of left ventricle relaxation, and the effect is greater with isoflurane.[124]

The cardiac status of the elderly patient is a significant factor in determining the response to inhalational anesthetics. For instance, healthy elderly surgical patients with well-controlled hypertension tolerate inhalational induction of general anesthesia with sevoflurane. Whether receiving sevoflurane as a rapidly delivered bolus (8% for 3 minutes) or in a graded manner (8% initially with 2% incremental decreases until reaching 2%), patients with good pump function tolerate the induction with no change in heart rate, no electrocardiographic evidence of ischemia, and moderate decreases in blood pressure. The decrease in blood pressure when using incremental decreases of sevoflurane compared with maintaining the same concentration throughout the induction was less than that encountered when using low-dose sevoflurane and propofol in combination.[125]

Blood pressure decreases significantly with the administration of inhalational anesthetics to patients with diminished cardiac function.[126] In patients with congestive heart failure, blood pressure and cardiac index decrease during isoflurane anesthesia. The decrease is greater with halothane in those patients with poor left ventricle function.[127] The catecholamine blocking effect of the inhalational agents may have a role in the hypotension encountered in these settings.

The inhalational anesthetics have a variable effect on heart rate. Isoflurane decreases systemic blood pressure in both young and old subjects. However, isoflurane decreases the cardiac index and heart rate in elderly subjects whereas it increases the heart rate and leaves the cardiac index unchanged in young individuals. Thus, iso-

flurane seems to maintain the cardiac index in younger patients through increases in heart rate whereas this does not happen in older patients. Sevoflurane produces a dose-dependent increase in heart rate when given to normal, healthy volunteers.[128] In contrast, the heart rate shows no significant change during induction with either 4% or 8% sevoflurane.[129] Halothane and enflurane have little effect on heart rate in elderly patients.[130] There is no difference in the heart rate during the initial period after induction of anesthesia when using halothane. With isoflurane anesthesia, elderly patients have a lower heart rate compared with younger subjects.[120,131]

Inhalational anesthetics also influence the cardiovascular system indirectly through actions on the autonomic nervous system. Rapid increases above 1 MAC in the inspired concentration of isoflurane and desflurane trigger transient sympathetic stimulation. There is a brief period of hypertension and tachycardia that is more pronounced with desflurane.[33] This action is apparently mediated through rapidly adapting airway receptors. Fentanyl and alpha- and beta-adrenergic blocking drugs easily block the effect.[132,133] Although this phenomenon was studied in subjects in their early twenties, elderly patients have a higher state of sympathetic nervous system activity and it is likely this action may be more pronounced.

Inhalational anesthetics may have a delayed inhibition of hemodynamic control. Patients having a carotid endarterectomy with isoflurane anesthesia required more phenylephrine for blood pressure support and needed more labetalol during emergence to manage hypertension than did patients receiving propofol for general anesthesia. More significantly, although there was no difference in hemodynamic stability between patients anesthetized with isoflurane or propofol, patients anesthetized with isoflurane experienced significantly more frequent myocardial ischemia.[134]

Volatile anesthetics typically cause peripheral vasodilatation. The expected consequence is greater blood flow if cardiac output can be maintained or increased. However, there is a distinct, age-related difference in peripheral blood flow between young (18–34 years) and healthy elderly (60–79 years) subjects during the induction of general anesthesia. When receiving either isoflurane or halothane in combination with 66% nitrous oxide, there is a slight difference in changes of heart rate or mean blood pressure between the age groups. The perfusion of skin and muscle, assessed by forearm blood flow, decreases along with the mean arterial blood pressure during anesthesia with halothane, and there is no age-related difference. However, with isoflurane anesthesia, the peripheral perfusion is maintained in young patients even though the blood pressure decreases whereas the perfusion decreases in the elderly (Figure 17-13).[135]

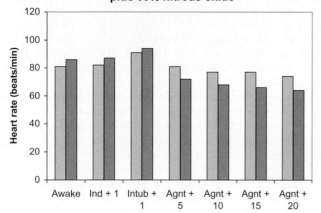

Heart rate during induction of anesthesia, isoflurane plus 66% nitrous oxide

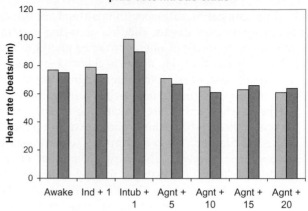

Heart rate during induction of anesthesia, halothane plus 66% nitrous oxide

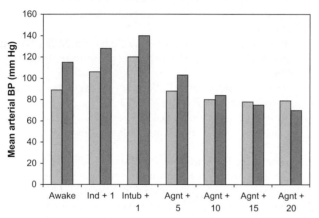

Mean arterial blood pressure during induction of anesthesia, isoflurane plus 66% nitrous oxide

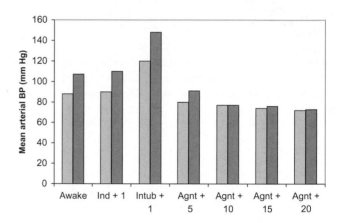

Mean arterial blood pressure during induction of anesthesia, halothane plus 66% nitrous oxide

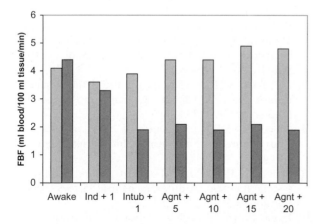

Forearm blood flow during induction of anesthesia, isoflurane plus 66% nitrous oxide

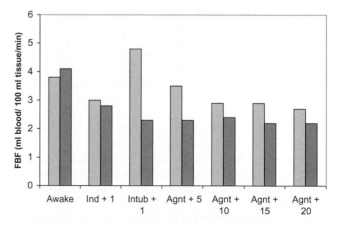

Forearm blood flow during induction of anesthesia, halothane plus 66% nitrous oxide

FIGURE 17-13. Heart rate, mean arterial blood pressure, and forearm blood flow measured following the induction of general anesthesia in healthy young and elderly subjects. Patients received isoflurane (0.8%–1.2%) or halothane (0.7%–1.0%) and nitrous oxide (66%) after induction with etomidate and endotracheal intubation. Little difference in the change of heart rate or blood pressure was found between subject groups. Forearm blood flow decreased in older and younger patients receiving halothane whereas it was much greater in young patients receiving isoflurane. Mean values are shown. Light gray bars = young (18–34 years), dark gray bars = elderly (60–79 years). Time units are in *minutes*. (Data from Dwyer and Howe.[135])

Summary

Much of the clinical literature on inhalational anesthetic agents during the past decade focused on trying to demonstrate the superiority of one agent over another. The clinical issue is not that one agent is clearly better than another in all instances. Each agent can control the response to surgical stimulation during general anesthesia. The issues that matter are which drug is best, given the particular disease or pathophysiology of the patient, and to what degree do we suppress consciousness and autonomic responses. The growing interest in the relationship of depth of anesthesia to long-term survival raises the possibility that we should use cardiovascular drugs as adjuncts to control heart rate and blood pressure.

Because of the limited number of publications describing how age affects anesthesia, extracting age-related data from studies that compare intravenous and inhalational agents is useful. In reviewing the anesthesia literature of the past decade, it is apparent there is a growing interest in the relationship between aging and general anesthesia. However, the limited knowledge regarding the influence age has on anesthesia is a cause for concern.

References

1. Luntz SP, Janitz E, Motsch J, Bach A, Martin E, Böttiger BW. Cost effectiveness and high patient satisfaction in the elderly: sevoflurane versus propofol anesthesia. Eur J Anesthesiol 2004;21:115–122.
2. Carpenter RL, Eger EI II, Johnson BH, et al. A new concept in inhaled anesthetic pharmacokinetics [abstract]. Anesth Analg 1984;64:197.
3. Carpenter RL, Eger EI II, Johnson BH, et al. Pharmacokinetics of inhaled anesthetics in humans: measurements during and after simultaneous administration of enflurane, halothane, isoflurane, methoxyflurane, and nitrous oxide. Anesth Analg 1984;65:575–582.
4. Weiskopf RB, Eger EI II. Comparing the costs of inhaled anesthetics. Anesthesiology 1993;79:1413–1418.
5. Coetzee JF, Stewart LJ. Fresh gas flow is not the only determinant of volatile agent consumption: a multi-centre study of low-flow anesthesia. Br J Anaesth 2002;88:46–55.
6. Avramov MN, Griffin JD, White PF. The effect of fresh gas flow and anesthetic technique on the ability to control acute hemodynamic responses during surgery. Anesth Analg 1998; 87:666–670.
7. Pump KK. Emphysema and its relation to age. Am Rev Resp Dis 1976;114:5–13.
8. Kitamura H, Sawa T, Ikezono E. Postoperative hypoxemia—the contribution of age to the maldistribution of ventilation. Anesthesiology 1973;36:244–252.
9. Ward RJ, Tolas AG, Benveniste RJ, Hansen JM, Bonica JJ. Effect of posture on normal arterial blood gas tensions in the aged. Geriatrics 1966;21:139–143.
10. Wahba WM. Influence of aging on lung function—clinical significance of changes from age twenty. Anesth Analg 1983;62:764–776.
11. Pontoppdan H, Geffin B, Lowenstein E. Acute respiratory failure in the adult. N Engl J Med 1972;287:690–698.
12. Crapo RO, Morris AH, Clayton PD, Nixon CR. Lung volumes in healthy nonsmoking adults. Bull Eur Physiopathol Respir 1982;18:419–425.
13. Turner J, Mead J, Wohl M. Elasticity of human lungs in relation to age. J Appl Physiol 1968;25:644–671.
14. Niewoehner DE, Kleinerman J. Morphologic basis of pulmonary resistance in the human lung and effects of aging. J Appl Physiol 1974;36:412–418.
15. Cerveri I, Zoia MC, Fanfulla F, et al. Reference values of arterial oxygen tension in the middle-aged and elderly. Am J Respir Crit Care Med 1995;152:934–941.
16. Eger EI II. Uptake and distribution. In: Miller RD, ed. Anesthesia. New York: Churchill Livingstone; 1990:85–104.
17. Lu CC, Tsai CS, Ho ST, et al. Pharmacokinetics of sevoflurane uptake into the brain and body. Anaesthesia 2003;58: 951–956.
18. Muravchick S. Anesthesia for the elderly. In: Miller RE, ed. Anesthesia. New York: Churchill Livingstone; 1990:1977–1978.
19. Guénard H, Marthan R. Pulmonary gas exchange in elderly subjects. Eur Respir J 1996;9:2573–2577.
20. Sorbini CAA, Grassi V, Solinas SE, et al. Arterial oxygen tension in relation to age in healthy subjects. Respiration 1968;25:3–13.
21. Kronenberg R, Hamilton FN, Gabel R, et al. Comparison of three methods for quantitating respiratory response to hypoxia in man. Respir Physiol 1972;16:109–125.
22. Eger EI II, Kellogg RH, Mines AH, et al. Influence of CO_2 on ventilatory acclimatization to altitude. J Appl Physiol 1968;24:607–615.
23. Kronenberg RS, Drage CW. Attenuation of the ventilatory and heart rate responses to hypoxia and hypercapnia with aging in normal men. J Clin Invest 1973;52:1812–1819.
24. Pedersen T, Eliasen K, Henriksen E. A prospective study of mortality associated with anaesthesia and surgery: risk indicators of mortality in hospital. Acta Anaesthesiol Scand 1990;34:176–182.
25. McLeskey CH. Anesthesia for the geriatric patient. In: Barash PG, ed. Clinical Anesthesia. Philadelphia: JB Lippincott; 1992:1353–1387.
26. Schocken DD. Epidemiology and risk factors for heart failure in the elderly. Clin Geriatr Med 2000;16: 407–418.
27. Senni M, Redfield MM. Heart failure with preserved systolic function. A different natural history? J Am Coll Cardiol 2001;38:1277–1282.
28. Evans TI. The physiological basis of geriatric general anesthesia. Anaesth Intensive Care 1973;1:319–322.
29. Hurley B, Roth S. Strength training in the elderly: effects on risk factors for age-related diseases. Sports Med 2000; 30:244–268.
30. Robergs R, Roberts S. Exercise Physiology: Exercise, Performance, and Clinical Applications. 1st ed. St. Louis: Mosby-Yearbook; 1997.

31. Dinenno FA, Seals DR, DeSouza CA, Tanaka H. Age-related decreases in basal limb blood flow in humans: time course, determinants and habitual exercise effects. J Physiol 2001;531:573–579.

32. Hagberg JM, Allen WK, Seals DR, Hurley BF, Ehsani AA, Holloszy JO. A hemodynamic comparison of young and older endurance athletes during exercise. J Appl Physiol 1985;58:2041–2046.

33. Weiskopf RB, Moore MA, Eger EI II, et al. Rapid increase in desflurane concentration is associated with greater transient cardiovascular stimulation than with rapid increase in isoflurane concentration in humans. Anesthesiology 1994;80:1035–1045.

34. Guo SS, Zeller C, Chumlea WC, Siervogel RM. Aging, body composition, and lifestyle: the Fels Longitudinal Study. Am J Clin Nutr 1999;79:405–411.

35. Hughes VA, Frontera WR, Roubenoff R, et al. Longitudinal changes in body composition in older men and women: role of body weight change and physical activity. Am J Clin Nutr 2002;76:473–481.

36. Arner P. Not all fat is alike. Lancet 1998;351:1301–1302.

37. Wissing H, Kulin I, Riebrock, Fuhr U. Pharmacokinetics of inhaled anesthetics in a clinical setting: comparison of desflurane, isoflurane and sevoflurane. Br J Anaesth 2000;84:443–449.

38. Stevens WC, Cromwell TH, Halsey MJ, et al. The cardiovascular effects of a new inhalational anesthetic, Forane, in human volunteers at a constant arterial carbon dioxide tension. Anesthesiology 1971;35:8–16.

39. Juvin P, Servin F, Giraud O, Desmonts JM. Emergence of elderly patients from prolonged desflurane, isoflurane, or propofol anesthesia. Anesth Analg 1997;85:647–651.

40. Haevner JE, Kaye AE, Lin B-K, King T. Recovery of elderly patients from two or more hours of desflurane or sevoflurane anaesthesia. Br J Anaesth 2003;91:502–506.

41. Hollenberg NK, Adams DF, Solomon HS, Rashid A, Abrams HL, Merrill JP. Senescence and the renal vasculature in normal man. Circ Res 1974;34:309–316.

42. Lindeman RD, Tobin J, Shock NW. Longitudinal studies on the rate of decline in renal function with age. J Am Geriatr Soc 1985;33:278–285.

43. Beck LH. The aging kidney: defending a delicate balance of fluid and electrolytes. Geriatrics 2000;55:26–28, 31–32.

44. Mazze RJ, Trudell JR, Cousins MJ. Methoxyflurane metabolism and renal dysfunction: clinical correlation in man. Anesthesiology 1971;35:247–260.

45. Aronson S. Renal function monitoring. In: Miller RD, ed. Anesthesia. Philadelphia: Churchill Livingstone; 2005:1489.

46. Crandell WB, Pappas SC, MacDonald A. Nephrotoxicity associated with methoxyflurane anesthesia. Anesthesiology 1966;27:591–607.

47. Baden JM, Rice SA. Metabolism and toxicity. In: Miller RD, ed. Anesthesia. New York: Churchill Livingstone; 1990:155–170.

48. FDA Prescribing Information: Sevoflurane. North Chicago, IL: Abbott Laboratories; Ref. 06–9230-RZ. Rev. June, 1995.

49. Cousins MJ, Mazze RI. Methoxyflurane nephrotoxicity: a study of the dose response in man. JAMA 1973;225:1611–1616.

50. Cittanova ML, Lelongt B, Verpont MC, et al. Fluoride ion toxicity in human kidney collecting duct cells. Anesthesiology 1996;84:428–435.

51. Kharasch ED, Armstrong AS, Gunn K, Artru A, Cox K, Karol MD. Clinical sevoflurane metabolism and disposition. II. The role of cytochrome P450 2E1 in fluoride and hexafluoroisopropanol formation. Anesthesiology 1995;82(6):1379–1388.

52. Kharason ED, Karol MD, Lanni C, Sawchuk R. Clinical sevoflurane metabolism and disposition. I. Sevoflurane and metabolite pharmacokinetics. Anesthesiology 1995;82:1369–1378.

53. Gentz BA, Malan TPJ. Renal toxicity with sevoflurane: a storm in a teacup? Drugs 2001;61:2155–2162.

54. Frink EJ, Malan TP, Isner J, et al. Renal concentrating function with prolonged sevoflurane or enflurane anesthesia in volunteers. Anesthesiology 1994;80:1019–1025.

55. Mazze RI, Sievenpiper TS, Stevenson J. Renal effects of enflurane and halothane in patients with abnormal renal function. Anesthesiology 1984;60:161–163.

56. Conzen PF, Nuscheler M, Melotte A, et al. Renal function and serum fluoride concentrations in patients with stable renal insufficiency after anesthesia with sevoflurane or enflurane. Anesth Analg 1995;81:569–575.

57. Koblin DD, Eger EI II, Johnson BH, et al. I-653 resists degradation in rats. Anesth Analg 1988;67:534–538.

58. Frink EJ Jr, Malan T, Morgan S, et al. Quantification of the degradation products of sevoflurane in two CO_2 absorbents during low-flow anesthesia in surgical patients. Anesthesiology 1992;77:1064–1069.

59. Eger EI II, Sturm DP. The absorption and degradation of isoflurane and I653 by dry soda lime at various temperatures. Anesth Analg 1987;66:1312–1315.

60. Munday I, Foden N, Ward P, et al. Sevoflurane degradation in a circle system at two different fresh gas flows. Anesthesiology 1994;81:A433.

61. Bito H, Ikede K. Closed-circuit anesthesia with sevoflurane in humans. Effects on renal and hepatic function and concentrations of breakdown products with soda lime in the circuit. Anesthesiology 1994;80:71–76.

62. Bito H, Ikeda K. Degradation products of sevoflurane during low-flow anaesthesia. Br J Anaesth 1995;74:56–59.

63. Kharasch ED, Frink EJ, Zager R, Bowdle TA, Artru A, Nogami WM. Assessment of low-flow sevoflurane and isoflurane effects on renal function using sensitive markers of tubular toxicity. Anesthesiology 1997;86:1238–1253.

64. Frink EJ Jr, Isner RJ, Malan TP Jr, Morgan SE, Brown EA, Brown BR Jr. Sevoflurane degradation product concentrations with soda lime during prolonged anesthesia. J Clin Anaesth 1994;6:239–242.

65. Bito H, Ikeda K. Renal and hepatic function in surgical patients after low-flow sevoflurane or isoflurane anesthesia. Anesth Analg 1996;82:173–176.

66. Tsukamoto N, Hirabayashi Y, Shimizu R, Mitsuhata H. The effects of sevoflurane and isoflurane anesthesia on renal tubular function in patients with moderately impaired renal function. Anesth Analg 1996;82:909–913.

67. Higuchi H, Adachi Y, Wada H, Kanno M, Satoh T. The effects of low-flow sevoflurane and isoflurane anesthesia

on renal function in patients with stable moderate renal insufficiency. Anesth Analg 2001;92:650–655.

68. Vestal RE. Drug use in the elderly: a review of problems and special considerations [review]. Drugs 1978;16:358–382.

69. Muravchick S. The aging patient and age related disease. ASA Annual Refresher Course Lecture #151. Park Ridge, IL: American Society of Anesthesiologists; 1987.

70. Carleden CM, Kaye CM, Parsons RL. The effect of age on plasma levels of propranolol and practolol in man. Br J Clin Pharmacol 1975;2:303–306.

71. Woodhouse KW, Mutch E, Williams FM, Rawlins MD, James OE. The effect of age on pathways of drug metabolism in human liver. Age Ageing 1984;13:328–334.

72. Rehder K, Forbes J, Alter H, et al. Halothane biotransformation in man: a quantitative study. Anesthesiology 1967; 28:711–715.

73. Carpenter RL, Eger EI II, Johnson BH, et al. The extent of metabolism of inhaled anesthetics in humans. Anesthesiology 1986;65:201–205.

74. Koblin D, Weiskopf R, Holmes MA, et al. Metabolism of I-653 and isoflurane in swine. Anesth Analg 1989;68:147–149.

75. Yasuda N, Lockhart S, Eger EI II, et al. Kinetics of desflurane, isoflurane, and halothane in humans. Anesthesiology 1991;74:489–498.

76. Cascorbi HF, Blake DA, Helrish M. Differences in biotransformation of halothane in man. Anesthesiology 1970; 32:119–123.

77. Holaday DA, Fiserova-Bergerova V, Latto IP, et al. Resistance of isoflurane to biotransformation in man. Anesthesiology 1975;43:325–332.

78. Koblin DD. Characteristics and implications of desflurane metabolism and toxicity. Anesth Analg 1992;75(4 Suppl): S10–S16.

79. Sutton TS, Koblin DD, Fuenke LD, et al. Fluoride metabolites after prolonged exposure of volunteers and patients to desflurane. Anesth Analg 1991;73:180–185.

80. Franks JJ, Kruskal JB, Holaday DA. Immediate depression of fibrinogen, albumin, and transferrin synthesis by halothane, isoflurane, sevoflurane and enflurane. Anesthesiology 1989;71:A238.

81. Johnes RM. Desflurane and sevoflurane: inhalation anaesthetics for this decade? Br J Anaesth 1990;65:527–536.

82. Saidman LJ, Eger EI II. Effect of nitrous oxide and of narcotic premedication on the alveolar concentration of halothane required for anesthesia. Anesthesiology 1964;25: 302–306.

83. deJong R, Eger EI II. MAC explained: AD_{50} and AD_{95} values of common inhalational anesthetics in man. Anesthesiology 1975;42:384–389.

84. Mapleson WW. Effect of age on MAC in humans: a meta-analysis. Br J Anaesth 1996;76:179–185.

85. Shüttler J, Ihmsen H. Population pharmacokinetics of propofol. A multicenter study. Anesthesiology 2000;92:727–738.

86. Guedel AE. Inhalation anesthesia: a fundamental guide. New York: Macmillan; 1937:61–62.

87. Gregory GA, Eger EI II, Munson ES. The relationship between age and halothane requirement in man. Anesthesiology 1969;30:488–491.

88. Stevens WC, Nolan WM, Gibbons RT, et al. Minimum alveolar concentrations (MAC) of isoflurane with and without nitrous oxide in patients of various ages. Anesthesiology 1975;42:197–200.

89. Gold MI, Abello D, Herrington C. Minimum alveolar concentration of desflurane in patients older than 65 years. Anesthesiology 1993;79:710–714.

90. Rampil J, Lockart S, Zwass M, et al. Clinical characteristics of desflurane in surgical patients: minimum alveolar concentration. Anesthesiology 1991;74:429–433.

91. Nakajima R, Nakajima Y, Ikeda A. Minimum alveolar concentration of sevoflurane in elderly patients. Br J Anesth 1993;70:273–275.

92. Lerou JGC. Nomogram to estimate age-related MAC. Br J Anaesth 2004;93:288–291.

93. Martin G, Glass PSA, Breslin DS, et al. A study of anesthetic drug utilization in different age groups. J Clin Anesth 2003;15:194–200.

94. Katoh T, Suguro Y, Kimura T, Ikeda K. Cerebral awakening concentration of sevoflurane and isoflurane predicted during slow and fast alveolar washout. Anesth Analg 1993;77:1012–1017.

95. Jones AG, Hunter JM. Anaesthesia in the elderly. Special considerations. Drugs Aging 1996;9:319–331.

96. Avram MJ, Krejcie TC, Henthorn TK. The relationship of age to disposition of thiopental and indocyanine green. Anesthesiology 1990;72:403–411.

97. Avram MJ, Sanghvi R, Henthorn TK, et al. Determinants of thiopental induction dose requirements. Anesth Analg 1993;76:10–17.

98. Kirkpatrick T, Cockshodt ID, Douglas EH, Nimmo WS. Pharmacokinetics of propofol (Diprivan) in elderly women. Br J Anaesth 1988;60:146–150.

99. Schwartz AE, Maustisho FE, Bachus WW, et al. Nimodipine decreases the minimum alveolar concentration of isoflurane in dogs. Can J Anesth 1991;38:239–242.

100. Nagasaka H, Yaksh TL. Pharmacology of intrathecal adrenergic agonists: cardiovascular and nociceptive reflexes in halothane-anesthetized rats. Anesthesiology 1990;73:1198–1207.

101. Johnston RR, White PF, Way WL, et al. The effect of levodopa on halothane anesthetic requirements. Anesth Analg 1975;54:178–181.

102. Miller RD, Way WL, Eger EI II. The effects of alpha-methyl-dopa, reserpine, guanethidine, and iproniazid on minimum alveolar anesthetic requirement (MAC). Anesthesiology 1968;29:1153–1158.

103. Gustafson Y, Berggren D, Brannstrom B, et al. Acute confusional states in elderly patients treated for femoral neck fracture. J Am Geriatr Soc 1988;36:525–530.

104. Lakatta EG. Diminished beta-adrenergic modulation of cardiovascular function in advanced age. Cardiol Clin 1986;4:185–200.

105. Virtanen K, Janne J, Frick MH. Response of blood pressure and plasma norepinephrine to propranolol, metoprolol and clonidine during isometric and dynamic exercise in hypertensive patients. Eur J Clin Pharmacol 1982;21: 275–279.

106. Duncan AK, Vittone J, Fleming KC, Smith HC. Cardiovascular disease in elderly patients. 1996;71:184–196.

107. Elliott HL, Sumner DJ, McLean K, Reid JL. Effect of age on the responsiveness of vascular alpha-adrenoceptors in man. 1982;4:388–392.

108. Rodeheffer RJ, Gersten Glith G, Brecker LC, et al. Exercise cardiac output is maintained with advancing age in healthy human subjects: cardiac dilation and increased stroke volume compensate for diminished heart rate. Circulation 1984;69:203–213.

109. Joris J, Honore P, Lamy M. Changes in oxygen transport and ventilation during laparoscopic cholecystectomy. Anesth Analg 1993;76:1067–1071.

110. Dhoste K, Lacoste L, Karayan J, et al. Haemodynamic and ventilatory changes during laparoscopic cholecystectomy in elderly ASA III patients. Can J Anaesth 1996;8:783–788.

111. Fox LG, Hein HAT, Gawey BJ, et al. Physiologic alterations during laparoscopic cholecystectomy in ASA III and IV patients. Anesthesiology 1993;79:A55.

112. Feig BW, Berger DH, Dupuis JF, et al. Hemodynamic effects of CO_2 abdominal insufflation (CAI) during laparoscopy in high-risk patients. Anesth Analg 1994;78:S109.

113. Safran D, Sgambati S, Orlando R III. Laparoscopy in high-risk cardiac patients. Surg Gynecol Obstet 1993;176:548–554.

114. Critchley LAH, Critchley JAJH, Gin T. Haemodynamic changes in patients undergoing laparoscopic cholecystectomy: measurement by transthoracic electrical bioimpedance. Br J Anaesth 1993;70:681–683.

115. Cunningham AJ, Turner J, Rosenbaum S, et al. Transoesophageal echocardiographic assessment of haemodynamic function during laparoscopic cholecystectomy. Br J Anaesth 1993;70:621–625.

116. Joris JL, Noirot DP, Legrand MJ, et al. Hemodynamic changes during laparoscopic cholecystectomy. Anesth Analg 1993;76:1067–1071.

117. McLaughlin JG, Bonnell BW, Scheeres DE, et al. The adverse hemodynamic effects of laparoscopic cholecystectomy. Surg Endosc 1995;9:121–124.

118. Roizen MF, Lampe GH, Sheiner LB, et al. Aging increase hemodynamic responses to induction and incision [abstract]. Anesth Analg 1985;64:275.

119. Hoffman WE, Miletich DJ, Albrecht RF. Cardiovascular and regional blood flow changes during halothane anesthesia in the aged rat. Anesthesiology 1982;56:444–448.

120. McKinney MS, Fee JP, Clarke RS. Cardiovascular effects of isoflurane and halothane in young and elderly patients. Br J Anaesth 1993;71:696–701.

121. Haldermann G, Schmid E, Frey P, et al. Wirkung von ethrane auf die kreislaufgrossen geriatrischer patienten. Anaesthesist 1975;24:343–346.

122. Martin WE, Freund FG, Hornbein RF, et al. Cardiovascular effects of halothane and halothane-nitrous oxide anesthesia during controlled ventilation. Anesthesiology 1969;30:346.

123. McKinney MS, Fee JPH. Cardiovascular effects of 50% nitrous oxide in older adult patients anesthetized with isoflurane or halothane. Br J Anaesth 1998;80:169–173.

124. Houltz E, Caidahl K, Adin C, et al. Effects of halothane and isoflurane on left ventricular diastolic function during surgical stress in patients with coronary artery disease. Acta Anaesthesiol Scand 1997;41:931–938.

125. Yamaguchi S, Ikeda T, Wake K, et al. A sevoflurane induction of anesthesia with gradual reduction of concentration is well tolerated in elderly patients. Can J Anesth 2003;50:26–31.

126. Kemmotsu O, Hashimoto Y, Shimosato S. Inotropic effects of isoflurane on mechanics of contraction in isolated cat papillary muscles from normal and failing hearts. Anesthesiology 1973;39:470–477.

127. Urzua J, Serra M, Lema G, et al. Comparison of isoflurane, halothane and fentanyl in patients with decreased ejection fraction undergoing coronary surgery. Anaesth Intensive Care 1996;24:579–584.

128. Malan TP, DiNardo JA, Isner RJ, et al. Cardiovascular effects of sevoflurane compared with those of isoflurane in volunteers. Anesthesiology 1995;83:918–928.

129. Walpole R, Logan M. Effect of sevoflurane concentration on inhalational induction of anesthesia in the elderly. Br J Anaesth 1999;82:20–24.

130. Hilgenberg JC. Inhalation and intravenous drugs in the elderly. Semin Anesth 1986;5:44–53.

131. Linde HW, Oh SO, Homi J, et al. Cardiovascular effects of isoflurane and halothane during controlled ventilation in older patients. Ancsth Analg 1975;54:70–104.

132. Weiskopf RB, Eger EI II, Noorani M, Daniel M. Repetitive rapid increases in desflurane concentration blunt transient cardiovascular stimulation in humans. Anesthesiology 1994;81:843–849.

133. Weiskopf RB, Eger EI II, Noorani M, Daniel M. Fentanyl, esmolol, and clonidine blunt the transient cardiovascular stimulation induced by desflurane in humans. Anesthesiology 1994;81:1350–1355.

134. Mutch WAC, White IWC, Donen N, et al. Haemodynamic instability and myocardial ischaemia during carotid endarterectomy: a comparison of propofol and isoflurane. Can J Anaesth 1995;42:577–587.

135. Dwyer R, Howe J. Peripheral blood flow in the elderly during inhalational anesthesia. Acta Anaesthesiol Scand 1995;39:939–944.

18
Relaxants and Their Reversal Agents

Cynthia A. Lien and Takahiro Suzuki

Whether or not to maintain neuromuscular block in patients, young or elderly, is very much a matter of debate[1] and is influenced by the type of anesthesia administered as well as the planned surgical procedure. Once the decision is made to administer a nondepolarizing neuromuscular blocking agent to an elderly patient, special consideration must be given to the potential for altered pharmacologic behavior in this patient population.

A number of factors that accompany aging may affect the effect of nondepolarizing neuromuscular blocking agents in the geriatric patient. Because of skeletal muscle denervation, geriatric patients have a decrease in generalized muscle strength and coordination. Many alterations in the neuromuscular junction accompany aging. Additionally, decreased total body fluid and lean body mass, as well as decreased kidney function, cardiac output, and splanchnic blood flow may all affect the pharmacodynamics and kinetics of neuromuscular blocking agents.

An increasing geriatric surgical population, coupled with constantly changing surgical trends and practices, mandates that nondepolarizing neuromuscular blocking agents, as well as anesthetics, are chosen based on their specific pharmacodynamic characteristics in aged patients.

Changes in the Structure of the Neuromuscular Junction

In people over the age of 60 years, the neuromuscular junction in skeletal muscle undergoes continuous degeneration and regeneration. The reorganization is primarily mediated through a reduction in the number of motor neurons in the spinal cord[2] and the ventral root fibers.[3] Moreover, the number of motor units composed of a motor neuron and the innervated muscle fibers seems to decrease with aging. Because reinnervation does not compensate for the progressive neurogenic process,

muscle fibers degenerate and are subsequently replaced with fat and fibrous tissue. A 25%–35% decrease in muscle mass is typically seen in the elderly[4] and is considered to be the result of both a loss of muscle fibers as well as a reduction in size of primarily type 2, or fast-twitch, fibers.[5] This is accompanied by a 50%–75% increase in body fat.[6] The loss of motor units is offset by an increase in the size of the motor unit. Because of this, an augmented twitch tension is evoked by stimulating a single motor nerve[7] in the aged.

Aging is accompanied by many structural changes at the neuromuscular junction. Preterminal axons are increased in number and a greater number of the axons enter into a single endplate. The distance between the preterminal axon and the motor endplate is increased. The motor endplate is composed of a greater number of smaller conglomerates of nicotinic acetylcholine receptors and is lengthened with increasing age. This is accompanied by a flattening of the folds of the endplate at the neuromuscular junction.[8]

Alterations in muscle anatomy and physiology extend beyond the neuromuscular junction in that extrajunctional acetylcholine receptors are frequently found in aged muscles.[9] This may be the result of a progressive denervation that accompanies aging. How these changes in the neuromuscular junction influence neuromuscular transmission in the elderly is not known. Proliferation of acetylcholine receptors, as is observed in disuse atrophy, leads to a relative resistance to neuromuscular blocking agents.[10] Elderly patients, however, are not resistant to the effects of neuromuscular blocking agents.

In animal experiments, age-related changes in acetylcholine storage and release at the neuromuscular junction have been found. In the neuromuscular junction of the diaphragm of aged rats, the acetylcholine content of a single motor nerve terminal is lower than that found in young adult rats. However, in these neuromuscular junctions, increased numbers of nerve terminals per endplate caused by terminal arborization contribute to the release of greater amounts of acetylcholine for each endplate.[11] This alteration in transmitter release is likely responsible for maintenance of normal neuromuscular transmission in the aged rats. Overall, however, advanced age is associated with a decrease in the amount of acetylcholine released.[8]

Despite all of the changes at the neuromuscular junction, changes in the pharmacodynamic behavior of the nondepolarizing neuromuscular blocking agents seem to be the result of alterations in their pharmacokinetics rather than altered interaction of the nondepolarizing compound and the motor endplate.

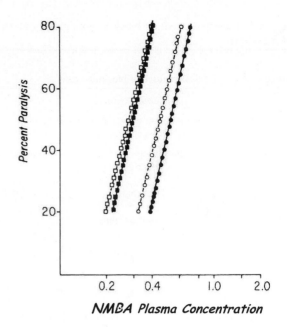

FIGURE 18-1. The relationship between plasma metocurine (o-o) and d-tubocurarine (□-□) in young and elderly patients and their depth of neuromuscular block. Values for the young are represented by the unfilled symbols (o and □) and those for the elderly by the filled symbols (● and ■). Differences between the young and elderly are not significant for either of the neuromuscular blocking agents. (Adapted with permission from Matteo et al.[15] Copyright © Lippincott Williams & Wilkins.)

Dose-Response Relationships in the Elderly

As the elderly become more sedentary and lose muscle mass, one would expect that there would be an upregulation of acetylcholine receptors, as is seen with denervation.[12] These physiologic changes would be expected to contribute to a relative resistance to neuromuscular blockers. With the decrease in lean body mass[13] and volume of distribution[14] that accompany aging, one would also expect that the dose required to establish neuromuscular block in geriatric patients would be less that that required in younger patients. Nondepolarizing neuromuscular blocking compounds are bulky, highly charged compounds that do not readily leave the central volume. This has been confirmed in elderly patients receiving either d-tubocurarine or metocurine.[15] Patients, young and elderly, received a single intravenous dose of the study compound and elderly patients were found to have both a decreased initial volume of distribution and volume of distribution. Results, with respect to volumes of distribution of other nondepolarizing compounds, however, are not consistent. Pharmacokinetic study of the intermediate-acting agent, vecuronium, in patients over the age of 70 years demonstrated that both the initial volume of distribution and the volume of distribution after a single intravenous dose of 0.1 mg/kg were indistinguishable from what was found in younger patients.[16]

The decrease in plasma proteins in the elderly would argue that bioavailability of drugs would be increased as less would be bound to proteins. However, nondepolarizing neuromuscular blocking agents are not highly protein bound[17] and the available free fractions of long-, intermediate-, and short-acting compounds have been shown, in vitro, to be the same in elderly and young adults.[18]

With the structural changes in the neuromuscular junction, already described in this chapter, it would not be unreasonable to expect that sensitivity to nondepolarizing compounds would be increased. This, however, has

not been found to be true. Duvaldestin[19] found that, in the case of the long-acting nondepolarizing compound pancuronium, there was no difference in the plasma concentration–response relationships in young and elderly patients. Similarly, both metocurine and d-tubocurarine have no difference between the plasma concentration–response relationships of the elderly and the young adult patients (Figure 18-1).[15] Similar results have been documented with the intermediate-acting nondepolarizing agents. Rupp et al.[20] found that the steady-state concentration of vecuronium at 50% neuromuscular block was the same in elderly and young adult patients. These results indicate that at the same plasma concentration of relaxant, elderly and young patients have the same degree of neuromuscular blockade, and sensitivity of the acetylcholine receptor is, therefore, not increased in geriatric patients.

Although alterations in pharmacokinetics influence the onset of effect and duration of action, the dose of relaxant that will generally produce 95% neuromuscular block is the same in elderly and young adults. This has been shown for the long-acting compounds pancuronium,[19] pipecuronium,[21] and doxacurium[22] as well as the intermediate-acting compounds vecuronium,[23] rocuronium,[24] and atracurium.[25]

TABLE 18-1. Onset of maximal block in young and elderly patients following administration of nondepolarizing neuromuscular blocking agents.

Reference	Neuromuscular blocking agent	Dose (mg · kg⁻¹)	Onset (minutes)	
			Elderly patients	Young adult patients
26	Succinylcholine	1	1.58 [0.12]	1.18 [0.13]
Short-acting nondepolarizing neuromuscular blocking agents				
52	Mivacurium	0.15	2.03 (0.53)	2.08 (0.82)
Intermediate-acting nondepolarizing neuromuscular blocking agents				
26	Vecuronium	0.1	4.92 [0.52]	3.70 [0.23]
59		0.1	3.52 (1.11)	2.57 (0.66)*
42	Rocuronium	0.6	4.5 (2.4)	4.1 (1.5)
43		1.0	1.33 (0.43)	1.04 (0.21)*
26	Cisatracurium	0.1	4.0	3.0*
50		0.1	3.4 (1.0)	2.5 (0.6)*
Long-acting nondepolarizing neuromuscular blocking agents				
21	Pipecuronium	0.07	6.9 (2.6)	4.5 (1.5)*
22	Doxacurium	0.025	11.2 (1.1)	7.7 (1.0)*

Note: Data are mean (SD) or [SEM].
*Statistically significant difference when compared with elderly patients.

Onset of Neuromuscular Block

For nondepolarizing neuromuscular blocking agents to exert their effect, they must be carried to the neuromuscular junction. The rate at which this is done is influenced by a number of factors including circulation to the muscles, and cardiac output. Once the nondepolarizing muscle relaxant arrives at the muscle, it needs to diffuse into the neuromuscular junction and bind with the acetylcholine receptor to cause neuromuscular blockade. In geriatric patients, although there are some differences as to the extent (Table 18-1), increased age is generally associated with a slower onset of neuromuscular block when doses of 2×ED₉₅ (2 times the dose that causes, on average, 95% neuromuscular block) or greater are administered. Differences in onset are more apparent when doses not causing complete neuromuscular block are examined[26] (Figure 18-2). With administration of these smaller doses of nondepolarizing compound, the time to the actual maximal effect can be measured. However, administration of the larger doses allows only for the determination of the time required to achieve 100% neuromuscular block. The greater time required for maximal effect may be attributable to a decreased cardiac output, although physically active, healthy geriatric patients may not have a decline in cardiac function.[27]

In a study in patients over the age of 65 years, receiving oxygen-nitrous oxide-isoflurane anesthesia, cisatracurium (0.1 mg/kg) was administered after induction of anesthesia and subsequent boluses of 0.025 mg/kg at recovery of twitch height to 25% in order to maintain neuromuscular block.[28] The authors found that onset of block after the administration of cisatracurium was slower

in elderly individuals than in young adults (3 versus 4 minutes, respectively). Pharmacodynamic modeling demonstrated that the biophase equilibration in the elderly was slower than in young adults (0.06 versus 0.071, respectively). The authors attributed the slower onset of neuromuscular block to the slower biophase equilibration in the elderly. The relative contributions of decreased cardiac

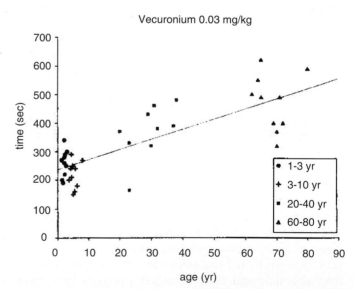

FIGURE 18-2. The onset of maximal neuromuscular blocking effect of vecuronium 0.03 mg/kg in four different age groups. Onset of maximal effect is faster in the children and slowest in the most aged subjects. p < 0.00001 by linear regression. (Reprinted with permission from Koscielniak-Nielsen et al.[26] Copyright © Lippincott Williams & Wilkins.)

output and slower biophase equilibration remain to be determined.

The slower onset of maximal clinical effect of non-depolarizing neuromuscular blocking agents in geriatric patients may result in relative overdosing of the muscle relaxant. Unwillingness to wait for onset of maximal effect of a given dose causes clinicians to administer either additional medication, or a larger dose at the outset to speed onset of block. This results in an increase in the duration of action of the drug because a larger total amount of drug has been administered. Furthermore, in the case of those compounds that are eliminated through hepatic and renal mechanisms, these larger doses and administration of subsequent doses result in cumulation so that each subsequent dose lasts longer than the previous one.[29] This occurs because after the initial dose of nondepolarizing compounds, such as pancuronium and vecuronium, recovery of neuromuscular function occurs as a result of distribution to sites other than the plasma rather than elimination of the relaxant from the body. With subsequent doses, the first dose is entering into its elimination phase and reentering the plasma. The drug effect, therefore, is a combination not only of the recently administered relaxant but also of a portion of the earlier dose as both contribute to plasma concentration. This effect is more pronounced with the long-acting pancuronium than with the intermediate-acting vecuronium.

Pharmacokinetics and Duration of Effect

Aging, even in healthy elderly patients, is accompanied by decreases in hepatic and renal blood flow and function. Because the majority of nondepolarizing neuromuscular blocking agents are eliminated through some combination of these means, alterations in pharmacokinetics and duration of effect are to be expected. Alterations in the pharmacodynamics of nondepolarizing compounds as a result of changes in the pharmacokinetics associated with the normal process of aging may be difficult to distinguish from concomitant disease processes.

Long-Acting Agents

Although there may be some differences in the actual percent of drug eliminated through splanchnic and renal mechanisms, the long-acting nondepolarizing agents depend largely on the kidney for their elimination from the plasma (Table 18-2). It is not surprising, therefore, that these compounds should have a longer duration of action in geriatric patients. As has been found in the

TABLE 18-2. Means of elimination of nondepolarizing neuromuscular blocking agents from the body.

Neuromuscular blocking agent	Means of elimination
Long-acting compounds	
Pancuronium	Kidney 85%, liver 15%
Pipecuronium	Kidney 90%, liver 10%
Doxacurium	Kidney 90%, liver 10%
d-Tubocurarine	Kidney 80%, liver 20%
Metocurine	Kidney 98%, liver 2%
Intermediate-acting compounds	
Vecuronium	Kidney 40%–50%, liver 50%–60%
Rocuronium	Kidney 10%, liver 70%
Atracurium	Kidney 10%–40%, Hofmann elimination 60%–90%
Cisatracurium	Kidney 16%, Hofmann elimination >75%
Short-acting compounds	
Mivacurium	Kidney <5%, plasma cholinesterase >95%

majority of studies with these agents, their prolonged duration of action can be attributed to a prolonged elimination half-life and a decreased clearance.

McLeod et al.[30] demonstrated that the clearance of pancuronium decreased with increasing age. In a later study, Duvaldestin et al.[19] studied the pharmacokinetics and dynamics of pancuronium in young adults and those older than 75 years. He found that the 10%–75% and 25%–75% recovery intervals were prolonged by at least 60% in the elderly. This could be attributed to a slower elimination of pancuronium from the plasma in elderly patients (Figure 18-3). Not surprisingly, the clearance of pancuronium was decreased from 1.8 in young adults to 1.2 mL/min/kg in patients of advanced age. Because the volume of distribution in the elderly was no different from that in younger adults, the decrease in clearance resulted in a doubling of the elimination half-life from 107 to 201 minutes.

Similar results have been found for metocurine and d-tubocurarine.[15] In this study, elderly patients were defined as being older than 70 years of age and young adults were between 29 and 59 years of age. The elderly patients had a significantly prolonged 25%–75% recovery interval. This could be attributed to a decreased volume of distribution and clearance as well as a markedly prolonged elimination half-life for both nondepolarizing neuromuscular blocking agents. The study results are summarized in Table 18-3.

Doxacurium, similar to the other long-acting neuromuscular blocking agents, is eliminated through the kidneys and, in patients with renal failure, its clearance is significantly decreased[31] and it has a longer duration of action.[32] Not surprisingly, therefore, the clinical duration of action[33] and interpatient variability[22] is increased in elderly patients. In a pharmacokinetic study of the

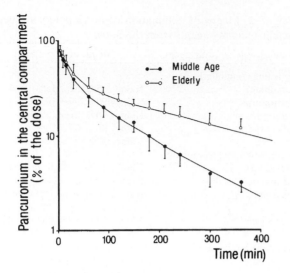

FIGURE 18-3. The elimination of pancuronium from the plasma after administration of a bolus dose. Pancuronium disappears from the plasma significantly more slowly in elderly patients than in middle-aged adults. (Reprinted with permission from Duvaldestin et al.[19] Copyright © Lippincott Williams & Wilkins.)

relaxant in elderly patients, however, the drug was found to not have a decreased clearance or prolonged elimination half-life.[22] This negative result may have been the result of differences in intraoperative fluid management of the young and elderly patients. The elderly patients received 1750 mL of intravenous fluid at the start of surgery whereas their younger counterparts received 1063 mL. In addition, the elderly patients sustained, on average, 5 times more blood loss than did the younger

patients so that total fluid replacement in the elderly was almost 6 L, whereas in the young it was 2500 mL. These differences would increase calculated volumes of distribution and lower the plasma concentration of drug measured in the elderly.

Similarly, pipecuronium has a prolonged duration of action and decreased clearance in patients with renal failure.[34] Despite this, the age-related decreases in renal function do not seem to cause the drug to have a prolonged duration of action or a decreased clearance.[21] In a study of 20 elderly and 10 young adults receiving nitrous oxide, fentanyl and droperidol anesthesia, patients received 70 µg/kg pipecuronium as a single intravenous bolus. The elderly patients developed, on average, a lesser degree of neuromuscular block with this dose than did the younger patients (95% versus 100%, respectively). Clearance of pipecuronium was the same in both groups and differences in elimination half-life (181 versus 154 minutes in the elderly and young, respectively) were not statistically different.

Intermediate-Acting Agents

In contrast to the dependence of the long-acting nondepolarizing compounds on the kidneys for their elimination, the intermediate-acting compounds are eliminated from the body primarily through other mechanisms (Table 18-2). These include hepatic elimination and Hofmann degradation. In addition to decreases in renal function and blood flow, aging is associated with decreases in hepatic blood flow and hepatocellular function.[35–37] One would, therefore, expect that compounds relying on this means for elimination from the body would have

TABLE 18-3. Pharmacokinetics of nondepolarizing neuromuscular blocking agents in geriatric patients.

Neuromuscular blocking agent	Patient age	$t_{1/2}\beta$ (minutes)	Cl (mL · kg^{-1} · min^{-1})	V_d (L · kg^{-1})	Reference
Vecuronium	Young	78 ± 21	5.6 ± 3.2	0.49 ± 0.02	16
	Elderly	125 ± 55*	2.6 ± 0.6*	0.44 ± 0.01	
	Young	70 ± 20	5.2 ± 0.8	0.24 ± 0.04	20
	Elderly	58 ± 10	3.7 ± 1.0*	0.18 ± 0.03*	
Atracurium	Young	15.7 ± 2.5	5.3 ± 0.9	0.10 ± 0.01	46
	Elderly	21.8 ± 3.3*	6.5 ± 1.1	0.19 ± 0.06*	
Cisatracurium	Young	21.5 ± 2.4	4.6 ± 0.8	0.11 ± 0.01	50
	Elderly	25.5 ± 3.7*	5.0 ± 0.9	0.13 ± 0.02*	
Pancuronium	Young	107 ± 24	1.81 ± 0.36	0.27 ± 0.06	19
	Elderly	201 ± 69*	1.18 ± 0.39*	0.32 ± 0.10	
Pipecuronium	Young	154 ± 61	2.5 ± 0.7	0.31 ± 0.07	21
	Elderly	181 ± 68	2.4 ± 1.0	0.39 ± 0.13	
d-Tubocurarine	Young	173 ± 38	1.71 ± 0.32	0.42 ± 0.06	15
	Elderly	268 ± 51*	0.79 ± 0.18*	0.28 ± 0.04*	
Metocurine	Young	269 ± 56	1.1 ± 0.16	0.45 ± 0.04	15
	Elderly	530 ± 83*	0.36 ± 0.08*	0.23 ± 0.03*	
Doxacurium	Young	86 ± 50	2.22 ± 1.09	0.15 ± 0.04	22
	Elderly	96 ± 20	2.47 ± 0.69	0.22 ± 0.08*	

$t_{1/2}\beta$ = half-life of elimination, Cl = plasma clearance, V_d = volume of distribution.
*There is a statistically significant difference compared with younger adults.

altered pharmacokinetics. In contrast, clearance by Hofmann elimination is independent of end-organ function and aging should have little impact on the pharmacokinetics of compounds eliminated primarily by this means.

Vecuronium was the first of the intermediate-acting nondepolarizing relaxants to be introduced into clinical practice. Although it is eliminated primarily in the bile,[38,39] 20%–25% of the relaxant is eliminated unchanged in the urine. Whether or not aging affects the pharmacokinetics of vecuronium has been much debated. The action of vecuronium in the elderly has been studied by four different groups of investigators.[16,20,39,40] d'Hollander and colleagues examined the rate of recovery from vecuronium-induced neuromuscular blockade in patients over the age of 60 years. These recovery rates were compared with those in patients under the age of 40 and those between 40 and 60 years of age. The 10%–25% and 25%–75% recovery intervals were significantly prolonged in the elderly patients compared with recovery intervals in younger patients. Additionally, less vecuronium was required to maintain 90% neuromuscular block for a period of 90 minutes in the elderly patients than it was in the younger controls.[39] McCarthy et al.[40] reported very similar results. They found that the duration of action was significantly prolonged in the elderly (39 versus 28 minutes) and the clinical duration of action was prolonged as well (69 and 45 minutes, respectively) after a bolus of 0.08 mg/kg vecuronium.

Rupp et al.[20] studied the pharmacokinetics and dynamics of vecuronium in elderly patients in whom an infusion had been discontinued once 70%–80% neuromuscular block had been achieved. In this study, patients older than 70 years had clearance and volume of distribution for vecuronium that were approximately 30% less than was found in younger adults. Elimination half-life and the 25%–75% recovery interval were not, in contrast, different from what was found in young adult controls. Lien et al.[16] used a different study design to determine the kinetics and dynamics of vecuronium in elderly patients. In this study, patients received a single intravenous bolus dose of vecuronium. Recovery was monitored and venous blood taken for determination of pharmacokinetics. Elderly patients (between 72 and 86 years of age) had 5%–25% and 25%–75% recovery intervals that were approximately 3 times longer than those in young adults. Clearance of vecuronium was half as fast in the elderly as it was in young adult patients (2.6 versus 5.6 mL·kg^{-1}, respectively) and elimination of the compound was slower in geriatric patients (78 and 125 minutes for young adult and elderly patients, respectively). The authors' conclusion that the prolonged duration of action of vecuronium in elderly patients is attributable to its decreased clearance in this patient population supports the findings of d'Hollander and colleagues[39] and is not inconsistent with the decreased clearance found by Rupp et al.[20]

Rocuronium is the other intermediate-acting nondepolarizing neuromuscular blocking agent that has a steroidal structure. Similar to vecuronium, it does not depend on the kidney for its primary means of elimination from the body. However, although it does not depend on the kidney solely for its elimination, clearance of rocuronium is decreased and its mean residence time is prolonged in patients with renal failure.[41] As with vecuronium, the behavior of this compound in aged patients has been studied by different groups of investigators.[24,42,43] In the case of rocuronium, however, the results are more similar across the studies. Baykara et al.[43] reported that the first response in the train-of-four response after administration of rocuronium, 1 mg/kg, was slower in the elderly than in young adults. Bevan et al.[24] found, in a study of repeat bolus doses of rocuronium, that the clinical duration of action and the 25%–75% recovery intervals were prolonged in elderly patients. With repeated doses of 0.1 mg/kg rocuronium administered at 25% recovery of twitch height, the duration of action became longer in the elderly patients but did not in the young adult control patients. Matteo et al.[42] studied the pharmacokinetics and pharmacodynamics of rocuronium in geriatric patients following a 0.6 mg/kg dose and found that in patients between the ages of 70 to 78 years, clearance was decreased by 27%. Not unexpectedly, the 25%–75% recovery interval was increased from 13 minutes in the young adults to 22 minutes in the elderly patients.

Atracurium depends on neither the kidney nor the liver as its primary means of elimination. Rather, it undergoes the base and temperature catalyzed process of Hofmann elimination (Table 18-2). This spontaneous degradation of the relaxant is not end-organ dependent. Therefore, the physiologic changes associated with aging should not affect the pharmacokinetics of atracurium and its duration of action should be unaffected by advanced age. As they had done with vecuronium, d'Hollander and colleagues[44] studied atracurium in patients over the age of 60 years. In this study, patients received an infusion of atracurium to maintain 90% depression of neuromuscular function for 90 minutes. The dose of relaxant required to maintain this depth of paralysis was calculated in the age groups studied (older than 60 years, 40–60 years, and younger than 40 years of age). There were no differences among the groups in terms of their 10%–25% and 25%–75% recovery intervals or the amount of relaxant necessary to maintain 90% twitch suppression.

Slight changes in the pharmacokinetics of atracurium in elderly patients, however, have been reported. Kent et al.[45] administered 0.6 mg/kg atracurium to elderly and young adult patients and found no difference in clearance and the volume of distribution between the two patient groups. There was, however, a small but significant difference in the elimination half-life. The elimination half-life of atracurium was prolonged by 15% in elderly patients, from 20 to 23 minutes. Kitts et al.[46] administered an infusion of atracurium to achieve 70% neuromuscular block. As described by Kent et al.,[45] elimination half-life was prolonged in the elderly. Because clearance was not affected by advanced age, the increase in elimination half-life was attributable to a larger volume of distribution in elderly patients. Most recently, Parker et al.[47] found that elimination half-life was prolonged and clearance decreased in elderly patients. The results of Kitts, Kent, and Parker support the finding by Fisher et al.[48] that in addition to Hofmann elimination, renal and hepatic mechanisms contribute to the elimination of the compound. Despite these pharmacokinetic differences in elderly patients, however, the dynamics of neuromuscular blockade with atracurium are not different in the young and elderly.[44,46]

Cisatracurium is one of the 10 isomers that comprise atracurium. Similar to atracurium, it is eliminated primarily through Hofmann elimination. Renal clearance accounts for 16% of its elimination from the body.[49] As with atracurium, small changes have been found in the pharmacokinetics of this compound in elderly patients. Ornstein et al.[50] described a prolongation of the half-life of 4 minutes (21.5 versus 25.5 minutes in young and elderly patients, respectively) and an increase in the volume of distribution (108 versus 126 mL·kg^{-1} in young and elderly patients, respectively) of cisatracurium in elderly patients. Clearance was unchanged by advanced age. Sorooshian et al.[28] also found that clearance was unaffected by advanced age, whereas volume of distribution in the elderly was larger. Both studies found no difference in recovery of neuromuscular function after administration of 0.1 mg/kg cisatracurium. In a later study, Pühringer et al.[51] also noted the lack of effect of small changes in pharmacokinetics of cisatracurium on the duration of action of the compound in the elderly. Patients received 0.15 mg/kg cisatracurium to induce neuromuscular blockade and 0.03 mg/kg boluses to maintain neuromuscular blockade. The clinical duration of action after the initial dose and the time to return to a train-of-four ratio of 0.8 following the last dose of cisatracurium were recorded. The recovery parameters were the same in young adults and those older than 65 years of age.

Short Duration of Action

Mivacurium is the only available nondepolarizing neuromuscular blocking agent with a short duration of action. Similar to succinylcholine, it is metabolized by plasma cholinesterase and is dependent on neither hepatic nor renal function for its elimination. Mivacurium has been shown to have a prolonged recovery in elderly patients.[52] In this study, patients received either a bolus of 0.15 mg/kg mivacurium and were allowed to recover or, following the bolus, were given an infusion to maintain 90% suppression of neuromuscular response to stimulation. All recovery parameters were prolonged by approximately 30% in elderly patients. The amount of mivacurium required to maintain neuromuscular blockade was also reduced (3.7 versus 5.5 μg/kg/min in the elderly and young, respectively). Goudsouzian et al.[53] also found that elderly patients required a lower infusion rate to maintain a stable depth of block. These results suggest that the pharmacokinetics of mivacurium are altered in elderly patients. The results of Østergaard et al. in a study of the kinetics of the compound do not explain the prolongation in recovery observed in the elderly.[54] They found that the half-life and clearances of the three isomers of mivacurium, cis-trans, trans-trans, and cis-cis, were not different in elderly patients. The volume of distribution of the relaxant, however, was larger in the elderly.

Plasma cholinesterase activity is reduced in the elderly[55] and mivacurium requirements are inversely related to plasma cholinesterase activity[56] in that patients with higher plasma cholinesterase activity require higher mivacurium infusion rates to maintain the desired depth of block than those patients with lower plasma cholinesterase activity. If mivacurium is to be used in geriatric patients, one can anticipate that lower infusion rates will be required to maintain a stable depth of neuromuscular block and, if administered with repeated boluses, longer dosing intervals would be appropriate.

Anticholinesterases

Because the duration of action of many nondepolarizing neuromuscular blocking agents is prolonged in the elderly, the impact of aging on the pharmacokinetics and pharmacodynamics of their antagonists is of interest. The three typically used anticholinesterases, edrophonium, neostigmine, and pyridostigmine, have prolonged durations of action and decreased clearances in the elderly (Table 18-4). The kinetics and dynamics of each in the elderly have been studied with vecuronium and many of the long-acting neuromuscular blocking agents.

Edrophonium

The clearance of edrophonium from the plasma depends primarily on the kidneys. Decreases in renal blood flow and glomerular filtration rate likely account for the altered pharmacokinetics of this compound in the elderly. As would be anticipated based on its means of elimination, the clearance of edrophonium (1 mg/kg) is decreased and its elimination half-life prolonged in the elderly.[57] In the study by Matteo et al.,[57] edrophonium was administered during an ongoing infusion of metocurine that was

TABLE 18-4. Pharmacokinetics of edrophonium, neostigmine, and pyridostigmine in the elderly and young adults.

Anticholinesterase	Patient group	$t_{1/2}\beta$ (minutes)	Cl (mL · kg^{-1} · min^{-1})	V_i (L · kg^{-1})	V_d (L · kg^{-1})
Edrophonium (1 mg · kg^{-1})[59]	Elderly	84.2 (17)*	5.9 (2)*	0.05 (0.02)	0.72 (0.3)
	Young	56.6 (16)	12.1 (4)	0.2 (0.2)	0.81 (0.3)
Neostigmine (0.07 mg · kg^{-1})[60]	Elderly	16.7 (0.8)	23.4 (5)	0.068 (0.018)*	0.566 (0.13)
	Young	18.5 (7)	33.5 (4)	0.1 (0.04)	0.549 (0.12)
Pyridostigmine (0.25 mg · kg^{-1})[68]	Elderly	157 (56)	6.7 (2.2)*	0.085 (0.06)	1.4 (0.4)
	Young	140 (60)	9.5 (2.7)	0.095 (0.046)	1.8 (0.7)

Note: Data are shown as mean (SD).

$t_{1/2}\beta$ = half-life of elimination, Cl = plasma clearance, V_i = initial volume of distribution, V_d = volume of distribution.

*There is a statistically significant difference compared with younger adults.

dosed to maintain 90% neuromuscular block before the administration of the anticholinesterase. Despite its altered pharmacokinetics, dosing adjustments are not required for antagonism of residual neuromuscular block. This has been demonstrated in two different dosing models. McCarthy et al.[58] demonstrated in a dose-response study that the dose of edrophonium required to antagonize 90% vecuronium-induced neuromuscular block, after a bolus administration of 0.08 mg/kg vecuronium, did not differ between the elderly and young adult patients. Similarly, Kitajima et al.[59] administered edrophonium, 0.75 mg/kg, to antagonize neuromuscular block that had been induced with vecuronium, 0.1 mg/kg. Edrophonium was administered when the train-of-four ratio had returned to 25%. The authors found that there was no difference in the time required for the train-of-four ratio to recover to 75% in elderly patients (over the age of 70 years) and young adults. Matteo et al.[57] evaluated the ability of 1 mg·kg^{-1} edrophonium to reverse a deep, steady-state block produced by continuous infusion of metocurine in the elderly and younger adult patients. They found that there was no significant difference in the time to the maximum effect of the anticholinesterase in the two study groups (elderly 2.1 versus younger 1.7 minutes). In this model, the plasma concentration of edrophonium at any given point in recovery was greater in the elderly patients than in the young adults.

Therefore, the change in the pharmacokinetic parameters of edrophonium in the elderly has no influence on its efficacy in antagonizing residual neuromuscular block in this patient population. Because the volume of distribution tends to be smaller and the clearance slower, the dose of edrophonium does not need to be adjusted to obtain the same degree of recovery as in younger adults.

Neostigmine

In a study designed similar to the kinetic studies of edrophonium in the elderly,[57] Young et al.[60] studied the pharmacokinetics and dynamics of neostigmine in this patient population. Neostigmine was administered to patients receiving a metocurine infusion to maintain 90% neuromuscular block. The authors found that there was a slight, but not statistically significant, decrease in clearance of the anticholinesterase in the elderly and a decreased initial volume of distribution.

Dose-response studies of neostigmine are not as consistent as those involving edrophonium. They have demonstrated that the dose of neostigmine required for antagonism of residual neuromuscular block in elderly patients is either similar to,[33] or greater[61] than, that required in younger adults. When neostigmine is used to antagonize doxacurium-induced block, there is no significant difference in the dose of neostigmine required to achieve recovery, within 10 minutes, to a train-of-four ratio of 0.7 from 25% spontaneous recovery of muscle strength (41.6 ± 5.8 in the elderly and 53.6 ± 7.5 µg·kg^{-1} in younger adults).[33] Furthermore, in a different study, neostigmine, 50 µg·kg^{-1}, administered as a bolus at 25% recovery of muscle strength after administration of doxacurium, accelerated recovery to a train-of-four ratio of 0.7 to the same degree in both patient populations (12.6 ± 7.3 in the elderly and 12.0 ± 6.7 minutes in younger adults).[62] It has also been reported, however, that the dose of neostigmine required to antagonize 90% vecuronium-induced block is greater in the elderly (31 µg·kg^{-1}) than in younger adults (19 µg·kg^{-1}).[61] Slower spontaneous recovery from vecuronium-induced block in geriatric patients during neostigmine-antagonized recovery may be a cause of their apparent greater requirement for neostigmine. That being said, because of its own decreased clearance in the elderly, the duration of action of neostigmine is prolonged in elderly patients.[63] In addition, the decreased initial volume of distribution of neostigmine[60] (Table 18-4) results in a greater plasma concentration of the anticholinesterase after bolus administration and may contribute to its prolonged duration of action. This is potentially advantageous because the duration of action of many nondepolarizing neuromuscular blocking agents is prolonged in the elderly.

Of note, the values reported for times to recovery to a train-of-four ratio of 0.7 are average values. As demonstrated by Kirkegaard et al.,[64] there is a substantial degree of interpatient variability in the time required for neostigmine antagonism cisatracurium-induced neuromuscular block. This interpatient variability in young adults becomes even more pronounced when attempting to achieve recovery to a train-of-four ratio of 0.9, which has been recommended as the new standard for adequacy of recovery.[65]

Pyridostigmine

Similar to neostigmine, pyridostigmine exhibits a prolonged duration of action in the elderly.[63,66] Approximately 75% of administered pyridostigmine is eliminated by the kidney[63] and its clearance is slower in patients with renal failure.[67] The reduced plasma clearance of pyridostigmine (Table 18-4) caused by age-related deterioration in renal function likely accounts for its prolongation of action.

Adverse Effects of Anticholinesterases in Geriatric Patients

The cardiac muscarinic effects of anticholinesterases include dysrhythmias, such as bradycardia and conduction defects. Especially in the geriatric patient population, a large percentage of which has preexisting cardiovascular disease, anticholinesterase administration creates a greater risk of cardiac dysrhythmias.[68] Of the anticholinesterases, neostigmine is more likely to cause dysrhythmias than pyridostigmine (35% versus 14%, respectively).[69] In any patient, antimuscarinic agents, such as atropine or glycopyrrolate, are administered with the anticholinesterase to counteract the bradycardic effects of the anticholinesterase. Depending on the dosing regimen, tachycardia, rather than bradycardia, is frequently observed. In patients with cardiovascular disease, the resultant increase in myocardial oxygen consumption may not be well tolerated and may lead to myocardial ischemia.

In addition, atropine is a tertiary amine and can, therefore, cross the blood–brain barrier. In the central nervous system, anticholinergic drugs are known to affect the central cholinergic pathway where they are a cause of deterioration in postoperative cognitive function.[70] Atropine has been shown to produce disorientation, hallucinations, and memory loss. Glycopyrrolate, which is a quaternary amine, does not readily cross the blood–brain barrier and postanesthetic arousal times after its administration with neostigmine are shorter than those after the administration of atropine and neostigmine.[71]

Outcome Studies

Reports of adverse outcome from residual neuromuscular blockade exist.[72–75] One prospective trial of patient outcome after general anesthesia and nondepolarizing relaxants has been done.[72] In this study, patients undergoing gynecologic, general, or orthopedic surgical procedures were randomly assigned to receive vecuronium, atracurium, or pancuronium. Muscle strength was determined in the postanesthesia care unit and patients were followed for several days for evidence of postoperative pulmonary complications. Elderly patients who received pancuronium were more likely to enter the postanesthesia care unit with a train-of-four ratio less than 0.7 than those receiving either of the intermediate-acting relaxants and the younger adult patients, regardless of the neuromuscular blocking agent they received. In addition, these patients were more likely to develop postoperative pulmonary complications than patients who had arrived to the postanesthesia care unit with a train-of-four ratio ≥0.7. This is not unexpected because residual neuromuscular block has been found to interfere with the coordination of swallowing[76,77] and the response of the carotid body chemoreceptor to hypoxia.[78]

Summary

Although age-related changes in hepatic, renal, and cardiac function slow the onset and clearance of many nondepolarizing neuromuscular blocking agents in geriatric patients, extensive changes at the neuromuscular junction do not increase sensitivity to these compounds. Decreased clearance mandates that neuromuscular block be maintained and subsequent doses administered only after documentation of return of muscle strength with a monitor of neuromuscular blockade. Except in rare cases, the clinician should anticipate having to pharmacologically antagonize residual neuromuscular block.

As the surgical population ages and surgical trends and practices evolve, neuromuscular blocking agents, like anesthetics, must be specifically chosen based not only on their pharmacokinetic and pharmacodynamic properties, but also on the basis of patient age.

References

1. Gueret G, Rossignol B, Kiss G, et al. Is muscle relaxant necessary for cardiac surgery? Anesth Analg 2004;99:1330–1333.
2. Tomlinson BE, Irving D. The numbers of limb motor neurons in the human lumbosacral cord throughout life. J Neurol Sci 1977;34:213–219.
3. Kawamura Y, Okazaki H, O'Brien PC, et al. Lumbar motoneurons of man. I. Numbers and diameter histograms of

alpha and gamma axons and ventral roots. J Neuropathol Exp Neurol 1977;36:853–860.

4. Young A, Stokes M, Crowe M. Size, and strength of the quadriceps muscles of old and young men. Clin Physiol 1985;5:145–154.

5. Lexell J, Taylor CC, Sjöström M. What is the cause of the ageing atrophy? Total number, size and proportion of different fiber types studied in whole vastus lateralis muscle from 15- to 83-year-old men. J Neurol Sci 1988;84:275–294.

6. Forbes GB, Reina JC. Adult lean body mass declines with age: some longitudinal observations. Metabolism 1970;19:653–663.

7. Doherty TJ, Brown WF. Age-related changes in the twitch contractile properties of human thenar motor units. J Appl Physiol 1997;82:93–101.

8. Frolkis VV, Martynenko OA, Zamostan VP. Aging of the neuromuscular apparatus. Gerontology 1976;22:244–279.

9. Oda K. Age changes of motor innervation and acetylcholine receptor distribution on human skeletal muscle fibres. J Neurol Sci 1984;66:327–338.

10. Martyn JA, White DA, Gronert GA, et al. Up-and-down regulation of skeletal muscle acetylcholine receptors. Effects on neuromuscular blockers. Anesthesiology 1992;76:822–843.

11. Smith DO. Acetylcholine storage, release and leakage at the neuromuscular junction of mature adult and aged rats. J Physiol 1984;347:161–176.

12. Gronert GA. Disuse atrophy with resistance to pancuronium. Anesthesiology 1981;55:547–549.

13. Novak LP. Aging, total body potassium, fat-free mass and cell mass in males and females between ages of 18–85 years. J Gerontol 1972;27:438–443.

14. Ritschel WA. Pharmacokinetic approach to drug dosing in the aged. J Am Geriatr Soc 1976;24:344–354.

15. Mattco RS, Backus WW, McDanicl DD, ct al. Pharmacokinetics and pharmacodynamics of d-tubocurarine and metocurine in the elderly. Anesth Analg 1985;64:23–29.

16. Lien CA, Matteo RS, Ornstein E, et al. Distribution, elimination and action of vecuronium in the elderly. Anesth Analg 1991;73:39–42.

17. Wood M. Plasma drug binding: implications for anesthesiologists. Anesth Analg 1986;65:786–804.

18. Cameron M, Donati F, Varin F. In vitro plasma protein binding of neuromuscular blocking agents in different subpopulations of patients. Anesth Analg 1995;81:1019–1025.

19. Duvaldestin P, Saada J, Berger JL, et al. Pharmacokinetics, pharmacodynamics, and dose-response relationships of pancuronium in control and elderly subjects. Anesthesiology 1982;56:36–40.

20. Rupp SM, Castagnoli KP, Fisher DM, et al. Pancuronium and vecuronium pharmacokinetics and pharmacodynamics of vecuronium in younger and elderly adults. Anesthesiology 1987;67:45–49.

21. Ornstein E, Matteo RS, Schwartz AE, et al. Pharmacokinetics and pharmacodynamics of pipecuronium (Arduan) in elderly surgical patients. Anesth Analg 1992;74:841–844.

22. Dresner DL, Basta SJ, Ali HH, et al. Pharmacokinetics and pharmacodynamics of doxacurium in young and elderly patients during isoflurane anesthesia. Anesth Analg 1990;71:498–502.

23. O'Hara DA, Fragen RJ, Shanks CA. The effects of age on the dose response curve of vecuronium in adults. Anesthesiology 1987;67:45–49.

24. Bevan DR, Fiset P, Balendran P, et al. Pharmacodynamic behavior of rocuronium in the elderly. Can J Anaesth 1993;40:127–132.

25. Bell PF, Mirakhur RK, Clarke RSJ. Dose-response studies of atracurium, vecuronium and pancuronium in the elderly. Anaesthesia 1989;44:925–927.

26. Koscielniak-Nielsen ZJ, Bevan JC, Popovic V, et al. Onset of maximum neuromuscular block following succinylcholine or vecuronium in four age groups. Anesthesiology 1993;79:229–234.

27. Rodeheffer RJ, Gerstenblith G, Becker LC, et al. Exercise cardiac output is maintained with advancing age in healthy human subjects: cardiac dilatation and increased stroke work compensate for a diminished heart rate. Circulation 1984;69:203–213.

28. Sorooshian SS, Stafford MA, Eastwood NB, et al. Pharmacokinetics and pharmacodynamics of cisatracurium in young and elderly adult patients. Anesthesiology 1996;84:1083–1091.

29. Fisher DM, Rosen JI. A pharmacokinetic explanation for increasing recovery time following larger or repeated doses of nondepolarizing muscle relaxants. Anesthesiology 1986;65:286–291.

30. McLeod K, Hull CJ, Watson MJ. Effects of ageing on the pharmacokinetics of pancuronium. Br J Anaesth 1979;51:435–438.

31. Cook RD, Freeman JA, Lai AA, et al. Pharmacokinetics and pharmacodynamics of doxacurium in normal patients and in those with hepatic or renal failure. Anesth Analg 1991;72:143–150.

32. Cashman JN, Luke JJ, Jones RM. Neuromuscular block with doxacurium (BW Λ938U) in patients with normal or absent renal function. Br J Anaesth 1990;64:186–192.

33. Koscielniak-Nielsen ZJ, Law-Min JC, Donati F, et al. Dose-response relations of doxacurium and its reversal with neostigmine in young adults and healthy elderly patients. Anesth Analg 1992;74:845–850.

34. Caldwell JE, Canfell PC, Castagnoli KP, et al. The influence of renal failure on the pharmacokinetics and duration of action of pipecuronium bromide in patients anesthetized with halothane and nitrous oxide. Anesthesiology 1989;70:7–12.

35. Bender AD. The effect of increasing age on the distribution of peripheral blood flow in man. J Am Geriatr Soc 1965;13:192–198.

36. Leithe ME, Hermiller JB, Magorien RD, et al. The effect of age on central and regional hemodynamics. Gerontology 1984;30:240–246.

37. Kato R, Vassanelli P, Frontino G, et al. Variation in the activity of liver microsomal drug-metabolizing enzymes in rats in relation to age. Biochem Pharmacol 1964;13:1037–1051.

38. Bencini AF, Scaf AHJ, Sohn YJ, et al. Hepatobiliary disposition of vecuronium bromide in man. Br J Anaesth 1986;58:988–995.

39. d'Hollander AA, Massaux F, Nevelsteen M, et al. Age-dependent dose-response relationship of Org NC45 in anaesthetized patients. Br J Anaesth 1982;54:653–656.

40. McCarthy G, Elliott P, Mirakhur RK, et al. Onset and duration of action of vecuronium in the elderly: comparison with adults. Acta Anaesth Scand 1992;36:383–386.

41. Cooper RA, Maddineni RK, Wierda JMKH, et al. Time course of neuromuscular effects and pharmacokinetics of rocuronium bromide (ORG 9426) during isoflurane anaesthesia in patients with and without renal failure. Br J Anaesth 1993;71:222–226.

42. Matteo RS, Ornstein E, Schwartz AE, et al. Pharmacokinetics and pharmacodynamics of rocuronium (Org 9426) in elderly surgical patients. Anesth Analg 1993;77:1193–1197.

43. Baykara N, Solak M, Toker K. Predicting recovery from deep neuromuscular block by rocuronium in the elderly. J Clin Anesth 2003;15:328–333.

44. d'Hollander AA, Luyckx C, Barvais L, et al. Clinical evaluation of atracurium besylate requirements for a stable muscle relaxation during surgery: lack of age-related effects. Anesthesiology 1983;59:237–240.

45. Kent AP, Parker CJ, Hunter JM. Pharmacokinetics of atracurium and laudanosine in the elderly. Br J Anaesth 1989;63:661–666.

46. Kitts JB, Fisher DM, Canfell PC, et al. Pharmacokinetics and pharmacodynamics of atracurium in the elderly. Anesthesiology 1990;72:272–275.

47. Parker CJ, Hunter JM, Snowdon SL. Effect of age, sex and anesthetic technique on the pharmacokinetics of atracurium. Br J Anaesth 1992;69:439–443.

48. Fisher DM, Canfell PC, Fahey MR, et al. Elimination of atracurium in humans: contribution of Hofmann elimination and ester hydrolysis vs. organ-based elimination. Anesthesiology 1986;65:6–12.

49. Kisor DF, Schmith VD, Wargin WA, et al. Importance of the organ-independent elimination of cisatracurium. Anesth Analg 1996;83:1065–1071.

50. Ornstein E, Lien CA, Matteo RS, et al. Pharmacodynamics and pharmacokinetics of cisatracurium in geriatric surgical patients. Anesthesiology 1996;84:520–525.

51. Pühringer FK, Heier T, Dodgson M, et al. Double-blind comparison of the variability in spontaneous recovery of cisatracurium- and vecuronium-induced neuromuscular block in adult and elderly patients. Acta Anesthesiol Scand 2002;46:364–371.

52. Maddineni VR, Mirakhur RK, McCoy EP, et al. Neuromuscular and haemodynamic effects of mivacurium in elderly and young adult patients. Br J Anaesth 1994;73;609–612.

53. Goudsouzian N, Charravorti S, Denman W, et al. Prolonged mivacurium infusion in young and elderly adults. Can J Anaesth 1997;44:955–962.

54. Østergaard D, Viby-Mogensen J, Pedersen NA, et al. Pharmacokinetics and pharmacodynamics of mivacurium in young adult and elderly patients. Acta Anaesthesiol Scand 2002;46:684–691.

55. Maddineni VR, Mirakhur RK, McCoy EP. Plasma cholinesterase activity in elderly and young adults. Br J Anaesth 1994;72:497.

56. Hart PS, McCarthy GJ, Brown R, Lau M, Fisher DM. The effect of plasma cholinesterase activity on mivacurium infusion rates. Anesth Analg 1995;80:760–763.

57. Matteo RS, Young WL, Ornstein E, et al. Pharmacokinetics and pharmacodynamics of edrophonium in elderly surgical patients. Anesth Analg 1990;71:334–339.

58. McCarthy GJ, Mirakhur RK, Maddineni VR, et al. Dose-responses for edrophonium during antagonism of vecuronium block in young and older adult patients. Anaesthesia 1995;50:503–506.

59. Kitajima T, Ishii K, Ogata H. Edrophonium as an antagonist of vecuronium-induced neuromuscular block in the elderly. Anaesthesia 1995;50:359–361.

60. Young WL, Backus W, Matteo RS, et al. Pharmacokinetics and pharmacodynamics of neostigmine in the elderly. Anesthesiology 1984;61:A300.

61. McCarthy GJ, Cooper R, Stanley JC, et al. Dose-response relationships for neostigmine antagonism of vecuronium-induced neuromuscular block in adults and the elderly. Br J Anaesth 1992;69:281–283.

62. De Mey JC, Rolly G, Blauwen ND. Doxacurium block is not influenced by age. J Clin Anesth 1995;7:453–456.

63. Young WL, Matteo RS, Ornstein E. Duration of action of neostigmine and pyridostigmine in the elderly. Anesth Analg 1988;67:775–778.

64. Kirkegaard H, Heier T, Caldwell JE. Efficacy of tactile-guided reversal from cisatracurium-induced neuromuscular block. Anesthesiology 2002;96:45–50.

65. Kopman AF, Yee PS, Neuman GG. Relationship of the train-of-four fade ratio to clinical signs and symptoms of residual paralysis in awake volunteers. Anesthesiology 1997;86:765–771.

66. Stone JG, Matteo RS, Ornstein E, et al. Aging alters the pharmacokinetics of pyridostigmine. Anesth Analg 1995;81:773–776.

67. Cronnelly R, Stanski DR, Miller RD, et al. Pyridostigmine kinetics with and without renal function. Clin Pharmacol Ther 1980;28:78–81.

68. Muravchick S, Owens WD, Felts JA. Glycopyrrolate and cardiac dysrhythmias in geriatric patients after reversal of neuromuscular blockade. Can Anaesth Soc J 1979;26:22–25.

69. Owens WD, Waldbaum LS, Stephen CR. Cardiac dysrhythmias following reversal of neuromuscular blocking agents in the geriatric patient. Anesth Analg 1978;57:186–190.

70. Simpson KH, Smith RJ, Davies LF. Comparison of the effects of atropine and glycopyrrolate on cognitive function following general anesthesia. Br J Anaesth 1987;59:966–969.

71. Baraka A, Yared JP, Karam AM, et al. Glycopyrrolate-neostigmine and atropine-neostigmine mixtures affect post-anesthesia arousal times differently. Anesth Analg 1980;59:431–434.

72. Berg H, Viby-Mogensen J, Roed Mortensen CR, et al. Residual neuromuscular block is a risk factor for postoperative pulmonary complications: a prospective, randomized and blinded study of postoperative complications after atracurium, vecuronium and pancuronium. Acta Anaesthesiol Scand 1997;41:1095–1103.

73. Lunn JN, Hunter AR, Scott DB. Anaesthesia-related surgical mortality. Anaesthesia 1983;38:1090–1096.

74. Cooper AL, Leigh JM, Tring IC. Admissions to the intensive care unit after complications of anesthetic techniques over 10 years. Anaesthesia 1989;44:953–958.

75. Tiret L, Nivoche Y, Hatton F, Desmonts JM, Vourch G. Complications related to anesthesia in infants and children: a prospective survey in 40,240 anaesthetics. Br J Anaesth 1988;61:263–269.

76. Eriksson LI, Sundman E, Olsson R, et al. Functional assessment of the pharynx at rest and during swallowing in partially paralyzed humans: simultaneous videomanometry and mechanomyography of awake human volunteers. Anesthesiology 1997;87:1035–1043.

77. Sundman E, Witt H, Olsson R, et al. The incidence and mechanisms of pharyngeal and upper esophageal dysfunction in partially paralyzed humans: pharyngeal videoradiography and simultaneous manometry after atracurium. Anesthesiology 2000;92:977–984.

78. Wyon N, Joensen H, Yamamoto Y, Lindahl SG, Eriksson LI. Carotid body chemoreceptor function is impaired by vecuronium during hypoxia. Anesthesiology 1998;89:1471–1479.

19
Management of Regional Anesthesia

Bernadette Veering

There has been a dramatic increase in the elderly population throughout the past century. In one century, the number of persons aged 65 years or older has increased three times. Patients aged 85 and older are the most rapidly growing age group. By 2030, up to 20% of Western populations will be more than 65 years of age.[1] This situation has led to a progressive increase in the number of surgical interventions in elderly people. It has been estimated that more than half of the population older than 65 years will require surgical intervention at least once during the remainder of their lives.[2]

Regional anesthesia is frequently used in elderly patients, especially during genitourologic and gynecologic procedures, orthopedic surgery, cataract extraction, and inguinal hernia repairs. Knowledge of the age-related effects is important with respect to the design of an optimal regional anesthetic regimen in elderly patients.

Age-Related Changes Relevant to Regional Anesthesia

Anatomic and physiologic changes, associated with advancing age, may affect the nerve block characteristics and the pharmacokinetics after administration of local anesthetics (Figure 19-1). A declining number of neurons, deterioration in myelin sheaths in the dorsal and ventral roots, changes in the anatomy of the spine, and intervertebral foramina may contribute to altered nerve block characteristics after a regional anesthetic procedure.[3,4] Furthermore, the number of axons in peripheral nerves decreases with advancing age, and the conduction velocity diminishes, particularly in motor nerves.[5,6] With increasing age, changes in the connective tissue ground substances may result in changes in local distribution, i.e., in the distribution rate of the local anesthetic from the site of injection (the epidural space) to the sites of action.[3]

With aging, the dura becomes more permeable to local anesthetics because of enlarged arachnoid villi.[7] Aging is possibly associated with a reduction of the total volume of cerebrospinal fluid (CSF) and with an increase of its specific gravity.[8,9]

Central Neural Blockade

Epidural Anesthesia

The spread of analgesia increases with advancing age after epidural administration of a fixed dose of a local anesthetic solution (Figure 19-2).[10–14] Recently, it was demonstrated that the spread of analgesia was also greater in elderly patients than in younger patients after epidural anesthesia with the relatively new long-acting local anesthetics ropivacaine and levobupivacaine.[15,16] Furthermore, elderly patients have a faster onset of analgesia in the caudad segments and the rate of regression of analgesia is prolonged. However, the total time for recovery from analgesia is not affected by age. The motor block profile associated with epidural anesthesia alters with age as well. With epidural ropivacaine and bupivacaine, an enhanced intensity of motor blockade is shown with advancing age.[15] With bupivacaine, the onset of motor blockade is faster in the oldest compared with the youngest patients.[11]

Elderly patients exhibit anatomic and physiologic changes that influence the clinical course during epidural anesthesia. (See section on age-related changes relevant to regional anesthesia.) In older patients, the longitudinal spread of the local anesthetic in the epidural space is promoted by sclerosis and calcification of the intervertebral foramina and a reduced fatty tissue content of the epidural space. A more compliant and less resistant epidural space with advancing age may also contribute to this enhanced spread in the elderly.[17] The clinical course of epidural anesthesia may be further influenced by a

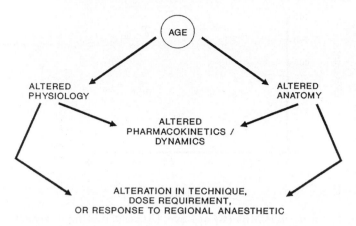

FIGURE 19-1. Factors that can modify epidural and spinal anesthesia in elderly patients.

shift of the site of action from a predominantly paravertebral site in the young to a subdural or transdural site in the elderly. Factors causing extensive spread are accelerated by arteriosclerosis and diabetes, both of which cause premature aging.[18]

Epinephrine is used frequently in the epidural test dose as a marker of intravascular injection. A given dose of epinephrine will not be totally reliable in older patients, because of decreased beta-adrenergic responsiveness.[19]

Patient-controlled epidural analgesia has been shown to be effective in elderly patients in the management of pain after major surgery.[20] Because elderly patients exhibit an increased sensitivity to opioids,[21] it has been suggested to reduce the bolus dose and infusion rate of opioids up to 50% when administered to the elderly. Patient-controlled epidural analgesia technique can be used only in elderly patients who can participate in self-medication, which excludes those with cognitive dysfunction.[22]

Spinal Anesthesia

Spinal anesthesia is frequently applied for lower abdominal, urologic, and lower limb surgery in older patients. The effect of age on the clinical profile of spinal anesthesia depends on the baricity of the injected solutions. With isobaric solutions, the effect of age on the maximal height of spinal analgesia is marginal.[23–25] With glucose-free 0.5% bupivacaine, which acts as a slightly hypobaric solution at body temperature, the spread of analgesia is unaltered with age.[23,24] However, with a solution of isobaric 2% mepivacaine, a slightly higher level of sensory analgesia has been found.[25] The caudad spread of analgesia as well as the development of motor blockade occurs

more rapidly in older patients during spinal anesthesia with glucose-free bupivacaine.[23,24] The effect of age on the spread of analgesia is more pronounced when hyperbaric solutions are used.[26–28] With a hyperbaric solution of bupivacaine, the level of analgesia increases with age, extending some 3–4 segments higher in elderly as compared to young adult patients. However, because of profound interindividual variability, the predictability of the analgesia levels that will be reached in an individual patient is low. In addition, a quicker onset time of motor block has been found in older patients. With both hyperbaric and glucose-free bupivacaine solutions, the duration of analgesia of the T12 dermatome is prolonged, which allows more time for operations on the lower abdominal or inguinal region in older patients. Addition of adjuvants to spinal solutions may prolong the duration of neural blockade. Addition of epinephrine to glucose-free bupivacaine solutions increases the duration of analgesia in elderly patients.[29] However, addition of clonidine is associated with prolongation of motor block.[30]

The effects of hypobaric spinal anesthetic solutions are probably less reliable in the elderly because of the higher average specific gravity and greater individual variation in the volume of CSF.

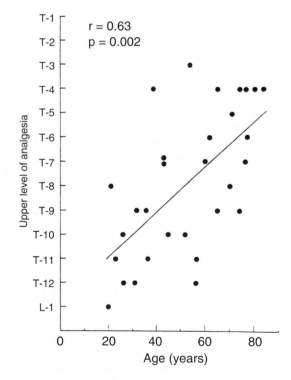

FIGURE 19-2. Relationship between the upper level of analgesia and age after epidural administration of 0.5% bupivacaine. (Reprinted with permission from Veering et al.[11] Copyright © Lippincott Williams & Wilkins.)

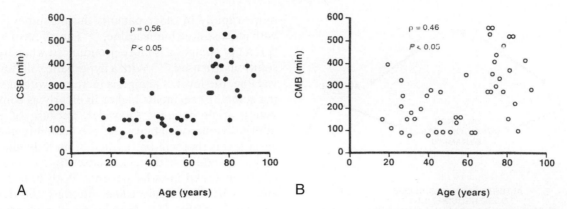

FIGURE 19-3. Duration of complete sensory block (CSB) **(A)** or motor block (CMB) **(B)** and age. (Reprinted with permission from Paqueron et al.[31] Copyright © Lippincott Williams & Wilkins.)

Peripheral Nerve Blockade

For peripheral blocks, the major physiologic changes are in the response of the nerves themselves to local anesthetics. By the age of 90 years, one third of the myelinated fibers have disappeared from peripheral nerves. In addition, conduction velocity, especially of the motor nerve, decreases with age.[6]

After administration of ropivacaine at a brachial plexus block, the duration of sensory block and motor block is greater than in younger patients (Figure 19-3).[31] Onset time of complete motor block is shorter in elderly patients. Further study is indicated to investigate the effect of age on the characteristics of other peripheral blocks.

Pharmacology

Regional anesthetic blocks are performed by injecting local anesthetic agents close to nerve trunks. Two quite separate processes simultaneously occur after injection. While there is a vascular uptake of the drug into the systemic circulation, which removes the drug from the injection site, the drug also diffuses directly to neural structures, where the therapeutic action occurs. This is the pharmacodynamic part. The uptake into the systemic circulation may lead to side effects.

Pharmacokinetics of Local Anesthetics

Changes in body composition and characteristics of tissues and organs within the body may have an impact on the rate and extent of systemic absorption, distribution, and elimination of local anesthetics used for regional anesthesia. Pharmacokinetic and/or pharmacodynamic changes, which may occur with increasing age, could alter the clinical profile of local anesthetics after a regional anesthetic procedure.

The effect of age on the pharmacokinetics of local anesthetics may be different in females than in males and may be influenced by concomitant diseases.

Systemic Absorption

Knowledge of the pharmacokinetics of local anesthetics is of importance in relation to the clinical profile, in particular, the duration of action, and in relation to the risk of systemic side effects and toxicity.[32] In this respect, both the systemic absorption, i.e., the uptake from the perineural site of administration into the blood, and the systemic disposition (distribution and elimination) must be considered. Peak plasma concentrations of lidocaine and bupivacaine after epidural or caudal administration change little, if at all, with increasing age.[11,33-35] However, the terminal half-life of bupivacaine increases after both epidural and subarachnoid administration, suggesting that the absorption rate of bupivacaine decreases with advancing age.[11,24,26]

Details on the absorption rate cannot be derived from the plasma concentration curves, unless a detailed description of the disposition is available. A stable isotope method allows simultaneous studies of the absorption and disposition.[36,37] Local anesthetics exhibit a biphasic absorption pattern, a fast initial absorption phase followed by a slower absorption phase after epidural and subarachnoid administration.[36-38] The initial fast absorption rate is a reflection of the high initial concentration gradient and the large vascularity of the epidural space. With spinal anesthesia, the initial absorption is much slower because the subarachnoid space has a poor perfusion. The slower second absorption phase is believed to occur from slow uptake of local anesthetics. Whereas a previous study on the systemic absorption and disposition kinetics of bupivacaine after epidural administration did not reveal an effect of age on the absorption kinetics,[12] a recent study demonstrated a significant effect on the rapid initial absorption kinetics of levobupivacaine after epidural administration.[16] After subarachnoid administration, the mean absorption has been shown to be shorter in elderly patients because of a faster late absorption rate.[28] Based on the faster absorption, one might expect a shorter duration of spinal and epidural anesthesia in older patients; however, this has not been demonstrated.

The epidural absorption studies with bupivacaine and levobupivacaine and the spinal absorption study with bupivacaine demonstrate an increased sensitivity in the elderly that does not seem to be related to the impairment of vascular absorption. Therefore, changes in the clinical profile with epidural and spinal anesthesia are best explained by anatomic considerations and possibly pharmacodynamic changes in the elderly rather than by pharmacokinetic changes in the elderly.

Systemic Disposition

Age-related changes in drug distribution may result from changes in body composition and/or changes in drug binding and tissue perfusion. As fatty tissue increases, the volume of distribution of lipophilic local anesthetics would be expected to increase.[39] Such an increase has been demonstrated for lidocaine.[40] However, others observed an unchanged volume of distribution of intravenously (IV) administered lidocaine.[41,42]

A second factor influencing distribution is the plasma binding of drugs. The main binding protein for local anesthetic agents is α_1-acid glycoprotein (AAG), an acute phase reactant protein.[43] The plasma protein binding of lidocaine tends to increase slightly with age.[44] However, age does not influence the serum protein binding of bupivacaine.[45] This is in keeping with the lack of effect of age on AAG concentrations.[46] Any effect of age on AAG concentrations is likely to be relatively small, and therefore age-related changes in protein binding and in volume of distribution of local anesthetic agents that bind to AAG are more likely related to other factors.[47,48]

Local anesthetics are predominantly eliminated by metabolism.[49] The effect of age on the metabolism and excretion of local anesthetics is related to changes in hepatic function. Decreases in hepatic mass, hepatic blood flow, and hepatic enzyme activity with advancing age may result in impairment of metabolism. For local anesthetics that exhibit a high rate of hepatic extraction (e.g., lidocaine), the rate-limiting step in metabolism is hepatic blood flow.[50] Accordingly, the decrease of liver blood flow is associated with a decline in clearance of lidocaine with advancing age.[51]

There is also a gradual decline in hepatic mass,[52] and, as a consequence, the clearance of local anesthetics with relatively low hepatic extraction ratios, which are mostly dependent on metabolizing hepatic enzyme activ-

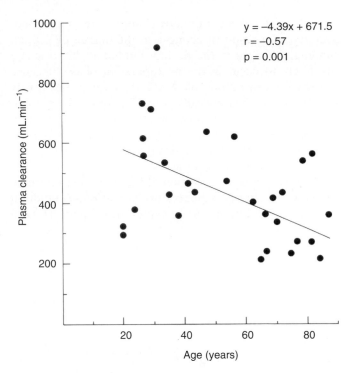

FIGURE 19-4. Relationship between total plasma clearance and age. (Reprinted with permission from Veering et al.[11] Copyright © Lippincott Williams & Wilkins.)

ity, may decrease with age. Total plasma clearance of bupivacaine has been found to decrease with increasing age after epidural and subarachnoid administration (Figure 19-4).[11,24,26,28]

Because bupivacaine has a relatively low hepatic extraction ratio, the observed age-related decline in clearance is likely the result of a change in drug-metabolizing hepatic enzyme activity and/or serum protein binding of bupivacaine, rather than from an alteration in the liver blood flow. However, age has not been shown to affect the protein binding of bupivacaine.[45] Therefore, the observed age-related decline in clearance probably reflects a concomitant decline in hepatic enzyme activity or capacity.

The altered pharmacokinetics in elderly patients (uncomplicated by disease) seem to be relatively unimportant with a single epidural injection. The local anesthetic doses need not be modified because of the resulting plasma concentrations.

However, taking into account the age-related decreased clearance of lidocaine and bupivacaine, administration of multiple intermittent injections or continuous epidural infusion of these local anesthetics for prevention of postoperative pain might lead to increased accumulation of these agents.[34] Consequently, the potential of developing side effects, including toxicity, might be enhanced.

Long-term epidural infusion of bupivacaine for the relief of postoperative pain has been shown to result in progressively increasing plasma concentrations.[53,54] This probably reflects a continuous change in the pharmaco-kinetics, as a result of changes in the degree of protein binding. Changes in the protein binding of bupivacaine are likely to occur in the postoperative phase, because plasma concentrations of AAG increase progressively during the first postoperative days.[55] It should be emphasized, however, that postoperative increases in total plasma concentrations are not accompanied by similar increases in the pharmacologically more relevant unbound (free) plasma concentrations.

However, the concentration of free unbound lidocaine increases in elderly patients during continuous epidural infusion of lidocaine for postoperative pain (Figure

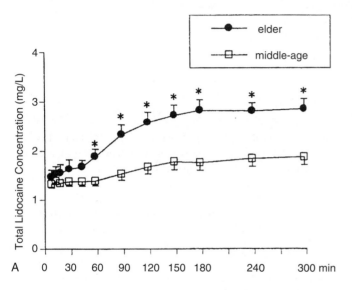

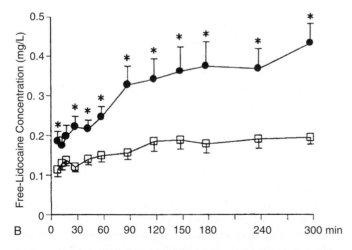

FIGURE 19-5. Mean plasma concentrations of total (A) and free (B) lidocaine after epidural administration to elderly or middle-aged male patients. *p < 0.05, compared with the middle-aged group. Bars represent standard errors. (Reprinted with permission from Fukuda et al.[56] Copyright © 2003. With permission from the American Society of Regional Anesthesia and Pain Medicine.)

19-5).[56] The upward trend of free lidocaine concentration in elderly patients is not caused by differences in AAG, but likely reflects a lower metabolic activity. The ratios of the total monoethylglycinexylidide (MEGX)/free lidocaine, which reflect the ability to metabolize lidocaine, were lower in the elderly group than in the middle-aged group. So caution must be exercised during continuous epidural infusion of lidocaine in geriatric patients.

Problems

Performing epidural and spinal anesthesia may be more difficult in elderly patients. It is often not easy to position the elderly patient appropriately because of the anatomic distortion, particularly curvature or rotation of the spine, that is found in many older people. The inability of the elderly patient to flex the back as much as the younger patient makes axial blockade difficult. Aging is frequently accompanied by an increase in the degree of lumbar lordosis often attributable to osteoporosis. Calcification of the interspinous ligaments and ligamentum flavum, the gradual stenosing of the intervertebral foramina in the elderly, make needle placement and advancement more complicated.

The most common complication of spinal anesthesia is postspinal headache. Although the incidence is largely related to the size of the needle used, the incidence is decreased with age, possibly because of a decreased elasticity of the cranial tissues.[57] Consequently, less CSF leaks away from the subarachnoid space in older patients. Decreasing pain sensibility with increasing age and a decrease in distensibility of pain-sensitive structures in the cranium are also considered to contribute.

Hypotension

Hypotension is the most common cardiovascular disturbance associated with central neural blockade with a particularly frequent incidence in the elderly. It occurs from decreases in systemic vascular resistance and central venous pressure from sympathetic block with vasodilatation and redistribution of central blood volume to lower extremities and splanchnic beds.[58] Hypotension after spinal anesthesia is a common problem, with an incidence of 15.3%–33%.[59,60] High levels of analgesia and old age seem to be the two main factors associated with the development of hypotension.[60] A greater spread of analgesia with epidural ropivacaine in elderly patients is accompanied with a higher incidence of hypotension and bradycardia (Figure 19-6).[15] This problem is a particularly important issue in elderly patients with cardiovascular disease such as hypertension, because the risk for ischemia secondary to hypotension is increased.[61,62] Moreover, morbidity and mortality rates in elderly patients

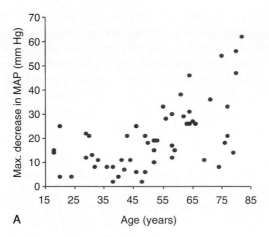
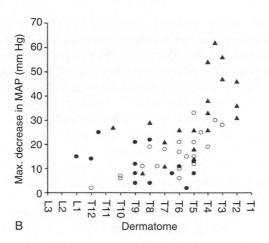
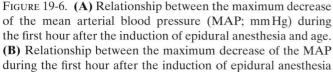
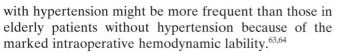

A · Age (years)

B · Dermatome

FIGURE 19-6. **(A)** Relationship between the maximum decrease of the mean arterial blood pressure (MAP; mm Hg) during the first hour after the induction of epidural anesthesia and age. **(B)** Relationship between the maximum decrease of the MAP during the first hour after the induction of epidural anesthesia and the highest level of analgesia for the three age groups (• = group 1, 19–40 years; o = group 2, 41–60 years; ▲ = group 3, >61 years). (Adapted with permission from Simon et al.[15] Copyright © Lippincott Williams & Wilkins.)

with hypertension might be more frequent than those in elderly patients without hypertension because of the marked intraoperative hemodynamic lability.[63,64]

Marked hypotension is especially harmful to elderly patients with limited cardiac reserve. Structural changes in the arterioles and changes in the autonomic nervous system with increasing age may contribute to substantial hypotension in elderly patients. The elderly have increased resting sympathetic nervous system activity and associated increased norepinephrine release from nerve terminals.[65,66] In addition, age-related baroreflex dysfunction may compromise arterial pressure homeostasis.[67] Hemodynamic instability after spinal anesthesia, therefore, might be exaggerated in the elderly because of larger decreases in systemic vascular resistance (Figure 19-7).[68]

Transthoracic electrical bioimpedance revealed that systolic blood pressure decreased by 25% as early as 6–9 minutes after the block, indicating that patients should be monitored immediately after subarachnoid block.[69]

Treatment of Hypotension in the Elderly

Common strategies used to prevent or reduce the incidence and severity of hypotension include IV fluid bolus and the use of vasopressors. Both prophylaxis and therapy should aim primarily at stabilizing or replenishing cardiac filling. Principally, this can be achieved either by increasing blood volume or by counteracting vasodilatation in the sympatholytic regions with vasoconstrictor agents. It is common practice to give IV fluids before and during

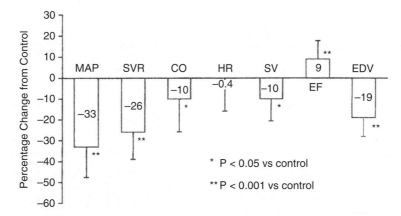

* P < 0.05 vs control

** P < 0.001 vs control

FIGURE 19-7. Hemodynamic response to high spinal anesthesia in elderly men with cardiac disease. Decrease in systemic vascular resistance (SVR) and no decreases in cardiac output (CO) were primarily responsible for the large decrease in mean arterial blood pressure (MAP). Heart rate (HR) was unchanged; therefore, the decrease in cardiac output was attributable to a decrease in stroke volume (SV). The decrease in stroke volume was less than the decrease in end-diastolic volume (EDV) because the ejection fraction (EF) increased. (Reprinted with permission from Rooke et al.[68] Copyright © Lippincott Williams & Wilkins.)

spinal anesthesia to prevent hypotension. In elderly patients, however, fluid preloading is not always effective.[70,71] Volume loading does not always prevent the decrease in systemic vascular resistance caused by spinal anesthesia but, in fact, may cause further decreases.[72] Irrespective of whether crystalloid, colloid, or no prehydration is used, a high incidence of hypotension follows spinal anesthesia in normovolemic elderly patients undergoing elective procedures. Additionally, the attenuated physiologic reserve in elderly patients seems to make them less able to increase cardiac output in response to volume loading.

Administration of a colloid preload during the induction phase of the block, usually about 7 mL/kg, has been recommended in elderly patients to compensate for any decrease in central venous pressure.[73,74] It should be emphasized, however, that rapid volume preloading constitutes a potential risk in older patients with limited cardiac reserve. At the same time, an alpha agonist should be used to reverse any decrease in vascular resistance.

The degree of hypotension correlates with the level of sympathetic block, which is generally two to four segments higher than the level of analgesia.[75] From a clinical point of view, it is, therefore, important to limit the level of sympathetic block. The rationale for combining local anesthetics with adjuvant drugs is to use lower doses of each agent and to preserve analgesia with fewer side effects. A "minidose" of 4 mg of bupivacaine in combination with 20 μg of fentanyl provided spinal anesthesia for surgical repair of hip fracture in the elderly.[76] The minidose combination caused dramatically less hypotension than 10 mg of bupivacaine and nearly eliminated the need for vasopressor support of blood pressure.

Changes in the technique of hyperbaric bupivacaine spinal anesthesia by injection of hyperbaric bupivacaine either at a lower L4-5 interspace than the usual (L3-4)

lumbar interspace[77] or different periods of sitting after injection had little, if any, influence on final analgesia levels and on hemodynamic changes in elderly patients.[78]

However, unilateral segmental spinal anesthesia may result in more restricted anesthetic spread with less hemodynamic variability. Unilaterality can be reliably produced with small doses of hyperbaric solutions and by prolonged lateral positioning.[79]

Continuous spinal anesthesia (CSA) is a technique that allows one to titrate local anesthetic solutions and thus reduce the dosage of local anesthetics, providing a more adequate analgesia with a lower level of sympathetic blockade and minimizing arterial hypotension and bradycardia.[80] Also, combined spinal-epidural technique (CSE) enables smaller intrathecal doses to be used with the option of topping up the epidural catheter if the block is inadequate. When hemodynamic stability is critical, CSE or CSA may be the techniques of choice for lower limb surgery in the elderly patients.

Hypothermia

As with general anesthesia, advanced age is associated with hypothermia during epidural and spinal anesthesia. This should be attributed to a variety of factors such as a physiologic decrease in basal metabolism, changes in the thermoregulatory center, and diminished muscular mass.[81–83] Also, elderly patients may be especially at risk of hypothermia because low core temperature may not initiate autonomic protective responses.

Advancing age and high-level spinal blockade are associated with a significant decrease of thermoregulatory threshold (Figure 19-8).[83] The shivering threshold is decreased in proportion with the level of spinal blockade because the vasomotor tone is inhibited below the

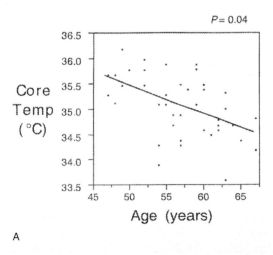

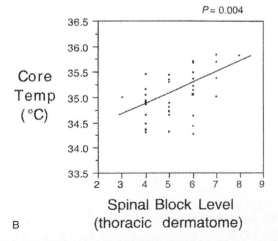

FIGURE 19-8. Advanced age (A) and high level of spinal block (B) were significant predictors of core hypothermia at admission to the postanesthesia care unit by linear regression.

(Reprinted with permission from Frank et al.[81] Copyright © Lippincott Williams & Wilkins.)

level of spinal block.[84,85] So the greater the proportion of the body that is blocked, the greater the level of thermoregulatory dysfunction that can be expected. Shivering and increase in oxygen demand further compromise patients, especially those with known cardiovascular diseases.

Controlling and monitoring body temperature in older patients and in those with high spinal blocks could decrease risk of hypothermia and its complications.

Sedation

Prompt and complete postoperative recovery of mental function is particularly important in elderly patients if the mental condition is already compromised by age-related disease or drug therapy.[22]

Elderly people are prone to confusion and are often sensitive to low doses of sedative drugs. Geriatric patients show an increased responsiveness for benzodiazepine compounds.[86] Therefore, smaller doses and more delayed increments must be used. Also, caution should be used when benzodiazepines are given as premedication in geriatric patients.

The pharmacokinetics and the pharmacodynamics of propofol change dramatically with age.[87] Elderly patients are more sensitive to the hypnotic and electroencephalographic effects of propofol than younger persons. Older patients require lower doses for any given effect, in many cases as little as 30% of the expected "standard" dose. Propofol infusion for sedation during spinal anesthesia resulted in a delayed recovery time in elderly patients compared with younger patients.[88] Elderly patients may require a more prolonged observation period after cessation of sedation with propofol.

Postoperative Cognitive Function

A proportion of mostly elderly orthopedic patients develop early postoperative cognitive dysfunction, confusion, and delirium, which are all nonspecific symptoms of central nervous system dysfunction.[89–91] This postoperative mental condition may persist for several days to several weeks and can result in increased morbidity, delayed functional recovery, and prolonged hospital stay. The mechanism of early postoperative confusion after orthopedic surgery and other operations is probably multifactorial.[92,93]

In most cases, recovery of cognitive function is prompt and complete within 1 week in elderly patients. Neither the choice of anesthetic technique nor the modality used for the management of postoperative pain seems to be an important determinant of postoperative confusion in elderly patients.[89,92,93]

The factors that likely explain the development of postoperative brain dysfunction are age, hospitalization, and extension and duration of surgery.

Beneficial Aspects of Regional Anesthesia

The use of both intraoperative and postoperative regional analgesic techniques provides physiologic benefits and may attenuate the pathophysiology that occurs after surgery.[94] Local anesthetic agents have the capability to block afferent and efferent signals to and from the spinal cord, thus suppressing the surgical stress response (Table 19-1).[95] The cascade of events unleashed during the stress response to surgical events can be blunted with epidural anesthesia.[95,96] One such effect is to decrease postoperative hypercoagulability. Epidural or spinal analgesia and anesthesia attenuates the hypercoagulable perioperative state by increasing fibrinolysis and decreasing coagulability.[97–99]

Regional anesthesia techniques provide excellent pain management, thus sparing the sedative effects of opioids and facilitating early postoperative mobilization for a faster convalescence.[96,100]

When compared with general anesthesia, intraoperative blood loss is reduced by spinal or epidural anesthesia, especially in patients undergoing hip replacement surgery.[101,102] This is attributed to lower venous pressures

TABLE 19-1. Effects of analgesic techniques on postoperative surgical stress responses.

Type of analgesia	Endocrine responses	Metabolic responses	Inflammatory responses
Systemic opioid (PCA or intermittent)	↓		
NSAID	↓		↓
Epidural opioid	↓		
Lumbar epidural local anesthetics (lower extremity surgery)	↓↓↓		
Thoracic epidural local anesthetics (abdominal surgery)	↓↓		

Source: Adapted with permission from Kehlet and Holte.[96] Copyright ® The Board of Management and Trustees of the *British Journal of Anaesthesia.* Reproduced by permission of Oxford University Press/*British Journal of Anaesthesia.*
PCA = patient-controlled analgesia, NSAID = nonsteroidal antiinflammatory drug, ↓ = small effect, ↓↓ = moderate effect, ↓↓↓ = major effect.

during central neural blockade compared with general anesthesia.

Compared with general anesthesia, epidural[103] and spinal anesthesia[104] are not associated with changes in arterial blood gases either during or after the operation, indicating a preservation of pulmonary gas exchange.[105]

Cardiovascular System

Thoracic epidural anesthesia (TEA) can produce a selective segmental blockade of the cardiac sympathetic nerves (T1–T5), with loss of chronotropic and inotropic drive to the heart.[58] Animal studies have been performed to test whether sympathetic block lessens ischemia.[106,107] Acute coronary occlusion during TEA resulted in redistribution of flow to the epicardium away from the endocardium, affecting beneficially collateral blood flow during myocardial ischemia.[106] Under the influence of TEA, the size of induced myocardial infarcts was smaller after experimental coronary occlusion in dogs.[107]

High TEA in humans improved an ischemia-induced left ventricular dysfunction; reduced electrocardiographic, echocardiographic, and angiographic signs of coronary insufficiency decreased the incidence of arrhythmias and provided relief of ischemic chest pain.[108–111]

These results show that TEA with an associated cardiac sympathetic blockade improves the oxygen supply–demand ratio.[112]

Pulmonary System

Thoracic and lumbar epidural anesthesia are often combined with general anesthesia in patients undergoing upper abdominal surgery, vascular surgery, and kidney surgery. Epidural anesthesia per se has little effect on respiration in patients with preexisting lung disease. Most of the respiratory changes associated with epidural anesthesia are directly attributed to motor block of the muscles of respiration.[58]

Perhaps the most profound effect of major abdominal and thoracic surgery on pulmonary function is a reduction in the functional residual capacity as a result of diaphragmatic dysfunction. This is caused by reflex inhibition of the phrenic nerve after major surgery, a decreased chest wall compliance, and pain-limited inspiration.[113]

Diaphragmatic activity increases after TEA, possibly because of the interruption of an inhibitory reflex of phrenic nerve motor drive, either related to direct deafferentation of visceral sensory pathways, or because of a diaphragmatic load reduction caused by increased abdominal compliance.[114,115]

Gastrointestinal System

A TEA over T12 is associated with splanchnic sympathetic nervous blockade, which results in reduced inhibitory gastrointestinal tone and increased intestinal blood flow.[94,116] Blood flow to the bowel is a critical factor for gastrointestinal motility. Intestinal sympathectomy also results in a contracted bowel because of vagal predominance. All these factors result in a faster digestive transit.[116,117] In addition, TEA improves microvascular perfusion of the small intestine.[118]

Outcome: Regional Versus General Anesthesia

Generally, geriatric patients have a decreased functional reserve of organ systems and thus become increasingly intolerant to surgical stress. Local anesthetics have the capability to block afferent and efferent signals to and from the spinal cord, thus suppressing the surgical stress response and spinal reflex inhibition of diaphragmatic and gastrointestinal function.

The question often asked is whether these mentioned beneficial aspects of regional anesthesia make a difference in the outcome of surgical patients. To demonstrate superiority of one anesthetic technique over another technique, one needs to look at outcome results.

Discrepancies exist between studies that have evaluated the early mortality, i.e., within 1 month, in elderly patients, after major orthopedic surgery under either regional (epidural or spinal) or general anesthesia (Table 19-2). Several studies on elderly patients undergoing hip

TABLE 19-2. Effect of anesthetic technique on postoperative mortality in elderly patients (age range: 60–90+).

| Author | Number of patients (reg/GA) | Method | Mortality (%) | | |
			7 days (reg/GA)	30 days (reg/GA)	1 year (reg/GA)
Sutcliffe[120]	383/950	Prospective		9.4/8.8	36.9/32.6
O'Hara et al.[119]	3129/6206	Retrospective	1.6/1.3	5.4/4.4	
Gilbert et al.[123]	430/311	Prospective			19.1/16.6
Urwin et al.[122]	1028/1005	Meta-analysis		6.4/9.4*	22.5/21

Reg = regional anesthesia, GA = general anesthesia.
*p < 0.05. Advantage regional anesthesia over general anesthesia.

fracture repair failed to reveal advantages of regional anesthesia compared with general anaesthesia.[119,120] With meta-analysis, it is possible to combine relevant data from several existing investigations in order to study the effect of specific techniques of anesthesia and to draw conclusions.[121] A systemic review of randomized trials showed that regional anesthesia for hip fracture surgery was associated with a reduced early mortality and incidence of deep vein thrombosis in comparison with general anesthesia.[122] The pattern of reduction in early mortality is possibly related to a decreased incidence of deep venous thrombosis. Long-term morbidity and mortality (2 months to 1 year) do not seem to be altered by the anesthetic type used during hip repair.[120,123]

Cardiac Outcome

Cardiac morbidity is the most common cause of death after major surgical procedures. The incidence of cardiovascular diseases is high in elderly surgical populations undergoing peripheral vascular surgery of the lower extremity. Because perioperative sympathetic activation has a causative role in the development of myocardial ischemia and infarction, inhibition of this activation would be expected to reduce cardiac morbidity.

There has been an ongoing discussion as to whether regional anesthesia is superior to general anesthesia in patients at cardiac risk. Discrepancies exist between studies that have evaluated this effect, because most studies are insufficiently powered to demonstrate clinically and statistically significant benefits.

The impact of anesthetic choice on cardiac outcome was studied in patients undergoing peripheral vascular surgery who had a likelihood of associated coronary artery disease.[124] In this study, patients were randomly assigned to be given general, epidural, or spinal anesthesia. There was no significant difference among groups in cardiovascular morbidity and overall mortality. In another study, patients were randomized to receive general anesthesia combined with postoperative epidural analgesia or general anesthesia with on-demand narcotic analgesia (PCA).[125] The rates of cardiovascular, infectious, and overall postoperative complications, as well as duration of intensive care unit (ICU) stay, were significantly reduced in the general anesthesia–postoperative epidural analgesia group. In addition, the incidences of graft occlusion were reduced. However, in a comparable study, no difference was found in the incidence of cardiac ischemia in patients scheduled for elective vascular reconstruction of the lower extremities.[126]

However, the need for reoperation for graft failure was reduced in the epidural group. Park et al.[127] observed in a large, multiinstitutional clinical trial that epidural plus general anesthesia and postoperative epidural analgesia improved the perioperative cardiac outcome of elderly patients undergoing abdominal aortic operations compared with that of general anesthesia alone and postoperative systemic opioid analgesia.

Beattie and colleagues[128] performed a meta-analysis to determine whether postoperative analgesia continued for more than 24 hours after surgery reduces postoperative myocardial infarction or in-hospital death. It seemed that thoracic epidural analgesia was superior to lumbar epidural analgesia in reducing postoperative myocardial infarction. These findings suggest that in high-risk cardiac patients, thoracic epidural postoperative analgesia is warranted and should be used more widely.

Early administration of continuous epidural analgesia was associated with a lower incidence of preoperative adverse cardiac events in elderly patients with hip fracture who had or were at risk for coronary artery disease.[129] Although the study group was small, the results warrant further study of preoperative analgesia in this population.

Coagulation

The risk and incidence of thromboembolic complications after lower body complications are lower in patients operated on under lumbar epidural and spinal anesthesia as compared with those given general anesthesia.[98,130,131] The mechanism is probably a combination of improved lower extremity blood flow, favorable changes in coagulation and fibrinolysis, inhibition of thrombocyte aggregation, and decreasing blood viscosity.[97–99,132] In addition, the systemic absorption of epidurally administered local anesthetics, improved pain control, and earlier mobility likely decrease the incidence of clot formation.[133]

Pulmonary Outcome

A major cause of postoperative complications is respiratory problems during the early postoperative recovery period.

Decreased intubation times and ICU stays in patients with epidural anesthesia and analgesia after major abdominal surgery in elderly patients have been reported.[129,134] A recent meta-analysis of 48 randomized controlled clinical trials assessed improvements in pulmonary outcomes comparing systemic opioids, epidural opioid, and epidural local anesthetic.[135] Compared with those who received systemic opioids, patients who received postoperative epidural analgesia with local anesthetics had a significant reduction in the incidence of pulmonary complications, atelectasis, and pneumonia and increase in the postoperative partial pressure of oxygen. So continuous epidural local anesthetic or local anesthetic–opioid mixtures have been demonstrated to improve outcome by controlling postoperative pain, permitting earlier extubation, and reducing length of stay.

Gastrointestinal Outcome

Postoperative ileus is a major surgical morbidity following abdominal surgery. As a consequence, the length of stay of elderly patients may be prolonged in the hospital. Colonic motility is inhibited for 48–72 hours. The most frequently accepted theory is that abdominal pain activates a spinal reflex arc that inhibits intestinal motility.[136–138]

Randomized clinical trials that investigated the recovery of gastrointestinal function after abdominal and other types of surgery have consistently shown that the use of postoperative thoracic epidural analgesia with a local anesthetic-based regimen compared with systemic opioid analgesia will allow earlier return of gastrointestinal function and even discharge from the hospital.[96,117,139]

Conclusion

This chapter has outlined several aspects of regional anesthesia in elderly patients. The general consensus is that elderly patients are more sensitive to local anesthetic agents and show altered clinical profiles. Older patients experience slightly higher levels of sensory and motor blockade after epidural and spinal anesthesia and are also at somewhat greater risk for arterial hypotension because of the sympatholytic consequences of acute peripheral autonomic blockade. Thus, bolus doses of local anesthetic should be reduced in elderly patients to limit the side effects.

Regional anesthesia offers several beneficial aspects to elderly patients, including reduced blood loss, better peripheral vascular circulation, suppression of the surgical stress response, and better postoperative pain control. The cardiac benefits of regional anesthesia have been especially attributed to TEA, particularly in patients with ischemic heart disease. Possibly postoperative thoracic epidural analgesia reduces cardiac morbidity in high-risk cardiac patients. Postoperative epidural analgesia can improve outcome after surgery by reducing pulmonary complications. Persistent age-related cognitive dysfunction seems not to be related to the history of an operation under general or regional anesthesia, suggesting the existence of other interacting etiologic factors. Regional anesthesia may reduce short-term mortality, especially in elderly patients undergoing hip fracture repair by a decrease in thromboembolism because of maintenance of relatively normal fibrinolysis. However, no conclusions can be drawn for longer-term mortality. There is evidence that epidural anesthesia facilitates earlier recovery by reducing ileus in abdominal surgical patients.

Nonetheless, large multicenter prospective randomized studies are required in elderly surgical patients to more definitively assess the impact of regional anesthesia on morbidity and mortality, ICU time, length of hospitalization, and cost of health care.

References

1. US Bureau of Census. Statistical Abstracts of the United States. 113th ed. Washington, DC: Department of Commerce; 1993.
2. Klopfenstein CE, Herrmann FR, Michel JP, et al. The influence of an aging surgical population on the anesthesia workload: a ten-year survey. Anesth Analg 1998;86:1165–1170.
3. Bromage PR. Epidural Analgesia. Philadelphia: WB Saunders; 1978:31–35.
4. Ferrer-Brechner T. Spinal and epidural anaesthesia in the elderly. Semin Anesth 1986;V:54–61.
5. Jacob JM, Love S. Qualitative and quantitative morphology of human sural nerve at different ages. Brain 1985; 108:897–924.
6. Dorfman LJ, Bosley TM. Age related changes in peripheral and central nerve conduction in man. Neurology 1979;29: 38–44.
7. Shanta TR, Evans JA. The relationship of epidural anesthesia to neural membranes and arachnoid villi. Anesthesiology 1972;37:543–557.
8. May C, Kaye JA, Atack JR, et al. Cerebrospinal fluid production is reduced in healthy aging. Neurology 1990;40: 500–503.
9. Greene NM. Physiology of Spinal Anaesthesia. 3rd ed. Baltimore: Williams & Wilkins; 1981:5.
10. Park WY, Balingit PE, MacNamara TE. Age and the epidural dose response in adult man. Anesthesiology 1982;56: 318–332.
11. Veering BT, Burm AGL, Van Kleef JW, et al. Epidural anesthesia with bupivacaine: effects of age on neural blockade and pharmacokinetics. Anesth Analg 1987;66: 589–594.
12. Veering BT, Burm AGL, Vletter AA, et al. The effect of age on the systemic absorption and systemic disposition of bupivacaine after epidural administration. Clin Pharmacokinet 1992;22:75–84.
13. Nydahl PA, Philipson L, Axelsson K, et al. Epidural anesthesia with 0.5% bupivacaine: influence of age on sensory and motor blockade. Anesth Analg 1991;73:780–787.
14. Hirabayashi Y, Shimizu R. Effect of age on extradural dose requirement in thoracic extradural anaesthesia. Br J Anaesth 1993;71:445–446.
15. Simon MJ, Veering BT, Stienstra R, et al. The effects of age on neural blockade and hemodynamic changes after epidural anesthesia with ropivacaine. Anesth Analg 2002;94: 1325–1330.
16. Simon MJG, Veering BT, Burm AGL, et al. The effect of age on the clinical profile and the systemic absorption and disposition of levobupivacaine following epidural anaesthesia. Br J Anaesth 2004;93:512–520.
17. Hirabayashi Y, Shimizu R, Matsuda J, et al. Effect of extradural compliance and resistance on spread of extradural analgesia. Br J Anaesth 1990;65:508–513.

18. Bromage PR. Exaggerated spread of epidural analgesia in arteriosclerotic patients. Dosage in relation to biological and chronological ageing. Br Med J 1962;2:1634–1638.

19. Guinard JP, Mulroy MF, Carpenter RL. Aging reduces the reliability of epidural epinephrine test doses. Reg Anesth 1995;20:193–198.

20. Mann C, Pouzeratte Y, Boccara G, et al. Comparison of intravenous or epidural patient-controlled analgesia in the elderly after major abdominal surgery. Anesthesiology 2000;92:433–441.

21. Scott JC, Stanski DR. Decreased fentanyl and alfentanil dose requirements with age. A simultaneous pharmacokinetic and pharmacodynamic evaluation. J Pharmacol Exp Ther 1987;240:159–166.

22. Jin F, Chung F. Minimizing perioperative adverse events in the elderly. Br J Anaesth 2001;87:608–624.

23. Pitkänen M, Haapaniemi L, Tuominen M, et al. Influence of age on spinal anaesthesia with isobaric 0.5% bupivacaine. Br J Anaesth 1984;56:279–284.

24. Veering BT, Burm AGL, Van Kleef JW, et al. Spinal anesthesia with glucose-free bupivacaine: effects of age on neural blockade and pharmacokinetics. Anesth Analg 1987;66:965–970.

25. Boss EG, Schuh FT. Der Einfluss des Lebensalters auf die Ausbreitung der Spinalanasthesie mit isobarem Mepivacain 2%. Anaesthesist 1993;42:162–168.

26. Veering BT, Burm AGL, Spierdijk J. Spinal anaesthesia with hyperbaric bupivacaine: effects of age on neural blockade and pharmacokinetics. Br J Anaesth 1988;60:187–194.

27. Racle JP, Benkhadra A, Poy JY, et al. Spinal analgesia with hyperbaric bupivacaine: influence of age. Br J Anaesth 1988;60:508–514.

28. Veering BT, Burm AGL, Vletter AA, et al. The effect of age on systemic absorption and systemic disposition of bupivacaine after subarachnoid administration. Anesthesiology 1991;74:250–257.

29. Racle JP, Benkhadra A, Poy JY, et al. Prolongation of isobaric bupivacaine spinal anesthesia with epinephrine and clonidine for hip surgery in the elderly. Anesth Analg 1987;66:442–446.

30. Racle JP, Benkhadra A, Poy JY, et al. Effects of increasing amounts of epinephrine during isobaric bupivacaine spinal anesthesia in elderly patients. Anesth Analg 1987;66:882–886.

31. Paqueron X, Boccara G, Bendahou M, et al. Brachial plexus nerve block exhibits prolonged duration in the elderly. Anesthesiology 2002;97:1245–1249.

32. Tucker GT. Pharmacokinetics of local anaesthetics. Br J Anaesth 1986;58:717–731.

33. Freund PR, Bowdle TA, Slattery JT, et al. Caudal anesthesia with lidocaine or bupivacaine: plasma local anaesthetic concentration and extent of sensory spread in old and young patients. Anesth Analg 1984;63:1017–1020.

34. Bowdle TA, Freund PR, Slattery JT. Age dependent lidocaine pharmacokinetics during lumbar peridural anesthesia with lidocaine hydrocarbonate or lidocaine hydrochloride. Reg Anesth 1986;11:123–127.

35. Finucane BT, Hammonds WD, Welch MB. Influence of age on vascular absorption of lidocaine from the epidural space. Anesth Analg 1987;66:843–846.

36. Burm AGL, Vermeulen NPE, Van Kleef JW, et al. Pharmacokinetics of lignocaine and bupivacaine in surgical patients following epidural administration. Simultaneous investigation of absorption and disposition kinetics using stable isotopes. Clin Pharmacokinet 1987;13:191–203.

37. Burm AGL, Van Kleef JW, Vermeulen NPE, et al. Pharmacokinetics of lidocaine and bupivacaine following subarachnoid administration in surgical patients: simultaneous investigation of absorption and disposition kinetics using stable isotopes. Anesthesiology 1988;69:584–592.

38. Emanuelsson BMK, Persson J, Alm C, et al. Systemic absorption and block after epidural injection of ropivacaine in healthy volunteers. Anesthesiology 1997;87:1309–1317.

39. Greenblatt DJ, Sellers EM, Shader RI. Drug disposition in old age. New Engl J Med 1982;306:1081–1108.

40. Nation RL, Triggs EJ, Selig M. Lignocaine kinetics in cardiac patients and aged subjects. Br J Clin Pharmacol 1977;4:439–448.

41. Cusson J, Nattel S, Matthews C, et al. Age-dependent lignocaine disposition in patients with acute myocardial infarction. Clin Pharmacol Ther 1985;37:381–386.

42. Cussack B, O'Malley K, Lavan J, et al. Protein binding and disposition of lignocaine in the elderly. Eur J Clin Pharmacol 1985;29:923–929.

43. Tucker GT, Boyes RN, Bridenbaugh PO, et al. Binding of anilide-type local anesthetics in human plasma. I. Relationships between binding, physicochemical properties and anesthetic activity. Anesthesiology 1970;33:287–303.

44. Davis D, Grossman SH, Kitchell BB, et al. The effects of age and smoking on the plasma binding of lignocaine and diazepam. Br J Clin Pharmacol 1985;19:261–265.

45. Veering BT, Burm AGL, Gladines MPRR, et al. Age does not influence the serum protein binding of bupivacaine. Br J Clin Pharmacol 1991;32:501–503.

46. Veering BT, Burm AGL, Souverijn JHM, et al. The effect of age on serum concentrations of albumin and α_1-acid glycoprotein. Br J Clin Pharmacol 1990;29:201–206.

47. Mather LE, Thomas J. Bupivacaine binding to plasma protein fractions. J Pharm Pharmacol 1978;30:653–654.

48. Tucker GT. Is plasma binding of local anesthetics important? Acta Anaesthesiol Belg 1988;39:147–150.

49. Tucker GT, Wiklund L, Berlin-Wahlen A, et al. Hepatic clearance of local anesthetics in man. J Pharmacokinet Biopharm 1977;5:11–22.

50. Wilkinson GR, Shand DG. A physiological approach to hepatic drug clearance. Clin Pharmacol Ther 1975;18:377–390.

51. Abernethy DR, Greenblatt DJ. Impairment of lidocaine clearance in elderly male subjects. J Cardiovasc Pharmacol 1983;5:1093–1096.

52. Wynne HA, Cope LH, Mutch E, et al. The effect of age upon liver volume and apparent liver blood flow in healthy man. Hepatology 1989;9:297–301.

53. Ross RA, Clarke JE, Armitage EN. Postoperative pain prevention by continuous epidural infusion. Anaesthesia 1980;35:663–668.

54. Veering BT, Burm AGL, Feyen MH, et al. Pharmacokinetics of bupivacaine during postoperative epidural infusion: enantioselectivity and role of protein binding. Anesthesiology 2002;96:1062–1069.

55. Aronson KF, Ekelund G, Kindmark CO, et al. Sequential changes of plasma proteins after surgical trauma. Scand J Clin Lab Invest 1972;29(Suppl 124):127–136.

56. Fukuda T, Kakiuchi Y, Masayuki M, et al. Free lidocaine concentrations during continuous epidural anesthesia in geriatric patients. Reg Anesth Pain Med 2003;28:215–220.

57. Gielen M. Post dural puncture headache (PDPH): a review. Reg Anesth 1989;14:101–106.

58. Veering BT, Cousins MJ. Cardiovascular and pulmonary effects of epidural anaesthesia. Anaesth Intensive Care 2000;28:620–635.

59. Tarkkila P, Isola J. A regression model for identifying patients at high risk of hypotension, bradycardia and nausea during spinal anesthesia. Acta Anaesthesiol Scand 1992;36:554–558.

60. Carpenter RL, Caplan RA, Brown DL, et al. Incidence and risk factors for side effects of spinal anesthesia. Anesthesiology 1992;76:906–912.

61. Juelsgaard P, Sand NP, Felsby S, et al. Perioperative myocardial ischaemia in patients undergoing surgery for fractured hip randomized to incremental spinal, single-dose spinal or general anaesthesia. Eur J Anaesthesiol 1998;15:656–663.

62. Racle JP, Poy JY, Haberer JP, et al. A comparison of cardiovascular responses of normotensive and hypertensive elderly patients following bupivacaine spinal anesthesia. Reg Anesth 1989;14:66–71.

63. Priebe HJ. The aged cardiovascular risk patient. Br J Anaesth 2000;85:763–778.

64. Rooke GA. Cardiovascular aging and anesthetic implications. J Cardiothorac Vasc Anesth 2003;17:512–523.

65. Korkuschko OW, Sarkisow KG, Schatilo WB, et al. Hemodynamic effects of stimulation of alpha 1-adrenoreceptors in healthy elderly and aged persons. Z Gerontol 1992;25:88–93.

66. Veith RC, Featherstone JA, Linares OA, et al. Age differences in plasma norepinephrine kinetics in humans. J Gerontol 1986;41:319–324.

67. Ebert TJ, Morgan BJ, Barney JA, et al. Effects of aging on baroreflex regulation of sympathetic activity in humans. Am J Physiol 1992;263:H789–803.

68. Rooke GA, Freund PR, Jacobsen AF. Hemodynamic response and change in organ blood volume during spinal anesthesia in elderly men with heart disease. Anesth Analg 1997;85:99–105.

69. Critchley LAH, Stuart JC, Short TG, et al. Haemodynamic effects of subarachnoid block in elderly patients. Br J Anaesth 1994;73:464–470.

70. Coe AJ, Revanas B. Is crystalloid preloading useful in spinal anaesthesia in the elderly? Anaesthesia 1990;45:241–243.

71. Buggy DJ, Power CK, Meeke R, et al. Prevention of spinal anaesthesia-induced hypotension in the elderly: i.m. methoxamine or combined hetastarch and crystalloid. Br J Anaesth 1998;80:199–203.

72. Critchley LAH. Hypotension, subarachnoid block and the elderly patient. Anaesthesia 1996;51:1139–1143.

73. Critchley LA, Short TG, Gin T. Hypotension during subarachnoid anaesthesia: haemodynamic analysis of three treatments. Br J Anaesth 1994;72:151–155.

74. Critchley LA, Conway F. Hypotension during subarachnoid anaesthesia: haemodynamic effects of colloid and metaraminol. Br J Anaesth 1996;76:734–736.

75. Chamberlain D, Chamberlain B. Changes in skin temperature of the trunk and their relationship to sympathetic block during spinal anesthesia. Anesthesiology 1986;65:139–143.

76. Ben-David B, Frankel R, Arzumonov T, et al. Minidose bupivacaine-fentanyl spinal anesthesia for surgical repair of hip fracture in the aged. Anesthesiology 2000;92:6–10.

77. Veering BT, Ter Riet PM, Burm AGL, et al. Spinal anaesthesia with 0.5% hyperbaric bupivacaine in elderly patients: effect of site of injection on spread of analgesia. Br J Anaesth 1996;77:343–346.

78. Veering BT, Immink-Speet TTM, Burm AGL, et al. Spinal anaesthesia with 0.5% hyperbaric bupivacaine in elderly patients: effects of duration spent in the sitting position. Br J Anaesth 2001;87:738–742.

79. Sumi M, Sakura S, Koshizaki M, et al. The advantages of the lateral decubitus position after spinal anesthesia with hyperbaric tetracaine. Anesth Analg 1998;87:879–884.

80. Favarel-Garrigues JF, Sztark F, Petitjan ME, et al. Hemodynamic effects of spinal anesthesia in the elderly: single dose versus titration through a catheter. Anesth Analg 1996;82:312–316.

81. Frank SM, Beattie C, Christopherson R, et al. Epidural versus general anesthesia, ambient operating room temperature, and patient age as predictors of inadvertent hypothermia. Anesthesiology 1992;77:252–257.

82. Wagner JA, Robinson S, Marinao RP. Age and temperature regulation of humans in neutral and cold environments. J Appl Physiol 1974;37:562–565.

83. Frank SM, El-Rahmany HK, Cattaneo CG, et al. Predictors of hypothermia during spinal anesthesia. Anesthesiology 2000;92:1330–1334.

84. Leslie K, Sessler DI. Reduction in the shivering threshold is proportional to spinal block height. Anesthesiology 1996;84:1327–1331.

85. Vassilieff N, Rosencher N, Sessler DI, et al. Shivering threshold during spinal anesthesia is reduced in elderly patients. Anesthesiology 1995;83:1162–1166.

86. Bell GD, Reeve PA, Moshiri M, et al. Intravenous midazolam for upper gastrointestinal endoscopy: a study of 800 consecutive cases relating dose to age and sex of patient. Br J Clin Pharmacol 1987;23:241–243.

87. Schnider TW, Minto CF, Shafer SL, et al. The influence of age on propofol pharmacodynamics. Anesthesiology 1999;90:1502–1516.

88. Shinozaki M, Usui Y, Yamaguchi S, et al. Recovery of psychomotor function after propofol sedation is prolonged in the elderly. Can J Anaesth 2002;49:927–931.

89. Wu CL, Hsu W, Richman JM, et al. Postoperative cognitive function as an outcome of regional anesthesia and analgesia. Reg Anesth Pain Med 2004;29:257–268.

90. Gustafson Y, Beggren D, Banstöm B, et al. Acute confusional states in elderly patients treated for femoral neck fracture. J Am Geriatr Soc 1988;36:525–530.

91. Williams-Russo P, Urquhart RN, Sharrock NE, et al. Postoperative delirium: predictors and prognosis in elderly orthopedic patients. J Am Geriatr Soc 1992;40:759–767.

92. Moller JT, Cluitmans P, Rasmussen LS, et al. Long-term postoperative cognitive dysfunction in the elderly. ISPOCD1 study. IOPOCD investigators. International Study of Post Operative Cognitive Dysfunction. Lancet 1998;351:857–861.

93. Canet J, Raeder J, Rasmussen LS, et al. Cognitive dysfunction after minor surgery in the elderly. Acta Anaesthesiol Scand 2003;47:1204–1210.

94. Liu S, Carpenter RL, Neal JM. Epidural anesthesia and analgesia. Their role in postoperative outcome. Anesthesiology 1995;82:1474–1506.

95. Kehlet H. Surgical stress: the role of pain and analgesia. Br J Anaesth 1989;63:189–195.

96. Kehlet H, Holte K. Effect of postoperative analgesia on surgical outcome. Br J Anaesth 2001;87:62–72.

97. Rosenfeld BA. Benefits of regional anaesthesia on thrombo-embolic complications following surgery. Reg Anesth 1996;21:S9–S12.

98. Donadoni R, Baele G, Devulder J, et al. Coagulation and fibrinolytic parameters in patients undergoing total hip replacement: influence of anaesthesia technique. Acta Anaesthesiol Scand 1989;33:588–592.

99. Rosenfeld BA, Beattie C, Christopherson R, et al. The Perioperative Ischaemia Randomized Anesthesia Trial Study Group: the effects of different anesthetic regimens on fibrinolysis and the development of postoperative arterial thrombosis. Anesthesiology 1993;79:435–443.

100. Wu CL, Caldwell MD. Effect of post-operative analgesia on patient morbidity. Best Pract Res Clin Anaesthesiol 2002;16:549–563.

101. Davis FM, McDermott E, Hickton C, et al. Influence of spinal and general anaesthesia on haemostasis during total hip arthroplasty. Br J Anaesth 1987;59:561–571.

102. Valentin N, Lomholt B, Jensen JS, et al. Spinal or general anaesthesia for surgery of the fractured hip? Br J Anaesth 1986;58:284–291.

103. Lundh R, Hedenstierna G, Johansson H. Ventilation-perfusion relationships during epidural analgesia. Acta Anaesthesiol Scand 1983;27:410–416.

104. McKenzie PJ, Wishart HY, Dewar KMS, et al. Comparison of the effects of spinal anaesthesia and general anaesthesia on postoperative oxygenation and perioperative mortality. Br J Anaesth 1980;52:49–55.

105. Catley D, Thornton C, Jordan C, et al. Pronounced, episodic oxygen desaturation in the postoperative period: its association with ventilatory pattern and analgesic regimen. Anesthesiology 1985;63:20–28.

106. Klassen GA, Bramwell RS, Bromage PR, et al. The effect of acute sympathectomy by epidural anesthesia on the canine coronary circulation. Anesthesiology 1980;52:8–15.

107. Davis RF, De Boer LWV, Maroko PR. Thoracic epidural anesthesia reduces myocardial infarct size after coronary artery occlusion in dogs. Anesth Analg 1986;65:711–717.

108. Blomberg S, Curelaru J, Emanuelsson H, et al. Thoracic epidural anaesthesia in patients with unstable angina pectoris. Eur Heart J 1989;10:437–444.

109. Blomberg S, Emanuelsson H, Kvirst H, et al. Effects of thoracic epidural anesthesia on coronary arteries and arterioles in patients with coronary artery disease. Anesthesiology 1990;73:840–847.

110. Blomberg S, Emanuelsson H, Ricksten SE. Thoracic epidural anesthesia and central hemodynamics in patients with unstable angina pectoris. Anesth Analg 1989;69:558–562.

111. Kock M, Blomberg S, Emanuelsson H, et al. Thoracic epidural anesthesia improves global and regional left ventricular function during stress-induced myocardial ischemia in patients with coronary artery disease. Anesth Analg 1990;71:625–630.

112. Meissner A, Rolf N, Van Aken H. Thoracic epidural anesthesia and the patient with heart disease: benefits, risks and controversies. Anesth Analg 1997;85:517–528.

113. Ford G, Whitelaw W, Rosenal T, et al. Diaphragm function after upper abdominal surgery in humans. Am Rev Respir Dis 1987;127:431–436.

114. Pansard JL, Mankikian B, Bertrand M, et al. Effects of thoracic extradural block on diaphragmatic electrical activity and contractility after upper abdominal surgery. Anesthesiology 1993;78:63–71.

115. Polaner DM, Kimball WR, Fratacci M, et al. Thoracic epidural anesthesia increases diaphragmatic shortening after thoracotomy in the awake lamb. Anesthesiology 1993;79:808–816.

116. Steinbrook RA. Epidural anesthesia and gastrointestinal motility. Anesth Analg 1998;86:837–844.

117. Lehman JF, Wiseman JS. The effect of epidural analgesia on the return of peristalsis and the length of stay after elective colonic surgery. Am Surg 1995;61:1009–1012.

118. Adolphs J, Schmidt DK, Mousa SA, et al. Thoracic epidural anesthesia attenuates hemorrhage-induced impairment of intestinal perfusion in rats. Anesthesiology 2003;99:685–692.

119. O'Hara DA, Duff A, Berlin JA, et al. The effect of anesthetic technique on postoperative outcomes of hip fracture repair. Anesthesiology 2000;92:947–957.

120. Sutcliffe AJ. Mortality after spinal and general anaesthesia for surgical fixation of hip fractures. Anaesthesia 1994;49:237–240.

121. Pedersen T, Moller A, Cracknell J. The mission of the Cochrane Anesthesia Review Group: preparing and disseminating systematic reviews of the effect of health care in anesthesiology. Anesth Analg 2002;95:1012–1018.

122. Urwin SC, Parker MJ, Griffiths R. General versus regional anaesthesia for hip-fracture surgery: meta-analysis of randomized trials. Br J Anaesth 2000;84:450–455.

123. Gilbert TB, Hawkes WG, Hebel JR, et al. Spinal anesthesia versus general anesthesia for hip fracture repair: a longitudinal observation of 741 elderly patients during 2-year follow-up. Am J Orthop 2000;29:25–35.

124. Bode RH, Lewis PL, Zarich SW, et al. Cardiac outcome after peripheral vascular surgery. Comparison of general and regional anesthesia. Anesthesiology 1996;84:3–13.

125. Tuman KJ, McCarthy RJ, Marck RJ, et al. Effects of epidural anesthesia and analgesia on coagulation and outcome after major vascular surgery. Anesth Analg 1991;73:696–704.

126. Christopherson R, Beattie C, Meinert CL, et al. Perioperative Ischemia Randomized Anesthesia Trial Study Group. Perioperative morbidity in patients randomized to epidural or general anesthesia for lower extremity vascular surgery. Anesthesiology 1993;79:422–434.

127. Park WY, Thompson JS, Lee KK. Effect on epidural anesthesia and analgesia on perioperative outcome. A randomized, controlled veterans affairs cooperative study. Ann Surg 2001;234(4):560–571.

128. Beattie SW, Badner NH, Choi P. Epidural analgesia reduces postoperative myocardial infarction: a metaanalysis. Anesth Analg 2001;93:853–858.

129. Matot I, Oppenheim-Eden A, Ratrot R, et al. Preoperative cardiac events in elderly patients with hip fracture randomized to epidural or conventional analgesia. Anesthesiology 2003;98:156–163.

130. Modig J, Borg T, Karlström G, et al. Thromboembolism after total hip replacement: role of epidural and general anesthesia. Anesth Analg 1983;62:174–180.

131. Modig J, Borg T, Bagge L, et al. Role of extradural and of general anaesthesia in fibrinolysis and coagulation after total hip replacement. Br J Anaesth 1983;55:625–629.

132. Modig J, Borg T, Karlström G, et al. Effect of epidural versus general anaesthesia on calf blood flow. Acta Anaesthesiol Scand 1980;24:305–309.

133. Borg T, Modig J. Potential anti-thrombotic effects of local anaesthetics due to their inhibition of platelet aggregation. Acta Anaesthesiol Scand 1985;29:739–742.

134. de Leon-Casasola OA, Parker BM, et al. Epidural analgesia versus intravenous patient-controlled analgesia: differences in the postoperative course of cancer patients. Reg Anesth 1994;19:307–315.

135. Ballantyne JC, Carr DB, deFerranti S, et al. The comparative effects of postoperative analgesic therapies on pulmonary outcome: cumulative meta-analyses of randomized, controlled trials. Anesth Analg 1998;86:598–612.

136. Smith J, Kelly K. Pathophysiology of postoperative ileus. Arch Surg 1977;112:203–209.

137. Holte K, Kehlet H. Postoperative ileus—a preventable event? Br J Surg 2000;87:1480–1493.

138. Kehlet H, Holte K. Review of postoperative ileus. Am J Surg 2001;182:3S–10S.

139. Lui SS, Carpenter RL, Mackey DC, et al. Effects of perioperative analgesic technique on rate of recovery after colon surgery. Anesthesiology 1995;83:757–765.

20
Fluid Management

Jessica Miller, Lee A. Fleisher, and Jeffrey L. Carson

It is imperative that anesthesiologists are well versed in modifications to fluid management for the elderly patient.[1] This chapter discusses the guiding principles in fluid management and the important alterations in kidney function and fluid homeostasis in the elderly patient. These concepts are built upon to provide recommendations for the perioperative period. Preoperative evaluation, assessment, and decision making in the intraoperative period are discussed below, including methods of monitoring intraoperatively, types of fluids to administer, and the use of blood transfusions. Special anesthetic challenges such as spinal anesthesia and fluid management are also included.

Fluid and Electrolyte Homeostasis

Understanding changes in fluid and electrolyte balance requires examining the major determinants of fluid regulation. Total body water decreases with age from 60%–65% in a young man to 50% by age 80.[2] Total body water is distributed as 67% extracellular fluid volume and 33% intracellular fluid volume. The cell wall separates extracellular fluid from intracellular fluid. Extracellular fluid volume is further divided into 75% interstitial fluid and 25% plasma. The cells making up the walls of arteries and veins and the capillary endothelium separate the extracellular compartment into interstitial and intravascular fluid. Water moves freely through cell walls and vessels. Ions such as sodium can pass freely across capillary endothelium, but sodium pumps driven by adenosine 5′-triphosphate maintain a concentration gradient across cells. Larger molecules such as albumin and colloids are unable to move across intact capillary endothelium, thus creating a colloid oncotic pressure. Movement of fluids between the extracellular and intracellular compartment is governed by the Starling equilibrium. Starling forces are composed of hydrostatic pressure, colloid oncotic pressure, and specific permeability coefficients:

$$J = K[Pc - Pt - r(C - T)]$$

where J = filtration rate out of capillary, K = filtration coefficient, Pc = capillary pressure, Pt = tissue fluid pressure, C = plasma colloid oncotic pressure, T = tissue colloid oncotic pressure, r = reflection coefficient.

Hydrostatic pressure in the capillaries drives movement of fluid from the capillary to the interstitial space. Elevated colloid oncotic pressure in intravascular fluid opposes hydrostatic pressure to maintain intravascular volume and a relatively dry interstitial compartment.

During surgery, capillary membrane permeability increases at the surgical site. Proteins move down their concentration gradient into the interstitial fluid, thus decreasing colloid oncotic pressure in the intravascular space. Administration of fluid in the perioperative period also decreases colloid oncotic pressure due to hemodilution.

Perioperative fluid distribution can be understood with the Starling equilibrium; however, alterations in endocrine and inflammatory mediators also affect fluid homeostasis. Surgical trauma results in an increased activity of antidiuretic hormone (ADH), aldosterone, and the renin-angiotensin system. Increased ADH secretion enhances water reabsorption in the kidney resulting in lowered plasma sodium concentration and a decrease in diuresis. Increased aldosterone and renin release results in sodium conservation and potassium excretion (Figure 20-1).[3] Further aspects of the stress response lead to increased cortisol secretion. Cortisol may be beneficial in counteracting inflammatory mediators and helping to maintain capillary integrity. Inflammatory mediators such as interleukin-6, tumor necrosis factor, substance P, and bradykinin may act as vasodilators and cause further increases in capillary permeability.[4]

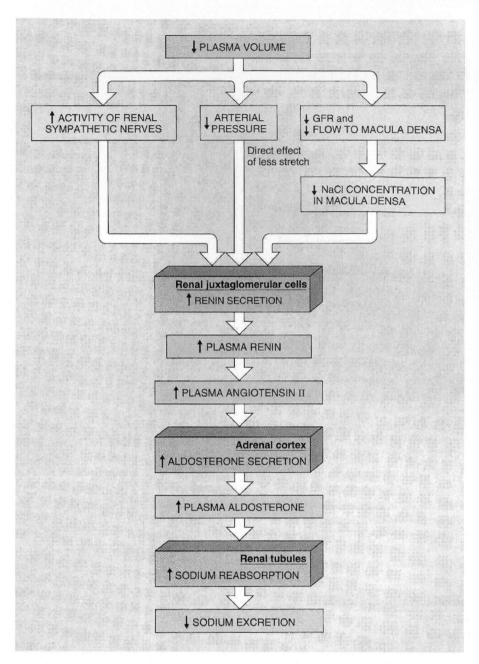

FIGURE 20-1. Pathways by which decreased plasma volume leads, via the renin-angiotensin system and aldosterone, to increased sodium reabsorption and hence decreased sodium excretion.

GFR = glomerular filtration rate. (Reprinted from Vander et al.[3] with permission of The McGraw-Hill Companies.)

These concepts can be applied to perioperative management of the elderly patient by understanding the evolution of these mechanisms with age. As mentioned, total body water decreases in the elderly to approximately 50% of body weight by the age of 80 years. Muscle mass is decreased by as much as 30% in the 80-year-old patient. The effect of a deceased total body water and decreased lean body mass results in a larger volume of distribution. Elderly patients have subtle alterations in the dynamic renal, endocrine, and hormonal elements that work to maintain homeostatic balance. These will be discussed in more detail below. These alterations in fluid homeostasis are magnified by the decrease in arterial distensibility, decreased baroceptor reflexes, and more sluggish homeostatic response to result in larger alterations in hemodynamic stability.[5]

Aging and Renal Function

An understanding of changes in renal sodium and water excretion is central to understanding fluid and electrolyte balance. The aged kidney is able to maintain stable volume and electrolyte status. Age has been shown to have no effect on basal plasma sodium and potassium concentrations, or maintenance of normal extracellular fluid volume. However, the aged kidney has less functional reserve and is slower to adapt to acute changes.

Changes in structure and function of the kidney with age affect fluid management, electrolyte homeostasis, drug metabolism, and pharmacokinetics. These changes have been well described; however, the methods of assessment of kidney function in aging individuals have received more attention recently. Early analysis of aging kidney function utilized cross-sectional studies. Attempts were made to exclude patients with overt renal disease; however, limitations in testing inevitably overlook subclinical renal disease. Comparison studies between active young individuals were frequently matched with institutionalized elderly individuals, thus not representing the segments of the elderly population that are residing and functioning in the community.[6,7] More recent studies have used longitudinal comparison of kidney function in carefully selected patients who lacked renal diseases, specifically patients who were deemed suitable for kidney donation.[8–10] Predictably, these studies showed less marked changes in kidney function than previous studies. The availability of this more accurate representation of changing kidney function is beneficial to overall understanding of clinical management; however, the frequent presence of comorbid diseases that affect kidney function cannot be overlooked in applying these principles to individual patient management.

Alterations in the kidney associated with aging include both structural and functional changes. Studies have indicated total and cortical renal mass decreases with age. Between the ages of 30 and 85 years, renal mass decreases by 20%–25%.[2] The decline in renal mass is relatively sparing of the medulla, with most loss occurring in the cortical area. The number of functioning glomeruli decreases proportionally with change in mass; however, the size of each remaining glomeruli increases. Global sclerosis of the glomeruli increases the proportion of sclerotic glomeruli from 5% in middle age to 10%–30% by the eighth decade. The length of the proximal convoluted tubule decreases in size with age, thus matching the decline in glomerular and tubular function seen in aging.[6]

Multiple studies have demonstrated that renal blood flow decreases with age.[11–13] Renal blood flow begins to decline after the fourth decade of life by approximately 10% per decade.[14] Further studies also showed a decrease in mean blood flow per unit mass with advancing age. When correlated with changes in flow rates, it has been deduced that the largest decreases in renal perfusion occur in the cortex, with relative sparing of flow to the deeper regions of the kidney. As flow decreases from the cortex, the juxtaglomedullary glomeruli receive more perfusion. Their preexisting increased filtration fraction compared with the cortex glomeruli may explain the increase in filtration fraction with aging.[6]

Glomerular filtration rate (GFR) is the predominant measure of renal function. Initial studies assessing nursing home residents resoundingly found that GFR decreased with age. GFR can be estimated to decrease approximately 1 mL/min/y.[15] Assessment of GFR in the elderly has been repeated using community-dwelling elderly in both cross-sectional and longitudinal studies. These studies also found a general decline in GFR, but also revealed more variations in GFR. Up to 30% of the elderly subjects had a stable GFR over a 20-year longitudinal study, suggesting that declining GFR is not inevitable.[11,15] Only explicit measurement of creatinine clearance could identify these patients, thus it should not be assumed the elderly patient has a decreased GFR.

Serum creatinine is relatively constant with age, reflecting the decrease in muscle mass with age that parallels the decrease in GFR. In clinical practice, a method of estimating GFR from creatinine clearance is helpful. The most frequently used formula is the Crockroft-Gault equation[16]:

$$\text{Creatinine clearance} = [K\,(140 - \text{age})\,(\text{weight in kg})]/[(72)\,(\text{serum creatinine concentration})]$$

$$K = 1.23 \text{ for men, } 1.03 \text{ for women,}$$
$$\text{creatinine clearance in } \mu\text{mol/min.}$$

The development of this formula may have been skewed by the use of validation on a small number of subjects, subjects of only one gender, and institutionalized individuals. A recent reevaluation of the accuracy of the Crockroft-Gault equation in comparison to a measured 24-hour creatinine clearance showed only a moderate correlation in the equation's estimates with the measured clearance in the elderly subgroup.[17,18] A more comprehensive study comparing the validity of several methods of estimating GFR found most equations underestimated creatinine clearance. In general, it is recommended that if an accurate measure of GFR is required, a 24-hour creatinine clearance should be measured. There is no one estimation method that accurately predicts GFR. For purposes needing less accuracy, the Crockroft-Gault equation is a reasonable guide. Clinical drug dosing in the elderly should maintain careful consideration of drugs cleared mainly by renal mechanisms.

Sodium Handling

Less is known about the ability of the aged kidney to process sodium (Tables 20-1 and 20-2). Studies have concluded that age significantly decreases the kidney's ability to conserve sodium. The aged kidney takes a longer period of time to reduce urinary excretion of sodium in response to a low-sodium diet when compared with a young person's kidney.[8] The decrease in renal blood flow and GFR does not explain this sluggish response. Other elements of the sodium conservation axis, such as the renin aldosterone system and atrial natriuretic peptide may be responsible. Several studies have shown that the renin aldosterone response to acute stimuli is slower with advancing age.[14,19,20]

The aged kidney seems to have impaired sodium excretion mechanisms. Mechanisms responsible for reduced sodium excretion may include a decrease in pressure-sensitive natriuresis, which may lead to salt-sensitive hypertension. An altered response to angiotensin II has also been investigated. The administration of sodium-rich fluids, dietary indiscretion, and radiocontrast dye must be considered with forethought into the possible negative effects of the resultant volume load.

The aged kidney's ability to alter its response to total body sodium is especially critical in the elderly. Older patients are more likely to experience confusion and loss of thirst sensation in periods of acute illness, which further aggravates the body's sluggish response to altered plasma sodium. Other studies have suggested that sodium losses have magnified effects on hemodynamic stability. A study by Shannon et al.[21] showed that a diuresis of 2 kg resulted in a 24 mm Hg decrease in systolic blood pressure upon changing from the supine to a standing position, a much larger effect than seen in younger patients.

Investigations into other aspects of fluid homeostasis have also been conducted. Studies have concluded that substantial declines in plasma renin activity occur with aging.[20] Plasma renin is decreased in the resting state, and ranges from a 40% to 60% decrease in stimulated conditions. Significant and consistent declines in plasma renin are found after the sixth decade. The effect of renin on angiotensin II release is technically difficult to study. Aldosterone is also depleted in elderly patients in the stimulated and basal states.[19] Atrial natriuretic peptide has shown to be increased in elderly patients with possible decreased end-organ responsiveness; at this time its full effect is not understood.

Renal diluting capacity is also shown to be affected by aging. A mild defect in renal diluting capacity occurs with age, which seems to be related to the decline in GFR. This puts the elderly patient at increased risk for dilutional hyponatremia in settings of stress, such as surgery, fever,

TABLE 20-1. Symptoms of hyponatremia.

Malaise
Nausea
Headache
Lethargy
Confusion
Obtundation
Stupor
Seizures
Coma

TABLE 20-2. Symptoms of hypernatremia.

Polyuria
Thirst
Altered mental status
Weakness
Neuromuscular irritability
Focal neurologic deficits
Seizures
Coma

or acute illness. Studies have found the decrease in plasma sodium level to be approximately 1 mEq/L per decade from a mean of 141 mEq/L in youth.[22] Hyponatremia in the inpatient is frequently iatrogenic, because of either fluid therapy or medications. Possibilities for medications—such as antidepressants, carbamazepine, clofibrate, and neuroleptics—to increase the secretion of ADH or enhancing the action of ADH at the tubule must also be considered. Hyponatremia is not a benign diagnosis because some studies have shown a twofold increase in mortality over age-matched control subjects.[2,22]

Hypernatremia developing in hospitalized elderly patients is most often attributable to surgery or febrile illness. Hypernatremia also has implications for mortality with a sevenfold increase in mortality compared with age-matched controls.[23]

Potassium Management

Maintaining proper kidney function is crucial to potassium homeostasis, because the kidney is the primary organ for potassium excretion. Elderly patients are more susceptible to hyperkalemia, given the decrease in aldosterone and reduction in GFR. Undergoing surgery, tissue breakdown, or trauma also increases the risk of hyperkalemia especially if acute renal failure is present. Elderly patients are at increased risk of gastrointestinal bleeding, causing increased potassium levels as a result of red blood cell breakdown. Comorbid conditions may be present that affect flow to distal tubular sites, thus decreasing the amount of sodium available to enable potassium secretion. Examples of tubular flow-reducing diseases include hypovolemia, postsurgical or gastrointestinal losses, and congestive heart failure.[24]

Other risk factors present in elderly patients that may contribute to the risk of hyperkalemia include use of medications that increase potassium. Many elderly patients are prescribed diuretics, which may include the potassium-sparing diuretics spironolactone, triamterene, and amiloride. Prescription of thiazide diuretics may prompt the physician to include potassium supplementation as well. Patients may also be managing hypertension with salt-lowering diets, which are frequently high in potassium salts. Angiotensin-converting enzyme inhibitors may cause hyperkalemia, because of reductions in aldosterone. Similarly, nonsteroidal antiinflammatory drugs can also result in a hyporeninemic hypoaldosterone state. Beta-blockers inhibit renin release in the kidney to cause hyperkalemia. Heparin blocks aldosterone synthesis in the adrenal gland, which may rarely cause elevated potassium. Trimethoprim-sulfamethazine acts similar to amiloride and inhibits the sodium channel in the apical membrane of the late distal tubule and collecting duct. This leads to a reduction of sodium and hydrogen transport into the urine.[24]

Regulation of Urinary Concentration

Closely related to the kidney's ability to process sodium is the kidney's ability to alter the concentration of the urine produced. A well-designed study by Rowe et al.[25] demonstrated that elderly patients were less able to significantly alter urine flow or urine osmolarity after 12 hours of dehydration. This study also detailed that the differences were not attributable to differences in solute intake or correlated to a decreased GFR in the elderly. Other contributing factors may include a decrease in the efficacy of the countercurrent exchange system resulting from a relative increase in the medullary blood flow, or a possible defect in solute transport from the tubule to the medulla. The role of vasopressin has been investigated more recently.[26,27] These studies have shown that the osmoreceptor sensitivity is increased with increasing age to result in a great amount of vasopressin released per increase in osmolarity. This would seem to be compensatory for the reduced ability of the kidney to concentrate urine. However, the osmoreceptor does not seem to have increased sensitivity to changes in volume and pressure, such as those induced with orthostatic changes. More recent studies have produced conflicting results and failed to find a difference in overall ability to excrete a water load.[28-30]

Another aspect of water handling is thirst. A study by Phillips et al.[31] found that the elderly had less sensation of thirst and exhibited less water intake after a 24-hour period of dehydration compared with younger individuals, despite increases in plasma osmolarity and greater decreases in body mass. This defect is attributed to a defect in an opioid-mediated thirst center in the central nervous system.

These altered physiologic responses are insignificant in maintaining daily homeostasis, but become increasingly important when access to free water is controlled. Treatment of electrolyte abnormalities is similar, regardless of age, but balancing comorbid conditions may complicate management. For instance, it has been shown that patients with Alzheimer's disease have a decreased ADH sensitivity. Patients treated with thiazide diuretics have impaired ability to increase free water clearance during water diuresis. It is worth noting that elderly persons may have a lag in return to normal mentation after severe electrolyte abnormalities, despite clinical normalization of lab indicators.

Acid-Base Abnormalities

Acid-base balance is well maintained in the elderly patient under normal conditions. However, acute illness often results in acidosis that may become exaggerated in the elderly. The aged kidney has a decrease in ammonia generation which acts to buffer about half of the acid excreted in the kidney. This increases the frequency of severe metabolic acidosis. Coexisting pulmonary disease may also limit the ability to excrete carbon dioxide.

Calcium, Phosphate, Magnesium

Studies have shown that, at any given plasma level of calcium, concentration of parathormone is increased. Poor dietary intake, medications, and coexisting disease may result in calcium, magnesium, and phosphorus deficiencies. The existence of renal disease and impaired ability to excrete electrolytes must be considered when initiating therapy.

Nutrition

Perioperative nutrition affects fluid and electrolyte management in the elderly patient. It is also well known that a malnourished patient has a much higher likelihood for postoperative morbidity and mortality, also increasing the chance that the anesthesiologist will be further involved in their postoperative critical care management. Nutrition strongly affects surgical recovery by delaying wound healing, increasing risk of anastomotic breakdown, infection, and even possible development of multi–organ system failure. Hypoalbuminemia affects plasma oncotic pressure, thus altering the distribution of intravascular fluids. Electrolyte abnormalities are common in the malnourished patient.

Debate exists about how best to identify and correct malnutrition. In theory, elective intervention can be preceded by preoperative supplemental nutrition. Parenteral nutrition carries the risk of infection, whereas enteral nutrition has the risk of aspiration pneumonia and invasive surgical placement. In a thorough meta-analysis of studies addressing preoperative parenteral nutrition, only severely malnourished patients demonstrated fewer noninfectious complications. Benefit was demonstrated if preoperative parenteral nutrition was provided for 7 days or more.[32]

Preoperative enteral nutrition studies demonstrate reduced postoperative mortality and decreased incidence of wound infections.[33–36] Difficulties encountered in implementing these therapies include the need to place nasogastric tubes or feeding tubes. Oral supplementation is less predictable in increasing calorie intake because of poor appetite, taste barriers, and limitations because of cost.

Postoperative nutrition is more practical because many surgeries cannot be delayed. Studies have shown a significant increase in morbidity and mortality if a patient receives only hypocaloric feeding for more than 14 days.[37] However, postoperative parenteral nutrition has been shown to increase morbidity in some studies mainly because of septic complications. Postoperative enteral nutrition supplementation has been shown to have very positive effects. Two studies of hip fracture repair in elderly women showed reduced length of hospital stay, shortened time to weight bearing, and more rapid return to independent mobility with the use of enteral supplementation.[38,39]

Clinical Implications

The renal response to surgery and anesthesia does not seem to significantly alter with age. GFR is known to be directly depressed by general anesthesia; however, this is not usually clinically significant. Decreases in cardiac output and blood pressure, frequently attributable to intravascular losses and hypothermia in surgery, will decrease renal blood flow. Appropriately assessing and maintaining intravascular volume has the most impact on renal function in the perioperative period. Recognition and treatment of hypovolemia has the potential to reduce incidence of organ dysfunction, postoperative morbidity, and death. The elderly patient is at much higher risk of developing acute renal failure because of the lack of functional reserve of the kidney. Incidence of developing postoperative renal failure can range from 0.1% to 50% after high-risk surgeries such as trauma, thoracic, or cardiovascular interventions, depending on the site of surgery. Acute tubular necrosis is the most common cause of acute perioperative renal failure (Table 20-3).

Mortality in patients with acute renal failure can be greater than 50%, and at least one fifth of all perioperative deaths in elderly surgical patients are attributable to acute renal failure. Patients with perioperative renal failure account for up to 50% of the patients needing acute dialysis.[40] Acute renal failure in the elderly increases morbidity and mortality, and also burdens the health care system with additional costs. Avoidance of complications resulting from inappropriate fluid management involves intervention at all stages of perioperative medicine.

TABLE 20-3. Risk factors of acute tubular necrosis.

Ischemic acute tubular necrosis
  Major surgery
  Trauma
  Severe hypovolemia
  Sepsis
  Extensive burns
Toxic acute tubular necrosis
  Exogenous: radiocontrast, cyclosporine, antibiotics (aminoglycosides), chemotherapy (cisplatin), organic solvents (ethylene glycol), acetaminophen, illegal abortifacients.
  Endogenous: rhabdomyolysis, hemolysis, uric acid, oxalate, plasma cell dyscrasia (myeloma)

Preoperative Evaluation

There are several clinical conditions that merit additional attention to fluid balance. Preexisting azotemia prompts the clinician to look for correctable conditions before the perioperative period. Classification of renal dysfunction perioperatively is frequently delineated as prerenal, intrarenal, and postrenal. Chronic disorders such as enterocutaneous fistulas and chronic diarrhea can produce fluid and electrolyte depletion. Patients with chronic fluid imbalances may not have the typical signs and symptoms such as postural hypotension and tachycardia, making them more difficult to diagnose. Other important risk factors for elderly patients to develop hypovolemia include female sex, age older than 85 years, diagnosis of more than four chronic medical conditions, taking more than four medications, and being confined to bed[39] (Table 20-4).

Physical examination remains important in diagnosing volume status. The most reliable clinical signs of hypovolemia are postural pulse increment and postural hypotension. A postural pulse increment of 30 beats/min or more has a specificity of 96%.[41] Postural hypotension is defined as a decrease in systolic blood pressure of more than 20mmHg after rising from supine to standing position. With age, the increment in pulse can be less than 30 in a hypovolemic individual; however, there is no absolute cutoff level to indicate hypovolemia. Postural hypotension can also be found in 11%–30% of normovolemic patients older than 65 years. Mild postural dizziness is not definitive for hypovolemia; however, inability to stand for vital signs because of severe dizziness is a reliable predictor of hypovolemia. Skin turgor is less sensitive in elderly patients because of a reduction in skin elastin with age. Decreased axillary sweating can indicate hypovolemia. Invasive measurements of filling pressure and cardiac output may also be useful, but must be balanced with the inherent risk of invasive monitoring.

Intraoperative Management

Intrinsic renal failure is common perioperatively with the use of aminoglycosides, contrast dyes, and postoperative

TABLE 20-4. Adjusted odds ratios and 95% confidence intervals for significant risk factors among severe cases of dehydration.

	Age (years)* >85/<85		Sex* Male/female	Mobility* Assistance/bedridden	
				Strata	
Age	—		9.9 (4.5–21.2)†	28.8† (9.2–93.8)	11.5† (2.9–45.2)
Female sex	38.1 (14.2–84.8)‡		—	22.6 (7.5–68.1)‡	
>4 chronic diseases	42.4 (16.8–106.4)‡		53.6 (21.1–140.2)‡	22.3† (7.2–67.6)	8.4† (3.8–18.6)
>4 medications	30.7 (12.7–74.0)‡		26.1 (11.3–61.6)‡	65.0 (10.3–410.1)‡	
Mobility:					
Assistance	11.5† (2.9–45.2)	36.0† (7.4–174.7)	22.6 (7.5–68.1)‡	—	
Bedridden	1.3 (3.9–17.9)‡		7.6 (3.6–16.1)‡	—	
Feeding status:					
Assistance	30.0 (11.9–74.3)‡		28.8 (11.5–71.6)‡	19.0† (3–122.0)	10.0† (2.7–37)
Tube	79.00† (10.4–601.6)	17.01† (5.4–52.9)	24.8 (9.3–67.1)‡	—	
Skilled care level	4.2 (1.9–9.8)‡		4.3 (1.9–9.4)‡	45.0† (6.5–310.9)	3.0† (1.3–7.2)
Winter	14.8 (6.4–34.9)‡		12.8 (5.5–28.8)‡	25.8† (8.3–74.4)	5.9† (2.7–13.3)

*Pooled where appropriate using χ^2 heterogeneity test. All are statistically significant at $p = 0.05$. Confidence intervals calculated using test-based interval estimation.
†Not pooled based on heterogeneity score.
‡Pooled, significant with 95% confidence intervals.
Source: Reprinted with permission from Lavizzo-Mourey et al.[39] Published by Blackwell Publishers Ltd.

effects of cardiac bypass. Certain surgeries have increased risk of postoperative renal failure, such as cardiac or aortic surgery, as well as any surgery involving large fluid shifts, trauma patients, or the biliary tract. The risk of postoperative renal dysfunction in open abdominal aortic aneurysm repair is increased in emergency surgery and in incidences of increased length of cross-clamp duration and sustained hypotension. Dislodgement of atheromatous emboli may also occur in aortic repair. The mechanism of renal dysfunction after biliary tract surgery is unknown, but associated risk factors include postoperative sepsis, prior renal insufficiency, and height of preoperative bilirubin concentration. Preventing muscle compression and breakdown must also be considered in lengthy surgeries to decrease myoglobinuria. Postrenal azotemia should also be suspected, because elderly patients may have prostatic hypertrophy or nephrolithiasis.[24,42]

Several papers have addressed the best methods for determining the need for fluid administration in perioperative patients. These studies link fluid balance with its effect on hemodynamic stability. The Starling curve describes the effect of volume loading on myocardial performance. Starling curves (Figure 20-2) illustrate the relationship between preload and cardiac output. Administration of a volume of fluid can increase preload and thus increase cardiac output. Beyond a certain amount of fluid administration, further increases in end-diastolic

volume can decrease ventricular function and cardiac output.

From a physiologic standpoint, fluid management can be guided by physical signs and symptoms of hemodynamic stability, or more quantitative methods such as information from esophageal Doppler monitors, central venous catheters, or pulmonary artery catheters. The standard measures of volume status in the anesthetized patient are blood pressure, heart rate, oxygen saturation,

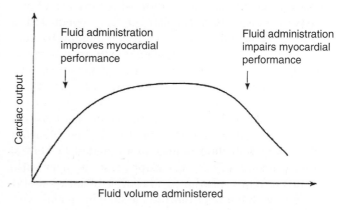

FIGURE 20-2. Effects of perioperative fluid therapy on the Starling myocardial performance curve. (Reprinted from Holte et al.[3] Copyright © The Board of Management and Trustees of the *British Journal of Anaesthesia.* Reproduced by permission of Oxford University Press/*British Journal of Anaesthesia.*)

and urine output. Interpretation of blood pressure and heart rate is frequently altered by many different variables in the perioperative patient, including sympathetic responses to surgical stimulus, anxiety and pain responses, and side effects of medications and anesthetic agents. Urine output is unreliable as well. Because of the depressive effects of general anesthesia, the common goal of 0.5 mL/kg/h of urine production is typically attained only with a fluid load. Meanwhile, studies have demonstrated that a low intraoperative urinary output did not correlate with development of renal failure, as long as hypovolemia was avoided.[43] Furthermore, excretion of a fluid excess of 1.5–2 L can take up to 2 days in healthy volunteers, which is an approximate indicator of the increased workload on the kidney with excessive fluid administration.[3]

A 2002 study[44] focused on the use of esophageal Doppler monitoring to guide fluid administration during the intraoperative period for moderate-risk surgical patients. The authors hypothesized that appropriate fluid resuscitation may decrease the extent of postoperative gastrointestinal dysfunction, reduce time to ability to tolerate oral intake, and ultimately reduce length of hospital stay. This prospective, single-blinded study compared fluid administration guided by esophageal Doppler, to administration guided by standard cardiovascular variables (blood pressure, heart rate, oxygen saturation), with significantly more hetastarch in the protocol group (847 ± 373 mL) compared with the control group (282 ± 470 mL). The study demonstrated a reduction in hospital stay in the Doppler-guided protocol group.

Several studies of perioperative fluid optimization targeted repair of proximal femoral fractures. This is a common procedure for elderly and frail patients, typically straightforward surgically, with outcome determined by medical comorbidities. Avoidance of hypovolemia is important; however, fluid overload is also of particular concern in this patient population with cardiac and pulmonary comorbidities. Sinclair et al.[45] conducted a randomized controlled trial of proximal femoral fracture repairs with fluid administration guided by an esophageal Doppler monitor that demonstrated reduction of hospital stay. Because of the data obtained from Doppler monitoring, the intervention group received a larger volume of colloid, with approximately equal amounts of crystalloid received in both groups. Venn et al.[46] concluded a similar study with fluid management guided by central venous pressure (CVP) or esophageal Doppler, also demonstrating a reduction in duration of hospital stay in patients with fluid optimization guided by quantitative strategies. The drawback of both of these studies is the small number of participants, only 130 total, which is inadequate to detect changes in early mortality or to detect particular subgroups that might especially benefit from guided fluid administration.[47]

The studies above describe guided fluid administration via goals for stroke volume or CVP, and assessment of changes in these variables in response to additional fluid boluses. Additional studies focused on using quantitative data to produce supranormal physiologic parameters and assess the effects on outcomes. Shoemaker et al.[48] in 1988 observed that survivors of high-risk surgery had increased hemodynamic and oxygen transport variables. They conducted a prospective randomized trial to determine if optimization of hemodynamic and oxygen transport variables to supranormal values would affect outcome. This study demonstrated that optimization to supranormal values with the use of pulmonary artery catheter data reduced complications, duration of hospitalization, decreased time in the intensive care unit (ICU), decreased duration of mechanical ventilation, and reduced hospital cost. The authors caution that use of supranormal physiologic parameters may be inappropriate for the elderly patient because of a possible limited capacity for physiologic compensation. Scalea et al.[49] showed an improvement in survival rate in patients older than 65 years when early hemodynamic monitoring was instituted within 2.2 hours from sustaining diffuse blunt trauma, and using this information to augment cardiac output. Although these approaches may be appropriate in younger patients with sepsis, they may lead to increased morbidity and mortality in the presence of multiple comorbidities. Therefore, more studies are needed in the elderly before such an approach is routinely adopted.

Discussion about the appropriate fluid to use in volume resuscitation continues for all perioperative patients. Use of crystalloid is supported by many practitioners for its economy. They cite colloid use as having potential alterations in coagulation factors and risk of adverse drug reactions. Colloid supporters cite the benefit of using a smaller amount of fluid to resuscitate a patient, which may lead to less tissue edema and fewer adverse consequences, such as pulmonary edema and bowel dysfunction. Recently there have been three meta-analyses focusing on the use of colloid versus crystalloid in patients requiring volume resuscitation and the effect on mortality (Tables 20-5 and 20-6). None of these studies has demonstrated a mortality benefit with the use of colloid. These conclusions have been criticized for their combination of heterogeneous populations, use of many types of solutions, and varying indications for use.[50–52] The SAFE study, which is the largest trial of its kind as of this writing, demonstrated no appreciable difference in outcomes with the use of either 4% albumin or normal saline for intravascular volume resuscitation.[53] The multicenter, randomized, double-blind 28-day study included a diverse cohort of 6997 ICU patients with analogous baseline characteristics. These results demonstrate that albumin and saline can be considered clinically comparable treatments. The choice of fluid for intravascular volume

Table 20-5. Summary of results of studies comparing colloid versus crystalloid for resuscitation in critically ill patients.

Review: Colloids versus crystalloids for fluid resuscitation in critically ill patients
Comparison: 01 colloid vs crystalloid (add-on colloid)
Outcome: 01 deaths

Study	Colloid n/N	Crystalloid n/N	Relative risk (fixed) 95% CI	Weight (%)	Relative risk (fixed) 95% CI
01 Albumin or PPF					
x Boldt 1986	0/1	0/1		0.0	Not estimable
x Boldt 1993	0/15	0/15		0.0	Not estimable
Boutros 1979	0/7	2/17		0.2	0.45 [0.02, 8.34]
x Gallagher 1985	0/5	0/5		0.0	Not estimable
Goodwin 1983	11/40	3/39		0.4	3.57 [1.08, 11.85]
Grundmann 1982	1/14	0/6		0.1	1.40 [0.06, 30.23]
Jelenko 1978	1/7	1/5		0.2	0.71 [0.06, 8.91]
Lowe 1977	3/77	4/94		0.5	0.92 [0.21, 3.97]
Lucas 1978	7/27	0/27		0.1	15.00 [0.90, 250.25]
Metildi 1984	12/20	12/26		1.4	1.30 [0.75, 2.25]
x Prien 1990	0/6	0/6		0.0	Not estimable
Rackow 1983	6/9	6/8		0.8	0.89 [0.48, 1.64]
SAFE 2004	726/3473	729/3460		95.0	0.99 [0.91, 1.09]
Shah 1977	2/9	3/11		0.4	0.81 [0.17, 3.87]
x Shires 1983	0/9	0/9		0.0	Not estimable
Tollofsrud 1995	0/10	1/10		0.2	0.33 [0.02, 7.32]
Virgilio 1979	1/15	1/14		0.1	0.93 [0.06, 13.54]
Woittiez 1997	8/15	4/16		0.5	2.13 [0.81, 5.64]
Zetterstrom 1981a	0/15	1/15		0.2	0.33 [0.01, 7.58]
Zetterstrom 1981b	2/9	0/9		0.1	5.00 [0.27, 91.52]
Subtotal (95% CI)	780/3783	767/3793		100.0	1.02 [0.93, 1.11]

Test for heterogeneity chi-square = 13.88 df = 14 p = 0.4584
Test for overall effect = 0.41 p = 0.7

Study	Colloid n/N	Crystalloid n/N	Relative risk (fixed) 95% CI	Weight (%)	Relative risk (fixed) 95% CI
02 Hydroxyethylstarch					
x Boldt 1993	0/30	0/15		0.0	Not estimable
x Boldt 2001	0/50	0/25		0.0	Not estimable
x Dehne 2001	0/45	0/15		0.0	Not estimable
x Lang 2001	0/21	0/21		0.0	Not estimable
Nagy 1993	2/21	2/20		12.0	0.95 [0.15, 6.13]
Prien 1990	1/6	0/6		2.9	3.00 [0.15, 61.74]
Rackow 1983	5/9	6/8		37.2	0.74 [0.36, 1.50]
x Sirieix 1999	0/8	0/8		0.0	Not estimable
Woittiez 1997	13/27	4/16		29.5	1.93 [0.76, 4.90]
Younes 1998	2/12	3/11		18.4	0.61 [0.12, 3.00]
Subtotal (95% CI)	23/229	15/145		100.0	1.16 [0.68, 1.96]

Test for heterogeneity chi-square = 3.71 df = 4 p = 0.4468
Test for overall effect = 0.55 p = 0.6

Study	Colloid n/N	Crystalloid n/N	Relative risk (fixed) 95% CI	Weight (%)	Relative risk (fixed) 95% CI
03 Modified gelatin					
x Boldt 1993	0/15	0/15		0.0	Not estimable
x Boldt 2001	0/25	0/25		0.0	Not estimable
Evans 1996	1/11	2/14		27.3	0.64 [0.07, 6.14]
x Ngo 2001	0/56	0/111		0.0	Not estimable
Tollofsrud 1995	0/10	1/10		23.3	0.33 [0.02, 7.32]
x Wahba 1996	0/10	0/10		0.0	Not estimable
Wu 2001	2/18	3/16		49.4	0.59 [0.11, 3.11]
Subtotal (95% CI)	3/145	6/201		100.0	0.54 [0.16, 1.85]

Test for heterogeneity chi-square = 0.13 df = 2 p = 0.9393
Test for overall effect = 0.98 p = 0.3

Study	Colloid n/N	Crystalloid n/N	Relative risk (fixed) 95% CI	Weight (%)	Relative risk (fixed) 95% CI
04 Dextran					
Dawidson 1991	1/10	1/10		1.5	1.00 [0.07, 13.87]
Hall 1978	18/86	16/86		24.7	1.13 [0.62, 2.06]
Karanko 1987	0/14	1/18		2.0	0.42 [0.02, 9.64]
x Modig 1983	0/14	0/17		0.0	Not estimable
x Ngo 2001	0/55	0/111		0.0	Not estimable
Tollofsrud 1995	0/10	1/10		2.3	0.33 [0.02, 7.32]
Vassar 1993a	21/89	11/85		17.4	1.82 [0.94, 3.55]
Vassar 1993b	49/99	20/50		41.1	1.24 [0.83, 1.83]
Younes 1992	7/35	7/35		10.8	1.00 [0.39, 2.55]
Subtotal (95% CI)	96/412	57/422		100.0	1.24 [0.94, 1.65]

Test for heterogeneity chi-square = 2.76 df = 6 p = 0.8379
Test for overall effect = 1.53 p = 0.13

```
        0.01      0.1        1        10       100
          favors colloid    favors crystalloid
```

Source: Reprinted with permission from Alderson.[51] Copyright Cochrane Library.

CI = confidence interval, PPF = plasma protein fraction, df = degrees of freedom; x = relative risk not estimable.

TABLE 20-6. Summary of results of studies comparing colloid versus crystalloid for resuscitation in critically ill patients.

Review: Colloids versus crystalloids for fluid resuscitation in critically ill patients
Comparison: 02 colloid and hypertonic crystalloid versus isotonic crystalloid
Outcome: 01 deaths

Study	Treatment n/N	Control n/N	Relative risk (fixed) 95% CI	Weight (%)	Relative risk (fixed) [95% CI]
01 Albumin or PPF					
Jelenko 1978	1/7	2/7		100.0	0.50 [0.06, 4.33]
Subtotal (95% CI)	1/7	2/7		100.0	0.50 [0.06, 4.33]
Test for heterogeneity chi-square = 0.00 df = 0					
Test for overall effect = 0.63 p = 0.5					
02 Hydroxyethylstarch					
Subtotal (95% CI)	0/0	0/0		0.0	Not estimable
Test for heterogeneity chi-square = 0.00 df = 0					
Test for overall effect = 0.0 p = 1.0					
03 Modified gelatin					
Subtotal (95% CI)	0/0	0/0		0.0	Not estimable
Test for heterogeneity chi-square = 0.00 df = 0					
Test for overall effect = 0.0 p = 1.0					
04 Dextran					
Chavez-Negrete 1991	1/26	5/23		2.9	0.18 [0.02, 1.41]
Mattox 1991	35/211	42/211		22.6	0.83 [0.56, 1.25]
Vassar 1990	12/23	13/24		6.8	0.96 [0.56, 1.65]
Vassar 1991	30/83	34/83		18.3	0.88 [0.60, 1.30]
Vassar 1993a	21/89	14/84		7.7	1.42 [0.77, 2.60]
Vassar 1993b	49/99	23/45		17.0	0.97 [0.68, 1.37]
Younes 1992	7/35	8/35		4.3	0.88 [0.36, 2.15]
Younes 1994	27/101	40/111		20.5	0.74 [0.49, 1.11]
Subtotal (95% CI)	182/667	179/616		100.0	0.88 [0.74, 1.05]
Test for heterogeneity chi-square = 5.79 df = 7 p = 0.565					
Test for overall effect = 1.41 p = 0.16					

0.01   0.1   1   10   100

Source: Reprinted with permission from Alderson.[51] Copyright Cochrane Library.
CI = confidence interval, PPF = plasma protein fraction, df = degrees of freedom.

resuscitation is ultimately governed by the clinician's preference and the patient's ability to tolerate the treatment. Specific studies addressing the use of colloid versus crystalloid exclusively in the elderly population have not been performed.

ments and creatinine clearance measurements are useful in patients with higher risk of postoperative acute tubular necrosis.

Postoperative Management

Postoperative management must include continued vigilance in fluid balance. Early resumption of oral intake should be encouraged. Fluid losses from all sites must be accurately accounted and carefully replaced. Insensible losses should be replaced, typically in the range of 500–1000mL/day in afebrile patients. Free water replacement is guided by serum sodium concentration. Third space losses, such as postoperative ileus, are deposits for extracellular fluids. Continued attention to the use of nephrotoxic drugs is imperative in maintaining renal function. Good urine output postoperatively is a good indication of renal function and fluid balance. Creatinine measure-

Special Situations: Regional Anesthesia

Regional anesthesia merits additional consideration when attempting appropriate fluid management in the perioperative period. Spinal anesthesia inhibits the release of norepinephrine of sympathetic efferent nerves at the vascular smooth muscle cells, the sinoatrial node, the atrioventricular node, and the muscle cells of the heart. The degree of sympathetic blockade is determined by the spread of local anesthetics in the intrathecal fluid. Studies have shown that sympathetic blockade extends several dermatomes above the level of sensory blockade, thus producing hypotension with even a modest degree of sensory inhibition.[54] The response to the effects of sympathetic blockade is sensed by the vagus nerve input to the baroreflex receptor; however, the subsequent response of the baroreflex is limited by the amount of vascular bed remaining for vasoconstriction.

Management of fluids during spinal anesthesia in the elderly can pose a conflict between competing physiologic concerns. The need to avoid hypotension is apparent, but the desire to limit fluid overload must also be considered. Additionally, it should be considered if the elderly have exaggerated responses to spinal anesthesia compared with younger patients. Elderly patients have increased sympathetic tone at rest, which may cause more dramatic changes in hemodynamics if vascular resistance is abruptly altered by spinal anesthesia. The aged heart is also less responsive to beta receptor stimulation triggered by the baroreflex to increase contractility and heart rate. In addition, this population may be especially sensitive to acute intravascular volume changes, because of a more preload-dependent aged ventricle with possible diastolic dysfunction.

Studies are limited that directly compare young and elderly patients. Young patients have an average of 10% decreases in vascular resistance and cardiac output. Elderly patients with a median block of T4 have an average 10% decrease in cardiac output, but a larger 26% decrease in systemic vascular resistance.[55] Hypotension with spinal anesthesia is prevalent, occurring in up to 60% of patients with sympathetic blockade higher than T7.[56] The appropriate treatment for this hypotension has been examined. Crystalloid preloading has been shown to have no effect on the incidence of hypotension in spinal anesthesia. Treatment with a vasopressor is appropriate if systolic blood pressure decreases by more than 25% of baseline, or below 90 mm Hg. Ephedrine is often used; however, it may be less effective in the elderly patient. A pure vasoconstrictor may seem appropriate because the primary mechanism of hypotension is decreased systemic vascular resistance. This may have adverse effects on coronary vascular resistance and afterload. Epinephrine can also be considered in small doses to provide some vasoconstriction, with minimal effect on blood pressure. Excessive tachycardia should be avoided. Fluid overload should also be avoided to reduce risk of adverse outcomes such as pulmonary edema, congestive heart failure, bowel dysfunction, and prolonged fluid retention. If hypotension is minimized, cardiac performance is minimally affected by spinal anesthesia and safe for patients with preexisting cardiac disease as well.[55] Currently, there is no best way to approach fluid management with regional anesthesia, and either additional fluid administration or use of vasopressors is appropriate.

Perioperative Transfusion in the Elderly

A discussion of fluid management should also take into account the need for repletion of blood products and the effect on fluid requirements. Blood transfusion is an extensively studied and discussed topic of medical care. Approximately 12 million units of red blood cells are transfused each year. Each unit of blood costs about $217 per patient, for a total cost of more than $2 billion a year. A large majority, 60%–70% of transfusions, occur in the perioperative period.[57] The need for rational decision making concerning blood transfusion is obvious. The following discussion will focus on transfusion of red blood cells.

Administration of blood-component therapy in a patient of any age must take into account the indications for the treatment, the risks, and the benefits of treatment. The objective of red blood cell transfusion is improvement of inadequate oxygen delivery. The use of perioperative transfusion assumes that surgical patients experience adverse outcomes as a result of diminished oxygen-carrying capacity, and that transfusion can prevent these adverse outcomes. The most serious effect of anemia and reduction of oxygen-carrying capacity is myocardial ischemia. Younger patients with less comorbidity may tolerate altered perfusion to less vessel-rich organs well; however, the elderly patient may have more significant long-term morbidity.

The decision to transfuse a patient in the perioperative period requires consideration of several factors. The National Heart, Lung, and Blood Institute Consensus Conference recommends considering the following: duration of anemia, intravascular volume, hemodynamic stability, extent of operation, probability for massive blood loss, and comorbidities such as impaired pulmonary function, decreased cardiac output, myocardial ischemia, cerebrovascular or peripheral vascular disease.[58]

Correlations between acute changes in intravascular volume and hemodynamic stability have been defined previously. The American College of Surgeons has classified hypovolemia caused by blood loss according to signs and symptoms.[59] Class I hemorrhage is a loss of up to 15% of blood volume and usually causes vasoconstriction and mild tachycardia. Class II hemorrhage is attributable to a loss of 15%–30% of blood volume, and produces tachycardia and decreased pulse pressure. Patients who are awake may exhibit anxiety or restlessness. Class III hemorrhage is attributable to 30%–40% of blood volume loss, and causes marked tachycardia, tachypnea, hypotension, and altered mental status. Class IV hemorrhage, occurring after loss of more than 40% of blood volume, results in marked tachycardia, hypotension, narrow pulse pressure, decreased urine output, and markedly depressed mental status.

Use of physical signs may be helpful perioperatively, but may not be as reliable for the anesthetized patient. Measurements of vital signs that typically indicate anemia or hypovolemia may be altered by the depressant effects of general anesthetics. Signs of organ ischemia under anesthesia can be subtle. Intraoperative myocardial ischemia is associated with tachycardia in only 26% of patients, and hypotension in less than 10%. Perioperative cardiac ischemia is often silent. Ischemic events may occur during a period of decreased monitoring in the postoperative period because of pain, fever, shivering, or physical activity. Invasive monitoring can provide additional parameters to measure blood volume, but introduce other risk factors. Blood pressure measurement, oxygen delivery, and oxygen extraction are global indicators, but are not representative of organ-specific oxygen delivery.

Estimation of surgical blood loss is routinely recorded by the anesthesiologist. Intraoperative blood loss is typically estimated by examining the surgical field, collected blood in suction containers, and the presence of sponges saturated with blood. These estimates are notoriously inaccurate. Laboratory evidence of hemorrhage is used to supplement decision making in the operative period. However, intercompartmental fluid shifts during surgery and the dilutional effects of crystalloid therapy can make intraoperative hemoglobin concentrations unreliable representations of clinical status.

The patient's ability to tolerate acute anemia is altered by general anesthesia as well. Most anesthetics decrease myocardial function, resulting in decreased blood pressure, cardiac output, stroke volume, peripheral vascular resistance, and oxygen consumption. Depression of the central nervous system also decreases cerebral metabolic demands. Hypothermia also reduces metabolic rate. Anesthetics may affect the body's ability to compensate for anemia by reducing the ability to augment cardiac output in response to hypovolemia. Decreased hepatic blood flow may inhibit the ability to metabolize lactic acid, thus worsening an acid-base abnormality due to decreased perfusion. Compensatory factors such as augmenting cardiac output may be inhibited by pharmacologic interventions, such as beta-blockade or use of calcium channel blockers. The complexity of these altera-

tions defies simple prediction for the need for blood transfusion therapy. Evidence-based evaluation of blood-component therapy and established guidelines are most helpful in making these difficult clinical decisions. The additional confounding factors of increased age and comorbidity make the issue increasingly complex.

The consideration of the risks of blood transfusion must also be balanced in the decision to transfuse. Frequently cited risks include nonhemolytic transfusion reaction, transfusion reactions, transmission of infectious disease, and possible effects of immunosuppression.

The initial recommendations concerning transfusion focused on calculations, stating that oxygen availability to tissues may be decreased when hemoglobin decreases below 10 g/dL. Clinical experience has repeatedly demonstrated that hemoglobin values less than 10 g/dL are well tolerated in the perioperative period. Other studies have demonstrated that cardiac output begins to increase dramatically as hemoglobin decreases below 7 g/dL. A recent study illustrates the effect of hemoglobin levels on mortality and morbidity in the perioperative period. A retrospective study by Carson et al.[60] examining 1958 patients, aged 18 and older, that declined blood products during the perioperative period found that overall mortality increased with decreasing hemoglobin. Also, patients with underlying cardiovascular disease defined as congestive heart failure, angina pectoris, or peripheral vascular disease, had a greater risk of death at any given hemoglobin concentration, compared with patients without cardiovascular disease (Table 20-7).

The mortality risk greatly increased when hemoglobin concentration decreased to below 10 g/dL. Risk of death was extremely high when hemoglobin concentration decreased below 5–6 g/dL.[60] This information is helpful in demonstrating the effect of anemia, but does not address a decrease in risk of death as a result of receiving transfusions. The most important randomized study in assessing blood transfusion therapy was the Transfusion Require-

TABLE 20-7. Adjusted odds ratio (95% confidence interval) for mortality and preoperative hemoglobin and decline in hemoglobin stratified by cardiovascular disease.

Preoperative hemoglobin (g/dL)	Decline <2.0 g/dL		Decline 2.0–3.9 g/dL		Decline ≥4.0 g/dL	
	No CVD	CVD	No CVD	CVD	No CVD	CVD
6.0–6.9	1.4 (0.5–4.2)	12.3 (2.5–62.1)	24.1 (3.1–195.8)	216.1 (19.3–240.4)	N/A	N/A
7.0–7.9	1.3 (0.6–3.3)	8.1 (2.2–31.2)	14.2 (2.6–81.2)	88.2 (11.8–656.4)	68.5 (4.5–1049.7)	N/A
8.0–8.9	1.3 (0.6–2.6)	5.3 (1.9–15.7)	8.3 (2.1–33.7)	36.0 (7.2–179.3)	29.4 (3.3–261–1)	N/A
9.0–9.9	1.2 (0.7–2.1)	3.5 (1.6–7.9)	4.9 (1.8–14.0)	14.7 (4.4–49.0)	12.6 (2.5–65.0)	37.2 (6.02–229.2)
10.0–10.9	1.1 (0.8–1.6)	2.3 (1.4–4.0)	2.89 (1.5–5.8)	6.0 (2.7–13.4)	5.4 (1.8–16.2)	11.2 (3.3–37.5)
11.0–11.9	1.1 (0.9–1.3)	1.5 (1.2–2.0)	1.7 (1.2–2.4)	2.5 (1.6–3.7)	2.3 (1.4–4.1)	3.3 (1.8–6.1)
≥12	Reference	Reference	Reference	Reference	Reference	Reference

Source: Reprinted from Carson et al.,[60] with permission from Elsevier.

N/A = odds ratio not calculated because no patients in this cell, CVD = cardiovascular disease.

Note: Odds ratios derived from logistic regression model including hemoglobin as a continuous variable (except ≥ 12 g/dL). Logistic regression model included preoperative hemoglobin by cardiovascular disease interaction, preoperative hemoglobin by decline in hemoglobin interaction, preoperative hemoglobin, cardiovascular disease, decline in hemoglobin, and APS + age score.

ments in Critical Care (TRICC) study.[61] This was the only randomized trial with adequate power to evaluate clinical outcomes of anemia and transfusion practices. A group of 833 volume-resuscitated patients in the ICU were randomized to a liberal or restrictive transfusion threshold level. The restrictive group received transfusions at a hemoglobin concentration less than 7g/dL and was maintained at a hemoglobin between 7 and 9g/dL. The liberal transfusion threshold group was transfused for hemoglobin concentrations less than 10g/dL and maintained between 10–12g/dL. The findings were not statistically significant; however, 30-day mortality was lower in the restrictive transfusion group. The restrictive transfusion group had a relative reduction in transfusion of 55%, which could result in significant cost savings. Further analysis identified a subgroup of patients that were younger than 55 years and less severely ill (as defined by APACHE II scores less than 20) in the restrictive transfusion strategy who were half as likely to die ($p < 0.02$) within the 30-day period, compared with the liberal transfusion strategy.[62] Another subgroup in this study consisted of 257 patients with ischemic heart disease. This group had a nonsignificant ($p = 0.3$) decrease in overall survival among those patients treated with the restrictive therapy regimen. Further investigation is required to determine groups that may benefit from a higher transfusion threshold, such as patients with cardiac disease, emphysema, more severe illness, cerebrovascular disease, trauma, and older patients. Patients with cardiac disease may be unable to tolerate compensatory responses to hypovolemia and anemia, such as increasing cardiac output and heart rate. Increasing chronotropy decreases coronary artery filling time and reduces blood flow to the endocardium at a time when metabolic demands are increased. As a result, myocardial ischemia may result at higher hemoglobin values of 20–30g/dL.

As yet, there are no randomized clinical trials that evaluated transfusion thresholds in patients with cardiovascular disease. Several observational studies have provided some insight but have come to different conclusions. In a group of 190 elderly patients undergoing radical retropubic prostatectomy, patients with a hematocrit of less than 28 were at a significantly higher risk of myocardial ischemia intraoperatively and postoperatively. Hematocrit levels also correlated with the duration of myocardial ischemic episodes.[63] Similarly, a group of 27 high-risk patients undergoing infrainguinal arterial bypass procedures, who were monitored for 80 hours postoperatively, were determined to have a higher risk of morbid cardiac events when hematocrit decreased to less than 28%.[64] A retrospective study of more than 78,000 Medicare patients older than 65 years admitted with acute myocardial infarction who received a blood transfusion had a decrease in short-term mortality when the patient's admission hematocrit was less than 33%. Lower hemoglobin values correlated with more frequent in-hospital events, such as heart failure, shock, and death and with increased length of hospital stay.[65] However, a recent analysis in 24,112 patients enrolled in three clinical trials with acute coronary syndrome came to the opposite conclusion.[66] Patients receiving blood transfusion had about a three- to fourfold higher risk of death and myocardial infarction than patients not receiving transfusion. Finally, a retrospective cohort study of 3783 patients with cardiovascular disease undergoing hip fracture repair found that postoperative transfusion at a hemoglobin of 8g/dL or higher did not influence mortality.[67] Thus, large clinical trials are needed to provide high-quality evidence to guide transfusion decisions in patients with cardiovascular disease.

There are few high-quality studies that establish the critical transfusion thresholds. The best evidence comes from the TRICC trial, which found a 7g/dL threshold was at least as safe, and may be preferable, to a 10g/dL threshold in critical care patients. Whether these results are applicable to geriatric patients undergoing surgery is unknown. Pending additional clinical trials, the best data suggest that a restrictive transfusion trigger (7g/dL) should be used in most patients. It is unclear whether a higher transfusion threshold, 9–10g/dL, should be used in patients with cardiovascular disease.

The American Society of Anesthesiologists evidence-based guidelines for transfusion therapy from 1994 are still relevant today. Selected recommendations as related to red blood cell transfusion are summarized below[57]:

1. Transfusion is rarely indicated at hemoglobin levels greater than 10g/dL, and is almost always indicated when hemoglobin is less than 6g/dL.

2. Transfusion of a patient with a hemoglobin concentration between 6–10g/dL is based on the patient's risk for complications as a result of inadequate oxygenation.

3. Use of a single hemoglobin "trigger" or other approaches that do not consider physiologic and surgical factors regarding oxygen delivery requirements is not recommended.

4. Preoperative autologous blood donation, intraoperative blood recovery, acute normovolemic hemodilution, and physiologic or pharmacologic measures to decrease blood loss may be beneficial. However, in our opinion, these methods have not been established to work, and their application is at least very limited. These methodologies result in cell salvage with significant blood loss, and normovolemic hemodilution has not been established to be effective, because it results in a need to make patients more anemic than can be tolerated.

5. Indications to transfuse autologous red blood cells may be more liberal than allogeneic red blood cells. We do not agree with this recommendation, because the risk of mislabeling may still lead to risks at transfusion.

Conclusion

The elderly patient is a challenge to the anesthesiologist because of the tremendous variability of their physiologic conditions. This is often combined with a limited ability to provide accurate clinical history. The goal of this discussion of fluid management in the elderly is to provide a summary of the known data concerning fluid management and patients in the perioperative period. These data can be combined with knowledge of a patient's comorbidities and used as a basis to inform clinical decision making for specific patients. Perhaps the most important and difficult concept for clinicians to grasp is that few generalizations will hold for all elderly patients, and careful observation and adaptability in treatment may prove most beneficial for the patient.

References

1. Liu LL, Leung JM. Perioperative complications in the elderly patient. Available at: http://www.asahq.org/clinical/geriatrics/perio_comp.htm. Accessed May, 2003.
2. Luckey A, Parsa C. Fluid and electrolytes in the aged. Arch Surg 2003;138:1055–1060.
3. Vander AJ, Sherman JH, Luciano DS. Human Physiology: The Mechanisms of Body Function. 6th ed. New York: McGraw-Hill; 1994:539.
4. Holte K, Sharrock NE, Kehlet H. Pathophysiology and clinical implications of perioperative fluid excess. Br J Anesth 2002;89(4):622–632.
5. Wei JY. Age and cardiovascular system. N Engl J Med 1992;327:1735–1739.
6. Epstein M. Aging and the kidney. J Am Soc Nephrol 1996;7:1106–1122.
7. Rowe JW. Clinical research on aging; strategies and directions. N Engl J Med 1977;297:1332–1336.
8. Epstein M, Hollenberg NK. Age as a determinant of renal sodium conservation in normal man. J Lab Clin Med 1976;87:411–417.
9. Hollenberg NK, Adams DF, Solomon HS, Rashid A, Abrams HL, Merrill JP. Senescence and the renal vasculature in normal man. Circ Res 1974;34:309–316.
10. Rowe JW, Andres R, Tobin JD, Norris AH, Shock NW. The effect of age on creatinine clearance in man: a cross sectional and longitudinal study. J Gerontol 1976;31:155–163.
11. Fliser D, Aeier M, Nowack R, Ritz E. Renal functional reserve in healthy elderly subjects. J Am Soc Nephrol 1993;3:1371–1377.
12. Faulstick D, Yeingst MJ, Oussler DA, Shock NW. Glomerular permeability in young and old subjects. J Gerontol 1962;17:40–44.
13. McDonald RK, Solomon DH, Shock NW. Aging is a factor in the renal hemodynamic changes induced by a standard pyrogen. J Clin Invest 1951;30:457–462.
14. Wesson LG. Renal hemodynamics in physiological states. In: Physiology of the Human Kidney. New York: Grune and Stratton; 1969:96–108.
15. Lindeman RD, Tobin JD, Shock NW. Longitudinal studies on the rate of decline in renal function with age. J Am Geriatr Soc 1985;33:278–285.
16. Crockroft DW, Gault MH. Prediction of creatinine clearance from serum creatinine. Nephron 1976;16:31–41.
17. Goldberg TH, Finkelstein MS. Difficulties in estimating glomerular filtration rate in the elderly. Arch Intern Med 1987;147:1430–1433.
18. Malmrose LC, Gray SL, Peiper CF, et al. Measured versus estimated creatinine clearance in a high functioning elderly sample: MacArthur Foundation study of successful aging. J Am Geriatr Soc 1988;36:437–441.
19. Crane MG, Harris JJ. Effect of aging on renin activity and aldosterone excretion. J Lab Clin Med 1976;87:947–959.
20. Weidmann P, Demyttenaere-Bursztein S, Maxwell MH, DeLima J. Effect of aging on plasma renin and aldosterone in normal man. Kidney Int 1975;8:325–333.
21. Shannon RP, Wei JY, Rosa RM, Epstein FH, Rowe JH. The effect of age and sodium depletion on cardiovascular response to orthostasis. Hypertension 1986;8:438–443.
22. Sunderam SG, Mankikar GD. Hyponatremia in the elderly. Age Aging 1983;12:77–80.
23. Snyder NA, Feigal DW, Ariff AI. Hypernatremia in elderly patients: a heterogenous, morbid and iatrogenic entity. Ann Intern Med 1987;107:309–319.
24. Beck LH. Changes in renal function with aging. Clin Geriatr Med 1998;14(2):199–209.
25. Rowe JW, Shock NW, DeFronzo RA. The influence of age on the renal response to water deprivation in man. Nephron 1976;17:270–278.
26. Helderman JH, Vestal RE, Rowe JW, Tobin JD, Andres R, Robertson GL. The response of arginine vasopressin to intravenous ethanol and hypertonic saline in man: the impact of aging. J Gerontol 1978;33:39–47.
27. Rowe JW, Minaker KL, Sparrow D, Robertson GL. Age-related failure of volume–pressure-mediated vasopressin release. J Clin Endocrinol Metab 1982;54:661–664.
28. Duggan J, Kilfeather S, Lightman SL. The association of age with plasma arginine vasopressin and plasma osmolality. Age Ageing 1993;22:332–336.
29. Frolkis VV, Golovchenko SF, Medved VI, Frolkis RA. Vasopressin and cardiovascular system in aging. Gerontology 1982;28:290–302.
30. Kirkland J, Lye M, Goddard C, Vargas E, Davies I. Plasma arginine vasopressin in dehydrated elderly patients. Clin Endocrinol 1984;20:451–456.
31. Phillips PA, Rolls BY, Ledingham JG, Forsling ML, Morton JJ, Crowe MJ. Reduced thirst after water deprivation in healthy elderly men. N Engl J Med 1984;311:753–759.
32. Howard L, Ashley C. Nutrition in the perioperative patient. Ann Rev Nutr 2003;23:263–282.
33. Flynn MB, Leightty FF. Preoperative outpatient nutritional support of patients with squamous cancer of the upper aerodigestive tract. Am J Surg 1987;154(4):359–362.
34. Foschi D, Cavagna G, Callioni F, Morandi E, Rovati V. Hyperalimentation of jaundiced patients on percutaneous trans hepatic biliary drainage. Br J Surg 196;73(9):716–719.
35. Shukla HS, Rao RR, Banu N, Gupta RM, Yaday RC. Enteral hyperalimentation in malnourished surgical patients. Ind J Med Res 1984;80:339–346.

36. Von Meyenfeldt MF, Meijerink WJHJ, Rouflart MMJ, Builmaassen MTHJ, Soeters PB. Perioperative nutritional support: a randomized clinical trial. Clin Nutr 1992;11:180–\186.

37. Sandstom R, Drott C, Hytlander A, et al. The effect of postoperative intravenous feeding (TPN) on outcome following major surgery evaluated in a randomized study. Ann Surg 1993;217:185–195.

38. Delmi M, Rapin CH, Bengoa JM, et al. Dietary supplementation in elderly patients with fractured neck of femur. Lancet 1990;335(8698):1013–1016.

39. Lavizzo-Mourey R, Johnson J, Stolley P. Risk factors for dehydration among elderly nursing home residents. J Am Geriatr Soc 1988;36:213–218.

40. Barlow I. Perioperative renal insufficiency and failure in elderly patients. Available at: www.asahq.org/clinical/geriatrics. Accessed 5/2003.

41. Mcgee S, Abernethy WB, Simel DL. Is this patient hypovolemic? JAMA 1999;281(11):1022–1029.

42. Beck LH. Perioperative renal, fluid, and electrolyte management. Clin Geriatr Med 1990;6(3):557–569.

43. Alpert RA, Roizen MF, Hamilton WK, et al. Intraoperative urinary output does not predict postoperative renal function in patients undergoing abdominal aortic revascularization. Surgery 1984;95:707–711.

44. Gan TJ, Soppitt A, Maroof M, et al. Goal-directed intraoperative fluid administration reduced length of hospital stay after major surgery. Anesthesiology 2002;97(4):820–826.

45. Sinclair S, James S, Singer M. Intraoperative intravascular volume optimisation and length of hospital stay after repair of proximal femoral fracture. Br Med J 1997;315(7113):909–912.

46. Venn R, Steele A, Richardson P, Poloniecki J, Grounds M, Newman P. Randomized controlled trial to investigate the influence of the fluid challenge on duration of hospital stay and perioperative morbidity in patients with hip fractures. Br J Anesth 2002;88:65–71.

47. Price JD, Sear JW, Venn RM. Perioperative fluid volume optimization following proximal femoral fracture. Cochrane Database Syst Rev 2004;(1):CD003004.

48. Shoemaker WC, Appel PL, Kram HB, Waxman K, Lee TS. Prospective trial of supranormal values of survivors as therapeutic goals in high risk surgical patients. Chest 1988;94:1176–1186.

49. Scalea TM, Simon HM, Duncan AO, et al. Geriatric blunt multiple trauma: improved survival with early invasive monitoring. J Trauma 1990;30(2):129–134.

50. Velanovich V. Crystalloid versus colloid fluid resuscitation: a meta-analysis of mortality. Surgery 1989;105(1):65–71.

51. Alderson P, Schierhout G, Roberts I, Bunn F. Colloids versus crystalloids for fluid resuscitation in critically ill patients. Cochrane Database Syst Rev 2000;(2):CD000567.

52. Bunn F, Alderson P, Hawkins V. Colloid solutions for fluid resuscitation. Cochrane Database Syst Rev 2003;(1): CD001319.

53. Finfer S, Bellomo R, Boyce N, et al. A comparison of albumin and saline for fluid resuscitation in the intensive care unit. NEJM 2004;350:2247–2256.

54. Rooke GA. Cardiovascular response to spinal anesthesia in the elderly. Available at: www.asahq.org/clinical/geriatrics. Accessed May 2003.

55. Rooke GA, Freund PR, Jacobson AF. Hemodynamic response and change in organ blood volume during spinal anesthesia in elderly men with cardiac disease. Anesth Analg 1997;85:99–105.

56. Coe AJ, Revanas B. Is crystalloid preloading useful in spinal anesthesia in the elderly? Anaesthesia 1990;45:241–243.

57. Nutall GA, Brost BC, Connis RT, et al. Practice Guidelines for Blood Component Therapy: a report by the American Society of Anesthesiologist Task Force on Blood Component Therapy. Anesthesiology 1996;84(3):732–747.

58. Perioperative red cell transfusion. Natl Inst Health Consens Dev Conf Consens Statement 1988;7(4):1–19.

59. American College of Surgeons, Committee on Trauma. Advanced Trauma Life Support Course Manual. Chicago: American College of Surgeons; 1989.

60. Carson JL, Duff A, Poses RM, et al. Effect of anemia and cardiovascular disease on surgical mortality and morbidity. Lancet 1996;348:1055–1060.

61. Herbert PC, Wells G, Blajchman MA, et al. A multicenter, randomized, controlled clinical trial of transfusion requirements in critical care. N Engl J Med 1999;340(6):409–417.

62. Ely EW, Bernard GR. Transfusions in critically ill patients. N Engl J Med 1999;340(6):467–468.

63. Hogue CW, Goudnough LR, Monk TG. Perioperative myocardial ischemic episodes are related to hematocrit level in patients undergoing radical prostatectomy. Transfusion 1998;38:924–931.

64. Nelson AH, Fleisher LA, Rosenbaum SH. Relationship between postoperative anemia and cardiac morbidity in high-risk vascular patients in the intensive care unit. Crit Care Med 1993;21:860–866.

65. Wei-Chih W, Rathore S, Wang Y, Radford M, Krumholz H. Blood transfusions in elderly patients with acute myocardial infarction. N Engl J Med 2001;345(17):1230–1236.

66. Rao SV, Jollis JG, Harrington RA, et al. Relationship of blood transfusion and clinical outcomes in patients with acute coronary syndromes. JAMA 2004;292(13):1555–1562.

67. Carson JL, Duff A, Berlin JA, et al. Perioperative blood transfusion and postoperative mortality. JAMA 1998;279(3):199–205.

21
Pain Management

Jack M. Berger

The United States senior population is expected to double over the next 30 years (www.agingstats.gov). According to the latest data from the National Center for Health Statistics, 40.3 million inpatient surgical procedures were performed in the United States in 1996, followed closely by 31.5 million outpatient surgeries. These statistics are from 1996 and although the ratio of outpatient to inpatient procedures may have changed in the past 10 years, the total number of surgical procedures per year has not diminished. And certainly, the elderly undergo a disproportionate number of surgical procedures compared with younger age groups. Therefore, acute pain secondary to surgery will continue to be a significant problem for physicians.

In addition, estimates are that 80%–85% of individuals over 65 years old have at least one significant health problem that predisposes them to pain. Epidemiologists at Brown University (reporting in JAMA, June 17, 1998) found that between 25%–40% of older cancer patients studied had daily pain. Among these patients, 21% between the ages of 65 and 74 received no pain medication at all. Of those 75–84 years old, 26% received no pain medication, and for those older than 85, 30% were left untreated.[1]

In northern California, Jury Verdict No. H205732–1 of the California Superior Court awarded $1.5 million to the family of an elderly lung cancer patient in a civil suit in which the physician was found liable for recklessness and elder abuse for failure to prescribe adequate pain medication. This resulted in California Assembly Bill 487 that now requires every physician in California to obtain 12 continuing medical education credits in pain management and palliative care in the next 3 years in order to renew their license. And so as much as providing adequate pain management is a moral obligation, inadequate pain management has become a liability.

There are about 1.5 million frail elderly residing in 20,000 nursing homes in the United States. Forty percent are over the age of 85 years. Forty-five percent to 85% may have pain as compared with 25%–50% of community-dwelling elderly.[2,3] A telephone poll conducted by Cooner and Amorosi from Louis Harris and Associates of New York City in 1997, revealed that more than half of older adults had taken prescription pain medications for longer than 6 months, and 45% had visited at least three physicians for their pain in the last 5 years.[4] New pain visits to physicians are most common in the 15- to 44-year-old group, whereas the lowest are in the elderly. Persistent pain complaints, however, are most common in the elderly, and pain is the most common symptom noted by the consulting physician.[5] Yet elderly people and young children are often perceived by the health care delivery system as being insensitive to pain. And therefore those who are most dependent on the health care system are most likely to receive the least optimal care for pain.

Pain is a highly subjective, variable sensory and emotional experience, with a pathophysiology composed of complex neuroanatomic and neurochemical processes.[6] Everyone has an intuitive idea of what pain is. Pain is always something that "hurts." But many things hurt. A broken arm hurts. This is an example of acute somatic pain. A heart attack hurts. This is ischemic pain. A kidney stone and appendicitis hurt, which are examples of visceral pain. An amputated leg may hurt; this is phantom limb pain. An individual may hurt in the arm or leg on the side affected by a stroke. Both of these are examples of central neuropathic pain. The death of a loved one "hurts." It is a "painful emotional experience" for which we use the same words of description as for physical injury. It is clear then that the perception of "pain" is always subjective and takes place in the brain. Tissue injury is perceived as nociception. But the site of the nociception does not necessarily correspond to the area of the body in which "the pain" is felt. Furthermore, the tissue injury may have actually healed while the perception of pain persists.

Three Pain Scenarios

It is quite clear from the above introduction that pain in the elderly follows one of three scenarios:

1. Acute pain results from surgery, cancer, fractures, medical conditions such as vascular ischemia, herpes zoster.

2. Chronic pain results from various persistent medical and physical conditions. Specific chronic pain syndromes that are known to affect the geriatric population disproportionately include: arthritis which may affect 80% of patients over 65, cancer, herpes zoster and postherpetic neuralgia, temporal arteritis, polymyalgia rheumatica, atherosclerotic peripheral vascular disease, diabetic neuropathy, and back pain syndromes.[6] In chronic pain states, there is often the absence of the "normal" physiologic indicators of acute pain such as tachycardia, hypertension, and diaphoresis. Yet, there may be hyperpathia, allodynia, and hyperalgesia in the absence of any physical findings of tissue injury:

- Allodynia is pain elicited by a nonnoxious stimulus (clothing, air movement, touch), mechanical (induced by light pressure), thermal (induced by a nonpainful cold or warm stimulus).
- Hyperalgesia is exaggerated pain response to a mildly noxious (mechanical or thermal) stimulus.
- Hyperpathia is delayed and explosive pain response to a noxious stimulus.

3. Finally, there are those who are suffering from persistent pain who then experience a new acute injury or exacerbation of their primary condition that is superimposed on their primary pain state.

Elderly patients present special problems with respect to treating pain in each of these three scenarios.

Depression, Anxiety, and Pain

Associations between pain and depression are well documented in elderly patients.[7,8] Studies show that elderly subjects who are anxious and/or depressed voice more localized pain complaints than their nonanxious and nondepressed counterparts. Furthermore, anxious and/or depressed individuals report more intense pain.[9] Clinical evidence suggests that cognitive impairment may be exacerbated by pain and/or its treatment, especially in the elderly. These patients may benefit dramatically from psychologic or psychiatric interventions. Common missed diagnoses or underdiagnosed diseases in the elderly that can cause pain are: endocrine disorders, neurologic disorders, major medical disorders including electrolyte imbalances, polypharmacy, dysphoria, sleep disturbances, and loss of appetite, etc.[6]

Assessment

Many older adults are afraid to report pain.[10,11] There is often fear of losing independence because of chronic illness. If an older adult fears that reporting pain will lead to a debilitating diagnosis that may cause nursing home placement or further loss of physical independence, he or she may be less likely to report it. Or the patient may fear additional procedures, diagnostic tests, or medication prescriptions that may result from reporting pain. For acute postoperative pain, this is less of a problem unless the patient has dementia or other condition that prevents direct communication.

Elderly patients may present special problems in obtaining an accurate pain history. Failures in memory, depression, and sensory impairments may hinder history-taking. They may tend to underreport symptoms because they expect pain associated with aging and their diseases, or because they just do not want to be a bother to anyone. The inability to be aware of, and to verbalize, one's emotional state is called alexithymia. Patients with chronic pain have been found to have a significant incidence (33%) of alexithymia. This may be a factor in causing geriatric patients to express emotional distress more often through somatic complaints because they have been found to be more alexithymic.[12]

Nociception Is Not Pain

Activity induced in the nociceptor and nociceptive pathways by a noxious stimulus is not pain, which is always a psychologic state. Although we appreciate that pain most often has a proximate physical cause, especially acute pain, activity in nociceptor systems is not equivalent to the experience of pain. The recognition that pain serves an important biologic function related to survival, raises the important question: To what extent do age-related changes in nociception affect the capacity of the pain experience to fulfill an "enteroceptive" function (such as thirst, hunger, and thermoception that constitute sensory indexes of the health of the body)?[13]

Age does not seem to affect success of traditional interventions for the treatment of pain. Assessment and intervention for pain in the elderly should begin with the assumption that all neurophysiologic processes subserving nociception are intact. That is to say, tissue injury produces the same intensity of stimulus in an elderly person as in a young person. There are data to suggest that there is impairment of Aδ fibers with aging and therefore of the early warning of tissue injury.[13] There are also data that suggest that widespread and substantial changes in structure, neurochemistry, and function occur in the dorsal horn of the spinal cord and central nervous system (CNS) with aging.[13]

Multiple studies report reductions in the descending inhibitory modulating systems for nociception in the elderly. Gibson and Ferrell[13] conclude that the reduced efficacy of endogenous analgesic systems might be expected to result in a more severe pain after prolonged noxious stimulation. It is also possible that documented decline in afferent transmission pathways could be offset by a commensurate reduction in the endogenous inhibitory mechanisms of older persons, with a net result of little or no change in the perceptual pain experience.[13] They further conclude that any deficit in endogenous analgesic response (which is stimulus intensity dependent) will become critical, thereby making it more difficult for persons of advanced age to cope with severe or persistent clinical pain conditions.[13]

Although there is controversy over whether the number and integrity of nociceptors decreases with age, *the position that age dulls the sense of pain is untenable*.[13] It is the processing of the nociceptive information that may be altered in the elderly, and the elderly may be more sensitive to the side effects of medications that are used to treat pain. These observations thereby give the impression that the elderly are less sensitive to pain. But no physiologic changes in pain perception in the elderly have been demonstrated according to a recent five-state study.[1] One would not assume that a surgical incision in an elderly patient will "hurt" less and therefore does not need to be treated. Likewise, anyone who has observed an elderly patient with acute herpes zoster certainly can attest to the excruciating pain that these unfortunate patients report.

Pathophysiology of Types of Pain

Somatic Pain

A noxious stimulus in the periphery activates nociceptors. This results in a release of pain-producing substances, e.g., prostaglandins, leukotrienes, and substance P. Impulses travel via Aδ and C fibers to the dorsal horn of the spinal cord. Somatic pain is well localized and gnawing. There is often associated tenderness and swelling. Examples include fractures, bone metastasis, and postoperative pain. This type of pain is usually opioid responsive.

Visceral Pain

When viscera are stretched, compressed, invaded, or distended, pain will result. The pain is poorly localized and may be referred. It is described as deep, squeezing, cramplike, or colicky. It is frequently associated with sympathetic and parasympathetic symptoms: nausea, diaphoresis, and hypotension. Examples include bowel obstruction and pancreatic cancer. This type of pain is also usually opioid responsive.

Neuropathic Pain

Injury to neural tissues or dysfunctional changes of the nervous system from trauma, compression, tumor invasion, or cancer therapies result in this form of pain. The pain may be associated with sensory and motor deficits, but not always. The quality of the pain is often described as burning, squeezing, lancinating, or electrical. There can be associated sleep and eating disturbances, and significant patient emotional suffering. Examples include brachial and lumbosacral plexopathy, postherpetic neuralgia, neuromas, complex regional pain syndrome, diabetic neuropathy, and radiculopathies. Neuropathic pain is associated with opioid tolerance, termed "apparent opioid resistance." That is, patients with neuropathic pain often require higher than expected doses of opioids to obtain pain relief and the pain relief is usually not complete.

Neuropathic Pain and Visceral Hypersensitivity

Injury of nerves innervating somatic structures enhances nociception from stimulation of viscera with convergent input from nearby dermatomes, suggesting that somatic neuropathic pain could be accompanied by an increased likelihood of visceral pain.[14] This raises the possibility that pain disorders such as fibromyalgia, chronic fatigue syndrome, chronic pelvic pain, and chronic interstitial cystitis all represent visceral hypersensitivity pain syndromes of neuropathic origin.

Medication Management

Little is known of the neurophysiologic relationships between pain and age-related degenerative brain diseases. However, Fine[15] has recently reviewed the issues of pharmacologic management of persistent pain in older patients. In general, pharmacodynamics (what the drug does to the patient) are unaffected in the normal aging process. The molecular action of morphine is the same in all animals, although dose requirements to produce the same effect may change with age. However, because centrally acting drugs may interact with a preexisting disease state, care must be taken when treating pain in patients with CNS disease such as parkinsonism, Alzheimer dementia, or stroke.

Pharmacokinetics (what the patient does to the drug) are frequently affected by aging processes, and disease states. Pharmacokinetic changes attributable to physical aging may complicate medication management. (See Chapter 15, The Pharmacology of Opioids.) There is decreased liver mass and blood flow, which prolongs opioid and acetaminophen metabolism. This is of concern, particularly with fixed combination drugs, such as hydrocodone or codeine with acetaminophen (Vicodin or Tylenol #3) and opioids with active metabolites (e.g., morphine to morphine-3-glucuronide or meperidine to normeperidine).

There is decreased renal function which increases the risk of nonsteroidal antiinflammatory drug (NSAID) nephrotoxicity and accumulation of metabolites of drugs such as meperidine. There is decreased plasma binding, which increases blood levels of active drugs, opioids, and NSAIDs [even the cyclooxygenase (COX)-2 specific inhibitors, such as Celebrex].

In the elderly, there is increased CNS sensitivity to opioids leading to enhanced sedation, analgesia, and side effects including delirium. But the experience of pain tends to counteract the sedative effects of opioids. Therefore, patients who have not received adequate doses of opioid analgesics and who are still experiencing pain do not suffer respiratory depression.[16]

In acute pain situations or in a "pain crisis," rapid titration of opioids in elderly patients is safe. In a study of 175 elderly patients versus 875 younger patients who were treated with intravenous (IV) morphine for postoperative pain in the postanesthesia care unit, there was no increased incidence of adverse side effects noted when a strict titration to pain level protocol was followed. It was not necessary to change the protocol according to age.[17]

The use of an opioid is the strategy of choice for rapid titration to pain relief in most clinical situations. Opioid side effects are usually manageable if frequent assessments are made. The elderly, of course, may require more frequent assessments and smaller incremental doses in order to manage side effects. The exact timing of interval assessments must be dictated by the needs of the individual case.

The management of an acute pain crisis involves immediate control of the pain, maintenance of analgesia, and long-term management. During the initial titration to pain relief, there is ample opportunity to evaluate the patient for the causes of the pain. The best way to gain control is to get the syringe and titrate to effect. The dose depends on the history of current use or whether the patient is opioid naïve. The choice of drug, e.g., 1–4 mg of morphine, 0.2–1 mg of hydromorphone (Dilaudid), 10–50 mg of meperidine (Demerol), or the equianalgesic IV dose based on the patient's P.O. breakthrough medication, is not as important.

Opioids reach maximum plasma levels in 10–15 minutes after IV bolus (excluding fentanyl and its congeners), so bolus doses every 10–15 minutes until the patient is comfortable, begins to become sedated, or has decreasing respiratory rate is the most effective method of opioid analgesic loading. An alternative method involves starting low, then doubling the dose every 30 minutes, until comfort is obtained, e.g., morphine 2, 4, 8, 16 mg, etc., with the effect being obtained in less than 90 minutes (range 4–215 minutes).[18] This second method may be more appropriate for the "younger elderly" as opposed to the "old elderly."

After loading the patient and obtaining comfort, maintenance dosing must be ordered. Intramuscular or IV bolus dosing by the nursing staff on a PRN basis is a poor choice. The dose required to make the patient comfortable can be used as an estimate of the 3-hour dose requirement for maintenance, e.g., when converting to IV patient-controlled analgesia (PCA).

Contraindications for IV PCA include patients who are unable to operate the device because of impaired mental status or physical limitations, and patients who are unwilling to use the technique, i.e., some patients do not want to push the button and want to be given their medication by the nurse. Patients with sleep apnea disorders pose a relative contraindication. Failure to achieve adequate analgesia without side effects after an appropriate trial is also a contraindication. If the patient chooses to have the nurse administer analgesia, it would still be advantageous to have a PCA set up, which would eliminate intramuscular injections that hurt and produce tissue injury in the elderly. Also, the medications can be titrated in small doses by the nurse to adequate analgesia.

Postsurgical Analgesia

Elderly patients undergo a high number of surgical interventions. The importance of adequate postoperative analgesia for reducing morbidity and mortality in the elderly is undisputed.[19] Epidural analgesia and IV PCA are both excellent postoperative techniques. Physicians are often reluctant to use PCA in older patients.[20,21] PCA was found to be effective in this population with the caveat that the patient is physically or mentally able to operate the machine.[22] Regional anesthetic techniques are excellent for the elderly. Although a fair amount of research has been published, data proving long-term benefit are lacking.[19]

In a study of elderly patients after abdominal surgery, IV PCA versus patient-controlled epidural analgesia (PCEA), the IV PCA group had general anesthesia with sufentanil, isoflurane, nitrous oxide, and atracurium for muscle relaxation. Postoperative loading was 5 mg of morphine followed by a morphine PCA of 1.5 mg, lockout 8 minutes. The epidural group had a T7–T11 catheter placed, depending on surgery level, which was activated with 2% lidocaine with epinephrine 5 μg/mL, dosed to T4 sensory level before induction of general anesthesia. A solution of 0.25% bupivacaine plus 1 μg/mL Sufenta was infused continuously throughout the surgery and continued postoperatively with a solution of 0.125% bupivacaine plus 0.5 µg/mL Sufenta at 3–5 mL/h with a 2- to 3-mL PCEA bolus and a lockout of 12 minutes.[23]

The authors concluded that PCEA with local anesthetic and opioid provided better pain control, improved mental status, and better bowel function return than did traditional IV PCA morphine after general anesthesia. Orthostatic and mobility deficits were not a problem with the PCEA adjustments.

Carli et al.,[24] in their study of 64 patients for elective colon surgery randomized to an IV PCA group or epidural group, found that epidural analgesia enhanced functional exercise capacity and health-related quality of life indicators after colonic surgery. In their study, the PCA group had anesthetics consisting of 250 µg of fentanyl, adjusted isoflurane, nitrous oxide, oxygen, and PCA morphine with no basal rate but a dose of 1–2 mg every 5 minutes. It was discontinued on day 3–4 if the verbal analog score was <3/10.

The epidural group had T8–9 catheters placed preoperatively and activated with 15–20 mL 0.5% bupivacaine to a sensory level of T4. General anesthesia was then induced and maintained with 100 µg of fentanyl, maintenance 0.4% end-tidal isoflurane, nitrous oxide, oxygen, and bolus doses of 5 mL 0.5% bupivacaine. Postoperatively, the epidural infusion was 4–15 mL/h of 0.1% bupivacaine and 2 µg/mL fentanyl and continued for 4 days.

The results indicated that the epidural group had improved outcomes for pain control, mobilization, gastrointestinal motility, and intake of protein and calories. This may be a function more of the local anesthetic, facilitating bowel function, thereby causing less nausea, and more willingness to eat. Decreased pain can also result in the same benefits, not just at rest but also with mobility, and less pain may ameliorate insulin sensitivity, hypercatabolism, and maintain muscle protein better. These benefits seemed to carry out to 6 weeks in the study of Health Related Quality of Life Indicators, leaving little doubt that epidural analgesia is even better than systemic opioids in the elderly.[24]

Opioid Therapy

Oral and transdermal medications should be used if possible. Opioids can be dissolved and put down a G-tube, and rectal preparations are available or can be compounded. Fast-onset and short-acting agents should be used for episodic pain, and long-acting agents for continuous pain. Meperidine and propoxyphene should be avoided in elderly patients because of a higher potential for CNS effects.[25] Nausea and constipation should be treated prophylactically.[4]

Opioid Addiction

The American Academy of Pain Medicine and American Pain Society define addiction as a compulsive disorder in which an individual becomes preoccupied with obtaining and using a substance for nonmedical reasons or reasons other than pain relief, the continued use of which results in a decreased quality of life. This does not seem to be a clinical issue in pain management for the elderly. Nonetheless, opioid phobia both on the part of the physician and the patient persists. It is even less of a problem in acute pain management postoperatively. Much of the problem is lack of knowledge about the differences among addiction, tolerance, physical dependence,[24] and pseudo-addiction as described by Weissman and Haddox.[26]

Any patient exposed to opioids for several days for the treatment of pain can experience withdrawal phenomena if the drug is stopped abruptly. This is not addiction and will occur with many different classes of drugs including beta-blockers, insulin, and various antihypertensive agents, etc. Likewise, the need to increase the dose of an opioid over time may be a measure of tolerance or worsening disease, neither of which equate with addiction. In pseudo-addiction, a patient who is prescribed an inadequate dose of an opioid may exhibit drug-seeking behavior in an attempt to obtain adequate analgesia. Drug seeking is frequently interpreted by medical staff as a sign of addiction. However, pseudo-addiction is an iatrogenically produced condition and careful monitoring of the patient will distinguish this from true drug addiction as defined above.

Titration of Opioids

So what is the correct dose of opioid analgesics? The "correct dose" is the dose that provides analgesia without producing intolerable and uncontrollable side effects. This was defined by Louis Lasagna and Henry Beecher in 1954.[27] The same principle holds today, some 50 years later. There is no ceiling effect with opioids. Opioids are not organ toxic. If the pupils are not pinpoint and if the patient is still in pain and is still free of side effects, the patient is not receiving too much.

Opioid Conversions

Patients who are treated with epidural opioids or IV PCA opioids in the hospital are rarely able to leave the hospital without the need for continued analgesic therapy. The pressure applied to physicians by Medicare, HMOs, and private insurers to reduce length of stay has made pain management a priority to allow earlier discharge. However, if this is to be accomplished successfully, physicians must have knowledge of equianalgesic equivalents. Equivalency charts can be found in many different texts. An excellent revised chart can be obtained from the Southern California Cancer Pain Initiative (sccpi@coh.org), and found in a relevant article by Gammaitoni and associates.[28] In the author's experience, some simple conversions for chronic administration include the following:

- IV morphine 10 mg = 30 mg orally.
- IV morphine 1 mg = hydromorphone 0.2 mg.
- Oral morphine 30 mg = hydromorphone 6 mg orally.
- Oral morphine 30 mg = oxycodone 15–20 mg orally.
- IV morphine 60 mg/day = morphine orally 180 mg/day = fentanyl transdermal patch of 100 μg/h.
- IV morphine 10 mg = hydrocodone 30 mg orally.

An example of a common mistake is the patient who is obtaining excellent pain relief from an IV PCA of 10 mg of morphine every 3 hours. The time for discharge arrives, and the PCA is discontinued; the substitution is hydrocodone/acetaminophen (Vicodin) 5 mg/500 mg tablets. The equivalency for analgesic effect for 10 mg of morphine IV is 30 mg of hydrocodone orally. Ten milligrams of morphine IV every 3 hours would be eight doses per day of 30 mg of hydrocodone or 48 tablets of hydrocodone/acetaminophen per day. Of course, this would be a lethal dose of acetaminophen. It is unlikely that any patient would actually take 48 tablets per day, but the normal prescription of 1 to 2 tablets every 6 hours PRN for pain might certainly be inadequate for someone requiring 10 mg of morphine IV every 3 hours.

It therefore behooves the physician managing the patient to convert the patient to an acceptable oral medication several days before discharge to ensure adequate pain control and lack of side effects. In converting from IV morphine to transdermal fentanyl, this author has found that 60 mg per day of IV morphine would require a 100 μg/h transdermal fentanyl patch, which would be changed every 72 hours. Because hydromorphone is approximately 5 times more potent than morphine, 60 mg per day of IV morphine would convert to 12 mg per 24 hours of hydromorphone and again equate to a transdermal fentanyl patch of 100 μg/h dose.

CYP 2D6 Enzyme and the Efficacy of Codeine and Codeine-Like Drugs

Codeine, dihydrocodeine (Synalgos DC), and hydrocodone (Vicodin, Lortab, etc.) are not active opioids. These opiates must be converted to morphine by the enzyme

TABLE 21-1. Medications that inhibit the enzyme CYP 2D6.

Amiodarone (Cordarone)
Fluoxetine (Prozac)
Haloperidol (Haldol)
Paroxetine (Paxil)
Propafenone (Rythmol)
Propoxyphene (Darvon)
Quinidine
Ritonavir (Norvir)
Terbinafine (Lamisil)
Thioridazine (Mellaril)

Source: Data from Supernaw.[29]

CYP 2D6 to become effective.[29,30] Approximately 20% of the population is genetically deficient in this enzyme and so would report a poor analgesic response when prescribed these medications. Furthermore, many medications also inhibit the action of CYP 2D6 that are frequently used by elderly patients; some of these are shown in Table 21-1.

Oxycodone is metabolized by CYP 2D6; therefore, patients who are deficient in this enzyme will have a greater effect from oxycodone medications.

Opioids for Neuropathic Pain and Broad-Spectrum Opioids

Many elderly patients suffer from neuropathic pain which is poorly responsive to opioid analgesics that act primarily at the μ opioid receptor (Table 21-2).[31] While affinity for μ, δ, and κ receptors of opiates are steric dependent, the affinity of "l" and "d" forms are nearly equal with respect to nonopiate receptor actions such as N-methyl-D-aspartate (NMDA) antagonist and blockage of reuptake of serotonin and noradrenaline. Multiple actions of the broad-spectrum opiates seem to be synergistic with respect to analgesic action, similar to using narrow-spectrum opiates in combination with an NMDA receptor antagonist and a tricyclic antidepressant. As listed in Table 21-3, the opioids that have dual actions both for opioid receptors and for NMDA receptors will be more effective for neuropathic pain than the narrow-spectrum opioids. The opioids in the gray-screened area

TABLE 21-2. Narrow-spectrum opioids acting only at opioid receptors.

Morphine
Hydromorphone
Codeine
Fentanyl
Sufentanil
Oxycodone
Buprenorphine

TABLE 21-3. Other actions of broad-spectrum opioids not at the opioid receptors.

Broad-spectrum opioids acting also as antagonists to N-methyl-D-aspartate receptors	Broad-spectrum opioids acting also as inhibitors of reuptake of serotonin and norepinephrine (similar to the tricyclic antidepressants)
Methadone	*Methadone*
Ketobemidone	Levorphanol
Dextropropoxyphene	Dextromethorphan
Dextromethorphan	*Dextropropoxyphene*
Meperidine (pethidine)	Tramadol
	Meperidine (pethidine)

are common to the effects of NMDA receptor antagonism and inhibition of reuptake of serotonin and norepinephrine.

Because dextropropoxyphene and meperidine both have metabolites that act in the brain of elderly patients and lead to confusion and even seizures, the only true broad-spectrum opioid analgesic available is methadone.

End-of-Life Care

For 67% of patients, the last place of care was an institution, with 38.4% dying in a hospital and 30.5% in a nursing home. Only 33% died at home; 49.3% of these were on home hospice care; 38.2% received no formal services; and 12.5% had home health care nursing services without hospice participation.[32]

Reporting on the degree of satisfaction of bereaved family members with the care their loved ones received, hospice care at home received the highest level of overall satisfaction with 71% of respondents. Twenty-five percent of all patients with pain or dyspnea did not receive "any" or "enough" treatment. Inadequate pain management was 1.6 times more likely in a nursing home setting or with home health services and 1.2 times more likely in a hospital than with home hospice.[33]

End-of-life pain management for patients who are being managed at home presents problems of assessment and administration of medication. Patients who are still able to swallow can be managed with oral medications. Rectal suppositories, transdermal medications, and transmucosal medications are available.

Kadian and Avinza are every-24-hour, single-dose sustained-release morphine preparations. Although their uptake properties differ, they both have the property of being packaged in a capsule that can be sprinkled as pellets onto applesauce or added to slurry for administration down an NG- or G-tube, while retaining the sustained-release characteristic. MS Contin is an every-12-hour sustained-release morphine preparation that

cannot be broken open. Doing so destroys the integrity of the sustained-release capsule; the patient receives the entire dose as an immediate-release preparation. OxyContin is a 12-hour sustained-release preparation of oxycodone that also cannot be opened or it too becomes an immediate-release preparation. There is currently no sustained-release preparation of hydromorphone or methadone. Fentanyl and buprenorphine are the only commercially available transdermal opioids.

It is important to remember that sustained-release medications are encouraged for patients who have continuous pain. But it must be remembered that activity will often increase the level of pain; patients must be prescribed rapid-onset, short-acting medications to be used for such breakthrough pain. Because patients vary tremendously in their requirements for pain medication, particularly in the senior population in which the margin for error is smaller, it is important to titrate patients with immediate-release medication to determine how to convert to sustained-release medication. Although sustained-release morphine is available in capsules that are recommended for every-12-hour dosing and every-24-hour dosing, the absorption characteristics will determine whether a particular patient experiences adverse effects such as nausea or sedation, or end of dose failure. It is sometimes necessary to lower the dose and change to every-8-hour or every-12-hour dosing.

Rarely in acute pain situations and more often in end-of-life care, patients' pain cannot be brought under control with opioid infusions alone. In such situations, optimum pain control with minimal side effects could be obtained with a combination solution of 1 mg/mL morphine and 1 mg/mL ketamine, with a lockout period of 8 minutes with an IV PCA.[34] These agents can both be given orally as well in the same ratio, e.g., 30 mg of immediate release morphine sulfate with 30 mg of ketamine every 3–4 hours.

Sedation of Terminally Ill

When patients are terminally ill and traditional analgesic regimens are unsuccessful at providing adequate analgesia and relief from suffering, the following solution can provide benefit[35]:

Ketamine (dissociative anesthetic, NMDA blocker) 2 mg/mL

Midazolam (benzodiazepine, reduces incidence of hallucinations, sedative effects, antianxiety) 0.1 mg/mL

Fentanyl (potent opioid, less nausea, less pruritus, less constipation, enhanced effect combined with ketamine/midazolam) 5 μg/mL

IV infusion should begin at 3–5 mL/h titrating to effect. Doubling the concentrations will allow reduction of the volume infused if needed. High concentrations can be used as subcutaneous infusion as long as the volume infused per hour remains less than 2 mL.

Nonsteroidal Antiinflammatory Analgesics

The antiprostaglandin effect of NSAIDs can be beneficial during the acute phase of soft tissue injury. This biochemical effect may control the inflammatory response to injury and provide pain relief. The duration of an NSAID's analgesic effect may be different from its antiinflammatory effect. The antiinflammatory effect may last longer than the analgesic effect.

Chronic inflammatory disease pain such as arthritis may warrant chronic NSAID therapy. But some authors have expressed concern that NSAIDs may actually interfere with the later stages of tissue repair and remodeling, where prostaglandins still help mediate debris cleanup. (This does not seem to be true for the COX-2 specific inhibitors.) Therefore, dosage, timing, and potential side effects of NSAIDs should be evaluated. It is not possible to predict patient response to a particular NSAID by chemical class or pharmacokinetics.[36]

Remember that COX-2 specific inhibitors do not affect platelet aggregation and therefore may pose a risk for myocardial infarction if a patient is taken off aspirin therapy. For the same reason, it is safe to continue COX-2 specific inhibitors with daily low-dose aspirin. COX-2 inhibitors also have a safer profile from the standpoint of gastrointestinal irritation, but care should still be taken in patients with borderline renal function. Baseline renal function tests should probably be obtained for elderly patients who are beginning a course of chronic coxib therapy or NSAID therapy. Drug holidays of 30–60 days every 4–6 months may also be advisable.

Tricyclic Antidepressants and Specific Serotonin Reuptake Inhibitors

Tricyclic antidepressants are often used as adjuvants in treating neuropathic pain because of their inhibition of reuptake of serotonin and norepinephrine. There is fear that antidepressants will cause cardiac arrhythmias. Tricyclic antidepressants are safe for cardiac patients, except for several months after a myocardial infarction or if a conduction defect or persistent dangerous arrhythmia is already present.[37]

Specific serotonin reuptake inhibitors (SSRIs) have safer cardiac profiles than tricyclic antidepressants. SSRIs are effective for depression. *SSRIs do not have analgesic effects like the tricyclics because they are only serotonin reuptake inhibitors and not norepinephrine reuptake*

inhibitors. Both are necessary to modulate neuropathic pain. Tricyclics are more effective for pain and for sleep but may also cause sedation, cognitive changes, and dizziness. Elderly patients taking tricyclic antidepressants are at risk for falling, resulting in hip or other fractures. Again, titration and frequent reassessment are the key to successful treatment. In addition, many newer classes of antidepressants provide inhibition of reuptake of norepinephrine and serotonin without the associated sedation.

Anticonvulsants for Neuropathic Pain

Gabapentin (Neurontin) is probably the most effective agent with the fewest side effects for the treatment of neuropathic pain. It is absorbed in the duodenum, not metabolized by the liver, not protein bound, excreted unchanged by the kidneys, and has no ceiling dose. It is nontoxic to the liver and kidney. The only significant side effects are sedation and cognitive impairment. Starting low and titrating to response again is the recommendation, but rapid titration upward is possible as tolerated. Oxcarbazepine (Trileptal), lamotrigine (Lamictal), and Topamax are also effective substitutes. And now pregabalin (Lyrica) is also available and FDA approved for use in treating both postherpetic neuralgic and diabetic neuralgia.

Evaluation by a psychiatrist may yield information about clinical depression resulting in emotional suffering perceived as pain versus sadness, frustration, and isolation in response to inadequately treated pain. This would be valuable information in making a choice of treating with an SSRI versus a tricyclic or other agent with both serotonin and norepinephrine reuptake inhibition effects.

With any of these medications, tricyclic or other antidepressants, anticonvulsants, etc., cognitive impairment caused by the medication must frequently be accepted or tolerated in the elderly in order to obtain pain relief.

Pain and Insulin Resistance

Acute, severe pain decreases insulin sensitivity. This would indicate that relief for acute pain is important for maintenance of normal glucose metabolism. Many elderly patients are diabetic, emphasizing the need for good pain relief.[38]

Regional Analgesia

Upper extremity surgeries are amenable to brachial plexus anesthesia and analgesia. Brachial plexus nerve blocks have a prolonged duration of action in the elderly, approximately 2.5 times longer. This would lead to a slower return of pain and therefore easier titration of postoperative medications.[39] However, elderly patients are frequently at risk for falls before surgery, so greater care must be taken in discharge criteria after a regional anesthetic to make sure they can maintain balance and that the caregiver with whom they will be discharged home is capable of protecting them from falls.

Common Pain Syndromes

Chronic lumbar pain as a result of degenerative arthritis is very common. Osteoarthritis is the most common cause of nociceptive pain in the elderly. Inflammatory pain does respond well to analgesics such as antiinflammatory medications and opioids. Cancer pain, myofascial pain syndromes, postherpetic neuralgia, diabetic polyneuropathy, radiculopathy or amyotrophy, trigeminal neuralgia, and central post-stroke pain (CPSP) syndrome are all common in the elderly. Furthermore, arthritis of the knee, hip, or shoulder are all common problems in the senior population, and surgical replacement is very advanced and highly successful. Diagnosis is easy and fairly certain to be correct.

CPSP is a neuropathic pain syndrome characterized by constant or intermittent pain in a body part occurring after stroke. It is associated with sensory abnormalities in the painful body part. The incidence of CPSP is 8% within the first year, but pain may appear up to 3 years after the stroke. Sixty-three percent of those who develop pain had onset within the first month.[40] Two thirds of those who develop pain experience moderate to severe pain. This 8% incidence of pain with 5% expressing moderate to severe pain is similar to other neuropathic pain syndromes such as phantom limb pain,[41] central pain in spinal cord injury,[42] and pain in diabetic neuropathy.[43]

Back Pain

About two thirds of adults have low back pain at some time. Of the 65 million people in the United States with low back pain, approximately 151,000 undergo fusion of the lumbar spine each year.[44] The number of spinal fusion surgeries is increasing annually, in part, according to Deyo and associates, because of widening indications, including the diagnosis of back pain made by discography.[45,46]

Because of the high rate of unsatisfactory results with open spinal surgery and the more tenuous physical condition of elderly patients to undergo and tolerate open spinal surgery, less-invasive techniques for treating discogenic pain have been developed. One such procedure is percutaneous diskectomy using coablation

technology. This is a percutaneous technique to reduce the volume of internally disrupted disk material.[47] Intrathecal drug delivery has also been effective for control of pain in unremitting low back pain and radicular pain.[48]

For chronic zygapophyseal joint (spinal facet joint) pain, radiofrequency neurotomy of the medial branch of the posterior spinal nerve ramus has been found to be effective in both the cervical and lumbar regions.[49,50]

Although low back pain is a fact of life for a substantial proportion of the population at all ages, the aged have a greater prevalence and experience greater impact on their quality of life than the remainder of the population. At the same time, they are underrepresented in research.[51] Treatment protocols are poorly defined in the elderly. History and a comprehensive evaluation are necessary for an appropriate strategy.[52]

Thoracic and Lumbar Compression Fractures

Epidural injections can be helpful for acute vertebral compression fractures, which are common in the elderly. Continuous epidural infusion of local anesthetic is also an option but requires hospitalization. Vertebroplasty is also an option. This involves a technique designed to consolidate pathologic vertebral bodies through the injection of orthopedic cement under fluoroscopic guidance.[53–55] This procedure has been shown to be safe in frail elderly patients and can improve quality of life.[56]

Spinal Stenosis

Neurogenic claudication is frequently a presenting symptom of lumbar spinal stenosis. The patient complains of pain in the legs with walking which is relieved with rest. Epidural injections can sometimes be helpful in early disease. In advanced disease if surgery is not an option, spinal infusion therapy may be helpful as an alternative.[57]

Herpes Zoster (AHZ, Shingles)

The word *herpes* stems from the Greek *herpein* which means "to creep," whereas *zoster* means "girdle." The disease infects 800,000 people in the United States each year, and the incidence increases with advancing age. The etiopathogenesis of herpes begins after chicken pox, when the varicella virus becomes dormant in a spinal nerve. When reduced cell-mediated immunity occurs, AHZ reactivates. Reactivation leads to infection down the nerve to the skin with the eruption of skin lesions. The inflammation can also travel to reach the spinal cord or the trigeminal brainstem complex.[58]

The first sign of shingles is intense pain or itching, even before the lesions erupt on the skin. It is only along one nerve on one side of the body. Treatment should start as soon as possible with antiviral medication, pain medication, and steroids. Steroids are safe in acute herpes zoster because it is an immunoglobulin G–mediated immune response.[58] Epidural injections usually are helpful only in the first 3 days after eruption. Subcutaneous infiltration of local anesthetic and long-acting steroid can provide relief and accelerate healing. Stellate ganglion sympathetic and superior cervical sympathetic ganglion local anesthetic blocks can be helpful for zoster of the face in the trigeminal distribution. Manabe and associates[59] demonstrated that continuous epidural infusion of local anesthetic can shorten the duration of zoster-associated pain.

Postherpetic Neuralgia

Usually this disease is defined as pain that extends beyond the normal healing period of 6 weeks to 2 months. The pain takes on the characteristics of neuropathic pain with allodynia, and hyperalgesia. The frequency of persistent pain is given in Table 21-4.[60] Aggressive therapy for acute herpes zoster will not prevent the development of postherpetic neuralgia. However, it will change the quality of the pain from the intense unsupportable pain syndrome to a more diffuse, deep aching pain that can be supported.[61]

Treatment options for postherpetic neuralgia have not significantly improved over the years. Analgesics, even traditional opioid analgesics, offer little relief. Methadone can be helpful if the patient can tolerate it. It is a difficult medication to titrate in the elderly. Spinal cord stimulation can be beneficial in about 50% of cases of postherpetic neuralgia if the virus has not affected the dorsal horn of the spinal cord. Lidocaine 5% topical patches have been found to reduce the symptoms of postherpetic neuralgia about 30%–40%. Kotani et al.[62] did report on the use of intrathecal methylprednisolone 60 mg administered with 3 mL of 3% lidocaine once per week for up to 4 weeks as being 70% effective in reducing pain.

TABLE 21-4. Persistent pain in postherpetic neuralgia as a function of age.

Age group	Percentage of patients with pain for <6 months	Percentage of patients with pain for >1 year
0–19	4	4
20–29	2	2
30–39	15	10
40–49	33	7
50–59	49	18
60–69	65	37
>70	74	48

Source: Reprinted with permission from de Moragas and Kierland.[60]

Case Examples

When assessing pain problems and making clinical decisions for therapy in the elderly, the situation is not always what it seems, and care must be taken to not go down the wrong path. Following are two cases that illustrate this problem.

Case 21-1. Lumbar Radiculopathy

A 67-year-old male physician presented with a sudden onset of back and leg pain, with a foot drop. A magnetic resonance imaging (MRI) scan showed a protruding disk with nerve root impingement corresponding to the side of the foot drop. The patient chose not go to a surgeon but instead requested that this author treat him with epidural steroid injection therapy. He received an initial lumbar epidural steroid injection followed by two caudal steroid injections over a 3-week interval. He experienced rapid resolution of all symptoms, including the foot drop, and returned to playing golf again with no return of the foot drop at 3 years after epidural injections. The MRI image is shown in Figure 21-1A (December 10, 2001). Figure 21-1B is a comparison MRI image (January 1, 1995) taken when the patient volunteered to have a scan done for a new scanner that needed calibration. The disk protrusion was present in 1995 but was asymptomatic until 2001. It is also clear that faced with the MRI image of 2001 along with pain and a foot drop, most neurosurgeons would have considered this a surgical emergency (Figure 21-2). It is clear that epidural steroid injections cannot dissolve away a disk protrusion. In this case, however, the problem was an acute nerve root irritation in the presence of a longstanding asymptomatic disk protrusion that did respond to epidural steroid injections.

Steroid injections are efficacious for different spine problems. Epidural steroid injections are being performed under image intensifier needle guidance both by the translaminar approach as well as the transforaminal approach to treat radiculitis and radiculopathy of the cervical as well as the lumbar nerve.[63–65]

Case 21-2. Excessive Treatment in a Missed Diagnosis

An 85-year-old woman who was healthy, ambulatory, and living independently, upon getting out of bed one morning, experienced a sudden onset of right hip pain radiating down her leg. Nothing was done for a week, but she was not able to bear weight on that leg. After a week, she went to her primary doctor who immediately ordered an MRI scan of her lumbar spine. Based on the results of that scan, she was referred to a pain clinic where she

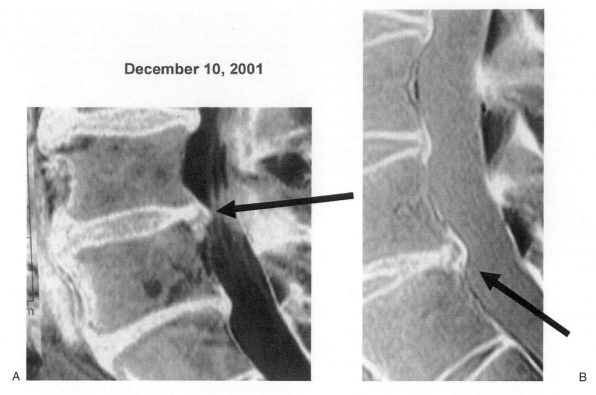

FIGURE 21-1. **A:** MRI from December 10, 2001. The patient was symptomatic of the disk protrusion at L4–5 (arrow). **B:** MRI from January 1, 1995. The patient was asymptomatic of the disk protrusion at L4–5 (arrow).

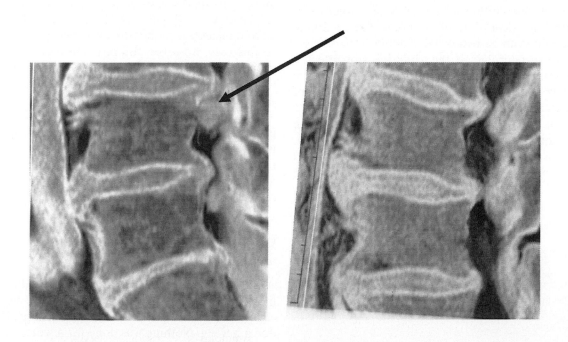

FIGURE 21-2. Significant disk protrusion noted (arrow).

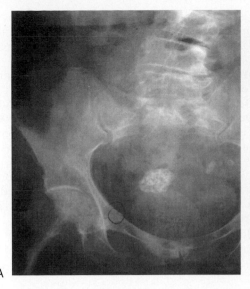
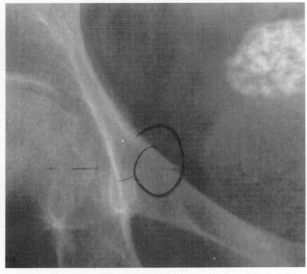

A   B

FIGURE 21-3. **A:** A-P X-ray of the lower lumber spine and pelvis showing extensive discogenic and vertebral body degeneration with scoliosis to the left, osteophytes and endplate abnormali- ties on the left. **B:** Magnified view of the right acetabulum showing the small fracture (circled in black). The patient never complained of back pain.

underwent a series of three translaminar lumbar epidural steroid injections and a left-sided L3 and S1 transforaminal epidural steroid injection without benefit. She continued to be unable to walk. Surgery was recommended for her back, but fortunately the patient declined. After 6 months, she was referred to this author. Upon taking the history and performing an examination, it was clear that the most likely diagnosis was a fracture of the right hip. The patient never complained of back pain and never complained of left-sided leg pain. Her pain was always emanating from her right hip. A plain X-ray was ordered by this author that revealed a fracture of the pelvis close to the acetabulum on the right side. It is a wonder in looking at the X-ray, however, that the patient never did suffer from back pain (Figure 21-3).

Conclusions

The major goal of geriatric care is often comfort and control of the symptoms of chronic disease.[3] The following guidelines are useful in approaching pain management in the elderly:

1. Always ask elderly patients about pain.
2. Accept the patient's word about pain and its intensity.
3. Never underestimate the potential effects of chronic pain on a patient's overall condition and quality of life.
4. Be compulsive in the assessment of pain. An accurate diagnosis will lead to the most effective treatment.
5. Treat pain to facilitate diagnostic procedures. Do not wait for a diagnosis to relieve suffering.
6. Use a combined approach of drug and nondrug strategies when possible.
7. Mobilize patients physically and psychosocially. Involve patients in their therapy.
8. Use analgesic drugs correctly. Start doses low and increase slowly. Achieve adequate doses and anticipate side effects.
9. Anticipate and attend to anxiety and depression.
10. Reassess responses to treatment. Alter therapy to maximize functional status and quality of life.

References

1. Cleeland C. Undertreatment of cancer pain in elderly patients. JAMA 1998;279(23):1914–1915.
2. Ferrell BA, Ferrell BR, Osterweil D. Pain in the nursing home. J Am Geriatr Soc 1990;38:409–414.
3. Ferrell BA. Pain management in elderly people. J Am Geriatr Soc 1991;39:64–73.
4. Chevlen E. Optimizing the use of opioids in the elderly population. Am J Pain Manage Suppl 2004;14(2):19S–24S.
5. Otis J, McGeeney B. Managing pain in the elderly. Clin Geriatr 2001;9:82–88.
6. Fine P. Difficulties and challenges in the treatment of chronic pain in the older adult. Am J Pain Manage 2004;14(2):2S–8S.
7. Parmelee PA, Katz IR, Lawton MP. The relation of pain to depression among institutionalized aged. J Gerontol 1991; 46:15–21.
8. Williamson G, Schulz RL. Pain, activity restriction, and symptoms of depression among community-residing elderly adults. J Gerontol 1992;47:367–372.
9. Casten R, Parmelee P, Kleban M, et al. The relationships among anxiety, depression, and pain in a geriatric institutionalized sample. Pain 1995;61:271–276.

10. Gaston-Johansson F, Johansson F, Johansson C. Pain in the elderly: prevalence, attitudes and assessment. Nurs Home Manage 1996;4(11):325–331.

11. Gaston-Johansson F, Johansson F, Johansson N. Undertreatment of pain in the elderly: causes and prevention. Ann Long-Term Care 1999;7(5):190–196.

12. Postone N. Alexithymia in chronic pain patients. Gen Hosp Psychiatry 1986;8:163–167.

13. Gibson S, Ferrell M. A review of age differences in the neurophysiology of nociception and the perceptual experience of pain. Clin J Pain 2004;20(4):227–239.

14. Shin S, Eisenach J. Peripheral nerve injury sensitizes the response to visceral distension but not its inhibition by the antidepressant Milnacipran. Anesthesiology 2004;100(3): 671–675.

15. Fine P. Pharmacological management of persistent pain in older patients. Clin J Pain 2004;20(4):220–226.

16. Zukerman LA, Ferrante FM. Nonopioid and opioid analgesics. In: Ashburn MA, Rice LJ, eds. The Management of Pain. New York: Churchill-Livingstone; 1998: 111–140.

17. Auburn F, Monsel S, Langeron O, et al. Postoperative titration of intravenous morphine in the elderly patient. Anesthesiology 2002;96(1):17–23.

18. Hagen NA, Elwood T, Ernst S. Cancer pain emergencies: a protocol for management. J Pain Symptom Manage 1997; 14(1):45–50.

19. Cook D, Rooke A. Priorities in perioperative geriatrics. Anesth Analg 2003;96:1823–1836.

20. Dyer C, Ashton C. Postoperative delirium: a review of 80 primary data-collection studies. Arch Intern Med 1995;155(5):461–465.

21. Gustafson Y, Berggren D, Brännström B, et al. Acute confusional states in elderly patients treated for femoral neck fracture. J Am Geriatr Soc 1988;36:525–530.

22. Gagliese L, Jackson M, Ritvo P, et al. Age is not an impediment to effective use of patient controlled analgesia by surgical patients. Anesthesiology 2000;93(3):601–610.

23. Mann C, Pouzeratte Y, Bocarra G, et al. Comparison of intravenous or epidural patient-controlled analgesia in the elderly after major abdominal surgery. Anesthesiology 2000;92(2):433–441.

24. Carli F, Phil M, Mayo N, et al. Epidural analgesia enhances functional exercise capacity and health related quality of life after colonic surgery. Results of a randomized trial. Anesthesiology 2002;97(3):540–549.

25. Jacox A, Carr DB, Payne R, et al. Management of cancer pain. Clinical practice guideline no. 9. AHCPR Publication No. 94–0592. Rockville, MD: Agency for Health Care Policy and Research, U.S. Department of Health and Human Services, Public Health Service; 1994.

26. Weissman DE, Haddox JD. Opioid pseudoaddiction—an iatrogenic syndrome. Pain 1989;36:363–366.

27. Lasagna L, Beecher H. Optimal dose of morphine. J Am Med Assoc 1954;156(3):230–234.

28. Gammaitoni A, Fine P, Alvarez N, et al. Clinical application of opioid equianalgesic data. Clin J Pain 2003;19(5):286–297.

29. Supernaw J. CYP2D6 and the efficacy of codeine-like drugs. Am J Pain Manage 2001;11(1):30–31.

30. Fishbain DA, Fishbain D, Lewis J, et al. Genetic testing for enzymes of drug metabolism: does it have clinical utility for pain medicine at the present time? A structured Review. Pain Med 2004;5(1):81–93.

31. Morley J. New perspectives in our use of opioids. Pain Forum 1999;8(4):200–205.

32. Quality of Life Matters Bulletin 2004;6(1). Published by Quality of Life Publishing Co. Tel: 1–877–513–0099.

33. Teno J, Clarridge B, Casey V, et al. Family perspectives on end-of-life care at the last place of care. JAMA 2004; 291(1):88–93.

34. Sveticic G, Gentilini A, Eichenberger U, et al. Combinations of morphine with ketamine for patient-controlled analgesia. A new optimization method. Anesthesiology 2003;98(5): 1195–1205.

35. Berger JM, Ryan A, Vadivelu N, et al. Use of ketamine-fentanyl-midazolam infusion for the control of symptoms in terminal life care. Am J Hosp Palliat Care 2000;17(2): 127–136.

36. Kellett J. Acute soft tissue injuries—a review of the literature. Med Sci Sports Exerc 1986;18:489–500.

37. Vieth R, Raskind M, Caldwell J, et al. Cardiovascular effects of tricyclic antidepressants in depressed patients with chronic heart disease. N Engl J Med 1982;306:954–959.

38. Greisen J, Juhl C, Grofte T, et al. Acute pain induces insulin resistance in humans. Anesthesiology 2001;95(3):578–584.

39. Paqueron X, Boccara G, Bendahou M, et al. Brachial plexus nerve block exhibits prolonged duration in the elderly. Anesthesiology 2002;97(5):1245–1249.

40. Andersen G, Vestergaard K, Ingeman-Nielsen M, et al. Incidence of central post-stroke pain. Pain 1995;61:187–193.

41. Jensen TS, Rasmussen P. Phantom pain. In: Wall PD, Melzack R, eds. Textbook of Pain. Edinburgh: Churchill-Livingstone; 1994:651–665.

42. Beri'c A, Dimitrijevi'c MA, Lindblom U. Central dysesthesia syndrome in spinal cord injury patients. Pain 1988;34: 109–116.

43. Melton LJ, Dyck PJ. Epidemiology. In: Dyck PJ, Thomas PK, Asbury AK, et al., eds. Diabetic Neuropathy. Philadelphia: Saunders; 1987:27–35.

44. Lipson S. Spinal-fusion surgery—advances and concerns. N Engl J Med 2004;350(7):643–644.

45. Deyo RA, Nachemson A, Mirza SK. Spinal-fusion surgery—the case for restraint. N Engl J Med 2004;350(7):722–726.

46. Cohen SP, Larkin TM, Barna SA, et al. Lumbar discography: a comprehensive review of outcomes studies, diagnostic accuracy, and principles. Reg Anesth Pain Med 2005;30(2):163–183.

47. Singh V, Piryani C, Liao K. Role of percutaneous disc decompression using coblation in managing chronic discogenic low back pain: a prospective, observational study. Pain Phys 2004;7:419–425.

48. Deer T, Chapple I, Classen A, et al. Intrathecal drug delivery for treatment of chronic low back pain: report from the national outcomes registry for low back pain. Pain Med 2004;5(1):6–13.

49. Faclier G, Kay J. Cervical facet radiofrequency neurotomy. Tech Reg Anesth Pain Manage 2000;4(3):120–125.

50. Dreyfuss P, Halbrook B, Pauza K, et al. Efficacy and validity of radiofrequency neurotomy for chronic lumbar zygapophysial joint pain. Spine 2000;25:1270–1277.

51. Manchikanti L. Chronic low back pain in the elderly: Part I. Am J Pain Manage 1997;7(3):104–117.

52. Manchikanti L. Chronic low back pain in the elderly: Part II. Am J Pain Manage 1997;7(4):133–145.

53. Mathis JM, Barr JD, Belkoff SM, et al. Percutaneous vertebroplasty: a developing standard of care for vertebral compression fractures. AJNR Am J Neuroradiol 2001;22: 373–381.

54. Sesay M, Dousset V, Liguoro D, et al. Intraosseous lidocaine provides effective analgesia for percutaneous vertebroplasty of osteoporotic fractures. Can J Anesth 2002;49:137–143.

55. Jensen ME, Evans AJ, Mathis JM, et al. Percutaneous polymethylmethacrylate vertebroplasty in the treatment of osteoporotic vertebral body compression fractures: technical aspects. Am J Neuroradiol 1997;18:1897–1904.

56. McKiernan F, Faciszewski T, Jensen R. Quality of life following vertebroplasty. J Bone Joint Surg 2004;86(12): 2600–2606.

57. Dougherty P, Staats P. Intrathecal drug therapy for chronic pain: from basic science to clinical practice. Anesthesiology 1999;91(6):1891–2003.

58. Toliver KT, Berger JM, Pardo ES. Review of herpes zoster. Semin Anesth 1997;16(2):127–131.

59. Manabe H, Dan K, Hirata K, et al. Optimum pain relief with continuous epidural infusion of local anesthetic shortens the duration of zoster-associated pain. Clin J Pain 2004; 20(5):302–308.

60. de Moragas JM, Kierland RR. The outcome of patients with herpes zoster. AMA Arch Derm 1957;75:193–196.

61. Pardo ES, Berger JM, Toliver KT. Post herpetic neuralgia. Semin Anesth 1997;16(2):132–135.

62. Kotani N, Kushikata T, Hashimoto H, et al. Intrathecal methylprednisolone for intractable postherpetic neuralgia. N Engl J Med 2000;343(21):1514–1519.

63. Abram S. Treatment of lumbosacral radiculopathy with epidural steroids: clinical concepts and commentary. Anesthesiology 1999;91(6):1937–1941.

64. Rowlingson J. Epidural steroids in treating failed back surgery syndrome. Anesth Analg 1999;88:240–242.

65. Fredman B, Nun M, Zohar E, et al. Epidural steroids for treating "failed-back surgery syndrome." Is fluoroscopy really necessary? Anesth Analg 1999;88:367–372.

22
Anesthesia Considerations for Geriatric Outpatients

Kathryn E. McGoldrick

During the past two decades, ambulatory anesthesia has matured and expanded. With ambulatory surgery currently accounting for almost 80% of all surgical procedures performed in the United States, it has become undisputedly the dominant mode of surgical practice in North America, as well as in many of the world's other developed nations. Several factors have contributed to the phenomenal growth of outpatient surgery, including economic pressures; technologic advances that allow minimally invasive surgery; and new, short-acting drugs and anesthetic agents that have dramatically improved our ability to prevent and treat postoperative nausea and vomiting (PONV)[1] and to manage postoperative pain. Nonetheless, ambulatory anesthesiologists cannot afford the luxury of resting on our laurels. To paraphrase the gifted poet, Robert Frost, we still have miles to go before we sleep. . . .

The elderly (≥65 years old) population is the fastest growing demographic segment in the United States as well as in many parts of the developed world. According to the 2000 census, there are 4.2 million Americans age 85 years or older, an increase of 30% since 1990. Those 75–84 years of age number 12.4 million, an increase of >20% since 1990. These realities have profound implications for clinicians, including anesthesiologists and surgeons. Aging, for example, increases the probability that an individual will require surgery. Whereas approximately 12% of those aged 45–60 years undergo surgery annually, this number increases to >21% in those aged ≥65 years.[2] Unfortunately, however, morbidity and mortality are increased in the geriatric population, with steep increases observed after age 75 years. Thus, an aging population has multifaceted implications for the practice of anesthesiology that are evident in the preoperative, intraoperative, and postoperative periods.

In 2000, Dr. Lee A. Fleisher, as the recipient of the first Society for Ambulatory Anesthesia (SAMBA) Outcomes Research Award, began an investigation of the impact of location of care and patient factors on the rate of complications and readmission after outpatient surgery.[3] Not surprisingly, the study determined that age in excess of 85 years, prior inpatient hospital admission within 6 months, invasive surgery, and surgical venue were predictive of unanticipated admission and other adverse outcomes, including death. These findings are suggestive that not all ambulatory facilities—i.e., hospitals, freestanding surgicenters, or office-based operating rooms—are created equal in terms of their ability to successfully manage complicated patients having lengthy, relatively invasive procedures. Clearly, this important work by Dr. Fleisher highlights two major challenges confronting anesthesiologists today: the exigencies and nuances of gerontologic anesthesia and the safety of office-based surgery.

In this context, it is important to appreciate that 15% of all elective surgeries performed in the United States in 2002 were conducted in offices. Indeed, office-based anesthesia is currently the fastest growing segment of anesthesia practice in our country. However, startling death rates associated with office-based anesthesia and surgery have been reported. The death rate for office-based surgery in Florida a few years ago was estimated at 1:8500, and it has been disclosed that the mortality for liposuction may be as high as 1:5000 procedures.[4] Vila and colleagues[5] reviewed all adverse incidents reported to the Florida Board of Medicine from April 2000 until April 2002. Despite the implementation of corrective-action measures by the Board of Medicine for office-based surgery in 2000, the investigators found a more than tenfold increase in rates of adverse incidents (66:100,000 versus 5.3:100,000) and death (9.2:100,000 versus 0.78:100,000) when comparing offices and ambulatory surgery centers, respectively. There are multiple reasons for these alarming findings, and most of them pertain to the lack of regulatory control that is characteristic of private offices, where it is not uncommon to have clerical staff administer sedative-hypnotics and opioids under the "guidance" of the operating physician (who often may be a dermatologist rather than a surgeon). Indeed, only a small minority of states have regulations pertaining to office-based surgery. Therefore, SAMBA and the American Society of Anesthesiologists (ASA) have joined together to ensure the same level of safety in offices as in hospitals or accredited surgicenters. To accomplish this goal, patients and procedures must be appropriately matched to venue, and anesthesia care must be delivered only by those with expertise in the specialty. Frail, complex elderly patients are inappropriate candidates for lengthy, relatively invasive surgical procedures performed in private offices.

Preoperative Evaluation

The preoperative evaluation of the geriatric patient characteristically is more complex than that of the younger patient because of the heterogeneity of seniors and the increased frequency and severity of comorbid conditions associated with aging. The process of aging is highly individualized. Different people age at varying rates and often in different ways. Typically, however, virtually all physiologic systems decline with advancing chronologic age. Nevertheless, chronologic age is a poor surrogate for capturing information about fitness or frailty.[6] Moreover, perioperative functional status can be difficult to quantitate because many elderly patients have reduced preoperative function related to deconditioning, age-associated disease, or cognitive impairment. Thus, it is challenging to satisfactorily evaluate the patient's capacity to respond to the specific stresses associated with anesthesia and surgery. How, for example, does one determine cardiopulmonary reserve in a patient severely limited by osteoarthritis and dementia? Even "normal" aging results in alterations in cardiac, respiratory, neurologic, and renal physiology that are linked to reduced functional reserve and ability to compensate for physiologic stress. Moreover, the consumption of multiple medications so typical of the elderly can alter homeostatic mechanisms.

Preoperative Testing

In the general population, there is strong consensus that most routine tests are not indicated. In the subset of geriatric patients, our knowledge is somewhat more limited. Nonetheless, a recent study on routine preoperative testing in more than 18,000 patients undergoing cataract surgery is worthy of comment. Patients were randomly assigned to undergo or not undergo routine testing (electrocardiogram, complete blood cell count, electrolytes, blood urea nitrogen, creatinine, and glucose).[7] The analysis was stratified by age and disclosed no benefit to routine testing for any group of patients. Similar conclusions were drawn in a smaller study of

elderly noncardiac surgical patients by Dzankic and colleagues.[8] Some physicians and lay people, however, misinterpreted the results of the study by Schein et al.,[7] believing that patients having cataract surgery need no preoperative evaluation. It is vital to note that all patients in this trial received regular medical care and were evaluated by a physician preoperatively. Patients whose medical status indicated a need for preoperative laboratory tests were excluded from the study. Because "routine" testing for the more than 1.5 million cataract patients in the United States is estimated to cost $150 million annually, the favorable economic impact of this "targeted" approach is obvious.

From these investigations and others, a few concepts emerge. First, routine screening in a general population of elderly patients does not significantly augment information obtained from the patient's history. Second, the positive predictive value of abnormal findings on routine screening is limited. Third, positive results on screening tests have modest impact on patient care.

The dearth of population studies of perioperative risk and outcomes specifically addressing the geriatric population can make selecting the most appropriate course of care challenging. Because age itself adds very modest incremental risk in the absence of comorbid disease, most risk-factor identification and risk-predictive indices have focused on specific diseases.[9-11] It is well known, for example, that normal aging produces structural changes in the cardiovascular system, as well as changes in autonomic responsiveness/control, that can compromise hemodynamic stability. The superimposition of such comorbid conditions as angina pectoris or valvular heart disease can further impair cardiovascular performance, especially in the perioperative period.

According to the guidelines of the American College of Cardiology and the American Heart Association for preoperative cardiac evaluation, the patient's activity level, expressed in metabolic units, is a primary determinant of the necessity for further evaluation, along with the results obtained from history and physical examination.[9] These findings are then evaluated in conjunction with due consideration for the invasiveness of the planned surgical procedure. Clearly, the goal of the preoperative evaluation should be the identification of major predictors of cardiac risk such as unstable coronary syndromes [for example, unstable angina or myocardial infarction (MI) <30 days ago], decompensated congestive heart failure, severe valvular disease, and significant arrhythmias. These patients have a prohibitive rate of perioperative morbidity and mortality, and are inappropriate candidates for elective outpatient surgery. In patients with intermediate clinical predictors (mild angina, previous MI >30 days ago, compensated or prior congestive heart failure, diabetes mellitus, or renal insufficiency), the invasiveness of the surgery and the functional status of the patient will have major roles in determining the nature and extent of preoperative testing or intervention. Importantly, no preoperative cardiovascular testing should be performed if the results will not change perioperative management. For those in whom further testing is warranted, there are several options including pharmacologic stress testing and dobutamine stress echocardiography. The use of perioperative betablockade in intermediate- or high-risk patients undergoing vascular surgery can be beneficial and may obviate the need for more invasive interventions.[12] However, there is a dearth of data pertaining to the use of perioperative betablockade in patients undergoing less-invasive outpatient surgery.

Given the heterogeneity of the elderly population, it is reasonable to examine more domains than just cardiopulmonary capacity. A multidimensional approach seems indicated and should include screening for mental status, depression, and alcohol abuse. We have recently come to appreciate that subtle forms of cognitive impairment can predispose to worsened cognitive outcome postoperatively. It is mandatory to appreciate that the elderly patient is at much greater risk for long-term functional compromise after the stress of surgery than is the younger patient. These potential complications include, but are not limited to, aspiration, postoperative delirium and cognitive dysfunction, adverse drug interactions, malnutrition, pressure ulcers, urosepsis, falls, and failure to return to ambulation or to home. Appropriate preoperative optimization may well pay dividends in terms of improving functional status after discharge.

Sleep Apnea

The prevalence of sleep disorders among the general American population is high. Sleep apnea has received increasing attention during the past few decades in tandem with the pandemic of obesity in the United States, as well as the accumulation of research linking obstructive sleep apnea (OSA) to cognitive, behavioral, cardiovascular, and cerebrovascular disease. OSA is defined as the cessation of airflow for >10 seconds during sleep despite persistent respiratory effort by the abdomen and rib cage. OSA is usually associated with a decrease in arterial oxygen saturation of >4%. Although there is no uniform definition of hypopnea, it is characterized by decreased airflow for 10 seconds during sleep and is associated with an oxyhemoglobin desaturation of 3% from baseline. It should be noted for the sake of completeness that the three types of sleep apnea are obstructive, central, and mixed. Central sleep apnea, a much rarer entity than OSA, is also known as Ondine's curse, an allusion to the mythologic man who was condemned by his rejected lover, a mermaid, to stay awake in order to breathe. Unlike OSA, respiratory efforts temporarily stop in central sleep apnea. Diagnosis is established during polysomnography.

Conservative estimates suggest that 2% of middle-aged women and 4% of middle-aged men are afflicted with this disorder.[13] Growing evidence points to a much higher incidence in the elderly.[14,15] Indeed, the prevalence of OSA is two- to threefold greater in older persons (>65 years) compared with those in middle age.[16] Some data actually suggest that OSA in elders is a condition distinct from that of middle age. Bixler and colleagues[17] reported that OSA is less severe in older compared with middle-aged persons, and suggested that central sleep apnea is more common than in younger counterparts. Interestingly, other data suggest that the associations of OSA with hypertension, sleepiness, and cognitive dysfunction are weaker in older versus middle-aged persons.[18]

Obesity is a critical independent causative/risk factor. The majority of people who have OSA are obese and the severity of the condition seems to correlate with the patient's neck circumference.[13] In the minority of patients who are nonobese, causative risk factors are craniofacial and orofacial bony abnormalities, nasal obstruction, and hypertrophied tonsils.[19,20]

The apnea/hypopneic index (AHI) is obtained by performing polysomnography. The number of apneic and hypopneic episodes per hour is recorded, and the patient is assigned a corresponding number. An AHI value between 5 and 14 is associated with mild OSA, 15–30 moderate, and >30 severe OSA.[21]

It is generally accepted that many patients with OSA have resultant daytime sleepiness associated with performance decrements and an increased incidence of work- and driving-related accidents. It has also been well established that patients with severe apnea suffer major health consequences, including premature death, as a result of their condition. Few absolute conclusions can be drawn at this time about the long-term consequences of mild to moderate OSA. However, recently published findings from the Sleep Heart Health Study,[22] the Copenhagen City Heart Study,[23] and others[24] demonstrate a firm association between sleep apnea and systemic hypertension, even after other important patient characteristics, such as age, gender, race, consumption of alcohol, and use of tobacco products are controlled for. Additionally, patients with OSA have been found to have disturbances in inflammatory and coagulation profiles as well as altered vascular responsiveness. Increased sympathetic tone and enhanced platelet aggregation may contribute to the greater incidence of MI and stroke noted in these patients.[25,26] A preoperative assessment of comorbid conditions should be undertaken to detect hypertension, dysrhythmias, previous MI, cerebrovascular disease, and biventricular failure. Polycythemia, electrocardiogram abnormalities including right and left ventricular hypertrophy, and cor pulmonale may be present secondary to

TABLE 22-1. Conditions often associated with sleep apnea.

- Obesity
- Cor pulmonale
- Systemic hypertension
- Dysrhythmias
- Pulmonary hypertension
- ↑ Platelet aggregation
- Right and/or left ventricular hypertrophy
- Inflammatory disturbances
- Polycythemia

pulmonary or systemic hypertension (Table 22-1). The physical examination of a patient with known or suspected OSA should include particular attention to neck circumference, Mallampati class, and signs of redundant oropharyngeal tissue.

In terms of pathophysiology, sleep apnea occurs when the negative airway pressure that develops during inspiration is greater than the muscular distending pressure, causing collapse of the airway. Obstruction can occur throughout the upper airway, above, below, or at the level of the uvula.[27,28] Because there is an inverse relationship between obesity and pharyngeal area, the smaller size of the upper airway in the obese patient causes a more negative pressure to develop for the same inspiratory flow.[28,29] Kuna and Sant'Ambrogio[28] have also postulated that there may be a neurologic basis for the disease in that the neural drive to the airway dilator muscles is insufficient or not coordinated appropriately with the drive to the diaphragm. Obstruction can occur during any sleep state, but is often noted during rapid eye movement sleep. Nasal continuous positive airway pressure (CPAP) can ameliorate the situation by keeping the pressure in the upper airway positive, thus acting as a "splint" to maintain airway patency.

The site(s) of obstruction can be determined preoperatively by such techniques as magnetic resonance imaging, computed tomography studies, and intraluminal pressure measurements during sleep.[30] Some studies suggest that the major site of obstruction in most patients is at the oropharynx, but obstruction can also occur at the nasopharynx, the hypopharynx, and the epiglottis.[31]

CPAP devices, at least in the recent past, were often not well tolerated by patients. However, many technologic advances have been made with positive airway pressure devices, making these gadgets more easily tolerated. Additionally, weight loss may improve OSA, and avoidance of alcohol and sedatives may have beneficial effects. Recently, atrial overdrive pacing has shown promising results in patients with central or OSA.[32] Interestingly, French investigators serendipitously observed that some patients who had received a pacemaker with atrial overdrive pacing to reduce the incidence of atrial dysrhythmias reported a reduction in breathing disorders after pacemaker implantation. These cardiologists, therefore,

initiated a study to investigate the efficacy of atrial overdrive pacing in the treatment of sleep apnea symptoms in consecutive patients who required a pacemaker for conventional indications. They found that atrial pacing at a rate 15 beats per minute faster than the mean nocturnal heart rate resulted in a significant reduction in the number of episodes of both central and obstructive apnea.[32] Postulating that enhanced vagal tone may be associated with (central) sleep apnea, the investigators acknowledged, however, that the mechanism of the amelioration of OSA by atrial overdrive pacing is unclear. Moreover, whether these unexpected findings are germane to the sleep apnea patient with normal cardiac function is uncertain. Gottlieb[33] has tantalizingly suggested that a central mechanism affecting both respiratory rhythm and pharyngeal motor neuron activity would offer the most plausible explanation for the reported equivalence in the improvement of central and OSA during atrial overdrive pacing. Do cardiac vagal afferents also inhibit respiration? Perhaps identification of specific neural pathways might also advance efforts to develop pharmacologic treatment for sleep apnea.

A variety of surgical approaches to treating sleep-related airway obstruction are available. They include classic procedures, such as tonsillectomy, that directly enlarge the upper airway, or tracheotomy to bypass the pharyngeal part of the airway, as well as more specialized procedures to accomplish the former objective. Examples include uvulopalatopharyngoplasty, lingualplasty, and maxillomandibular osteotomy and advancement. Many OSA patients can be managed effectively with one or a combination of therapies.

Few definitive data exist to guide perioperative management of patients with OSA. Therefore, it is not surprising that many anesthesiologists question whether OSA patients are appropriate candidates for ambulatory surgery. The risks of caring for these challenging patients in the ambulatory venue are further amplified by the unfortunate fact that 80%–95% of people with OSA are undiagnosed[34]; they have neither a presumptive clinical and/or a sleep study diagnosis of OSA. This is disconcerting because these patients may suffer perioperatively from life-threatening desaturation and postoperative airway obstruction.

Recently, the ASA Task Force on Perioperative Management of Patients with Obstructive Sleep Apnea published practice guidelines intended to assist in the perioperative management of these challenging patients.[35] The task force members commented that the literature is insufficient to offer guidance regarding which patients with OSA can be safely managed on an outpatient basis, as well as the appropriate time for discharge of OSA patients from the surgical facility. The consultants agreed, however, that procedures typically performed on an outpatient basis in non-OSA patients may also be safely performed on an outpatient basis in patients at increased risk for perioperative OSA when local or regional anesthesia is administered. The consultants were equivocal concerning whether superficial procedures may be safely performed during general anesthesia in outpatients with OSA, and they believe that airway surgery should not be performed on an outpatient basis in patients with OSA. Moreover, the capabilities of the outpatient facility are critical, and the availability of emergency difficult airway equipment, respiratory care equipment, radiology and clinical laboratory facilities, and a transfer agreement with an inpatient facility should be in place if an outpatient facility assumes responsibility for outpatient surgery in OSA patients.[35]

The serious and thoughtful ongoing debate about whether OSA patients should undergo surgery as outpatients suggests there is no one-size-fits-all solution.[34] In deciding a management strategy, it is important to consider the patient's body mass index and neck circumference, the severity of the OSA, the presence or absence of associated cardiopulmonary disease, the nature of the surgery, and the anticipated postoperative opioid requirement (Table 22-2). It seems reasonable to expect that OSA patients without multiple risk factors who are having relatively noninvasive procedures under local or regional anesthesia (carpal tunnel repair, breast biopsy, knee arthroscopy, etc.) typically associated with minimal postoperative pain may be candidates for ambulatory status. However, those individuals with multiple risk factors, those with severe OSA, or those OSA patients having airway surgery, most probably will benefit from a more conservative approach that includes postoperative admission and careful monitoring. It is imperative to appreciate that these patients are exquisitely sensitive to the respiratory depressant effects of opioids and other central nervous system (CNS) depressants. Additionally, the risk of prolonged apnea is increased for as long as 1 week postoperatively.

It is important not to be lulled into a false sense of security simply because general anesthesia is not involved. Certainly, the use of regional anesthesia may not necessarily obviate the need for securing the airway, and may even require emergency airway intervention if excess sedative-hypnotics or opioids are administered. Regardless of the type of anesthesia selected, sedation should be administered judiciously. These patients frequently have

a difficult airway, and often it is more difficult to ventilate them via a mask than it is to intubate them, although the latter may also prove challenging. Moreover, it is important to be aware that the American Sleep Apnea Association[36] notes that "It may be fitting to monitor sleep apnea patients for several hours after the last doses of anesthesia, longer than non-sleep apnea patients require and possibly through one full natural sleep period." Notably, the ASA guidelines indicate that patients with OSA should be monitored for a median of 3 hours longer than their non-OSA counterparts before discharge from the facility. Additionally, they indicated that monitoring of patients with OSA should continue for a median of 7 hours after the last episode of airway obstruction or hypoxemia while breathing room air in an unstimulating environment.[35]

When confronted with an especially challenging OSA patient requiring general anesthesia, a judicious approach may include awake fiberoptic intubation, administering very low-dose, short-acting narcotics, short-acting muscle relaxants, and a low solubility inhalational agent, and infiltrating the surgical site with a long-acting local anesthetic. Extubation should be performed only when the patient is without residual neuromuscular blockade and fully awake, using a tube changer or catheter, and CPAP should be available postoperatively. Elevation of the head of the bed to 30 degrees may facilitate pulmonary excursion. In the postanesthesia care unit (PACU), it is prudent to have a more prolonged period of observation and monitoring in patients with OSA, and it is, therefore, helpful to schedule the procedure early in the day. If no problems occur in the PACU, and the patient has returned to baseline with satisfactory analgesia, the patient is discharged to home. However, if episodes of desaturation or obtundation have occurred, or if analgesia is problematic, it is prudent to admit these high-risk patients to a telemetry ward or intensive care unit because the challenge of maintaining the airway will extend well into the postoperative period. Respiratory events after surgery in OSA patients may occur at any time.

General Principles of Intraoperative Management

General Anesthesia

Because of pulmonary changes (discussed elsewhere in this book) (Table 22-3), it is imperative to appreciate that desaturation occurs faster in older adults. Additionally, elderly patients are more vulnerable to desaturation-related cardiac events. Therefore, proper preoxygenation is critical. Benumof[37] points out that maximal preoxygenation is achieved with 8 breaths of 100% O_2 within 60 seconds with an oxygen flow of 10 L/min.

TABLE 22-2. Factors affecting perioperative management of obstructive sleep apnea.

• Severity of obstructive sleep apnea (apnea/hypopnea index)
• Body mass index and neck circumference
• Comorbid conditions
• Surgical invasiveness
• Anticipated postoperative opioid requirement

Advanced age is clearly associated with a reduction in median effective dose requirements for all agents that act within the CNS regardless of whether these drugs are administered via the oral, parenteral, or inhalational route. Indeed, the median effective dose equivalent for inhalation anesthetics decreases linearly with age, such that the "typical" 80-year-old will require only about two thirds of the anesthetic concentration required to produce comparable effects in a young adult. This reduction in anesthetic requirement is agent-independent and probably reflects fundamental neurophysiologic changes in the brain, such as reduced neuron density or altered concentrations of neurotransmitters.

Elderly patients require less propofol (and other agents) for induction, and it is also important to appreciate that the concurrent use of midazolam, ketamine, and/or opioids with propofol synergistically increases the depth of anesthesia. Moreover, even with an appropriate dose reduction of propofol, hypotension is common. Less hypotension has been reported with appropriately titrated administration of mask sevoflurane for induction compared with a propofol infusion.[38] Interestingly, gender differences have been described in the pharmacokinetics of propofol given by continuous infusion in elderly patients,[39] but data in this area have been inconsistent.

The time required for clinical recovery from neuromuscular blockade is markedly increased in older adults for nondepolarizing agents that undergo organ-based clearance from plasma, but is minimally different for atracurium, cisatracurium, or mivacurium because they undergo hydrolysis in plasma. The likelihood of postoperative pulmonary complications after long-acting muscle relaxants increases with advanced age, and it is not unusual for patients who meet rigorous extubation criteria in the operating room to deteriorate in the PACU. Therefore, it seems advisable to administer a short- or intermediate-acting muscle relaxant to any elderly patient for whom extubation is planned at the end of the surgical procedure (Table 22-4).

In planning an expeditious emergence, the anesthesiologist should be aware that end-tidal gas monitoring significantly underestimates the brain concentration of the more soluble agents. Failure to appreciate this hyster-

TABLE 22-3. Pulmonary changes associated with aging.

- Reduced chest wall compliance, elastic recoil, and maximal minute ventilation
- Increased work of breathing
- Increased closing volume
- Reduced forced expiratory volume in 1 second
- Increased ventilation-perfusion mismatch, diffusion block, and anatomic shunt
- Progressive decline in arterial oxygen tension
- Disproportionately high incidence of postoperative respiratory complications

TABLE 22-4. Recommendations for geriatric outpatients having general anesthesia.

- Appropriate preoxygenation
- ↓↓ Dose of anesthetic agents
- Prevent hypotension by maintaining euvolemia and carefully titrating appropriate agents
- Select shorter-acting drugs, including neuromuscular blockers
- ? Role of bispectral index monitoring
- Transport to postanesthesia care unit with oxygen
- Maintain normothermia and provide adequate analgesia

esis effect leads to prolonged emergence. Moreover, MAC_{awake} is more favorable if the vaporizer is turned down gradually rather than turned off abruptly.[40] Not surprisingly, it has been reported that use of shorter-acting drugs (propofol, desflurane, sevoflurane), in conjunction with bispectral index (BIS) monitoring, can provide more rapid emergence in geriatric patients and facilitate PACU bypass.[41] Whether this approach will have a favorable effect on longer-term outcomes remains to be determined. Interestingly, a recent study reported that advancing age and deeper intraoperative anesthetic levels are associated with higher first-year death rates, and the authors recommended keeping the BIS level under general anesthesia close to 60 rather than in the 40 range.[42] Additionally, because of the abnormalities in gas exchange characteristic of the elderly, it is recommended that they be transported to the PACU with 2–4 L/min of oxygen via nasal cannula, even after relatively minor ambulatory surgery.[43]

Regional Anesthesia

When one considers selection of anesthetic technique, it is important to appreciate that there are no controlled, randomized studies in elderly patients to show that regional anesthesia is superior to general anesthesia for ambulatory surgery. Indeed, neuraxial, plexus, or nerve blocks in the elderly may be associated with an increased risk of persistent numbness, nerve palsies, and other neurologic complications. Additionally, it has recently been demonstrated that age is a major determinant of duration of complete motor and sensory blockade with peripheral nerve block, perhaps reflecting increased sensitivity to conduction failure from local anesthetic agents in peripheral nerves in the elderly population.[44] That said, peripheral nerve blocks offer some appealing features, especially in terms of postoperative pain control. Clonidine is a valuable adjunct because it enhances both local anesthetic and narcotic efficacy, and its addition to the local anesthetic mixture may afford some hemodynamic advantages compared with epinephrine. However, one should select a dose of clonidine that will not produce postoperative sedation or hypotension. When administering central neuraxial blockade to elderly patients, it is important to remember that a given dose will produce a higher level of block in seniors and is typically accompanied by a greater incidence and degree of hypotension and bradycardia as well as a longer duration of anesthesia.[45] Sedation requirements are dramatically reduced under conditions of central neuraxial block.[46] Sensory input to the brain is attenuated and the BIS_{50} is shifted to a higher index. Although recent data have supported a relaxation of the requirements for voiding before discharge after outpatient neuraxial blockade with short-acting drugs for low-risk surgical procedures in low-risk patients, it is important to appreciate that elderly patients do not meet these criteria.[47] Currently, it seems that elderly (≥ 70 years) patients who received neuraxial block, regardless of the duration of the block, should be required to demonstrate ability to void before discharge.

Monitored Anesthesia Care

Monitored anesthesia care with intravenous sedation has become increasingly important in the ambulatory venue for a variety of cogent reasons. Advances in surgical technology have enabled many procedures to be performed through an endoscope rather than a surgical incision, and these procedures that previously required general or major regional anesthesia can now be accomplished with local anesthesia plus sedation. Similarly, technologic advances in the expanding area of diagnostics have created an augmented demand for monitored anesthesia care. Additionally, demographic shifts have seen a steady growth in the proportion of geriatric patients with coexisting medical conditions that benefit from minimally invasive surgical and anesthetic techniques. Finally, as patients become more knowledgeable "consumers," they frequently request anesthetic techniques that will obviate the side effects associated with general or neuraxial anesthesia and that will facilitate the most rapid return to their normal activities. Monitored anesthesia care nicely dovetails with these exigencies.

Monitored anesthesia care is typically selected for patients who require supervision of vital signs and administration of sedative/anxiolytic drugs to supplement local infiltration or regional anesthesia, or to provide sedation during uncomfortable or unpleasant diagnostic procedures. In everyday clinical practice, monitored anesthesia care usually connotes an anesthetic state ranging from conscious sedation to deep sedation. However, it is imperative to appreciate that sedation is a continuum, and it is not always possible to predict how an individual patient will respond to a given dose of drug.

The major objective of outpatient anesthesia is to provide a balance between patient comfort and patient safety while preventing hemodynamic or respiratory instability, or delay in recovery. Sedation techniques encompass the use of sedatives, hypnotics, analgesics, and subanesthetic concentrations of inhalational anesthetics alone or in combination to supplement local or regional anesthesia. These classes of drug, when combined, confer three important components of sedation: amnesia, anxiolysis, and analgesia.

It is essential to appreciate that the technique of sedation is as much an art as a science, and facility is gained best through experience, sensitivity, and proper patient and surgeon selection. Monitored anesthesia care is recommended for patients who fear or reject general anesthesia or who are at increased risk because of age or certain coexisting medical conditions. Monitored anesthesia care must be used with caution, however, for extremely anxious, impaired, or uncooperative patients. Similarly, monitored anesthesia care is not a panacea for certain types of medical problems. For example, patients with severe coronary artery disease or certain morbidly obese patients might be managed with a greater degree of control under general anesthesia. Additionally, the surgeon must be comfortable operating on an awake patient and must be capable of working gently and with alacrity. The outpatient procedures that lend themselves to management with monitored anesthesia care include arthroscopy, biopsies, blepharoplasty and other types of superficial skin procedures, bronchoscopy, carpal tunnel repair and other types of upper extremity surgery, cataract extraction as well as retina and vitrectomy surgery, cystoscopy, dilatation and curettage, dental surgery, gastrointestinal endoscopy, insertion of lines and shunts, herniorrhaphy, rhinoplasty, and rhytidectomy. Similarly, many diagnostic cardiologic and radiologic procedures are conducted smoothly and expeditiously under monitored anesthesia care.

Agents frequently used for monitored anesthesia care, either alone or in combination, include midazolam, propofol, fentanyl, and remifentanil. Interpatient variability is marked with midazolam, and it is important to appreciate that some patients may be exquisitely sensitive to its pharmacologic effects. Indeed, when midazolam initially was introduced to clinicians, reports soon began to circulate of deaths from unrecognized airway obstruction, apnea, and hypoxia predominantly in older patients with concomitant respiratory or cardiovascular disease. The package insert was appropriately revised to include warnings about the necessity of careful monitoring, ability to manage the airway, and immediate availability of emergency resuscitation equipment. It is imperative to appreciate that midazolam depresses the slope of the carbon dioxide response curve, and attenuates the ventilatory response to hypoxia. Apnea is not uncommonly encountered. The apparent steepness of the dose-response curve seen with midazolam underscores the necessity for meticulous titration and careful monitoring. In geriatric or debilitated patients, elimination is slower and the dose should be adjusted downward. Moreover, effects are synergistic with narcotics. Indeed, when combined with barbiturates, narcotics, or propofol, the dose of midazolam should be reduced by at least 25% in young, healthy patients. This dose reduction should be much more marked (i.e., ≥50%) initially in elderly and frail individuals. Although flumazenil may have limited ability to reverse benzodiazepine-induced respiratory depression,[48] it is thought to have efficacy in reversing the benzodiazepine component of apnea associated with administration of midazolam-opioid combinations.[49] Because the half-life of flumazenil is approximately only 1 hour, the potential for resedation exists and has been reported. Therefore, it is incumbent upon clinicians to monitor patients carefully for at least 2 hours after administration of flumazenil.

Propofol possesses a short context-sensitive half-life and a high plasma clearance that produce a rapid, clear-headed awakening when used as the sole agent even after a prolonged continuous infusion. Propofol does, however, cause a dose-dependent reduction in arterial blood pressure and it should be used with caution, if at all, in hypovolemic patients. The respiratory effects of low-dose propofol are moderate. To avoid the unwanted hemodynamic side effects associated with relative overdosage, it is critical to reduce initial doses by approximately 40% in the elderly, even for conscious sedation.[50] Additionally, it is important to appreciate that recovery of psychomotor function after propofol sedation is prolonged in geriatric patients.[51]

Remifentanil, the most recently introduced opioid and an ultrashort-acting fentanyl analog, has a truncated onset, resembling that of alfentanil, and a high metabolic clearance. Its most relevant advantage, however, is its brief context-sensitive half-life (approximately 3 minutes) that is independent of the duration of the infusion. Remifentanil's high lipid solubility and relatively high unbound un-ionized fraction at physiologic pH result in peak effect compartment concentration within 1–2 minutes after bolus administration.[52,53] Likewise, distribution and widespread esterase metabolism of remifentanil allow for early offset and return of spontaneous ventilation.[54] Although remifentanil is unique among the opioids in terms of its metabolism and brief context-sensitive half-life, remifentanil shares the typical opioid-related side effects of bradycardia and potential to produce chest wall rigidity and nausea/vomiting.

Nuances pertaining to dosing of remifentanil merit discussion. Elderly patients require less remifentanil because of altered pharmacokinetics and pharmacodynamics that involve a substantial reduction in central compartment volume and clearance, and reduction in median effective concentration and the equilibration between plasma and its effect compartment.[55] It has also been reported that adjusting pharmacokinetic models to lean body mass improve model performance.[55,56] These results suggest that the dosing of remifentanil should be adjusted to the lean body mass and that geriatric patients require as much as 50%–70% dosage reduction.

Remifentanil has been used effectively by bolus injection for intensely stimulating procedures of brief duration, such as awake laryngoscopy.[57] Because of the relative absence of residual opioid effect, prudent use of remifentanil requires adjunctive analgesics to maintain satisfactory postoperative analgesia after painful procedures. This is often accomplished with a combination of nonopioid analgesics given well in advance of remifentanil discontinuation, often at or before induction or toward the completion of surgery. Examples of this multimodal approach to analgesia include preoperative oral administration of an appropriate nonsteroidal antiinflammatory drug followed by infiltration of the wound with local anesthetic.

It is, perhaps, easy to be lulled into a false sense of security when one is involved in "only" a monitored anesthesia care anesthetic for a healthy patient. This misperception, combined with the production pressures inherent in contemporary clinical practice, can lead to tragic outcomes. Unfortunately, the literature is replete with reports of adverse events associated with sedation techniques.[58-60] Some of these catastrophes reflect performance in remote locations with inadequate monitoring and sedation administered by individuals not thoroughly trained in monitoring, pharmacology, airway management, and resuscitation.

Even in the skilled hands of an experienced anesthesiologist, monitored anesthesia care can be challenging. Patients expected to be most susceptible to the effects of these medications are those at the extremes of age, the obese, those given additive or synergistic drug combinations, and those with cardiopulmonary, renal, or hepatic disease.

According to data from the Food and Drug Administration, midazolam was implicated in at least 80 deaths during gastrointestinal endoscopy, which occurred mainly in the absence of monitoring by an anesthesiologist.[58] Respiratory events were responsible for the majority of the incidents, and most patients had also received an opioid.

In a study by Cohen of 100,000 anesthetics, monitored anesthesia care morbidity was 208/10,000, higher than that associated with either general anesthesia or regional techniques.[61] In fact, during the 1990s, monitored anesthesia care medicolegal claims became more common, accounting for 6% of the cases in the Closed Claims database.[62] Sixty-five percent of the monitored anesthesia care patients involved were older, sicker (ASA physical status 3–5) outpatients. In contradistinction to most ambulatory claims that tend to involve rather minor types of injuries in healthier patients,[63] the monitored anesthesia care claims reflected more severe injuries, with death (39%) and brain damage (15%) common. Moreover, payments were high (similar to that for general anesthesia), and the mechanism of injury was often respiratory (25%) or cardiovascular (14%). It is troubling that litigation from monitored anesthesia care–related injury increased during the 1990s, despite the use of pulse oximetry and other respiratory monitoring. The sine qua non of safety is that the provider must have a profound respect for the continuum from anxiolysis to unconsciousness. Adherence to uniform standards is critical. Patients receiving monitored anesthesia care should benefit from the same level of preoperative, intraoperative, and postoperative vigilance as patients receiving general or regional anesthesia. Therefore, it is imperative that patients be monitored appropriately by qualified personnel who are knowledgeable about pharmacokinetics and pharmacodynamics, especially in the gerontologic population, and who are experienced in airway management and resuscitation. The recent development of ultrashort-acting drugs such as remifentanil, new techniques of administration (e.g., patient-controlled sedation and target-controlled infusions), and monitoring devices such as the BIS may further optimize intraoperative conditions and expedite recovery, thereby enhancing the safety, efficiency, and cost-effectiveness of ambulatory surgery.

Pain Management Pitfalls

Many elderly individuals suffer from acute or chronic pain and increasingly seek treatment for their condition. Depression is common in the elderly and is especially likely to be encountered in the geriatric patient with chronic pain. Given the increased prevalence of pain management options and facilities that became available in the 1990s, it is not surprising that the overall percentage of chronic pain management claims in the Closed Claims increased from 2%–3% in the 1970s and 1980s to 10% in the 1990s. The overwhelming majority (97%) of pain litigation in the claims database involved invasive procedures such as blocks, injections, ablative procedures, and insertion and/or removal of implantable pumps or stimulators.[64] Although nerve injury and pneumothorax were the most common adverse outcomes in pain management claims, devastatingly serious injuries involving brain damage occurred also.

Nerve injury was the most common complication of invasive pain management procedures; tragically, half of the 63 nerve injury claims involved spinal cord injury. Epidural hematoma was a common mechanism of spinal cord injury. Therefore, the anesthesiologist should have a high index of suspicion concerning any unexpected motor or sensory findings after performance of neuraxial blockade, and should carefully monitor patients for an extended time after performance of the procedure.

Twenty-one percent of pain management claims were related to pneumothorax, which was associated primarily with intercostal nerve blocks, trigger point injections, and stellate ganglion blocks. Interestingly, in nearly two thirds (64%) of chronic pain management claims, the injury became apparent only after discharge from the treatment facility. Because this temporal association was noted in some of the cases of pneumothorax, it is important to instruct patients about the signs and symptoms of pneumothorax after intercostal nerve blocks, stellate ganglion blocks, trigger point injections, and brachial plexus blocks. Additionally, it is critical to be vigilant with implantable device procedures in which pump programming errors, drug overdose, and concomitant use of other CNS depressants can result in death or brain damage.

Postoperative Management

Most surgical morbidity and mortality occur in the postoperative period.[65] This incontrovertible fact has multifaceted implications for management of the geriatric outpatient.

Postoperative Respiratory Insufficiency

Postoperative hypoxemia may occur in 20%–60% of elderly surgical patients.[66] As highlighted previously, gerontologic patients have an increased alveolar-arterial gradient, reduced respiratory muscle strength, and blunted hypoxic and hypercarbic drives at baseline. Additionally, there is progressive loss of airway reflexes with age, and apnea and periodic breathing after administration of narcotics are more common.[67,68] Postoperative pain, atelectasis, and shivering further increase the likelihood of respiratory complications. The supine position during recovery increases the transpulmonary shunt, making hypoxemia more likely. Finally, orthopedic, upper abdominal, and intrathoracic procedures, which are common in elderly persons, have an independent effect in exacerbating postoperative hypoxemia and other respiratory complications.[69,70] Fortunately, these types of procedures—with the possible exception of laparoscopic cholecystectomy and minor orthopedic interventions—are not performed on patients in the ambulatory setting. Nonetheless, as ambulatory surgical centers become increasingly more inundated with patients, continued pressure is applied to truncate the time to discharge. Clearly, such tactics may not be in the best interests of our geriatric patients who should be observed carefully for signs of hypoxemia or apnea.

The anesthesiologist must be mindful of the risk of postoperative aspiration in the elderly surgical patient. Because of alterations in pharyngeal function, diminished cough, and a higher incidence of gastroesophageal reflux, elderly patients have an accentuated risk of aspiration.[71,72] This risk is compounded by the effects of anesthesia, sedatives, and narcotics, as well as by such interventions as endotracheal intubation, nasogastric tube placement, and upper abdominal or neck surgery.[73–75] Most probably, pharyngeal manipulation alters sensation, motor function, and the protective reflexes that prevent aspiration. The duration of this effect after extubation is often presumed to be a function of the duration of endotracheal intubation or other forms of pharyngeal trespass. If so, this may offer some reassurance to the ambulatory anesthesiologist. Nonetheless, although the incidence of perioperative aspiration is low and is rarely associated with clinically important pneumonitis or pneumonia,[76] the risk for aspiration extends well beyond the immediate postoperative period. Clearly, additional research is needed in the areas of restoration of pharyngeal and tracheal reflexes, as well as the advancement of feeding after surgery in the elderly.[77] It seems prudent for the ambulatory anesthesiologist to alert the geriatric patient and family members to this potential hazard and to adjust oral intake accordingly for 24–48 hours postoperatively.

Hypothermia

Because of altered autonomic function, perioperative hypothermia is prevalent in both young and elderly surgical patients, but it is more frequent, pronounced, and prolonged in the elderly who have compromised ability to regain thermoregulatory control quickly.[78] Adverse consequences of postoperative hypothermia include cardiac ischemia, arrhythmias, increased blood loss, wound infection, decreased drug metabolism, and prolonged hospitalization.[79] Indeed, it has been shown that maintaining normothermia decreases cardiac morbidity by 55%.[80]

Postoperative Pain

Postoperative pain increases the risk of adverse outcome in elderly patients by contributing to cardiac ischemia, tachycardia, hypertension, and hypoxemia. Effective analgesia can decrease the incidence of myocardial ischemia and pulmonary complications, accelerate recovery, promote early mobilization, shorten hospital stay, and reduce medical care costs. However, postoperative pain control often is inadequate in the elderly[81] because of concerns about drug overdose, adverse response, drug interactions, and other issues. Pain control is further complicated by the fact that the patient's perception and expression of pain often are affected by changes in mental status. Current postoperative analgesic techniques include the use of opioids by various routes, nonsteroidal antiinflammatory drugs, local anesthetic techniques (neuroax-

ial, intraarticular, peripheral nerve block, etc.), and nonpharmacologic (transcutaneous or percutaneous electrical nerve stimulation, acupuncture, acupressure, etc.) methods. Preemptive, multimodal approaches are favored to minimize the risk of such opioid-related side effects as hypoxemia, constipation, and pruritus. A balanced analgesic technique combining opioids, nonopioids, and local anesthetic agents is recommended.

Clearly, the elderly person is extremely vulnerable to drug interactions and has an enhanced probability of respiratory depression, urinary retention, ileus, constipation, and postoperative falls. The likelihood of these complications can be influenced by the selection of analgesics and, possibly, the route of administration.[82–85] Drugs such as clonidine, dexmedetomidine, or the nonsteroidal antiinflammatory agents may have a valuable role in reducing side effects attributable to opioids. It is imperative to be cognizant of the investigation by Bates and colleagues[86] demonstrating that analgesics are the class of drugs associated not only with the highest number of adverse events, but also with the greatest number of preventable adverse events. Other significant offenders are sedatives and antibiotics.

Postoperative Atrial Fibrillation

In terms of cardiac function, it is well known that geriatric patients have decreased beta-adrenergic responsiveness, and they experience an increased incidence of conduction abnormalities, bradyarrhythmias, and hypertension. Fibrotic infiltration of cardiac conduction pathways and replacement of myocardial elastic fibers render the elderly individual vulnerable to conduction delay and to atrial and ventricular ectopy. Indeed, it is well known that postoperative atrial arrhythmias, and atrial fibrillation (AF) and flutter specifically, are seen in 6.1% of elderly patients undergoing noncardiothoracic surgery and in 10%–40% of patients after cardiothoracic operations.[87–90] Although it has been firmly established that older age (>60 years) is the strongest predictor of postoperative AF, a recent investigation found that a greater preoperative heart rate (≥74 beats per minute) is also independently associated with postoperative AF.[91] This suggests that a lower vagal tone before surgery may be a contributing trigger of this arrhythmia. Interestingly, AF occurred at a median of 69 hours after surgery. Because reliance on atrial "kick" is critically important for older adults, should we prophylactically treat high-risk patients to prevent postoperative AF? If so, should we use rate control or rhythm control drugs? These are unanswered questions and offer inviting opportunities for important research. However, given the types of procedures that are typically conducted on an ambulatory basis, geriatric outpatients may be at less risk for this complication than their inpatient counterparts.

Postoperative Cognitive Impairment

Reports of postoperative cognitive deterioration in elderly patients surfaced more than a century ago, and anesthesia had often been implicated as a possible cause or contributing factor. Although improvements in surgical techniques and anesthetic agents and methods have led to improved outcomes in the elderly, a troubling proportion of these patients experience postoperative cognitive impairment.[92-95] The implications of this abrupt cognitive decline are devastating because affected individuals often become dependent and withdraw from society. Sadly, our knowledge about the CNS effects of anesthetics on the aging brain is rather primitive. However, the previously described age-associated changes imply that the aging CNS has reduced functional reserve, similar to the heart, lungs, and kidneys. Perhaps this putative reduction in brain functional reserve renders the elderly more likely to develop postoperative cognitive disturbances.

The syndromes of postoperative cognitive impairment can be classified into two main categories: postoperative delirium and postoperative cognitive dysfunction (POCD).[96] Although postoperative delirium and POCD may have similar predisposing factors, they are not equivalent syndromes. Delirium is defined as an acute change in cognitive function that develops over a brief period of time, often lasting for a few days to a few weeks, and frequently has a fluctuating course. Onset is typically on the first to third postoperative day, and the patient's confusion tends to wax and wane. Prospective studies have cited an incidence of delirium that ranges from 3% to >50% and is dependent on the type of surgery, the patient's preoperative physical and cognitive status, and the age of the patient.[96] The etiology of delirium is probably multifactorial and may include drug intoxication or withdrawal, drug interaction, anticholinergic agents, metabolic disturbances, hypoxia, abnormal carbon dioxide levels, sepsis, inadequate analgesia, and organic brain disease.[97] Curiously, the incidence of postoperative confusion is similar regardless of whether spinal, epidural, or general anesthesia is used.[93] It has been postulated that postoperative delirium may be associated with failure of CNS cholinergic transmission.[98] It has also been suggested that pain, sleep deprivation, sensory deprivation or overload, and an unfamiliar environment may contribute to delirium. Recently, the use of melatonin to treat delirium has produced some benefit, presumably by resetting the circadian sleep–awake cycle of older surgical patients.[99] Postoperative delirium is common in the elderly and its incidence may be reduced by protocol-driven perioperative treatment. Marcantonio and colleagues,[100] in a study of orthopedic inpatients, reported a reduction in postoperative delirium by one third, and of severe delirium by half, by adherence to multifaceted

recommendations that included elimination or minimization of benzodiazepines, anticholinergics, antihistaminics, and meperidine. Additionally, systolic blood pressure was kept more than two thirds of baseline or >90 mm Hg, oxygen saturation was maintained at >90% (preferably >95%), hematocrit was maintained at >30%, early mobilization was encouraged, and appropriate environmental stimuli were provided. Because ambulatory patients return home to a familiar environment postoperatively where appropriate stimuli and support are available, one suspects that the incidence of delirium may be less in outpatients than in their hospitalized counterparts.

POCD is defined as a "deterioration of intellectual function presenting as impaired memory or concentration."[101] The clinical features of this disorder range from mild forgetfulness to permanent cognitive impairment. We have much to learn about the pathogenesis and prevention of POCD. A current hypothesis is that the etiology is multifactorial and may include impaired preoperative cognitive status, as well as intraoperative events related to the surgery itself (e.g., microemboli), and anesthetic agents/depth. Additionally, physiologic and sociologic consequences of hospitalization and surgery may have a role.

Moller and colleagues[92] in a multinational study evaluated cognitive function in patients aged 60 years or older after *major* abdominal and orthopedic surgery. These investigators found that approximately 25% of the patients had measurable cognitive dysfunction a week after their surgery and 10% had cognitive changes 3 months postoperatively. This finding contrasted with a 3% incidence of cognitive deterioration 3 months later in healthy control subjects in the same age range who did not undergo anesthesia and surgery. Interestingly, despite extensive monitoring, neither hypoxemia nor hypotension correlated with the occurrence of prolonged cognitive dysfunction. The identified risk factors for early POCD were increasing age and duration of anesthesia, low education level, a need for a second operation, postoperative infection, and respiratory complications. The only risk factor for late POCD was age. Although the incidence of late POCD was 14% for patients ≥70 years, this rate decreased to only 7% for patients between the ages of 60 to 70 years.

An additional large, prospective study conducted by Monk and colleagues[95] evaluated the relationship of age to POCD. Using the same methodology as the first multinational study,[92] Monk and colleagues reported that cognitive decline occurred in 16% of patients aged 60 years or older at 3 months after major noncardiac surgery, but was present in only 3%–5% of younger patients.[94] This study also determined that rates of cognitive decline were higher in those ≥70 years compared with younger elderly patients. Interestingly, anesthetic technique does not seem to matter; there is no difference between regional and general anesthesia in the incidence of cognitive impairment 3–6 months postoperatively even though short-term recovery may be better with regional anesthesia.[93,102]

There are few prospective studies on long-term cognitive outcomes after *outpatient* surgery, but an analysis of cognitive recovery after major and minimally invasive surgery exists. Monk classified the type of surgical procedure as minimally invasive (laparoscopic or superficial surgery), major intraabdominal surgery, or orthopedic surgery.[95] The incidence of POCD was significantly greater for patients undergoing major or orthopedic procedures compared with minimally invasive surgery. Because outpatient surgery is usually minimally invasive, these results suggest that outpatients may have a better cognitive outcome than patients who require hospitalization. The International Study of Postoperative Cognitive Dysfunction group recently conducted a longitudinal study comparing the incidence of POCD after inpatient versus outpatient surgery in patients older than 60 years.[103] At 7 days after surgery, the incidence of POCD was significantly lower in the outpatient group, but this difference was not detected 3 months later. These results suggest that elderly outpatients have better cognitive outcomes at discharge than elderly inpatients, but we currently have no explanation for the difference. Possible explanations for the improved early outcome in outpatients include the healthier status of patients who qualify for outpatient surgery, the briefer surgical and anesthesia times, the minimally invasive nature of most outpatient procedures, or avoidance of hospitalization.

Although we have much to learn about postoperative delirium and cognitive decline, it is clear that subclinical decrements in functional status may become evident during the perioperative period. Indeed, if a cognitive deficit is noted preoperatively, it may be a harbinger of further postoperative decline. The data on the predictive value of preoperative cognitive status[104] and the ability of that assessment to result in successful intervention (as may be the case with delirium)[100,105] offer compelling reasons to conduct a simple, brief mental status examination as part of the preoperative interview.

It is important to understand that full return of cognitive function to preoperative levels may require several days, even after ambulatory surgery in young, healthy patients.[97,106] Indeed, Lichtor et al.[107] have suggested that even young adults may be sleepy for 8 hours after receiving intravenous sedation with midazolam and fentanyl, and the elderly outpatient with balance disturbances or age-related gait impairment may be at high risk of falling because of residual drowsiness. Moreover, Monk et al.[95] have reported that POCD is detected with psychometric testing in 34% of young (aged 18–39 years), 35% of middle-aged (40–59 years), and 40% of elderly (aged ≥60 years) patients 1 week postoperatively. Similarly,

Johnson[108] has reported a 19.6% incidence of POCD at 1 week postoperatively in patients aged 40–60 years. This rate decreased to 6.2% at 3 months.

Nonetheless, it remains unclear which patient populations are most vulnerable and what the causative factors might be for the serious problem of POCD. As mentioned, there seems to be no difference in the incidence of POCD whether regional or general anesthesia is administered.[93,102,109] Hopefully, future studies will lead to a clearer definition of the incidence, mechanisms, and prevention of POCD.

Other Postdischarge Concerns

Although the Aldrete guidelines offer a satisfactory paradigm to determine when an inpatient is fit for discharge from the PACU to an overnight bed, or when an outpatient is able to bypass phase I recovery and go directly to a step-down unit, the Aldrete criteria are inadequate to assess fitness for discharge to home in an ambulatory patient. To that end, Chung[110] has developed a modified postanesthesia discharge scoring system (PADSS) that addresses this need. Whereas the Aldrete score focuses on activity (ability to move the extremities), respiration, blood pressure, level of consciousness, and color, the modified PADSS assesses such additional and germane parameters as ability to ambulate without dizziness, nausea and vomiting, pain, and surgical bleeding (Table 22-5).

Typically, PONV and pain are two of the most common reasons for unanticipated admission after planned outpatient surgery.[111] Apfel and colleagues[112] have shown that the four most relevant risk factors for predicting PONV are female gender, previous PONV or motion sickness, nonsmoking status, and postoperative opioid use. The

TABLE 22-5. Modified postanesthesia discharge scoring system.

Vital signs	2 = within 20% of baseline
	1 = 20%–40% of baseline
	0 = 40% of baseline
Ambulation and mental status	2 = steady gait, no dizziness
	1 = walks with assistance
	0 = none/dizziness
Nausea and vomiting	2 = minimal
	1 = moderate
	0 = severe
Pain	2 = minimal
	1 = moderate
	0 = severe
Surgical bleeding	2 = minimal
	1 = moderate
	0 = severe

Source: Reprinted from Chung,[110] with permission from Elsevier.
Note: Total postanesthesia discharge scoring system score is 10; score ≥9 considered fit for discharge.

Sinclair score requires a probability calculation based on the same first three factors as well as the age of the patient and the duration and type of surgery.[113] Fortunately, the risk of PONV is said to decrease 17% with each decade after age 50.

Transient, subclinical hearing loss is not uncommon after spinal anesthesia.[114,115] The pathophysiology is thought to involve movement of perilymph from the ear into the subarachnoid space as cerebrospinal fluid leaks out. The perilymph enters the subarachnoid space via the cochlear aqueduct; the resultant increase in endolymphatic pressure in the ear is thought to contribute to the diminished hearing. It has been demonstrated that the rate of mild hearing loss after spinal anesthesia varies inversely with the patient's age. A recent investigation disclosed that both the incidence and degree of hearing loss were increased in patients aged ≤30 years.[115] Perhaps cerebrospinal fluid leakage after dural puncture occurs more frequently and more extensively in the young, and possibly this phenomenon also accounts for the much greater incidence of postdural puncture headache in the young.

It is imperative that elderly outpatients be discharged from an outpatient surgery facility only if accompanied by an escort, and a competent individual should remain with the patient for at least 24 hours postoperatively. Geriatric patients are at higher risk for drowsiness, confusion, falls, urinary retention, and adverse drug interactions than their younger counterparts. Clinicians should provide the patient and his or her caregiver with clear, written postoperative instructions about administration of medications, activities to be avoided, and the phone number to be called should problems or questions arise.

Summary

Elderly patients are uniquely vulnerable and particularly sensitive to the stresses of hospitalization and surgery/anesthesia in ways that are only partially understood. Preoperatively a thoughtful assessment of organ function and reserve is required. Efforts to identify the "best" intraoperative anesthetic agent or technique or approach for the elderly continue, but it seems that no anesthetic agent or technique is unequivocally superior for all conditions or circumstances. Therefore, clinicians should strive to maintain homeostasis, to avoid drug cocktails—especially long-acting benzodiazepines and anticholinergics—to administer short-acting drugs, maintain normothermia and euvolemia, and provide adequate postoperative analgesia. When possible, a case might be made for encouraging ambulatory surgery because of its typically brief duration, relatively noninvasive approach, and its ability to allow elderly patients to recover in their familiar, supportive home environment.

References

1. McGoldrick KE. Postoperative nausea and vomiting. In: Afifi A, Rosenbaum S, eds. Problems in Anesthesia. Vol 12, No. 3. PACU and Anesthetic Management. Philadelphia: Lippincott Williams & Wilkins; 2000:274–286.
2. Ergina P, Gold S, Meakins J. Perioperative care of the elderly patient. World J Surg 1993;17:192–198.
3. Fleisher LA, Pasternak LR, Herbert R, Anderson GF. Inpatient hospital admissions and death after outpatient surgery in elderly patients. Arch Surg 2004;139:67–72.
4. Rao RB, Ely SF, Hoffman RS. Deaths related to liposuction. N Engl J Med 1999;340:1471–1475.
5. Vila H, Soto R, Cantor AB, Mackey D. Comparative outcomes analysis of procedures performed in physician offices and ambulatory surgery centers. Arch Surg 2003;138:991–995.
6. Silverstein JH. Geriatric anesthesia enters a new age. ASA Newslett 2004;68:6, 22.
7. Schein OD, Katz J, Bass EB, et al. The value of routine preoperative medical testing before cataract surgery. N Engl J Med 2000;342:168–175.
8. Dzankic S, Pastor D, Gonzalez C, Leung JM. The prevalence and predictive value of abnormal preoperative laboratory tests in elderly surgical patients. Anesth Analg 2001;93:301–308.
9. Eagle KA, Berger PB, Calkins H, et al. ACC/AHA guideline update for perioperative cardiovascular evaluation for noncardiac surgery. J Am Coll Cardiol 2002;39:542–553.
10. Goldman L. Cardiac risks and complications of noncardiac surgery. Ann Intern Med 1983;98:504–513.
11. Liu LL, Leung JM. Predicting adverse postoperative outcomes in patients aged 80 years or older. J Am Geriatr Soc 2000;48:405–412.
12. Poldermans D, Boersma E, Bax JJ, et al. The effect of bisoprolol on perioperative mortality and myocardial infarction in high-risk patients undergoing vascular surgery. N Engl J Med 1999;341:1789–1794.
13. Young T, Palta M, Dempsey J, et al. The occurrence of sleep-disordered breathing among middle-aged adults. N Engl J Med 1993;328:1230–1235.
14. Carskadon MA, Dement WC. Respiration during sleep in the aged human. J Gerontol 1981;36:420–423.
15. Strollo PJ Jr, Rogers RM. Obstructive sleep apnea. N Engl J Med 1996;334:99–104.
16. Young T, Skatrud J, Peppard PE. Risk factors for obstructive sleep apnea in adults. JAMA 2004;219:2013–2016.
17. Bixler EO, Vgontzas AN, Ten Have T, et al. Effects of age on sleep apnea in men: prevalence and severity. Am J Respir Crit Care Med 1998;157:144–148.
18. Young T, Peppard PE, Gottlieb DJ. Epidemiology of obstructive sleep apnea. Am J Respir Crit Care Med 2002;165:1217–1239.
19. Helfaer MA, Wilson MD. Obstructive sleep apnea, control of ventilation, and anesthesia in children. Pediatr Clin North Am 1994;41:131–151.
20. Loadsman JA, Hllman DR. Anaesthesia and sleep apnoea. Br J Anaesth 2001;86:254–256.
21. American Academy of Sleep Medicine Task Force. Sleep-related breathing disorders in adults: recommendations for

syndrome definition and measurement techniques in clinical research. Report of the American Academy of Sleep Medicine Task Force. Sleep 1999;22:667.

22. Nieto FJ, Young TB, Lind BK et, al. Association of sleep-disordered breathing, sleep apnea, and hypertension in a large community-based study: Sleep Heart Health Study. JAMA 2000;283:1829–1836.

23. Nymann P, Backer V, Dirksen A, Lange P. Increased diastolic blood pressure associated with obstructive sleep apnea independently of overweight [abstract]. Sleep 2000; 23:A61.

24. Bixler EO, Vgontzas AN, Lucas T, et al. The association between sleep-disordered breathing and cardiovascular abnormalities [abstract]. Sleep 2000;23:A59.

25. Grote L, Kraiczi H, Hedner J. Reduced alpha- and beta$_2$-adrenergic vascular response in patients with obstructive sleep apnea. Am J Respir Crit Care Med 2000;162:1480–1487.

26. Shamsuzzaman AS, Somers VK. Fibrinogen, stroke, and obstructive sleep apnea: an evolving paradigm of cardiovascular risk. Am J Crit Care Med 2000;162:2018–2020.

27. Hudgel DW. Mechanisms of obstructive sleep apnea. Chest 1992;101:541–549.

28. Kuna ST, Sant'Ambrogio G. Pathophysiology of upper airway closure during sleep. JAMA 1991;266:1384–1389.

29. Beydon L, Hassapopoulos J, Quera MA, et al. Risk factors for oxygen desaturation during sleep after abdominal surgery. Br J Anaesth 1992;69:137–142.

30. Boudewyns AN, DeBacker WA, Van de Heyning PH. Pattern of upper airway obstruction during sleep before and after uvulopalatopharyngoplasty in patients with obstructive sleep apnea. Sleep Med 2001;2:309–315.

31. Catalfumo FJ, Golz A, Westerman ST, et al. The epiglottis and obstructive sleep apnoea syndrome. J Laryngol Otol 1998;112:940–943.

32. Garrigue S, Bordier P, Jais P, et al. Benefit of atrial pacing in sleep apnea syndrome. N Engl J Med 2002;346:404–412.

33. Gottlieb DJ. Cardiac pacing—a novel therapy for sleep apnea? [editorial]. N Engl J Med 2002;346:444–445.

34. Benumof JL. Obstructive sleep apnea in the adult obese patient: implications for airway management. J Clin Anesth 2001;13:144–156.

35. ASA Task Force on Perioperative Management of Patients with Obstructive Sleep Apnea. Practice guidelines for the perioperative management of patients with obstructive sleep apnea. Anesthesiology 2006;104:1081–1093.

36. American Sleep Apnea Association: sleep apnea and same day surgery. Washington, DC: American Sleep Apnea Association; 1999. www.sleepapnea.org/sameday/html.

37. Benumof J. Preoxygenation: best method for both efficacy and efficiency [editorial]. Anesthesiology 1999;91:603–605.

38. Kirkbride DA, Parker JL, Williams GD, Buggy DJ. Induction of anesthesia in the elderly ambulatory patient: a double-blind comparison of propofol and sevoflurane. Anesth Analg 2001;93:1185–1187.

39. Vuyk J, Oostwouder CJ, Vletter AA, Burm AGL, Bovill JG. Gender differences in the pharmacokinetics of propofol in elderly patients during and after continuous infusion. Br J Anaesth 2001;86:183–188.

40. Katoh T, Suguro Y, Kimura T, Ikeda K. Cerebral awakening concentration of sevoflurane and isoflurane predicted during slow and fast alveolar washout. Anesth Analg 1993; 77:1012–1017.

41. Fredman B, Sheffer O, Zohar E, et al. Fast-track eligibility of geriatric patients undergoing short urologic procedures. Anesth Analg 2002;94:560–564.

42. Weldon BC, Mahla ME, van der Aa MT, Monk TG. Advancing age and deeper intraoperative anesthetic levels are associated with higher first year death rates [abstract]. Anesthesiology 2002;96:A1097.

43. Mathes DD, Conaway MR, Ross WT. Ambulatory surgery: room air versus nasal cannula oxygen during transport after general anesthesia. Anesth Analg 2001;93: 917–921.

44. Paguerson X, Boccara G, Bendahou M, Coriat P, Riou B. Brachial plexus nerve block exhibits prolonged duration in the elderly. Anesthesiology 2002;97:1245–1249.

45. Simon MJG, Veering BT, Stienstra R, van Kleek JW, Burm AGL. The effects of age on neural blockade and hemodynamic changes after epidural anesthesia with ropivacaine. Anesth Analg 2002;94:1325–1330.

46. Pollock JE, Neal JM, Liu SS, et al. Sedation during spinal anesthesia. Anesthesiology 2000;93:728–734.

47. Mulroy MF, Salinas FV, Larkin KL, Polissar NL. Ambulatory surgery patients may be discharged before voiding after short-acting spinal and epidural anesthesia. Anesthesiology 2002;97:315–319.

48. Mora CT, Torjman M, White PF. Sedative and ventilatory effects of midazolam infusion: effect of flumazenil reversal. Can J Anaesth 1995;42:677–684.

49. Rouiller M, Forster A, Gemperle M. Evaluation de l'efficacité et de la tolerance d'un antagoniste des benzodiazepines (Ro 15–1788). Ann Fr Anesth Reanim 1987; 6:1–6.

50. Kazema T, Takeuchi K, Ikeda K, et al. Optimal propofol plasma concentration during upper gastrointestinal endoscopy in young, middle-aged, and elderly patients. Anesthesiology 2000;93:662–669.

51. Shinozaki M, Usui Y, Yamaguchi S, et al. Recovery of psychomotor function after propofol sedation is prolonged in the elderly. Can J Anaesth 2002;49:927–931.

52. Egan TD. The clinical pharmacology of the new fentanyl congeners. Anesth Analg 1997;84(Suppl):31–38.

53. Bailey PL, Egan TD, Stanley TH. Intravenous opioid anesthesia. In: Miller RD, ed. Anesthesia. 5th ed. Philadelphia: Churchill Livingstone; 2000:273–376.

54. Egan TD. Remifentanil pharmacokinetics and pharmacodynamics: a preliminary appraisal. Clin Pharmacokinet 1995;29:80–94.

55. Minto CF, Schnider TW, Egan TD, et al. Influence of age and gender on the pharmacokinetics and pharmacodynamics of remifentanil. Anesthesiology 1997;86:10–23.

56. Egan TD, Huizinga B, Gupta SK, et al. Remifentanil pharmacokinetics in obese versus lean patients. Anesthesiology 1998;89:562–573.

57. Johnson KB, Swenson JD, Egan TD, et al. Midazolam and remifentanil by bolus injection for intensely stimulating procedures of brief duration: experience with awake laryngoscopy. Anesth Analg 2002;94:1241–1243.

58. Food and Drug Administration. Warning re-emphasized in midazolam labeling. FDA Drug Bull 1986;27:5.

59. Coté CJ, Notterman DA, Karl HW, et al. Adverse sedation events in pediatrics: a critical incident analysis of contributing factors. Pediatrics 2000;105:805–814.

60. Coté CJ, Karl HW, Notterman DA, et al. Adverse sedation events in pediatrics: analysis of medications used for sedation. Pediatrics 2000;106:633–644.

61. Cohen MM, Duncan PG, Tate RB. Does anesthesia contribute to operative mortality? JAMA 1988;260:2859–2863.

62. Domino KB. Trends in litigation in the 1990s: MAC claims. ASA Newslett 1997;61:15–17.

63. Posner KL. Liability profile of ambulatory anesthesia. ASA Newslett 2000;64(6):10–12.

64. Fitzgibbon DR, Posner KL, Domino KB, Caplan RA, Lee LA, Cheney FW. Chronic pain management: American Society of Anesthesiologists closed claims project. Anesthesiology 2004;100:98–105.

65. Pedersen T, Eliasen K, Henriksen E. A prospective study of risk factors and cardiopulmonary complications associated with anaesthesia and surgery: risk indicators of cardiopulmonary morbidity. Acta Anaesthesiol Scand 1990;34:144–155.

66. Moller JT, Wittrup M, Johansen SH. Hypoxemia in the postanesthesia care unit: an observer study. Anesthesiology 1990;73:890–895.

67. Arunasalam K, Davenport HT, Painter S, Jones JG. Ventilatory response to morphine in young and old subjects. Anaesthesia 1983;38:529–533.

68. Pontoppidan H, Beecher HK. Progressive loss of protective reflexes in the airway with advance of age. JAMA 1960;174:2209–2213.

69. Seymour DG, Vaz FG. A prospective study of elderly general surgical patients. II. Postoperative complications. Age Ageing 1989;18:316–326.

70. Pedersen T, Viby-Mogensen J, Ringsted C. Anaesthetic practice and postoperative pulmonary complications. Acta Anaesthesiol Scand 1992;36:812–818.

71. Aviv JE. Effects of aging on sensitivity of the pharyngeal and supraglottic areas. Am J Med 1997;103:74S–76S.

72. Marik PE. Aspiration pneumonitis and aspiration pneumonia. N Engl J Med 2001;344:665–671.

73. de Larminat V, Montravers P, Dureuil B, Desmonts JM. Alteration in swallowing reflex after extubation in intensive care unit patients. Crit Care Med 1995;23:486–490.

74. Hogue CW Jr, Lappas GD, Creswell LL, et al. Swallowing dysfunction after cardiac operations. Associated adverse outcomes and risk factors including intraoperative transesophageal echocardiography. J Thorac Cardiovasc Surg 1995;110:517–522.

75. Mitchell CK, Smoger SH, Pfeifer MP, et al. Multivariate analysis of factors associated with postoperative pulmonary complications following general elective surgery. Arch Surg 1998;133:194–198.

76. Warner MA, Warner ME, Weber JG. Clinical significance of pulmonary aspiration during the perioperative period. Anesthesiology 1993;78:56–62.

77. Cook DJ. Geriatric anesthesia. In: Solomon DH, LoCicero J III, Rosenthal RA, eds. New Frontiers in Geriatric Research. New York: American Geriatrics Society; 2004:9–52.

78. Vaughan MS, Vaughan RW, Cork RC. Postoperative hypothermia in adults: relationship of age, anesthesia, and shivering to rewarming. Anesth Analg 1981;60:746–751.

79. Leslie K, Sessler DI, Bjorksten AR, Moayeri A. Mild hypothermia alters propofol pharmacokinetics and increases the duration of action of atracurium. Anesth Analg 1995;80:1007–1014.

80. Frank SM, Higgins MS, Breslow MJ, et al. The catecholamine, cortisol, and hemodynamic responses to mild perioperative hypothermia: a randomized clinical trial. Anesthesiology 1995;82:83–93.

81. Jones JS, Johnson K, McNinch M. Age as a risk factor for inadequate emergency department analgesia. Am J Emerg Med 1996;14:157–160.

82. Petros JG, Alameddine F, Testa E, et al. Patient-controlled analgesia and postoperative urinary retention after hysterectomy for benign disease. J Am Coll Surg 1994;179:663–667.

83. Petros JG, Mallen JK, Howe K, et al. Patient-controlled analgesia and postoperative urinary retention after open appendectomy. Surg Gynecol Obstet 1993;177:172–175.

84. Carpenter RL, Abram SE, Bromage PR, Rauck RL. Consensus statement on acute pain management. Reg Anesth 1996;21:152–156.

85. Carpenter RL. Gastrointestinal benefits of regional anesthesia/analgesia. Reg Anesth 1996;21:13–17.

86. Bates DW, Cullen DJ, Laird N, et al. Incidence of adverse drug events and potential adverse drug events: implications for prevention. ADE Prevention Study Group. JAMA 1995;274:29–34.

87. Polanczyk CA, Goldman L, Marcantonio ER, et al. Supraventricular arrhythmias in patients having noncardiac surgery: clinical correlates and effect on length of stay. Ann Intern Med 1998;129:279–285.

88. Amar D, Roistacher N, Burt M, et al. Clinical and echocardiographic correlates of symptomatic tachydysrhythmias after noncardiac thoracic surgery. Chest 1995;108:349–354.

89. Aranki SF, Shaw DP, Adams DH, et al. Predictors of atrial fibrillation following coronary artery bypass graft surgery: current trends and impact on hospital resources. Circulation 1996;94:390–397.

90. Mathew JP, Parks R, Savino JS, et al. Atrial fibrillation following coronary artery bypass graft surgery: predictors, outcomes, and resource utilization. JAMA 1996;276:300–306.

91. Amar D, Zhang H, Leung DHY, et al. Older age is the strongest predictor of postoperative atrial fibrillation. Anesthesiology 2002;96:352–356.

92. Moller JT, Cluitmans P, Rasmussen LS, et al. Long-term postoperative cognitive dysfunction in the elderly: ISPOCD1 study. Lancet 1998;351:857–861.

93. Williams-Russo P, Sharrock NE, Mattis S, Szatowski TP, Charlson ME. Cognitive effects after epidural vs. general anesthesia in older adults. JAMA 1995;274:44–50.

94. Dodds C, Allison J. Postoperative cognitive deficit in the elderly surgical patient. Br J Anaesth 1998;81:449–462.

95. Monk TG, Garvin CW, Dede DE, van der Aa MT, Gravenstein JS. Predictors of postoperative cognitive

dysfunction following major surgery [abstract]. Anesthesiology 2001;95:A50.

96. Moller JT. Cerebral dysfunction after anaesthesia. Acta Anaesthesiol Scand 1997;110(Suppl):13–16.

97. O'Keefe ST, Chonchubhair AN. Postoperative delirium in the elderly. Br J Anaesth 1994;73:673–687.

98. Marcantonio ER, Juaraz G, Goldman L, et al. The relationship of postoperative delirium with psychoactive medication. JAMA 1994;272:1518–1522.

99. Hanania M, Kitain E. Melatonin for the treatment and prevention of postoperative delirium. Anesth Analg 2002; 94:338–339.

100. Marcantonio ER, Flacker JM, Wright RJ, Resnick NM. Reducing delirium after hip fracture: a randomized trial. J Am Geriatr Soc 2001;49:516–522.

101. Rasmussen LS, Larssen K, Houx P, et al. The assessment of postoperative cognitive dysfunction. Acta Anaesthesiol Scand 2001;45:275–289.

102. Rasmussen LS, Johnson T, Kuipers HM, et al. Does anaesthesia cause postoperative cognitive dysfunction? A randomized study of regional versus general anaesthesia in 438 elderly patients. Acta Anaesthesiol Scand 2003;47: 260–266.

103. Canet J, Raeder J, Rasmussen LS, et al. for the ISPOCD2 group. Cognitive dysfunction after minor surgery in the elderly. Acta Anaesthesiol Scand 2003;47:1204– 1210.

104. Inouye SK. Predisposing and precipitating factors for delirium in hospitalized older patients. Dement Geriatr Cogn Disord 1999;10:393–400.

105. Inouye SK, Bogardus ST Jr, Charpentier PA, et al. A multicomponent intervention to prevent delirium in hospitalized older patients. N Engl J Med 1999;340:669–676.

106. Tzabar Y, Asbury AJ, Millar K. Cognitive failure after general anaesthesia for day-case surgery. Br J Anaesth 1996;76:194–197.

107. Lichtor JL, Alessi R, Lane BS. Sleep tendency as a measure of recovery after drugs used for ambulatory surgery. Anesthesiology 2002;96:878–883.

108. Johnson T. Postoperative cognitive dysfunction in middle-aged patients. Anesthesiology 2002;96:1351–1357.

109. Wu CL, Hsu W, Richman JM, Raja SN. Postoperative cognitive function as an outcome of regional anesthesia and analgesia. Reg Anesth Pain Med 2004;29:257–268.

110. Chung F. Are discharge criteria changing? J Clin Anesth 1993;5(Suppl):66S.

111. Gold BS, Kitz DS, Lecky JH, Neuhaus JM. Unanticipated admission to the hospital following ambulatory surgery. JAMA 1989;262:3008–3010.

112. Apfel CC, Läärä E, Koivuranta M et al. A simplified risk score for predicting postoperative nausea and vomiting: Conclusions from cross-validations between two centers. Anesthesiology 1999;91:693–700.

113. Sinclair DR, Chung F, Mezei G. Can postoperative nausea and vomiting be predicted? Anesthesiology 1999;91:109–118.

114. Wang LP, Fog J, Boe M. Transient hearing loss following spinal anaesthesia. Anaesthesia 1987;42:1258–1263.

115. Gultekin S, Ozcan S. Does hearing loss after spinal anesthesia differ between young and elderly patients? Anesth Analg 2002;94:1318–1320.

Part IV
Anesthesia for Common Surgical Procedures in the Aged

23
Sedation and Monitoring

Sheila R. Barnett

Sedation is often required for patients undergoing minor procedures. The increased availability of newer medications with short duration, rapid onset, and minimal side effects has led patients and physicians to expect comfort, amnesia, and good "operating" conditions for a multitude of minimally invasive procedures. Given the increase in the elderly population, it is not surprising that there has also been a marked increase in procedures performed in extremely old patients. The skillful administration of sedation and analgesia for interventional procedures may allow these very elderly patients to avoid more invasive surgery and the consequent associated morbidity of surgery and prolonged hospitalization.[1]

What Is Meant by the Term Sedation?

Both the American Society of Anesthesiologists (ASA) and the Joint Commission on Accreditation of Healthcare Organization describe four levels of sedation, from minimal or anxiolysis to general anesthesia[2,3] (Table 23-1).

Minimal sedation or anxiolysis refers to a controlled state of diminished consciousness wherein the ability to respond to moderate verbal stimuli and the ability to maintain a patent airway are retained.[4,5] There is little impact on the cardiopulmonary status. Although this is popularly referred to as *conscious sedation* by many nonanesthesia specialties, the ASA task force recommends the use of *sedation and analgesia* rather than conscious sedation.[2]

Moderate sedation or analgesia is a drug-induced state during which a patient may be less responsive than with anxiolysis but still respond to verbal commands appropriately, although sometimes requiring simultaneous light tactile stimulation. Spontaneous respiration is maintained and cardiovascular parameters are unchanged.

Deep sedation or analgesia is a drug-induced condition whereby the patient may be difficult to awaken but will respond purposefully to painful stimuli. With deep sedation, spontaneous respiration may not be adequate, and the patient may not be able to maintain a patent airway without assistance. Although controversial, in general, the ASA and many hospitals recommend the presence of anesthesia-trained personnel if deep sedation is anticipated or required to complete a procedure.[2] At a minimum, deep sedation requires the immediate availability of an individual trained in cardiopulmonary resuscitation and airway management.

Sedation is a continuum of consciousness, and the practitioner providing sedation should be ready to respond appropriately to the next-higher level of sedation in addition to being comfortable at the current sedation level. This is particularly relevant when sedation is administered by nonanesthesiologists such as dental practitioners, radiologists, dermatologists, cardiologists, and gastroenterologists.[4,6–10]

Why Is Sedation a Particular Concern in Elderly Patients?

The geriatric population is a heterogeneous group, and chronologic age does not always parallel physiologic age. Older patients present with multiple comorbidities, numerous medications, and less physiologic reserve.[5,11] They can be more sensitive to the sedative and depressant effects of the drugs used for sedation and are at increased risk from additive side effects when combinations of medications are administered. Although brief episodes of hypotension or desaturation may be insignificant in a young patient, the same episodes in an elderly frail patient may result in serious consequences, such as cardiac ischemia and arrhythmias[12] (Table 23-2).

TABLE 23-1. Sedation depth.

Minimal	Patient responds appropriately to normal-volume verbal cues, through voice or action. The response is immediate.
Moderate	Patient responds purposefully to verbal or light tactile stimulus. The response is either verbal or physical. For example, opening eyes, turning head in a given direction, appropriate change in position.
Deep	The patient does not respond to either verbal or tactile stimulus, but responds appropriately to painful stimuli.

Comorbid Conditions

Elderly patients carry a large burden of disease: In a recent study examining preoperative health status in elderly patients, more than 84% of 544 patients had at least one comorbid condition, with 30% of patients having three or more preoperative health conditions and 27% with two.[11] Disability restricting mobility is also prevalent: 73% of people older than 80 years have at least one disability. These conditions have an impact on the delivery of sedation and may limit the options available for sedation.

Cardiac conditions such as angina, hypertension, and congestive heart failure are all prevalent among elderly patients.[13-15] The high incidence of coronary artery disease places older patients at high risk for myocardial ischemia during awake procedures, especially if the procedure is painful and/or anxiety provoking and it proves difficult to relieve the pain/anxiety without resorting to unacceptable levels of sedation. Similarly, hemodynamic instability, particularly hypotension, is more likely in older patients because of their sensitivity to hypovolemia and the increased sympathetic tone that could be reduced by sedation. However, hypotension is not a likely result if stage II sedation is not exceeded.[2,16]

Age-related pulmonary changes[17] also affect the administration of sedation; changes in lung and chest wall compliance predispose the older patient to atelectasis with associated hypoxia that may not be amenable to treatment with supplemental oxygen. Hypercarbia may also develop and produce hypoxia (if not on supplemental oxygen) and may produce undesired hypertension and tachycardia.

TABLE 23-2. Considerations for sedation in the elderly.

1. Presence of multiple comorbidities: coronary disease, arrhythmias; prior cerebrovascular accidents
2. Positioning challenges
3. Chronic pain especially of the back and spine
4. Prevalence of chronic hypoxia and the need for home oxygen
5. Hearing and vision impairments that interfere with communication
6. Dementia and cognitive dysfunction

Renal disease may require alternations in medication dosing, and uremia can render patients very sensitive to the effects of sedation, especially the apneic side effects of narcotics. With the obesity epidemic in the United States, diabetes is becoming more prevalent and is very common in older patients. Glucose control can be problematic, and associated diabetic gastroparesis may result in a full stomach, even after 8 hours of fasting.

Central nervous system aging renders older patients more sensitive to sedatives and analgesics, and patients with mild cognitive dysfunction are at particular risk for agitation and confusion with even small amounts of sedatives.

Challenges Encountered During Administration of Sedation

There are certain issues that are uniquely relevant to elderly patients that may impinge on the sedation plan[5,18,19] (Table 23-3).

Positioning

The accelerated loss of subcutaneous and intramuscular fat observed with aging may result in bony prominences that are at risk from skin breakdown and predispose elderly patients to accidental injury from seemingly benign positions. The loss of skin elasticity and slow healing further contribute to complex skin wounds and shearing injuries. Chronic pain, especially back pain, may limit the ability of an elderly patient to attain or maintain certain positions for long periods of time. Vertebrobasilar insufficiency may predispose an older patient to unexpected cerebral ischemia with neck extension; this may be particularly important if manipulation of the airway or neck is required. Cardiopulmonary compromise may occur secondary to positioning. For instance, the prone position or Trendelenburg may be less well tolerated in the elderly patient with significant cardiac disease.

TABLE 23-3. Practical considerations for the administration of sedation in elderly patients.

- Allow extra time to explore the preoperative history including medications and comorbidities.
- Provide written instructions in large type.
- Provide extra copy of instructions to caretaker if applicable.
- Allow extra time for changing clothes at the beginning and end of the procedure.
- Be prepared to provide additional assistance transferring to and from procedure table.
- Postoperative recovery facilities with monitoring should be available in the event of a slow postoperative recovery.

Communication

Diminished visual acuity, blindness, deafness, or impaired hearing make it more difficult to communicate during a procedure. Furthermore, many common procedures such as colonoscopies and endoscopies take place in a darkened endoscopy suite, further reducing the sensory input to the older patient. Any written information should be easy to read, and extra copies should be available for patient's family, especially if the patient has any cognitive or communication issues.

Administering Sedation

More than 10 million gastrointestinal procedures are performed in the United States and Canada annually,[20] and the volume of procedures conducted by gastroenterologists in the United States has increased almost twofold in the past 15 years. Individual endoscopists may perform between 9 and 15 esophagogastroduodenoscopies and 22 colonoscopies per week. Colonoscopy is generally an unpleasant procedure associated with considerable discomfort. It is possible to perform colonoscopies with no sedation, but widespread use of sedation is well known to many patients, and most expect the option of safe sedation.[21,22] Endoscopic management of biliary disease in the elderly may be particularly advantageous,[23] and skillful administration of sedation is a vital component for these procedures, which may be complex and at times uncomfortable.[24,25]

Results from a survey of sedation practices among 1500 gastroenterologists demonstrated that 98% of gastroenterologists routinely used sedation of some type, more than 70% routinely administered oxygen, almost 99% monitored blood pressure and saturation, whereas capnography remained relatively infrequent and was monitored in only 3% of respondents. With respect to drug administration, the endoscopist was responsible for making decisions regarding sedation doses in 78% of cases unless propofol was used, in which case anesthesia personnel were responsible in almost 70% of the cases.[20]

This section particularly addresses the issues of sedation with respect to gastroenterology procedures.[24,25] The administration of sedation to an elderly patient involves

TABLE 23-4. Predictors of difficult sedation.

History of:
Substance abuse
Heavy alcohol use
Chronic narcotic use
Difficulty with previous sedation case
Anticipated prolonged or complex procedure

TABLE 23-5. General anesthesia recommendations.

General anesthesia is recommended in patients who are:

- Obtunded
- Intoxicated
- Septic
- Have active hematemesis
- Have significant cognitive impairment—e.g., dementia or are unable to cooperate secondary to confusion or anxiety
- At high risk from aspiration—e.g., obesity, reflux, or ascites
- Unable to lie still secondary to pain, confusion, or other medical conditions

a preprocedure assessment and formulation of a plan, including monitoring, ensuring availability of resuscitative equipment, and an appropriate choice of drugs.[5,26,27]

Preprocedure Evaluation

Before administering sedation, an assessment of the patient's overall health including an estimate of the patient's reserve function of major organ systems is needed. At a minimum, this should include a medical history, a comprehensive list of medications, and a brief physical examination including an airway assessment. One of the guiding principles for the successful administration of sedation is cooperation; preprocedure assessment should include an evaluation of the patient's ability to cooperate at baseline. Patients who cannot cooperate because of dementia, sensory issues such as hearing or visual loss, or who are in extreme pain or disabled from arthritis and prior strokes and so on may not be suitable sedation candidates, and a deep sedation or a general anesthetic may be required.[2,5,24,25]

Sedation History

A history of sedation and anesthesia is invaluable. Difficulties with prior procedures under sedation, substance and alcohol abuse, and extensive pain medication use have been shown to predict difficulty in sedation administration. In addition, technically difficult or lengthy procedures also predict difficulty with sedation. In these instances, it may be preferable to schedule elective procedures for deep sedation or general anesthesia[2,5,24,25] (Tables 23-4 and 23-5).

Consent

The patient should understand and agree with the specific plan for sedation and the risks involved. When the patient is significantly disabled or dependent, it is important to involve caregivers early. Aside from consent issues in these patients, caregivers are likely to be needed in the postprocedure care of the patient. Frequently, the surgical consent will include permission for sedation during the procedure, and separate consent for sedation is not always needed; however, specifics will depend on local administration and regulations within the hospital or facility.

Preoperative Fasting Guidelines

Both the ASA and the American Society for Gastrointestinal Endoscopy (ASGE) recommend restricting solid foods for 6–8 hours and allowing only clear liquids until 2–3 hours before the procedures. In the elderly person, it is useful to establish who is receiving these instructions and who is responsible to enforce them. In the more frail or demented patient, adherence with fasting guidelines is particularly important because it can be difficult to predict the reaction to sedation and there may be a need for conversion to a deeper sedation or a general anesthesia.[24,25]

Monitoring

Guidelines for monitoring have been developed by the ASA and ASGE.[28] At a minimum, all sedated patients must be monitored throughout the procedure for level of consciousness. Standard monitoring includes heart rate monitoring via pulse oximetry, noninvasive blood pressure at regular intervals, respiratory rate, and oxygen saturation, and in the elderly population, electrocardiography is also recommended. Postprocedure vital signs should also be monitored periodically during the recovery period until the effects of all medications have worn off and the patient is ready for discharge.

The presence of a pacemaker requires the availability of a magnet if cautery is contemplated. Patients with a significant cardiac history, ongoing angina, congestive heart failure, or oxygen-dependent lung disease have almost no reserve function. These patients may not be suitable candidates for sedation because they may require additional monitoring.

Patients may maintain normal oxygen saturation despite significant hypoventilation and hypercapnia, and monitoring of ventilation is advisable whenever deep sedation is contemplated, especially during long procedures. Capnography[28] can be used to monitor ventilation and to detect early increases in carbon dioxide. However, the role for routine capnography is not clear and probably unnecessary in most instances of routine (nonpropofol) conscious sedation. Similarly, the bispectral index monitor has been used to assess the level of sedation in patients receiving propofol for sedation; however, the utility has yet to be determined.[29]

It should be recognized that clinical monitoring of the elderly patient may be more demanding than that of the younger patient. During the procedure, a dedicated individual should be able to supervise the patient. This individual should not be performing the procedure but rather should be continuously monitoring the patient for responsiveness, cooperation, and vital signs. Because by definition a sedated patient should be responsive at all times, communication with the patient is one of the most valuable monitoring methods.

Emergency Resuscitation

When administering sedation, emergency resuscitative equipment should be available, and those providing sedation should ideally be trained in basic and advanced life support. Minimal emergency equipment should include dedicated oral suction, oxygen, a bag-valve-mask device, an oral airway, and reversal agents.[30,31]

Oxygen

Elderly patients with limited reserve function are predisposed to hypoventilation and hypoxemia; this may be exacerbated by cardiopulmonary and other diseases. Studies in gastroenterology have described episodes of desaturation during endoscopic and colonoscopic procedures in both sedated and nonsedated patients[32,33] emphasizing the vulnerability of these patients. Supplemental oxygen provided via nasal cannula at 4 L/min has been successful in abolishing or attenuating episodes of desaturation. As stated, monitoring of ventilation is indicated because oxygen may mask the development of hypercapnia in sedated patients, especially those receiving supplemental narcotics.[2,24,28]

Medications

Intravenous administration of medications is preferable to oral or intramuscular administration because it provides a more immediate effect and allows for more precise dosing. In addition, the presence of an intravenous line can be used to administer reversal or resuscitative drugs if needed. The time taken for the effect of a drug to peak can be slower in the elderly patient, and lengthening the interval between incremental doses in the older patient is recommended. Combinations of medications can allow a reduction in individual doses needed to produce the effect. However, in the older person, there is a potential for exaggerated effects; this can be minimized through dose reduction and interval extension. Some of the drugs used most frequently are combinations of midazolam, fentanyl, and meperidine.[3,20,24,25,30]

Midazolam is the preferred benzodiazepine: it has a fast onset, is short acting, and has few residual effects. In contrast, the longer-acting benzodiazepines such as diazepam and lorazepam may provide equally good sedative effects, but may result in prolonged sedation.[22,34,35]

Advanced age is associated with an increased central sensitivity to midazolam,[36] and the doses recommended are an initial bolus of 0.5–1 mg followed by incremental doses of 0.25–0.5 mg during the procedure.

The narcotics remifentanil, fentanyl, and meperidine are popular choices for sedation and are frequently combined with midazolam. Fentanyl is a relatively short-acting opioid that has been used for many years to provide sedation. As with all opioids, postoperative nausea is a risk, and this may preclude its use in certain instances. The respiratory depressant effects of fentanyl may be exaggerated by midazolam, and doses should be reduced when the combination is used. In the elderly, fentanyl doses range from 12.5 to 50 µg, titrating to effect and closely monitoring for respiratory depression. The extreme short duration of remifentanil is particularly advantageous for infusions, although, as with other opioids, the risk of postoperative nausea may limit its value.[37] The combination of remifentanil and propofol may provide better sedation, pain relief, and toleration of colonoscopies compared with the administration of midazolam, fentanyl, and propofol.[35] However, the overall benefits of these and other combinations have not been adequately investigated at this point to make a single recommendation, and there are clearly multiple approaches to sedation that are acceptable.[37–39]

Meperidine is also popular for sedation in the younger generation, but in older patients it is best avoided because of its relatively long action, toxic metabolites, and the potential for central nervous system side effects.

Dexmedetomidine is an alpha2 receptor agonist that has some significant advantages over the classic sedative choices. It is a relatively new agent currently approved for administration in the intensive care unit for sedation. A major advantage is the lack of respiratory depression with significant sedation and analgesia; however, it can cause significant hypotension. When compared with a propofol infusion, dexmedetomidine may cause slightly more hypotension and sedation, but it does have narcotic-sparing qualities that may be of value in frail elderly patients. The role of dexmedetomidine continues to be explored.[40,41]

Propofol

Although in general the ASA discourages the use of propofol by nonanesthesia personnel,[2,30,35] propofol is clearly gaining popularity for sedation by nonanesthesiologists[23] (Table 23-6). Advantages of propofol are its rapid action and fast clearance that make it an attractive choice for sedation. However, caution is required in elderly patients in whom administration may also result in abrupt hypotension and severe respiratory depression. One study investigated the recovery of psychomotor function in elderly compared with young patients after propofol

TABLE 23-6. Administration of propofol for sedation: general recommendations.

- Anesthesiology-trained personnel recommended for deep-sedation administration
- Provision for a dedicated individual for the administration of sedating medication
- Individuals administering propofol should:
    Be trained in advanced cardiac life support
    Have experience in airway management
- Monitoring of vital signs is required
- Emergency resuscitation equipment should be immediately available

infusions. The authors compared 15 elderly patients, mean age 72 years, with 15 young patients, mean age 38. Both groups received continuous propofol infusions for approximately 140 minutes. Immediate recovery time to opening eyes was similar in each group, but the elderly patients had a much prolonged complete recovery of psychomotor function as tested using the Tieger's dot test.[42] Although the study numbers are small, this study emphasizes the potential for prolonged effects of medications in the elderly patient, even when the agent is regarded as of very short duration.

Several protocols using propofol delivery have been developed by gastroenterology services with success. In these trials, low-dose propofol given by endoscopists provided a good level of low sedation and optimal operating environments for the procedure. It is important to note that in these studies individuals received specific training in propofol administration, and emergency equipment was extensive.[23,39]

In a survey conducted on gastroenterologists, propofol was used by about 25% of endoscopists, anesthesia providers were involved in 28% of endoscopies, and only 7.7% of endoscopists reported using propofol themselves in their practices. In contrast, European studies suggest the use of propofol by endoscopists may be as high as 34%. Interestingly, when questioned, more than 40% of endoscopists would choose propofol for their own procedure. The reasons they stated for preferring propofol was speed of onset and recovery, and satisfaction.[20]

Propofol for sedation is also popular among emergency room physicians where it is often the drug of choice for brief procedures such as cardioversions, fracture reductions, and dislocations. Overall, the role of propofol by nonanesthesiologists is still unresolved and varies substantially across the nation.[43–46]

Another new trend emerging in endoscopy studies is patient-controlled sedation (PCS). Lee et al.[47] randomized patients to receive either PCS or intravenous sedation. They found that in general the incidence of hypotension was lower in the PCS group and the patients recovered faster. Although this is obviously not feasible in the demented or cognitively fragile elderly patient,

patient autonomy may lead to less medication usage and high satisfaction.

Reversal Agents

Although reversal issues are not unique to the elderly, it is advisable to have naloxone, a selective opioid reversal agent, and flumazenil, a benzodiazepine antagonist, immediately available if narcotics and benzodiazepines are being administered. Many elderly patients take chronic opioid therapy for pain,[5,15] and administration of naloxone should be done cautiously because it may result in a catecholamine surge and subsequent hypertension and tachycardia. The initial dose to reverse narcotic respiratory depression is frequently less than a full dose of 0.4 mg; in the elderly patient, an even smaller initial dose may be sufficient. Flumazenil will reverse the sedative and psychomotor effects of midazolam but not any narcotic respiratory depression. Usually naloxone should be administered first if respiratory depression is the primary issue after combination therapy. Sedative protocols using routine reversal of benzodiazepines have been described but these have not been popular in the United States.[48,49]

Scheduling and Information

The geriatric patient may have limited mobility and other issues that may result in the need for extra time to change and transfer from a chair to a stretcher. Therefore, additional time in between cases and arrangements to help with dressing and so on should be allotted.

All instructions should be written avoiding medical jargon and available in large easy-to-read print. In addition to preoperative instructions, written information should be given to patients and/or caregivers before discharge that clearly states what to expect postoperatively, whom to contact with questions, and how to arrange for emergency help if needed.

Adverse Events

Aspiration

With advanced age, the pharyngeal reflexes are diminished, and elderly patients are at increased risk from aspiration. For this reason, fasting guidelines should be adhered to and the level of sedation kept to a minimum when possible. The age-related reduction in pharyngeal sensitivity compared with younger patients is an advantage when performing a simple upper endoscopy, and the elderly patient may not require any sedation. When sedation is required, aspiration risk is increased, and in the frail elderly patient aspiration can be a morbid event.[18,21]

Cardiopulmonary Events

These are the most serious of all adverse events and include hypoxemia, hypoventilation, arrhythmias, airway obstruction, and hypotension. Fortunately, the incidence of serious complications is uncommon: results from two large studies looking at more than 30,000 patients reported complication rates of 2–5 per 1000 patients.[19,20,50] The complications ranged from mild hypoxemia to cardiac ischemia. More recently, Rodriguez-Gonzzalez et al.[1] looked retrospectively at 159 ERCPs (range 1–5 per patient) performed in patients over the age of 90 years at their institution. This included 126 very elderly patients with a mean age of 92 years, ranging from 90 to 101 years; some had more than one procedure. Forty-two percent of patients had significant chronic conditions—mostly diabetes mellitus and coronary artery disease. All patients underwent a procedure performed under local pharyngeal anesthesia, and 99% received supplemental intravenous sedation. The most frequently administered medication was midazolam, which was given in 96% of patients; meperidine was administered in 4%. In addition, hyoscine-N-butylbromide was given in 75% and glucagon in 25% of patients. Overall, the procedures were well tolerated in 92% of patients, and no patient experienced a direct complication from the sedation. The procedure was suspended for anatomic reasons in only nine or 5.7% of cases. Four patients went to surgery subsequently because of inadequate endoscopic interventions and all four died postoperatively. Although this was an unusually healthy group of 90-year-olds, this study supports the importance of skillful sedation. It is evident from the data that the mortality with biliary surgery can be high in very elderly patients, and avoidance of a surgery may be beneficial.[1,23]

Elderly patients can become significantly dehydrated easily, especially in hot climates or if they are taking diuretic and antihypertensive medications. Patients that have had fluid restricted or received bowel preparations may demonstrate significant orthostatic hypotension when standing up for the first time after a procedure, so care should be taken when getting these patients up to ambulate. A careful plan for postoperative hydration should be discussed with the patient and the caretaker.

Hypoxemia

Hypoxia is more common in individuals receiving a combination of medications such as midazolam and fentanyl or midazolam and meperidine. Longer procedures such as endoscopic retrograde cholangiopancreatographies (ERCPs) are also more likely to be associated with hypoxic episodes, and supplemental oxygen is recommended. As discussed above, hypoventilation may be underappreciated, especially in long procedures in patients with chronic obstructive pulmonary disease, dementia, and in patients receiving combined sedation with benzodiazepines and narcotics. In these instances, monitoring of end-tidal carbon dioxide may be merited, but this is not universally available or clearly stated in any guidelines.[5,24,25]

Summary

In general, administration of sedation to elderly patients undergoing minimally invasive procedures is safe.

Eye Surgeries in the Elderly

Cataract extraction is a classic example of an invaluable surgery performed with minimal sedation. One and a half million cataract surgeries are performed annually in the United States, and the annual Medicare expenditure is in excess of $3.4 billion.[51,52] In general, these are very low-risk outpatient surgeries,[53] but the complications related to the procedure can be devastating and may result in significant visual disability and even blindness.[54] An anesthesia care provider is frequently involved in the sedation and monitoring of these cases.[55]

Cataracts

More than 20 million people (17.5%) over age 40 years have a cataract in at least one eye, and 6.1 million (5%) have pseudoaphakia/aphakia (prior cataract surgery) in the United States. By 2020, it is estimated that 30 million Americans will have a cataract and 9.5 million pseudophakia/aphakia.[56,57] The majority of cataracts in the United States are senile or age-related cataracts and a major cause of blindness. The exact pathogenesis of cataracts is not completely understood; however, the current evidence suggests that a photoxidative mechanism has a major role. The normal crystalline lens is composed of a very complex structure consisting of specialized cells arranged in a highly ordered manner; the high content of the cytoplasmic protein provides the transparency critical to the functioning lens. During aging, the epithelial cells are not shed as they are in other structures, and there is a gradual buildup of protein and pigment, forming the basis of the cataract. Risk factors include aging, smoking, alcohol consumption, sunlight, low education, and diabetes mellitus.[58]

TABLE 23-7. Most common causes of blindness.

1. Cataract
2. Macular degeneration
3. Glaucoma
4. Diabetes mellitus

TABLE 23-8. Causes of cataracts.

1. Aging
2. Smoking
3. Alcohol
4. Sunlight exposure
5. Diabetes mellitus
6. Steroids

Nuclear cataracts are the type that usually occurs with aging and may themselves cause further eye problems such as glaucoma. Phacolytic glaucoma occurs when a mature cataract liquefies and leaks out of the capsule into the anterior chamber, resulting in inflammation and clogging of the trabecular network with subsequent increased intraocular pressure. Phacomorphic glaucoma occurs when large cataracts push forward resulting in a narrowing of the angle and subsequent narrow-angle glaucoma.[55,58]

The only known treatment for cataracts at this time is surgery, and fortunately, 90% of patients undergoing first-time cataract surgery have improved visual acuity and satisfaction at 4-month follow-up[59-61] (Tables 23-7 and 23-8).

Modern Cataract Surgery

All cataract surgery involves removal of the cataract; key advances in the field have been the development of small foldable implantable lenses and the development of phacoemulsification techniques. Nowadays, patients can be in and out of the hospital within a few hours and experience immediate improvement of sight[59,60,62-65] (Table 23-9).

Intracapsular cataract extraction (ICCE) refers to the total extraction of the opacified lens and the capsule; a new lens is then inserted into the anterior chamber. This technique is less common nowadays, although it may still be used for selected complex cases. Extracapsular cataract extraction (ECCE) refers to the procedure during which the lens is removed but the capsule is left intact. This procedure is more technically challenging but advantageous because the capsule supplies support for the implantable lens. Both ICCE and ECCE procedures require relatively large incisions.[62-64]

TABLE 23-9. Complications of cataract surgery.

1. Astigmatism
2. Wound leak or dehiscence
3. Prolapsed iris
4. Flat anterior chamber
5. Expulsive rupture of choroidal vessels
6. Strabismus

Today, the most popular approach to cataract extraction in the United States is phacoemulsification.[62] Under an operating microscope, ultrasonically driven oscillating needles are inserted through a tiny incision and used to emulsify the lens. At the same time, a continuous irrigation/aspiration system is used to remove the tiny pieces of shattered opacified lens. Foldable implantable lenses are inserted through the small incision. These tiny incisions frequently do not require sutures for closure, allowing for a rapid surgery and recovery. Occasionally, mature cataracts are extremely hard and difficult to break up using standard phacoemulsification techniques; in these instances, the procedure may be prolonged or alternative techniques such as ICCE or ECCE may be required.[53,62,65,66]

Indications for Surgery

Not all cataracts require immediate surgery. The key indication for surgery is visual impairment accompanied by deterioration in general function secondary to failing eyesight, and a promising surgical prognosis for recovery of vision. Generally, prognosis depends on the presence or absence of other ocular comorbidities, such as glaucoma or retinopathy. Phacomorphic glaucoma and follow-up of diabetic retinopathy through regular funduscopic examinations are other indications for cataract extraction. In older patients, even those with dementia, correction of vision may improve quality of life and allow for more independence.[67,68]

Preoperative Evaluation for Cataract Surgery

As stated, cataract surgery is very low risk, especially as many surgeons are now performing these surgeries using phacoemulsification techniques under topical anesthesia with minimal sedation. Unfortunately, the preoperative assessment in these patients can still be problematic because patients have complicated histories and multiple illnesses. The preoperative assessment will need to identify patients that may need additional anesthesia, such as those with unstable medical conditions or conditions that may prohibit the patient from lying still during the procedure such as severe cardiopulmonary disease.[69,70]

The value of preoperative laboratory testing has been questioned, and a recent prospective trial evaluated more than 18,000 cataract patients who were randomly assigned to either the preoperative routine testing group or the no-testing group.[69] At the time of the preoperative assessment, the testing group received routine tests including blood count and chemistries. In contrast, the no-testing group only underwent testing if there was a change in their medical history or physical examination that suggested the need for testing at the time of the visit. After the procedure, there was no difference in the surgical complications and the postoperative or intraoperative

events in either group, which was approximately 31.3 events per 1000 patients. The authors suggested that routine laboratory testing was not indicated; however, it is important to recognize that all patients did receive a preoperative history and physical examination. In general, a history and physical examination before cataract surgery, possibly as part of a routine physical visit, are beneficial because these patients have complex medical histories. In most instances, a baseline electrocardiogram within 6–12 months is also recommended in the event of a dysrhythmia or other cardiac event during the case.

Anticoagulation and Cataract Surgery

Controversy surrounds the relative risks of discontinuing anticoagulant or antiplatelet medications for cataract surgery versus continuing these medications. Several studies have not found any increase in hemorrhagic complications when aspirin or warfarin are continued during cataract surgery.[71–75] A more recent, large cohort study[33] in 2003 examined the impact of continuing or discontinuing aspirin or warfarin in patients undergoing cataract surgery in the United States and Canada.[74] Data on more than 19,000 patients undergoing cataract surgery were included. Twenty-four percent (4517) of patients took aspirin, and 4% were taking warfarin or warfarin and aspirin. A small percentage of patients (22.5%) discontinued aspirin for 2 weeks, and 28% had stopped warfarin 4 days before surgery. The incidence of adverse events was extremely low in all cases. There was no difference in the incidence of thrombotic events in individuals who continued aspirin (1.49/1000 surgeries) versus those who discontinued aspirin (1/1000 surgeries). Similarly, there was no increase in ocular hemorrhage between patients who continued or discontinued warfarin.

It is likely from the available evidence that anticoagulant and antiplatelet medication can be continued safely during the perioperative period. The decision to withhold the medication should take into account the reason the patient is taking the medication, the type of anesthesia planned (local versus regional), and whether the patient is monocular or not. The decision should be made in conjunction with the patient's primary physician. If a decision to stop the anticoagulants is agreed upon, there should be a clear timeline for the postoperative reinstatement of the medications, including who is responsible for follow-up.

Anesthesia for Cataract Surgery

Recent surveys suggest that local and intracameral anesthesia are the preferred anesthetic techniques, although there are areas in this country and the world where regional techniques are still routinely used[65,76–78] (Table 23-10). This section describes the different types of anesthesia as well as the relative merits of each approach.

TABLE 23-10. Common anesthetic options for cataract surgery.

1. Retrobulbar block
2. Peribulbar block
3. Sub-Tenon's block
4. Topical anesthesia
5. Topical anesthesia with intracameral injection

Regional Orbital Anesthesia

Regional anesthesia for eye surgery provides dense ocular anesthesia and akinesia; this may be advantageous in complex or prolonged cases. Retrobulbar and peribulbar blocks are the most common regional techniques described.[79] The successful regional block requires a block of the optic nerve and the ciliary ganglion. Blockade of the ciliary ganglion results in a fixed, mid-position pupil. The surgery may also require paralysis of the orbicularis oculi muscle to prevent blinking; this muscle is innervated by the seventh fascial nerve.

Retrobulbar and Peribulbar Anesthesia

The retrobulbar and peribulbar blocks are similar. The retrobulbar block involves the injection of local anesthetic agent behind the orbit within the muscular cone. The needle is introduced at the junction of the lateral and middle two thirds of the lower lid above the inferior orbital rim. As the needle pierces the orbital septum, it remains parallel to the orbit floor; after reaching the globe equator, the needle is redirected upward to the apex of the orbit. The operator may feel a pop as the needle traverses the bulbar fascia, entering the muscle cone. Between 2 to 4 mL of local anesthetic is injected inside the cone of muscles, close to the optic nerve. During the injection, an awake patient is instructed to look straight ahead (a primary gaze), minimizing the chance of an intraneural injection. The peribulbar block is very similar; the needle is introduced as described for the retrobulbar block. However, the needle is kept parallel and lateral to the rectus muscle, and no effort is made to enter the bulbar fascia. As the needle reaches the equator, the local anesthetic is injected, i.e., around the muscle cone, not inside. For the peribulbar block, a larger volume of anesthetic is required to allow diffusion—generally 4–6 mL. Additionally, it may take closer to 20 minutes to achieve the desired anesthesia. The peribulbar block may be accompanied by a second injection of 3–5 mL of local anesthetic injected medially in the superomedial orbit. A blunt-tipped needle of less than 31 mm in length is recommended to reduce the chance of a globe or neural puncture.[76–79]

Sub-Tenon's block is a combination block. Topical anesthesia is applied to the conjunctiva, and one quadrant of the sclera is exposed to reveal Tenon's capsule surrounding the sclera. A blunt catheter or needle is inserted into the sub-Tenon's space, and local anesthetic is infused. This provides excellent anterior anesthesia, but topical anesthesia is required for the cornea and conjunctiva. There is a small risk of global puncture with this type of injection, but in general, complications are lower than those described for retrobulbar blocks.[76,79]

Monitoring and Sedation

During the placement of the orbital block, the patient's electrocardiogram, blood pressure, and oxygen saturation should be monitored.[80] It is important that the patient remains still during the injection, and this may be achieved by the administration of short-acting sedative medication accompanied by supplemental oxygen. Multiple drug regimens have been described, and low-dose propofol (30–50 mg) is probably the medication of choice, offering excellent conditions with few side effects and a short duration.[81–83] Midazolam is also frequently used, but, as a solo agent, may not provide a deep enough plane of sedation to prevent movement during the injection. Short-acting narcotics can be used but most prefer to avoid narcotics because of an increased risk of postoperative nausea and vomiting.[84] Combinations of a benzodiazepine, such as midazolam, and ketamine may result in improved patient cooperation,[85] but it is not clear if there are true advantages over low-dose propofol. The role for dexmedetomidine in cataract surgery has yet to be established. A recent double-blind study comparing the use of midazolam to dexmedetomidine for sedation in cataract surgery under peribulbar block found that patient satisfaction was slightly higher with dexmedetomidine. This advantage was offset by greater reductions in blood pressure and longer recovery time with delayed discharge compared with the midazolam group.[40]

In contrast to the requirements for block placement, minimal sedation during the case is generally sufficient, and short-acting anxiolysis with midazolam is the most popular choice. Various protocols have been described including patient-controlled administration of propofol.[86,87] However, the data so far do not show any particular advantage, and indeed the combination of midazolam and propofol often resulted in undesirable head movement. Furthermore, any sedation must be balanced against the potential downside of disorientation and lack of cooperation in the patient during the procedure.

Side Effects and Complications of Intraorbital Anesthesia

Complications from intraorbital anesthesia are uncommon but the effects may be devastating, resulting in permanent visual damage or blindness (Table 23-11). Although the overall complication rate is less than 0.5%, this still has the potential to affect thousands of patients

TABLE 23-11. Complications of retrobulbar anesthesia.

1. Retrobulbar hemorrhage
2. Globe perforation
3. Neural injection of optic nerve
4. Vascular injection
5. Central retinal artery or vein occlusion
6. Brainstem anesthesia

because of the huge number of patients undergoing cataract surgery. The most significant adverse events are described below.

Orbital hemorrhage occurs in 0.1%–1.7% of retrobulbar and 0.072% of peribulbar blocks. Hemorrhage occurs as a result of the inadvertent puncture of the ophthalmic artery as it crosses the optic nerve. Immediate signs of hemorrhage include proptosis, subconjunctival hemorrhage, and increased orbital pressure. Initial treatment is direct intermittent pressure to the eye. If the globe relaxes back (retropulsion) and intraocular pressure is normal, cataract surgery may be continued. If increased intraocular pressure or proptosis persists, then a lateral canthotomy is performed. Retinal perfusion should be confirmed using the ophthalmoscope. If the intraocular pressure remains increased despite a patent canthotomy, then aqueous suppressants may be added.

Globe perforation is most common with a retrobulbar block, but may also occur during a peribulbar or sub-Tenon's block; the incidence varies from 0% to 0.75% of blocks performed. Major risk factors for perforation include inexperience by the operator and staphyloma of the eye. The visual damage after a globe perforation will depend on the presence or absence of a retinal detachment and vitreous hemorrhage[58,76] (Table 23-12).

Optic nerve damage is very rare after a retrobulbar injection.

Central Nervous System Complications

The optic nerve sheath communicates directly with cerebrospinal fluid, and inadvertent injection of local anesthesia into the sheath may result in immediate brainstem anesthesia. Similarly, intraarterial injection of local anesthesia may cause central nervous system toxicity and seizures. Acute vascular injury may result from damage to the central retinal artery or vein; this may lead to significant injury.

TABLE 23-12. Factors increasing risk of globe rupture.

• Uncooperative patient
• Long eye axial length >26mm
• Staphyloma
• Long needle used for the block

Topical Anesthesia for Ocular Surgery

Topical anesthesia, mostly with lidocaine or tetracaine eye drops, has become very popular with surgeons and patients.[53,88] In a survey from 1999, the American Society of Cataract and Refractive Surgery found that topical anesthesia was used by 45% of respondents. Caseload was a factor contributing to choice. Surgeons performing five or fewer cases per month favored regional anesthesia, whereas surgeons performing more than 50 cases per month preferred topical anesthesia. Eighty-one percent of surgeons using local anesthesia used a combination of topical and intracameral injection,[82] which involves a small incision and installation of local anesthesia into the anterior chamber. The intracameral injection reduces the discomfort during manipulation of the lens. Some patients may still require small amounts of midazolam or similar medications during the surgery.[80,89,90]

Advantages of Topical Anesthesia

There are several advantages to topical anesthesia (Table 23-13). The patient avoids the risk of retrobulbar hemorrhage and other complications, is able to see immediately, and the postoperative recovery is very speedy. Even complex cataract surgery may be performed under topical anesthesia. Jacobi et al.[88] found that surgical complications in complex surgeries were not different between patients receiving topical versus retrobulbar anesthesia. Patient satisfaction with the different techniques has been questioned. In the study on complex surgeries, Jacobi et al. found greater patient satisfaction for topical over retrobulbar anesthesia (p=0.01). However, Boezaart et al.[78] questioned elderly patients (mean age 71 years) having cataract surgery and found that 70% of patients preferred the block over the local anesthetic. Interestingly, 98% did not remember the insertion of the block, a positive benefit of sedation with the block. In general, patient satisfaction is high with both techniques; however, the rapid postoperative recovery ultimately makes the topical approach very appealing to patients and physicians.

The Role of the Anesthesiologist

Several surveys have provided conflicting data on the need for an anesthesiologist during cataract surgeries.

TABLE 23-13. Advantages of topical versus regional block.

1. Eliminates risk of retrobulbar hemorrhage
2. Reduces risk to the optic nerve and other structures
3. Minimizes risk of strabismus postoperatively
4. Very short recovery time with immediate sight

Rosenfield et al.,[80] in a study of 1006 patients, found that in one third of cases an intervention by an anesthesia team was required and that the need for an intervention was unpredictable. The lack of predictability is perhaps one of the strongest arguments for anesthesia involvement. The International Cataract Surgery Outcomes Study surveyed ophthalmologists in the United States, Canada, Denmark, and Spain from 1993 to 1994.[90] They found that in the United States 78% of surgeons used phacoemulsification for the cataract removal. In this survey, they found only 14% used topical for the anesthesia, 46% used retrobulbar, and 38% used peribulbar blocks. Most blocks (79%) were performed by the surgeon, although in 78% of cases an anesthesiologist was present. All patients were monitored: 97% with electrocardiogram, blood pressure, and oxygen saturation. The low rate of topical anesthesia may reflect the sampling era because more recent results support topical anesthesia. Furthermore, the international study had a high rate of anesthesia involvement. In an in-depth analysis of anesthesia management during cataract surgery, Reeves et al.[91] found preferences for an anesthesiologist, sedation, and a block for the surgery. However, these results were highly dependent on the selection of a relatively small expert panel. In contrast, the results of more recent surveys of ophthalmologists favor topical anesthesia. Thus, although not universal, anesthesiologists are still frequently involved in monitoring the patient during the cataract surgery.

Special Situations

There are some special circumstances in the elderly patient that may require alternative approaches. For instance, demented or uncooperative patients may require more sedation or even general anesthesia. Chronic pain patients may be unable to lie flat and be tolerant of medications. Occipital pain has been described during the procedure necessitating additional medications. In patients with significant cardiopulmonary disease, supplemental oxygen may be required during the case, and several instances of hypercapnia have been described.[92,93] The anesthesiologist should be prepared to respond to the variable needs of this population.

Postoperative

A cataract extraction is an outpatient procedure. Patients generally follow up with the ophthalmologist the next day. All patients should receive instructions from the ophthalmologist's office before discharge. In patients receiving blocks, an eye patch is common, and vision will take longer to return.[94] These patients may require additional help at home during convalescence.

Conclusions

Elderly patients should be offered the opportunity to undergo procedures and simple surgeries under sedation with minimal risk. Skillful administration of sedation may help avoid more morbid and complex surgeries and improve outcomes. Sedation in the older patient is safe, but requires additional vigilance and patience.

References

1. Rodriguez-Gonzzalez FJ, Naranjo-Rodriguez A, Mata-Tapia I, Chicano-Gallardo M, Puente-Gutierrez JJ, López-Vallejos P. ERCP in patients 90 years of age and older. Gastrointest Endosc 2003;58:220–225.
2. Practice Guidelines for Sedation and Analgesia by Non Anesthesiologists. Task force on sedation and analgesia. Anesthesiology 1996;84:459–471.
3. Gullo A. Sedation and anesthesia outside the operating room: definitions, principles, critical points and recommendations. Minerva Anestesiol 2005;71:1–9.
4. Arepally A, Oechsle D, Kirkwood S, Savader SJ. Safety of conscious sedation in interventional radiology. Cardiovasc Intervent Radiol 2001;24:185–190.
5. Modifications in endoscopic practice for the elderly. Gastrointest Endosc 2000;52(6):849–851.
6. Calderini E. Recommendation for anesthesia and sedation in non-operating room locations. Minerva Anestesiol 2005; 71:11–20.
7. Manninen PH, Chan ASH, Papworh D. Conscious sedation for interventional neuroradiology: a comparison of midazolam and propofol infusion. Can J Anaesth 1997;44: 26–30.
8. Otley CC, Nguyen TH. Safe and effective conscious sedation administered by dermatologic surgeons. Arch Dermatol 2000;136:1333–1335.
9. Parlak M, Parlak I, Erdur B, Ergin A, Sagiroglu E. Age effect on efficacy and side effects of two sedation and analgesia protocols on patients going through cardioversion: a randomized clinical trial. Acad Emerg Med 2006;13: 493–499.
10. Jackson DL, Johnson BS. Conscious sedation for dentistry: risk management and patient selection. Dent Clin North Am 2002;46:767–780.
11. Leung JM, Dzankic S. Relative importance of preoperative health status versus intraoperative factors in predicting postoperative adverse outcomes in surgical patients. J Am Geriatr Soc 2001;49:1080–1085.
12. Oei-Lim VL, Kalkman CJ, Bartelsman JF, Res JC, van Wezel HB. Cardiovascular responses, arterial saturation and plasma catecholamines concentration during upper gastrointestinal; endoscopy using conscious sedation with midazolam or propofol. Eur J Anaesthesiol 1998;15: 535–543.
13. Elveback LR, Connolly DC, Melton LJ. Coronary heart disease in residents of Rochester, Minnesota. VII. Incidence 1950–1982. Mayo Clin Proc 1986;61:896–900.
14. Gerstenblith G, Fleg JL, Van Tosh A, Weisfeldt M, Lakatta EG. Stress testing redefines the prevalence of coronary

artery disease in epidemiologic studies. Circulation 1980; 62:111–308.

15. Muravchik S, Geroanesthesia: Principles for Management of the Elderly Patient. St. Louis, MO: Mosby-Year Book; 1997.

16. Christe C, Janssens JP, Armenian B, Herrmann F, Vogt N. Midazolam sedation for upper gastrointestinal endoscopy in older persons: a randomized, double blind, placebo-controlled study. J Am Geriatr Soc 2000;48:1398–1403.

17. Smetana G. Preoperative pulmonary evaluation. N Engl J Med 1999;340:937–944.

18. Clarke GA, Jacobson BC, Hammett RJ, Carr-Locke DL. The indications, utilization and safety of gastrointestinal endoscopy in an extremely elderly patient cohort. Endoscopy 2001;33(7):580–584.

19. Waring J, Baron T, Hirota W, Goldstein J, Jacobson B, Leighton J, et al. Guidelines for conscious sedation and monitoring during gastrointestinal endoscopy. American Society for Gastrointestinal Endoscopy. Gastrointest Endosc 2003; 58(3):317–322.

20. Cohen LB, Wecsler JS, Gaetano JN, Benson AA, Miller KM, Durkalski V, et al. Endoscopic sedation in the United States: results form a nationwide survey. Am J Gastroenterol 2006;101:967–974.

21. Lukens FJ, Loeb DS, Machicao VI, Achem SR, Picco MF. Colonoscopy in octogenarians: a prospective outpatient study. Am J Gastroenterol 2002;97:1722–1725.

22. Morrow JB, Zuccaro G, Conwell DL, Vargo JJ, Dumot JA, Karafa M, et al. Sedation for colonoscopy using a single bolus is safe, effective and efficient: a prospective, randomized double blind trial. Am J Gastroenterol 2000;95:2242–2247.

23. Heuss LT, Schnieper P, Drewe J, Pflimlin E, Beglinger C. Safety of propofol for conscious sedation during endoscopic procedures in high risk patients—a prospective controlled study. Am J Gastroenterol 2003;98:1751–1757.

24. Sedation and monitoring of patients undergoing gastrointestinal endoscopic procedures. Gastrointest Endosc 1995; 42(6):626–629.

25. Faigel DO, Baron TH, Goldstein JL, Hirota WK, Jacobson BC, Johanson JF. Guidelines for the use of deep sedation and anesthesia for GI endoscopy. American Society of Gastrointestinal Endoscopy. Gastrointest Endosc 2002; 56(5):613–617.

26. Abraham N, Wieczorek P, Huang J, Mayrand S, Fallone CA, Barkun AN. Assessing clinical generalizability in sedation studies of upper GI endoscopy. Gastrointest Endosc 2004; 60:28–33.

27. Abraham N, Barkun A, Larocque M, Fallone C, Mayrand S, Baffis, V. Predicting which patients can undergo upper endoscopy comfortably without conscious sedation. Gastrointest Endosc 2002;56:180–189.

28. Silverman W, Chotiprasidhi P, Chuttani R, Liu J, Petersen B, Taitelbaum G. Monitoring equipment for endoscopy. Gastrointest Endosc 2004;59:761–765.

29. Chen SC, Rex DK. An initial investigation of bispectral monitoring as an adjunct to nurse-administered propofol sedation for colonoscopy. Am J Gastroenterol 2004;99: 1081–1086.

30. Heuss LT, Schnieper P, Drewe J, Pflimlin E, Beglinger C. Conscious sedation with propofol in elderly patients: a prospective evaluation. Aliment Pharmacol Ther 2003;17: 1493–1501.

31. Bhardwaj G, Conlon S, Bowles J, Baralt J. Use of midazolam and propofol during colonoscopy: 7 years of experience. Letter Am J Gastroenterol 2002;97:495–496.

32. Wang CY, Ling LC, Cardosa MS, Wong AKH, Wong NW. Hypoxia during upper gastrointestinal endoscopy with and without sedation and the effect of pre-oxygenation on oxygen saturation. Anaesthesia 2000;55:654–658.

33. Yano H, Iishi H, Tatsuta M, Sakai N, Narahara H, Omori M. Oxygen desaturation during sedation for colonoscopy in elderly patients. Hepatogastroenterology 1998;45:2138–2141.

34. Erb T, Sluga M, Hampl KF, Ummenhofer W, Schneider MC. Preoperative anxiolysis with minimal sedation in elderly patients: bromazepam or clorazepate-dipotassium? Acta Anaethesiol Scand 1998;42:97–101.

35. Rudner R, Jalowoecki P, Kawecki P, Gonciarz M, Mularczyk A, Patelenz M. Conscious sedation analgesia/sedation with remifentanil and propofol versus total intravenous anesthesia with fentanyl, midazolam, and propofol for outpatient colonoscopy. Gastrointest Endosc 2003;57:667–673.

36. Jacobs JR, Reves JG, Marty J, White WD, Bai SA, Smith LR. Aging increases pharmacodynamic sensitivity to the hypnotic effects of midazolam. Anesth Analg 1995;80: 143–148.

37. Akcaboy ZN, Akcaboy EY, Albayrak D, Altinoren B, Dikmen B, Gogus N. Can remifentanil be a better choice than propofol for colonoscopy during monitored anesthesia care? Acta Anaesthesiol Scand 2006;50:736–741.

38. Koshy G, Nair S, Norkus EP, Hertan HI, Pitchumoni CS. Propofol versus midazolam and meperidine for conscious sedation in GI endoscopy. Am J Gastroenterol 2000;95: 1476–1479.

39. Cohen LB, Hightower CD, Wood DA, Miller KM, Aisenberg J. Moderate level sedation during endoscopy: a prospective study using propofol. Meperidine/fentanyl and midazolam. Gastrointest Endosc 2004;58:795–803.

40. Alhashemi JA. Dexmedetomidine vs. midazolam for monitored anaesthesia care during cataract surgery. Br J Anaesth 206;96:722–726.

41. Arain SR, Ebert JE. The efficacy, side effects, and recovery characteristics of dexmedetomidine versus propofol when used for intraoperative sedation. Anesth Analg 2002;95: 461–465.

42. Shinozaki M, Usui Y, Yamaguchi S, Okuda Y, Kitajima T. Recovery of psychomotor function after propofol sedation is prolonged in the elderly. Can J Anaesth 2002;49:927–931.

43. Frank LR, Strote J, Hauff SR, Bigelow SK, Fay K. Propofol by infusion protocol for ED procedural sedation. Am J Emerg Med 2006;24:599–602.

44. Burton JH, Miner JR, Shipley ER, Strout TD, Becker C, Thode HC. Propofol for emergency department procedural sedation and analgesia: a tale of three centers. Acad Emerg Med 2006;13:24–30.

45. Heuss LT, Drewe J, Schnieper P, Tapparelli CB, Pflimlin E, Beglinger C. Patient controlled versus nurse administered

sedation with propofol during colonoscopy. A prospective randomized trial. Am J Gastroenterol 2004;99:511–518.

46. Heuss LT, Schnieper P, Drewe J, Pflimlin E, Beglinger C. Risk stratification and safe administration of propofol by registered nurses supervised by gastroenterologist: a prospective observational study of more than 2000 cases. Gastrointest Endosc 2003;57:664–671.

47. Lee DW, Chan AC, Sze TS, Ko CW, Poon CM, Chan KC. Patient controlled sedation versus intravenous sedation for colonoscopy in elderly patients: a prospective randomized controlled trial. Gastrointest Endosc 2002;56:629–632.

48. Mazzon D, Germanà B, Poole D, Celato M, Bernardi L, Calleri G. Conscious sedation during endoscopic retrograde cholangiopancreatography: implementation of SIED-SIAARTI-ANOTE guidelines in Belluno Hospital. Minerva Anestesiol 2005;71:101–109.

49. Harrison SJ, Mayet J. Cardioversion and the use of sedation. Heart 2004;90:1374–1376.

50. Walker JA, McIntyre RD, Schleinitz PF, Jacobson KN, Haulk AA, Adesman P. Nurse administered propofol sedation without anesthesia specialists in 9152 endoscopic cases in an ambulatory surgery center. Am J Gastroenterol 2003; 98:1744–1750.

51. Busbee BG, Brown MM, Brown GC, Sharma S. Incremental cost-effectiveness of initial cataract surgery. Ophthalmology 2002;109:606–613.

52. Steinberg EP, Javitt JC, Sharkey PD, Zuckerman A, Legro MW, Anderson GF, et al. The content and cost of cataract surgery. Arch Ophthalmol 1993;111:1041–1049.

53. Hutchisson B, Nicoladis CB. Topical anesthesia—a new approach to cataract surgery. AORN J 2001;74:340–350.

54. Powe NR, Schein OD, Gieser SC, Tielsch JM, Luthra R, Javitt J, et al. Synthesis of the literature on visual acuity and complications following cataract extraction with intraocular lens implantation. Arch Ophthalmol 1994;112: 239–252.

55. Woodcock M, Shah S, Smith RJ. Clinical review: recent advances in customizing cataract surgery. BMJ 2004;328:92–96.

56. Eye Diseases Prevalence Research Group. Prevalence of cataract and pseudophakia/aphakia among adults in the United States. Arch Ophthalmol 2004;122:487–494.

57. Solomon DH, Locicero J, Rosenthal RA. New Frontiers in Geriatric Research. New York: Americas Geriatrics Society; 2004:177–202.

58. Kohnen T, Koch DD, eds. Cataract and Refractive Surgery. Essentials in Ophthalmology (Series). Berlin: Springer-Verlag; 2005:1–36, 123–132.

59. Steinberg EP, Tielsch JM, Schein OD, Javitt JC, Sharkey P, Cassard SD, et al. National study of cataract surgery outcomes. Ophthalmology 2004;101:1131–1141.

60. Tielsch JM, Steinberg EP, Cassard SD, Schein OD, Javitt JC, Legro MW, et al. Preoperative Functional Expectations and Postoperative Outcomes among Patients Undergoing First Eye Cataract Surgery. Arch Ophthalmol 1995;113: 1312–1318.

61. Schein OD, Steinberg EP, Cassard SD. Predictors of outcome in patients who underwent cardiac surgery. Ophthalmology 1995;102:817–823.

62. Minassian DC, Rosen P, Dart JK, Reidy A, Desai P, Sidhu M, et al. Extracapsular cataract extraction compared with small incision surgery by phacoemulsification: a randomized trial. Br J Ophthalmol 2001;85:822–829.

63. Schein OD, Bass EB, Sharkey P, Luthra R, Tielsch JM, Javitt JC, et al. Cataract Surgical Techniques. Arch Ophthalmol 1995;113:1108–1112.

64. Powe NR, Tielsch JM, Schein OD, Luthra R, Steinberg EP. Rigor of research methods in studies of the effectiveness and safety of cataract extraction with intraocular lens implantation. Arch Ophthalmol 1944;112:228–238.

65. Vander JF, Gault JA. Ophthalmology Secrets. 2nd ed. Philadelphia: Hanley and Belfus; 2002:1–7, 8–11, 189–204.

66. Jaffe NS. History of cataract surgery. Ophthalmology 1996; 103(8):S5–S16.

67. Appollonio I, Carabellese C, Magni E, Frattola L, Trabucchi M. Sensory impairments and mortality in an elderly community population: a six-year follow-up study. Age Ageing 1995;24:30–36.

68. Keller BK, Morton JL, Thomas VS, Potter JF. The effect of visual and hearing impairments on functional status. J Am Geriatr Soc 1999;47:1319–1325.

69. Schein OD, Katz J, Bass EB, Tielsch JM, Lubomski LH, Feldman MA, et al. The value of routine preoperative medical testing before cataract surgery. N Engl J Med 2000;342:168–175.

70. Bass EB, Steinberg EP, Luthra R, Schein OD, Tielsch JM, Javitt, JC, et al. Do ophthalmologists, anesthesiologist, and internists agree about preoperative testing in healthy patients undergoing cataract surgery? Arch Ophthalmol 1995;113:1248–1256.

71. Gainey SP, Robertson DM, Fay W, Ilstrup D. Ocular surgery on patients receiving long-term warfarin therapy. Am J Ophthalmol 1989;108:142–146.

72. McMahan LB. Anticoagulants and cataract surgery. J Cataract Refract Surg 1988;14:569–571.

73. Hall DL, Steen WH, Drummond JW, Byrd WA. Brief notes: anticoagulants and cataract surgery. Ophthalmic Surg 1988; 19:221–222.

74. Katz J, Feldman MA, Bass EB, Lubomski LH, Tielsch JM, Petty, BG, et al. Risks and benefits of anticoagulant and antiplatelet medication use before cataract surgery. Ophthalmology 2003;110:1748–1788.

75. Fry RA. Anticoagulants and local anaesthesia for eye surgery. Anaesth Intensive Care 2000;28:709.

76. Dutton JJ. Anatomic considerations in ophthalmic anesthesia. Surv Ophthalmol 2001;46:172–178.

77. Roman S, Auclin F, Ullern M. Topical versus peribulbar anesthesia in cataract surgery. J Cataract Refract Surg 1996; 22:1121–1124.

78. Boezaart A, Berry R, Nell M. Topical anesthesia versus retrobulbar for cataract surgery: the patients' perspective. J Clin Anesth 2000;12:58–60.

79. Ripart JR, Lefrant JY, de La Coussaye JE, Prat-Pradal D, Vivien B, Eledjam JJ. Peribulbar versus retrobulbar anesthesia for ophthalmic surgery. Anesthesiology 2001; 94:56–62.

80. Rosenfeld SI, Litinsky SM, Snyder DA, Plosker H, Astrove AW, Schiffman J. Effectiveness of monitored anesthesia care in cataract surgery. Ophthalmology 1999;106:1256–1261.

81. Habib NE, Balmer HG, Hockind G. Efficacy and safety of sedation with propofol in peribulbar anaesthesia. Eye 2002; 16:60–62.

82. Bosman YK, Krige SJ, Edge KR, Newstead J, DuToit PW. Comfort and safety in eye surgery under local anesthesia. Anaesth Intensive Care 1998;26:173–177.

83. Malhoutra SK, Dutta A, Gupta A. Monitored anesthesia in elderly ophthalmic elderly patients. Lancet 2002;359:532.

84. Mandelcorn M, Taback N, Mandelcorn E, Ananthanarayan C. Risk factors for pain and nausea following retinal and vitreous surgery under conscious sedation. Can J Ophthalmol 1999;34:281–285.

85. Rosenberg JK, Raymond C, Bridge PD. Comparison of midazolam/ketamine with methohexital for sedation during peribulbar block. Anesth Analg 1995;81:173–174.

86. Janzen PRM, Hall WJ, Hopkins PM. Setting targets for sedation with a target controlled propofol infusion. Anaesthesia 2000;55:666–669.

87. Pac-Soo CK, Deacock S, Lockwood G, Carr C, Whitwam JG. Patient-controlled sedation for cataract surgery using peribulbar block. Br J Anaesth 1996;77:370–374.

88. Jacobi PC, Dietlein TS, Jacobi FK. Comparative study of topical vs. retrobulbar anesthesia in complicated cataract surgery. Arch Ophthalmol 2000;118:1037–1043.

89. Harman DM. Combined sedation and topical anesthesia for cataract surgery. J Cataract Refract Surg 2000;26:109–113.

90. Nørregaard JC, Schein OD, Bellan L, Black C, Alonso J, Bernth-Petersen P, et al. International variation in anesthesia care during cataract surgery. Arch Ophthalmol 1997; 115:1304–1308.

91. Reeves SW, Friedman DS, Fleisher LA, Lubomski LH, Schein OD, Bass EB. A decision analysis of anesthesia management for cataract surgery. Am J Ophthalmol 2001; 132:528–536.

92. Risdall JE, Geraghty EF. Oxygenation of patients undergoing ophthalmic surgery under local anaesthesia. Anaesthesia 1997;52:489–500.

93. Schlager A. Accumulation of carbon dioxide under ophthalmic drapes during eye surgery: a comparison of three different drapes. Anaesthesia 1999;54:683–702.

94. Shelswell NL. Perioperative patient education for retinal surgery. AORN J 2002;75:801–807.

24
Total Hip Replacement, Joint Replacement, and Hip Fracture

Idit Matot and Shaul Beyth

Surgical treatment of hip fracture is a well-known medical emergency in the elderly. Similar to arthroplasty, this operation is performed to acutely restore function and decrease pain. Although the anatomic approach, instrumentation, and final mechanical results of hip fracture repair are similar to what occurs with hip arthroplasty, major differences between the two patient populations exist and create differences in perioperative management.

Background

Total Hip and Knee Arthroplasty

Joint replacement is one of the most rewarding procedures in the field of orthopedic surgery in general. It is indicated in individuals with a painful, disabling arthritic joint that is no longer responsive to conservative treatment. For these patients, it may provide improvement in the quality of life. Focusing on the frequently replaced weight-bearing joints, i.e., hip and knee, it should be noted that in addition to complete primary joint replacement, a whole new field of reconstructive surgery has evolved around the implantation of prostheses that includes, but is not limited to, partial arthroplasty, revision procedures for failed implants, computer-assisted surgery, and minimally invasive surgery.

Patients coming for elective joint replacement surgery are highly motivated and in most cases mentally prepared to undergo major surgery in order to regain daily functions. These patients undergo a thorough preoperative evaluation and preparation including relevant specialist evaluation, revision of medications, autologous blood donation, and preparation from a rehabilitation facility for the postoperative period.

Elective total hip or knee arthroplasty (THA/TKA) is considered a relatively safe orthopedic procedure. Known complications after these procedures, not related to the implants used, include thromboembolism, postoperative anemia, infection, fractures, and death. However, despite the low incidence of mortality after total joint arthroplasty, a significant number of deaths occur given the extensive number of procedures being performed. The specific risk has been reported to be as low as 0.1% and as high as 3%.[1] Compared with THA, the risk of perioperative death after TKA is considerably lower. Preexisting comorbidities and the American Society of Anesthesiologists physical status classification are significantly related to the incidence of postoperative death in patients undergoing elective hip or knee arthroplasty.[2] Also, total joint arthroplasty performed for fracture or malignancy has a higher risk of mortality.[3,4] Other patient health-independent factors that are associated with a significantly increased mortality include: age more than 70 years, revision (as compared with primary) surgery, use of a cemented prosthesis, and simultaneous bilateral arthroplasty.[4] Recognition of these risk factors and implementation of appropriate measures may enable the orthopedic team to reduce perioperative mortality after major lower extremity surgery.

The preoperative medical status of the patient may be even more important to outcome than the risks of the surgical procedure. Patients with preexisting cardiac or respiratory disease have decreased physiologic reserve and are at greater risk of morbidity and mortality, specifically cardiorespiratory collapse after an embolic load, hypoxemia as a result of ventilation/perfusion mismatch during lateral decubitus position, and myocardial ischemia or infarct, which may be prompted by intra- or postoperative blood loss, hypotension, and/or tachycardia. Measures to consider include optimizing medical therapy of patients who have a history of cardiac or pulmonary problems; avoiding bilateral one-stage TKA in patients who are ill or elderly; vigilant anesthetic monitoring, especially around the times of surgical interventions that are known to be associated with marrow and fat embolization; and the use of vasopressor agents during episodes of hypotension. Modifications in surgical technique and implant choice to reduce marrow and fat embolization may also be appropriate in some high-risk patients. The use of prophylactic antibiotics decreases infection rate to less than 1%. Administration of antibiotics 30 minutes before skin incision or, during revision arthroplasty, after samples for bacterial culture are obtained, is recommended.

Hip Fracture Surgery

Fractures of the hip, which most frequently occur in the elderly, are associated with a very high mortality. With increasing life expectancy, these injuries are on the increase and will thus continue to be a substantial workload for trauma departments. Impaired balance and coordination, leading to frequent falls, paired with a high prevalence of osteoporosis make the elderly particularly prone to incur this fracture. Operative treatment of hip fractures is usually straightforward, but postoperative recovery and rehabilitation are fraught with complications. One-year mortality after hip fracture surgery is remarkably high, around 26%, with a range of 14%–36% reported in the literature. It is highest during the first 6 months after injury, and after the first year it approaches that of unoperated patients of matching age and sex.[5]

The reported in-hospital mortality rates range from 1.4% to 12%.[6-8] The principal causes of in-hospital death after hip fracture are cardiac failure and myocardial infarction, which occur early after the fracture, peaking at 2 days, bronchopneumonia, which accounts for the majority of late deaths, and pulmonary embolism, which peaks in the second week after injury. The overall incidence of perioperative myocardial ischemia in elderly patients undergoing hip fracture surgery has been reported to be 35%–42%.[9,10] Preoperative placement of an epidural catheter with provision of effective analgesia has recently been shown to reduce the preoperative incidence of adverse cardiac outcomes in high-risk patients with neck of femur fracture.[9,10] Mortality from bronchopneumonia and pulmonary embolism after hip fracture may be reduced by early surgical intervention, early mobilization, antibiotics, and prophylactic anticoagulation.[5,8,11]

Unlike patients scheduled for joint arthroplasty, patients with hip fracture are routinely admitted to the emergency room without prior preparation or evaluation. These patients should be considered as requiring urgent treatment. Thus, perioperative management should be oriented toward adequate pain control, multidisciplinary consultation, if needed, and optimal monitoring and risk-reduction within a given time frame. The issue that the anesthesiologist must consider in the preoperative evaluation and clearance for urgent surgical treatment of a hip fracture is the timing of surgery. In most studies, patients wait on average 1.5–3.5 days between admission and surgery.[5,11-16] Results of studies of the optimal timing of surgery are contradictory. Whereas some studies reported an increased mortality if patients had surgery within 24 hours, the majority have demonstrated a clear advantage of early surgical intervention. The current prevailing recommendation is that patients who are medically fit for surgery should be operated on the day of admission[16] because delays serve to increase morbidity, mortality, and resource utilization.[14-16] In two recent studies, longer waiting time increased the risk for developing deep vein thrombosis and pulmonary embolism, atelectasis, pneumonia,[11] and decubitus ulcer formation.[16] Nevertheless, sufficient time should be taken to study and prepare patients with significant comorbidities. For these patients, preoperative epidural analgesia may prove to be most helpful.[10]

It is important to note that, although the two categories of hip fracture surgeries (THA and hip fracture stabilization) aim to improve ambulation, they differ in both patient characteristics (as noted above) and in the expected end result. For arthroplasty, the expected surgical outcome is functioning "better than before," whereas the anticipated result of procedures for hip fractures is functioning "as close to before (the fracture)" as possible.

Surgical Procedure

Total Hip and Knee Arthroplasty

Arthroplasty of both hip and knee joints is a procedure aimed to improve patients' ambulation by means of replacing damaged and worn-out joint components with prosthetic devices. Inherently, these procedures involve surgical removal of articulating surfaces together with the subchondral bone, implantation of the substitute parts, and fixation of those components.

Hip

There are several prosthetic devices available, most of which share a few basic characteristics:

1. After surgical dislocation from the acetabulum, the arthritic femoral head and a portion of the femoral neck are resected and replaced with an intramedullary stemmed component, anchored to its place using a premade space reamed through the soft spongious bone ("press-fit") and/or cement surrounding the stem.

2. If the acetabulum needs replacement, the damaged articulating cartilage is reamed and the prosthetic acetabular component is attached to its place, using the same techniques as above. It can then be further supported by screws and/or bone graft.

3. No matter which surgical approach to the joint has been used (anterior, posterior, or lateral), the two artifi-

cial joint components are fit together ("reduction" of a "dislocated joint") at the very last stages of the operation. This step is best assisted by muscle relaxation. Dislocation may occur shortly after surgery if the muscle tone that keeps the joint in place is not restored.

Knee

This procedure begins with a knee joint arthrotomy. The distal femur and the proximal tibia are shaped using measured templates to fit the size of the available prosthetic parts. These parts are later attached to the bones, covering the exposed surfaces. Shaping of the bony ends is accompanied by bleeding, especially from the trabecular bone. Although fitting of the prosthesis leads to hemostasis, the bleeding from trabecular bone is not always fully controlled. Blood loss from trabecular bone may therefore proceed after surgery and is halted because of clot formation and/or tamponade effect of the hematoma. Close monitoring of hematocrit and hemoglobin levels is thus essential in the postoperative period.

The patella may be replaced either completely or partially, or may not be replaced at all. Also, the new prosthetic components may be either cemented or uncemented, depending on the findings and the surgeons' preferences.

Hip Fractures

Several procedures are accepted today in the management of hip fractures, depending primarily on the type of fracture and the patient's concurrent diseases (Figure 24-1).

Extracapsular Fractures

The vast majority of these fractures will unite after proper reduction and fixation. Both extra- and intramedullary systems are used to treat pertrochanteric and subtrochanteric fractures. The newest devices are introduced through minor skin incisions from a lateral aspect approach to the thigh and require not more than an hour for a skilled team.

Intracapsular Fractures

Because the retrograde blood supply to the head of the femur is often compromised after displaced femoral neck fractures, the degree of displacement dictates the nature of surgical procedure:

- Minimally and nondisplaced intracapsular fractures are usually stabilized in their position by percutaneous introduction of cannulated screws into the femoral neck and head through the fracture line. This is a minimally invasive procedure that results in minor systemic effect.
- Displaced intracapsular fractures, often termed "subcapital" or "femoral neck" fractures, are often treated

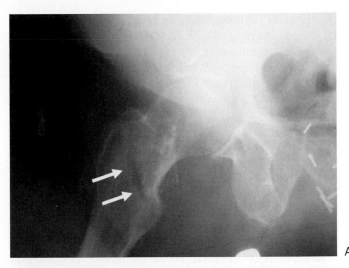

A

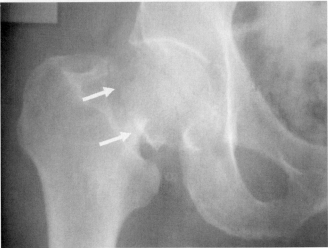

B

FIGURE 24-1. **(A)** Intertrochanteric femoral fracture. Fracture line extends from greater to lesser trochanters, external to hip joint capsule. **(B)** Femoral neck fracture. Fracture line extends from medial to lateral cortex of the proximal femur, within the hip joint capsule ("sub-capital" fracture).

by prosthetic replacement of the femoral side of the hip joint (hemiarthroplasty), because of the above-mentioned risk of femoral head necrosis after compromise of its blood supply. From the anesthesiologist's point of view, the surgical procedure itself is almost identical to that of complete hip joint replacement.

Anesthetic Management

Anesthetic Technique

The choice of anesthetic technique is a complex medical decision that depends on many factors, including patient characteristics (e.g., comorbidity, age), type of surgery performed, and risks of the anesthetic techniques. Assessment of the risks of the anesthetic technique should include consideration of technical factors (airway, establishment of regional blocks, invasive monitoring), anesthetic agent toxicities, incidence of critical intraoperative and postoperative events, and postoperative treatment of pain.[6]

Anesthesia for Hip Fracture Repair

In recent years, regional anesthesia has been used more frequently in hip fracture patients. In 1981–1982, general anesthesia was used in 94.8% of patients, whereas in 1993–1994, general anesthesia was used in only 49.6% of patients.[6]

Few studies have compared the outcome of patients administered general versus regional anesthesia for hip fracture surgery. The largest retrospective analysis that included 9425 hip fracture patients reported that the type of anesthesia did not seem to influence morbidity or overall mortality.[6] This finding suggests that unadjusted differences in outcome between general anesthesia and regional anesthesia are mainly a result of concomitant disease and not of any protective effect of one anesthetic technique versus another. As might be predicted from clinical practice, the authors found that older patients and those who were sicker were more likely to be receiving a regional anesthetic. Intraoperative hypotension and the use of vasopressors were more frequent in the regional anesthesia group than in the general anesthesia group. The results of this study are in agreement with two earlier meta-analyses[13,17] that included randomized controlled trials that evaluated the outcome of hip fracture surgery up to 1 month postoperatively. The authors were unable to identify any difference in long-term mortality or blood loss attributable to the use of either regional or general anesthesia. However, there was a clearly reduced incidence of deep vein thrombosis in the regional anesthesia group. Subsequent large, single-center observational studies[12,18] also did not identify meaningful differences in cardiopulmonary morbidity or mortality attributable to the choice of the anesthetic technique in hip surgery patients. A similar conclusion was reached in the 2002 Cochrane Library review.[19,20]

In the past few years, there has been a growing interest in peripheral nerve blockade in orthopedic patients. Such techniques are used more and more often not only to provide anesthesia but also for postoperative analgesia after limb surgery. Various nerve blocks have been used to reduce pain after hip fracture. The 2002 Cochrane Library review[21] summarized the data from eight randomized trials involving 328 patients. Three trials related to placement of a nerve block (lateral cutaneous, femoral, triple, psoas) preoperatively and the remaining five to perioperative insertion. Nerve blocks resulted in lower reported pain levels and reduced consumption of pain medications (parenteral and oral) during the periopera-

tive period. No clinical benefits beyond these reductions could be demonstrated.

Neuraxial Anesthesia for Total Knee or Hip Arthroplasty

Regional anesthesia may be of benefit to patients undergoing major joint surgery. A retrospective study found that the use of neuraxial anesthesia compared with general anesthesia in patients having elective total knee or hip replacements was associated with a lower rate of intensive care unit admission postoperatively.[22] In addition, intraoperative blood loss and transfusion requirements were significantly lower in patients who received neuraxial anesthesia or lumbar plexus block.[23–26] Neuraxial anesthesia and analgesia were associated with a reduction in thromboembolic complications.[27–29] Also, postoperative confusional state was reported to be less frequent in a group of patients who had epidural anesthesia compared with those patients who had surgery under general anesthesia.[30] Others[31,32] have failed to find an advantage of general versus regional anesthesia in all outcome measurements (magnitude or pattern of postoperative cognitive dysfunction and incidence of major cardiovascular complications) except that epidural anesthesia was associated with more rapid achievement of postoperative in-hospital rehabilitation goals. The largest benefit of regional anesthesia and analgesia is its role in providing adequate pain control for rehabilitation. This topic is discussed in depth in the section on postoperative analgesia.

Intraoperative Monitoring

With advances in both anesthetic and surgical techniques, the need for invasive intraoperative monitoring in medically fit patients has diminished. Nevertheless, several stages in the intraoperative period can cause significant hemodynamic and respiratory alterations. Therefore, in high-risk patients or procedures (complex or revision surgery), the use of an arterial line for continuous hemodynamic and blood gas monitoring may be useful. Intraoperative transesophageal echocardiography may detect fat embolization and monitor intraoperative volume status and cardiac function.[33] In high-risk patients undergoing bilateral procedures, pulmonary artery pressure monitoring may also be of benefit, both as a diagnostic and a prognostic tool.[34] Although more invasive monitoring improves detection of pulmonary embolization and its sequelae, there is no evidence to suggest that these interventions improve outcome in fat emboli syndrome.

Positioning

The lateral decubitus positioning, which is frequently used for THA and displaced intracapsular fractures

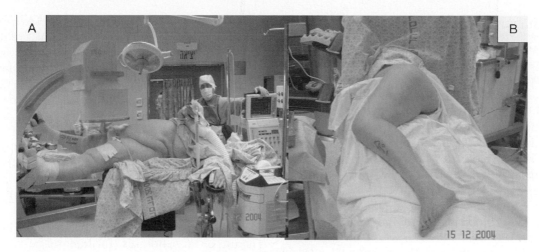

FIGURE 24-2. Positioning of the patient on the fracture table for fracture of hip surgery **(A)** or in the lateral decubitus position for total hip arthroplasty **(B)** should be performed carefully because of potential morbidities.

(Figure 24-2), requires special attention to pressure points, hemodynamic stability, and oxygenation. A low axillary roll is placed under the chest and lower shoulder to prevent brachial plexus stretching and axillary artery occlusion of the dependent side. Padding of the nonoperated (dependent) hip and leg is important, as well as padding of the nondependent leg and hand to prevent injury to the femoral, popliteal, and pudendal nerve, the brachial plexus, and the ulnar nerve. The head and neck should be aligned properly and supported to avoid injury to the cervical spine, ears, and eyes. Positioning into the lateral decubitus may cause brief hypotension, especially if the patient is hypovolemic. It may also result in hypoxemia, which results from increased degree of ventilation/perfusion mismatch: the nondependent lung is well ventilated but poorly perfused and the dependent lung is poorly ventilated but well perfused.[35]

Cement

Polymethylmethacrylate bone cement prepared in a liquid methylmethacrylate monomer is widely used to anchor prostheses in joint replacement surgery. Multiple adverse effects have been associated with the use of polymethylmethacrylate cement.[36,37] Hypoxemia, pulmonary hypertension, right ventricle failure, cardiac arrest, and sudden death are well-recognized complications during THA and to a lesser degree after TKA. Although incompletely understood, these complications have been in part attributed to formation of microemboli and activation of the complement system, resulting in triggering of the inflammatory cascade, which in turn leads to increased vascular endothelial permeability.[38,39] The increase of intramedullary pressure caused by the mechanical compression of the femoral canal during the insertion of the prosthetic stem is the most decisive pathogenic factor for the development of embolism. The thin-walled vessels in the medullary cavity are easily disrupted by focal application of compressive loads, allowing the intravasation of bone marrow, fat, and bone debris and the embolization through the venous system located along the linea aspera and through the metaphyseal vessels. Migration of bone marrow into the draining veins activates the coagulation system. Occlusion of lung capillaries by these emboli causes an increased arteriovenous shunt and alveolar hypoperfusion.[40–44] In addition, the methylmethacrylate cement causes direct vasodilatation leading to transient hypotension.

The progressive decrease of serious intraoperative cardiorespiratory complications in the past few decades has been attributed to the constant improvement of anesthesiologic and surgical techniques. To prevent hypoxemia intraoperatively, 100% oxygen administration during cementing and prosthesis insertion in patients at risk has been recommended anecdotally although there are no prospective studies confirming the usefulness of this maneuver.[34] Fluid therapy to prevent hypovolemia is also recommended, because canine studies have shown that acute hemodynamic changes during prosthesis insertion and fat embolism may be aggravated in hypovolemic states.[45] Maintenance of perfusion pressure with vasoconstrictors to preserve right heart perfusion and function and to avoid fluid loading may be preferable in patients with preexisting heart disease with congestive symptoms. Modifications of surgical techniques aimed at prevention of embolism, e.g., by venting of the femoral shaft and lavage of the medullary canal (to minimize increases in intramedullary pressure and the amount of fatty bone marrow present), and increased use of total condylar components from long-stemmed prostheses (that obviate the need for extensive intramedullary manipulation) may be most effective at reducing the incidence of these complications.

Blood Management

The likelihood of major intra- and postoperative blood loss and resultant transfusion of blood components is high in lower extremity joint replacement and hip fracture surgery. TKA, for example, can be associated with major blood loss. Lotke et al.[46] concluded in their study that the mean calculated total blood loss in TKA was approximately 1.5 L. In TKA the total blood loss is composed of "visible" blood loss (from the surgical field and wound drainage) and "hidden" blood loss (into the tissues). The latter can account for up to 50% of total blood loss.[47] Blood management should be aimed at addressing the total blood loss and underestimation ought to be avoided.

In several series over the past decade,[48–51] 32%–85% of the operated patients received allogeneic blood. The frequency of allogeneic blood transfusion varied with respect to the type of operative procedure (revision THA and bilateral TKA were associated with the highest prevalence of such transfusions) and with a baseline hemoglobin level of 130 g/L or less. Concerns about the risks associated with allogeneic blood transfusion led to the development of a variety of blood conservation techniques intended to minimize the need for allogeneic transfusion. These include preoperative donation of autologous blood, acute normovolemic hemodilution, blood salvage, hypotensive anesthesia, improvements in tissue hemostasis, and pharmacologic agents such as preoperative use of erythropoietin and intraoperative use of antifibrinolytics.[52] Several studies have confirmed the use of these techniques to reduce allogeneic blood transfusion; however, their use is based on hospital resources and on the anesthesiologist and surgeon preferences. In addition to reducing the need for and exposure to allogeneic blood, the potential for less blood loss may translate into less swelling, improved range of motion, and earlier return to function. The anesthesiologist should be thoroughly acquainted with these blood conservation techniques and remember that all methods come with varying amounts of risk and cost. Also, the use of regional anesthesia may reduce the risk of transfusion in lower extremity arthroplasties.[23–26]

Postoperative Analgesia

For lower limb orthopedic surgery, postoperative pain is a major problem. Peripheral nerve blocks with or without a catheter are the techniques of the new millennium.[53] For acute pain management after major lower limb surgery, continuous femoral nerve blockade has been advocated as an alternative to epidural analgesia or intravenous opiate administered by patient-controlled analgesia (PCA).[54–62] Both epidural analgesia and continuous femoral nerve blockade are more effective than intravenous PCA in patients undergoing THA. Both provide effective postoperative pain control, reduce opiate requirements and associated side effects, and improve functional recovery. The advantage of a femoral nerve block in this major joint surgery seems to be the analgesic effect on pain during mobilization. Similar results have been obtained after TKA.[55–58] Moreover, as was confirmed by Ganapathy et al.[59] and Chelly et al.,[57] compared with intravenous PCA, continuous femoral nerve blockade reduced the length of hospital stay and the frequency of serious complications while conveniently avoiding the risk of epidural hematoma associated with the use of anticoagulant. Thus, a continuous femoral nerve block should be considered after proximal lower limb surgery. The use of PCA boluses (for femoral nerve block), with or without low basal infusion rate after TKA or THR,[60,61] significantly reduces the local anesthetic consumption and therefore the risk of local anesthetic toxicity and increases patient satisfaction. It has been argued that femoral nerve block does not consistently produce anesthesia of the obturator nerve. The addition of an obturator nerve block has been therefore recommended to improve the quality of postoperative analgesia after total knee replacement.[62] The need for addition of a sciatic nerve block to a femoral nerve block is controversial. Whereas Allen et al.[58] reported that it does not further improve analgesic efficacy, Davies et al.[63] showed that combined femoral and sciatic blocks offer a practical alternative to epidural analgesia for unilateral knee replacements. Others suggested posterior lumbar plexus block for postoperative analgesia after TNA.[64,65]

Both clonidine and opioids have been used to supplement the analgesic effect of local anesthetics in peripheral nerve blocks. The addition of opioids to local anesthetic solution to maintain continuous nerve blockade has been debated because Picard et al.[66] failed to show any positive effect of opioids. A detailed discussion of the different peripheral nerve block techniques is beyond the scope of this chapter. For further discussion, the reader is referred to Internet resources, including the New York Society for Regional Anesthesia Web site (http://www.nysora.com), the Peripheral Regional Anesthesia Web site (http://www.nerveblocks.net), or the RegionalBlock.com Web site (http://www.regionalblock.com).

Specific Considerations

Venous Thromboembolism, Anticoagulation, and Neuraxial Anesthesia

Patients who undergo major lower extremity orthopedic surgery are among those considered to be at greatest risk for venous thromboembolism. Data suggest a deep vein thrombosis rate as high as 40%–84% when prophylaxis is not administered to patients undergoing TKA, a rate of 45%–57% after THA, and a rate of 36%–60% in patients receiving hip fracture surgery.[67] Clinically detected pulmonary embolism occurs in 2%–10% of patients with deep vein thrombosis who have had knee or hip arthroplasty. The incidence of fatal pulmonary embolism is 1%–2%. Thromboembolism can occur in vessels in the pelvis, thigh, and calf. Most thrombi probably develop in the deep veins of the calf and subsequently extend into the thigh, but isolated thrombi in the pelvis or deep femoral veins can also develop. Unfortunately, after knee or hip arthroplasty, deep vein thrombosis is clinically asymptomatic in 70%–80% of patients who experience clinically significant pulmonary emboli.[68] Therefore, thromboprophylaxis has become a worldwide standard practice for preventing complications during and after major lower extremity orthopedic surgery. Recently, the American College of Chest Physicians (ACCP) published its recommendation for prophylaxis for patients undergoing TKA, THA, and hip fracture surgery.[69] Either a low-molecular-weight heparin or an adjusted-dose warfarin is recommended for prophylaxis in THA and TKA (grade IA) and hip fracture surgery (grade IB). The ACCP also suggested that low-molecular-weight heparin is significantly more effective than warfarin in preventing asymptomatic and symptomatic in-hospital venous thromboembolism because of the more rapid onset of anticoagulant activity with low-molecular-weight heparin than with warfarin. Nevertheless, regimens for deep vein thrombosis prophylaxis are frequently institution- and surgeon-specific. Anesthetic techniques that enhance lower extremity blood flow and minimize the hypercoagulable state may be advantageous in the management of patients undergoing lower extremity surgery. Clearly, the incidence of intraoperative thrombosis formation is reduced with the use of central neuraxis techniques when compared with general endotracheal anesthesia without other active interventions.[27–29,70] Epidural anesthesia may prevent the development of the hypercoagulable state without impairing the coagulation process as measured by the platelet-mediated hemostasis time and the clotting time. Possible explanations include: central neuraxial blockade-induced sympathectomy, prolonged exposure to high systemic blood levels of local anesthetic, and the antiinflammatory effects of local anesthetics.[70]

The introduction of new anticoagulants and antiplatelet agents, the complexity of balancing thromboembolic with hemorrhagic complications, and the evolving indications for regional anesthesia/analgesia have raised concern over the issue of neuraxial anesthesia in caring for surgical orthopedic patients. Spinal/epidural hematoma is a rare but potentially catastrophic complication of spinal or epidural anesthesia, the incidence of which was estimated to be less than 1 in 150,000 epidural and less than 1 in 220,000 spinal anesthetics.[71] Risk factors include the intensity of the anticoagulant effect, epidural (versus spinal) technique, traumatic needle/catheter placement, sustained anticoagulation in an indwelling neuraxial catheter, catheter removal during therapeutic levels of anticoagulation, increased age, female gender, concomitant use of anticoagulant or antiplatelet medications, length of therapy, and twice-daily low-molecular-weight heparin administration.[72] Decreased weight and concomitant hepatic or renal disease may also exaggerate the anticoagulant response and theoretically increase the risk. The onset of symptoms immediately postoperatively is uncommon. Immediate diagnosis of spinal hematoma is critical because the reported time to progress from new neurologic deficits to complete paralysis was approximately 15 hours, and complete neurologic recovery was unlikely if more than 8 hours elapsed between the development of paralysis and surgical intervention.[73] Therefore, any new or progressive neurologic symptoms occurring in the presence of epidural analgesia warrant immediate discontinuation of the infusion (with the catheter left in situ) to rule out any contribution from the local anesthetic or volume effect.[71] Radiographic imaging, preferably magnetic resonance imaging, should be obtained as soon as possible as well as consultation with a neurosurgeon to determine the urgency of surgery.

When the American Society of Regional Anesthesia convened for the first Consensus Conference on Neuraxial Anesthesia and Anticoagulation in April 1998, 45 cases of spinal hematoma were associated with low-molecular-weight heparins, 40 of which involved a neuraxial anesthetic. Recently, recommendations for perioperative management of patients receiving low-molecular-weight heparin thromboprophylaxis were published[74] based on the consensus statements developed during the Second American Society of Regional Anesthesia Consensus Conference on Neuraxial Anesthesia and Anticoagulation.[72] Perioperative management of patients receiving low-molecular-weight heparins requires coordination and communication. Time intervals between neuraxial needle placement and administration of low-molecular-weight heparins must be maintained[74]; preoperatively, 10–12 hours should elapse after the last thromboprophylaxis dose of low-molecular-weight heparin (enoxaparin 40mg or dalteparin 5000U/kg every 24 hours), whereas higher doses require delays of at least 24 hours. Postoperatively, indwelling neuraxial catheters should be removed at least 10–12 hours after the last dose of low-molecular-weight heparin, and subsequent dosing of the drug should take place at least 2 hours after catheter removal. Other anticoagulants or antiplatelet medications should be avoided when low-molecular-weight heparins are used. In contrast to nonsteroidal antiinflammatory drugs and aspirin, which in and of themselves do not seem to present significant risk to patients for developing spinal-epidural hematomas, current practice is to have patients discontinue clopidogrel for a week and 14 days for ticlopidine before performing a neuroaxial block.[72,74] Platelet GP IIb/IIIa inhibitors exert a profound effect on platelet aggregation. After administration, the time to normal platelet aggregation is 24–48 hours for abciximab and 4–8 hours for eptifibatide and tirofiban. Neuraxial techniques should be avoided until platelet function has recovered. As experience grows with the newer antithrombotic and/or antiplatelet agents, guidelines will be revised. Herbal drugs, by themselves, seem to represent no added significant risk for the development of spinal hematoma in patients having epidural or spinal anesthesia.

The decision to perform neuraxial blockade on patients receiving thromboprophylaxis must be made on an individual basis, while weighing the risk of spinal hematoma from needle or catheter placement against the benefits gained. The anesthesiologists taking care of these patients are expected to be familiar with the updated recommendations for management of this patient population.

Tourniquet-Related Complications

The arterial tourniquet is widely used in lower extremity surgery to reduce blood loss and provide good operating conditions. The local and systemic physiologic effects and the anesthetic implications were recently reviewed.[75] Use of arterial tourniquet can be associated with complications ranging from the minor and self-limiting to the debilitating and even fatal. Localized complications result from either tissue compression beneath the cuff or tissue ischemia distal to the tourniquet. Pressure-related injuries to the underlying skin, nerve, muscle, and blood vessels are dependent on both the duration and pressure of tourniquet inflation. Systemic effects are related to the inflation or deflation of the tourniquet. Most tourniquet-related complications occur as a result of equipment failure or improper use and are thus easily avoided with good clinical practice. Tourniquet failure can result in over-pressurization, causing tissue injury, or under-pressurization, causing loss of hemostasis. Improper cuff application can result in bruising, blistering, friction burns to skin, and chemical burns from spirit solutions leaking under the tourniquet.[76] Results are conflicting from studies comparing postoperatively measured blood loss, operating time, need for blood transfusion, postoperative pain, analgesia requirement, and knee flexion in patients undergoing TKA with or without the use of tourniquet. Whereas some authors reported that operations without the use of a tourniquet cause a greater blood loss and need for blood transfusion,[77] others show no difference in operating time or total blood loss and/or blood transfusion. Furthermore, not using a tourniquet seems to be associated with significantly less postoperative pain,

earlier knee flexion, fewer superficial wound infections, and fewer deep vein thromboses.[78–80] These latter studies question the routine use of a tourniquet during TKA.

Local Effects

High tourniquet pressures directly under the cuff and prolonged ischemia are implicated in many cases of nerve and muscle damage, respectively. Arterial injury and skin damage are uncommon complications but may occur in patients with peripheral vascular disease and frail skin. Nerve compression causes intraneural microvascular abnormalities and edema formation, and these subsequently compromise local tissue nutrition, resulting in axonal degeneration.[81] Intracellular creatine phosphate and adenosine 5′-triphosphate are depleted in muscles after 2 and 3.5 hours of ischemia, respectively, resulting in prolonged metabolic recovery of the muscle.[81,82] After tourniquet release, reperfusion injury of the limb ensues, with edema and microvascular congestion that lead to the "post-tourniquet syndrome," the most common and least appreciated morbidity associated with tourniquet use.[83] This syndrome is characterized by stiffness, pallor, weakness without paralysis, and subjective numbness of the extremity without objective anesthesia. Nerve injuries associated with the use of tourniquets range from paresthesia to complete paralysis, but most nerve lesions heal spontaneously in <6 months, and only rarely does a permanent neurologic deficit occur.[84] The use of a tourniquet causes a marked decrease in force production in the muscles beneath and distal to the tourniquet. The loss of muscle power was found to be proportional to the tourniquet occlusion pressures, and recovery takes weeks to months. Use of lower inflation pressures may minimize complications after the use of tourniquets and hasten postoperative recovery.[83] Only a few cases of rhabdomyolysis directly related to tourniquet use have been reported, three of which were associated with unusually long ischemic times or high tourniquet pressures.[85]

Systemic Effects

Limb exsanguination and tourniquet inflation result in an increase in circulating blood volume and systemic vascular resistance. This leads to a transient increase in central venous pressure and systolic blood pressure.[86,87] Tourniquet inflation also results in increased heart rate and blood pressure, which frequently leads the anesthesiologist to increase the depth of anesthesia. This clinical syndrome is often referred to as "tourniquet pain." A cutaneous neural mechanism is thought to be responsible for tourniquet pain, and the hypertension is mediated by a humoral response to the pain. Tourniquet pain and the associated hypertension is observed less often during spinal or epidural anesthesia, but it occurs despite adequate sensory anesthesia of the dermatome underlying the tourniquet.[88,89] These changes are often resistant to analgesic drugs and increased depth of anesthesia, and are described in detail below.

After deflation of the tourniquet and reperfusion of the ischemic limb, central venous pressure and arterial blood pressure decrease as a result of a shift of intravascular volume back into the limb, aggravated by postischemic reactive hyperemia and the acute effects of ischemic metabolites released into the systemic circulation. In selected cases, acute blood loss complicates the picture.[90]

Because of the efflux of hypercapnic venous blood from an ischemic area into the systemic circulation and increase in cardiac output, deflation of the tourniquet is associated with a transient increase in end-tidal carbon dioxide tension. The increase in carbon dioxide tension is associated with an increase in cerebral blood volume. Precautions should therefore be taken in treating patients with increased intracranial pressures (e.g., polytrauma patients with head injury), and hyperventilation to normocapnia immediately after tourniquet deflation can help prevent increased cerebral blood flow velocity and intracranial pressure.[91–93] Modest increases in arterial plasma potassium and lactate concentrations, together with metabolic and respiratory acidosis, are observed for up to half an hour after tourniquet release, but are of minor clinical significance.[94]

Embolic phenomena (showers of fat, marrow, and thrombovascular emboli reaching the heart and lungs) after tourniquet release during TKA have been very well described. According to Berman et al.,[95] immediately after tourniquet release, echogenic material is seen in the hearts of all patients. Although well tolerated by most, this phenomenon may lead to cardiac arrest or fat embolism syndrome (discussed in the next section) in some patients.[95–98]

The pharmacokinetics of anesthetic drugs may be modified by the use of an arterial tourniquet. Drugs administered before inflation of the tourniquet cuff may be sequestered in the isolated limb, then redistributed systemically after tourniquet deflation; drugs administered after tourniquet inflation may have altered pharmacokinetics because of a reduced volume of distribution. However, except for antibiotics, which should be administered before tourniquet inflation, the effect of tourniquet inflation or deflation on pharmacokinetics of drugs is of limited clinical importance.[99]

Recommendations in the literature for both safe tourniquet time and reperfusion intervals vary. Most authors suggest that tourniquet inflation should be for the shortest period possible, with an upper limit of 2 hours in healthy patients.[75] The elderly, trauma patients, and those with peripheral vascular disease are probably more susceptible to muscle injury. For surgical procedures longer than 2 hours, the tourniquet should be deflated every 2

hours to allow 10 minutes of reperfusion of the muscles beneath and distal to the tourniquet cuff.[81] Because nerve damage results primarily from direct pressure beneath the cuff, use of the lowest pressure that causes arterial occlusion is recommended. Tourniquet pressures more than 40.0–46.7 kPa (300–350 mm Hg) should rarely be necessary to produce a bloodless field in normotensive patients with compliant vessels. However, in patients with atherosclerosis and the morbidly obese or hypertensive patients, higher pressures may be required. Common sense suggests that tourniquet pressure should be based on the patient's systolic blood pressure, with the tourniquet inflated to a pressure of approximately 150 mm Hg above the systolic pressure.[100,101]

Fat Embolism

Fat embolism occurs in almost all lower extremity trauma and intramedullary surgery, in particular, intramedullary nailing of long bones, hip arthroplasty, and knee arthroplasty. Fat emboli syndrome, however, is a severe multisystem manifestation of embolization that develops in 10%–20% of these patients.[102–106] Overall mortality varies between 7%–20%,[107,108] and long-term morbidity is usually attributable to neurologic dysfunction.[109]

The diagnosis of fat emboli syndrome is clinical, usually one of exclusion. A high index of suspicion is required for early clinical diagnosis in at-risk patients. Patients may present with intraoperative cardiorespiratory collapse after femoral reaming,[107] insertion of intramedullary alignment guide[107] or cemented prosthesis,[108] or after tourniquet release.[103] Hypotension, respiratory dysfunction with hypoxia, tachycardia, neurologic changes that may present as diffuse encephalopathy and/or focal abnormalities, petechiae that are distributed on the upper body (chest, neck, and conjunctivae), lipuria, and even electromechanical dissociation may also be presenting signs. These may develop in the postoperative period.

Laboratory tests should include arterial blood gas, complete blood count to identify anemia or thrombocytopenia, and a coagulation profile.[109] Any other treatable causes of neurologic dysfunction, e.g., toxic, metabolic, or infectious, must be excluded.[110] Urinalysis may reveal fat globules, but this is nonspecific. The electrocardiogram may be normal, reflect right heart strain, or may reveal ischemia. The chest radiograph is nonspecific, with diffuse fluffy bilateral infiltrates and opacities consistent with increased capillary permeability and edema.[33]

Treatment is essentially supportive, consisting of cardiovascular and respiratory resuscitation and stabilization.[33] No specific drug therapy is currently recommended. Small prospective randomized controlled studies of steroid prophylaxis in patients with long bone fractures have indicated both a decrease in the development of fat emboli syndrome and a decreased incidence of hypoxemia in steroid-treated groups compared with controls.[103,104]

Summary

1. Elective THA/TKA is a relatively safe orthopedic procedure. Known complications include thromboembolism, postoperative anemia, infection, fractures, and death. Fat emboli syndrome is an uncommon but devastating complication with relatively high mortality rate and long-term morbidity, which is usually attributable to neurologic dysfunction. Preexisting comorbidities and the American Society of Anesthesiologists physical status classification are significantly related to the incidence of postoperative death. In contrast, fractures of the hip, which most frequently occur in elderly women, are associated with a very high mortality. Major causes are cardiac morbidity, bronchopneumonia, and pulmonary embolism. Patients who are medically fit for surgery should be operated on the day of admission. Perioperative management should be oriented toward adequate pain control and multidisciplinary consultation, if needed. Patients undergoing major lower extremity orthopedic surgery should receive prophylaxis with antibiotics and anticoagulants to reduce the risk of infection and deep vein thrombosis. The decision to perform neuraxial blockade on patients receiving thromboprophylaxis should therefore take into account recent recommendations for management of this patient population.

2. The choice of anesthetic technique is a complex medical decision that depends on many factors. For hip fracture patients, the type of anesthesia does not seem to influence significantly morbidity or overall mortality. For THA/TKA, there is evidence to suggest that regional anesthesia may be of benefit because it was associated with a lower rate of intensive care unit admission postoperatively, reduced intraoperative blood loss and transfusion requirements, and was associated with a lower incidence of thromboembolic events. For all lower extremity operations, regional analgesia and anesthesia provide better pain control for the rehabilitation period.

3. Special attention during the operation should be given to positioning of the patient, blood loss and transfusion requirements, blood pressure control, fluid management, careful monitoring and management during cement insertion and possible associated complications, and to tourniquet-related complications.

4. For lower limb orthopedic surgery, postoperative pain is a major problem. Peripheral nerve blocks with or without a catheter are the techniques of choice.

References

1. Harris WH, Sledge CB. Total hip and total knee replacement. N Engl J Med 1990;323:725–731.
2. Rauh MA, Krackow KA. In-hospital deaths following elective total joint arthroplasty. Orthopedics 2004;27(4):407–411.
3. Dearborn JT, Harris WH. Postoperative mortality after total hip arthroplasty. An analysis of deaths after two thousand seven hundred and thirty-six procedures. J Bone Joint Surg Am 1998;80:1291–1294.
4. Parvizi J, Sullivan TA, Trousdale RT, et al. Thirty-day mortality after total knee arthroplasty. J Bone Joint Surg Am 2001;83:1157–1161.
5. Morrison RS, Chassin MR, Siu AL. The medical consultant's role in caring for patients with hip fracture. Ann Intern Med 1998;128:1010–1020.
6. O'Hara D, Duff A, Berlin JA, et al. The effect of anesthetic technique on postoperative outcomes on hip fracture repair. Anesthesiology 2000;92:947–957.
7. Myers AH, Robinson EG, Van Natta ML, et al. Hip fracture among the elderly: factors associated with inhospital mortality. Am J Epidemiol 1991;134:1128–1137.
8. Perez JV, Warwick CP, Case CP, et al. Death after proximal femoral fracture—an autopsy study. Injury 1995;26(4):237–240.
9. Scheinin H, Virtanen T, Kentala E, et al. Epidural infusion of bupivacaine and fentanyl reduces perioperative myocardial ischaemia in elderly patients with hip fracture—a randomized controlled trial. Acta Anaesthesiol Scand 2000;44:1061–1070.
10. Matot I, Oppenheim-Eden A, Ratrot R, et al. Preoperative cardiac events in elderly patients with hip fracture randomized to epidural or conventional analgesia. Anesthesiology 2003;98(1):156–163.
11. Casaletto JA, Gatt R. Post-operative mortality related to waiting time for hip fracture surgery. Injury 2004;35(2):114–120.
12. Sutcliffe AJ, Parker M. Mortality after spinal and general anaesthesia for surgical fixation of hip fracture. Anaesthesia 1994;49:237–240.
13. Sorenson RM, Pace NL. Anesthetic techniques during surgical repair of femoral neck fractures. A meta-analysis. Anesthesiology 1992;77:1095–1104.
14. Zuckerman JD, Skovron ML, Koval KJ, et al. Postoperative complications and mortality associated with operative delay in older patients who have a fracture of the hip. J Bone Joint Surg Am 1995;77(10):1551–1556.
15. Rogers FB, Shackford SR, Keller MS. Early fixation reduces morbidity and mortality in elderly patients with hip fractures from low impact falls. J Trauma 1995;39(2):261–265.
16. Grimes JP, Gregory PM, Noveck H, et al. The effect of time-to-surgery on mortality and morbidity in patients following hip fracture. Am J Med 2002;112:702–709.
17. Urwin SC, Parker MJ, Griffiths R. General versus regional anaesthesia for hip fracture surgery: a meta-analysis of randomized trials. Br J Anaesth 2000;84:450–455.
18. Gilbert TB, Hawkes WG, Hebel JR, et al. Spinal anesthesia versus general anesthesia for hip fracture repair: a longitudinal observation of 741 elderly patients during 2-year follow-up. Am J Orthop 2000;29:25–35.

19. Lien CA. Regional versus general anesthesia for hip surgery in older patients: does the choice affect patient outcome? J Am Geriatr Soc 2002;50:191–194.

20. Parker MJ, Handoll HH, Griffiths R. Anaesthesia for hip fracture surgery in adults. Cochrane Database Syst Rev 2001(4):CD000521.

21. Parker MJ, Griffiths R, Appadu BN. Nerve blocks (subcostal, lateral cutaneous, femoral, triple, psoas) for hip fractures. Cochrane Database Syst Rev 2002(1): CD001159.

22. Kaufmann SC, Wu CL, Pronovost PJ, et al. The association of intraoperative neuroaxial anesthesia on anticipated admission to the intensive care unit. J Clin Anesth 2002; 14:432–436.

23. McQueen DA, Kelly HK, Wright TF. A comparison of epidural and non-epidural anesthesia and analgesia in total hip or knee arthroplasty patients. Orthopedics 1992; 15:169–173.

24. Modig J, Karistrom G. Intra- and post-operative blood loss and haemodynamics in total hip replacement when performed under lumbar epidural versus general anaesthesia. Eur J Anaesthesiol 1987;4:345–355.

25. Twyman R, Kirwan T, Fennelly M. Blood loss reduced during hip arthroplasty by lumbar plexus block. J Bone Joint Surg Br 1990;72:770–771.

26. Stevens RD, Van Gessel E, Flory N, et al. Lumber plexus block reduces pain and blood loss associated with total hip arthroplasty. Anesthesiology 2000;93:115–121.

27. Mitchell D, Friedman RJ, Baker JD, et al. Prevention of thromboembolic disease following total knee arthroplasty. Epidural versus general anesthesia. Clin Orthop Relat Res 1991;(269):109–112.

28. Modig J, Borg T, Karistrom G, et al. Thromboembolism after total hip replacement: role of epidural and general anesthesia. Anesth Analg 1983;62:174–180.

29. Hollmann MW, Wieczorek KS, Smart M, et al. Epidural anesthesia prevents hypercoagulation in patients undergoing major orthopedic surgery. Reg Anesth Pain Med 2001; 26(3):215–222.

30. Laskin RS. Total knee replacement in patients older than 85 years. Clin Orthop 1999;367:43–49.

31. Williams-Russo P, Sharrock NE, Haas SB, et al. Randomized trial of epidural versus general anesthesia: outcomes after primary total knee replacement. Clin Orthop 1996; 331:199–208.

32. Williams-Russo P, Sharrock NE, Mattis S, et al. Cognitive effects after epidural vs general anesthesia in older adults. A randomized trial. JAMA 1995;274(1):44–50.

33. Jenkins K, Chung F, Wennberg R, et al. Fat embolism syndrome and elective knee arthroplasty. Can J Anaesth 2002;49:19–24.

34. Enneking FK. Cardiac arrest during total knee replacement using a long-stem prosthesis. J Clin Anesth 1995; 7:253–263.

35. Hedenstierna G, Mebius C, Bygdeman S. Ventilation-perfusion relationship during hip arthroplasty. Acta Anaesthesiol Scand 1983;27:56–61.

36. Fallon KM, Fuller JG, Morley-Forster P. Fat embolization and fatal cardiac arrest during hip arthroplasty with methylmethacrylate. Can J Anaesth 2001;48:626–629.

37. Ereth MH, Weber JG, Abel MD, et al. Cemented vs. noncemented total hip arthroplasty: embolism, hemodynamics, and intrapulmonary shunting. Mayo Clin Proc 1992; 67:1066–1074.

38. Bengtson A, Larsson M, Gammer W, et al. Anaphylatoxin release in association with methylmethacrylate fixation of hip prostheses. J Bone Joint Surg Am 1987;69A:46–49.

39. Dahl OE, Garvik LJ, Lyberg T. Toxic effects of methylmethacrylate monomer on leucocytes and endothelial cells in vitro. Acta Orthop Scand 1994;65:147–153.

40. Breed AL. Experimental production of vascular hypotension, and bone marrow and fat embolism with methylmethacrylate cement. Traumatic hypertension of bone. Clin Orthop 1974;102:227–244.

41. Tronzo RG, Kallos T, Wyche MQ. Elevation of intramedullary pressure when methylmethacrylate is inserted in total hip arthroplasty. J Bone Joint Surg 1974;56A:714–718.

42. Pitto RP, Kößler M. The relevance of the drainage along the linea aspera for the reduction of fat embolism in cemented total hip replacement. J Bone Joint Surg 1997; 79B(Suppl II):169–170.

43. Wenda K, Runkel M, Degreif J, et al. Pathogenesis and clinical relevance of bone marrow embolism in medullary nailing. Injury 1993;24(Suppl 3):73–81.

44. Woo R, Minster GJ, Fitzgerald RH Jr, et al. Pulmonary fat embolism in revision hip arthroplasty. Clin Orthop 1995; 319:41–53.

45. Berman AT, Price HL, Hahn JF. The cardiovascular effects of methylmethacrylate in dogs. Clin Orthop 1974; 100:265–269.

46. Lotke PA, Faralli VJ, Orenstein EM, et al. Blood loss after total knee replacement. J Bone Joint Surg Am 1999;73A: 1037–1040.

47. Sehat KR, Evans R, Newman JH. How much blood is really lost in total knee arthroplasty? Correct blood loss management should take hidden loss into account. Knee 2000;7(3):151–155.

48. Toy PT, Kaplan EB, McVay PA, et al. Blood loss and replacement in total hip arthroplasty: a multicenter study. The Preoperative Autologous Blood Donation Study Group. Transfusion 1992;32(1):63–67.

49. Bierbaum BE, Callaghan JJ, Galante JO, et al. An analysis of blood management in patients having a total hip or knee arthroplasty. J Bone Joint Surg Am 1999;81(1):2–10.

50. Churchill WH, McGurk S, Chapman RH, et al. The Collaborative Hospital Transfusion Study: variations in use of autologous blood account for hospital differences in red cell use during primary hip and knee surgery. Transfusion 1998;38(6):530–539.

51. Halm EA, Wang JJ, Boockvar K, et al. Effects of blood transfusion on clinical and functional outcomes in patients with hip fracture. Transfusion 2003;43(10):1358–1367.

52. Tenholder M, Cushner FD. Intraoperative blood management in joint replacement surgery. Orthopedics 2004;27(6 Suppl):S663–668.

53. Singelyn FJ, Capdevila X. Regional anaesthesia for orthopaedic surgery. Curr Opin Anaesthesiol 2001;14:733–740.

54. Singelyn F, Gouverneur JM. Postoperative analgesia after total hip arthroplasty: IV PCA with morphine, patient-controlled epidural analgesia, or continuous "3-in-1 block":

a prospective evaluation by our acute pain service in more than 1300 patients. J Clin Anesth 1999;11:550–554.

55. Capdevila X, Barthelet Y, Biboulet P, et al. Effects of perioperative analgesic technique on the surgical outcome and duration of rehabilitation after major knee surgery. Anesthesiology 1999;91:8–15.

56. Singelyn F, Deyaert M, Joris D, et al. Effects of intravenous patient-controlled analgesia with morphine, continuous epidural analgesia, and continuous three-in-one block on postoperative pain and knee rehabilitation after unilateral total knee arthroplasty. Anesth Analg 1998;87:88–92.

57. Chelly J, Greger J, Gebhard R, et al. Continuous femoral blocks improve recovery and outcome of patients undergoing total knee arthroplasty. J Arthroplasty 2001;16:436–445.

58. Allen H, Liu S, Ware P, et al. Peripheral nerve blocks improve analgesia after total knee replacement surgery. Anesth Analg 1998;87:93–97.

59. Ganapathy S, Wasserman R, Watson J, et al. Modified continuous femoral three-in-one block for postoperative pain after total knee arthroplasty. Anesth Analg 1999;88:1197–1202.

60. Singelyn F, Gouverneur JM. Extended "three-in-one" block after total knee arthroplasty: continuous versus patient-controlled techniques. Anesth Analg 2000;91:176–180.

61. Singelyn F, Vanderelst P, Gouverneur JM. Extended femoral nerve sheath block after total hip arthroplasty: continuous versus patient-controlled techniques. Anesth Analg 2001;92:455–459.

62. Macalou D, Trueck S, Meuret P, et al. Postoperative analgesia after total knee replacement: the effect of an obturator nerve block added to the femoral 3-in-1 nerve block. Anesth Analg 2004;99:251–254.

63. Davies AF, Segar EP, Murdoch J, et al. Epidural infusion or combined femoral and sciatic nerve blocks as perioperative analgesia for knee arthroplasty. Br J Anaesth 2004;93(3):368–374.

64. Kaloul I, Guay J, Cote C, et al. The posterior lumbar plexus (psoas compartment) block and the three-in-one femoral nerve block provide similar postoperative analgesia after total knee replacement. Can J Anaesth 2004;51:45–51.

65. Mansour N, Bennetts F. An observational study of combined continuous lumbar plexus and single-shot sciatic nerve blocks for post-knee surgery analgesia. Reg Anesth Pain Med 1996;21:287–291.

66. Picard P, Tramer M, McQuay H, et al. Analgesic efficacy of peripheral opioids (all except intra-articular): a qualitative systematic review of randomized controlled trials. Pain 1997;72:309–318.

67. Geerts WH, Heit JA, Clagett GP, et al. Prevention of venous thromboembolism. Chest 2001;119:132–175.

68. Haas S. Deep vein thrombosis: beyond the operating table. Orthopedics 2000;23(Suppl 6):S629–S632.

69. Sixth American College of Chest Physicians (ACCP) Consensus Conference on Antithrombotic Therapy. Chest 2004;126(3 Suppl).

70. Hollman MW, Durieux ME. Local anesthetics and the inflammatory response: a new therapeutic indication? Anesthesiology 2000;93:858–875.

71. Horlocker TT. What's a nice patient like you doing with a complication like this? Diagnosis, prognosis and prevention of spinal hematoma. Can J Anaesth 2004;51:527–534.

72. Horlocker TT, Wedel DJ, Benzon H, et al. Regional anesthesia in the anticoagulated patient: defining the risks (The Second ASRA Consensus Conference on Neuraxial Anesthesia and Anticoagulation). Reg Anesth Pain Med 2003;28(3):172–197.

73. Vandermeulen EP, Van Aken H, Vermylen J. Anticoagulants and spinal-epidural anesthesia. Anesth Analg 1994;79:1165–1177.

74. Horlocker TT. Thromboprophylaxis and neuroaxial anesthesia. Orthopedics 2003;26(2):243–248.

75. Kam PC, Kavanagh R, Yoong FF. The arterial tourniquet: pathophysiological consequences and anaesthetic implications. Anaesthesia 2001;56(6):534–545.

76. Carter K, Shaw A, Telfer ABM. Tourniquets for surgery: safety aspects. J Med Eng Technol 1983;7:136–139.

77. Vandenbussche E, Duranthon LD, Couturier M, et al. The effect of tourniquet use in total knee arthroplasty. Int Orthop 2002;26(5):306–309.

78. Tetro AM, Rudan JF. The effects of a pneumatic tourniquet on blood loss in total knee arthroplasty. Can J Surg 2001;44(1):33–38.

79. Abdel-Salam A, Eyres KS. Effects of tourniquet during total knee arthroplasty. A prospective randomised study. J Bone Joint Surg Br 1995;77(2):250–253.

80. Jarolem KL, Scott DF, Jaffe WL, et al. A comparison of blood loss and transfusion requirements in total knee arthroplasty with and without arterial tourniquet. Am J Orthop 1995;24(12):906–909.

81. Newman RJ. Metabolic effects of tourniquet ischaemia studied by nuclear magnetic resonance spectroscopy. J Bone Joint Surg Br 1984;66:434–440.

82. Wilgis EFS. Observations on the effects of tourniquet ischaemia. J Bone Joint Surg Am 1971;53:1343–1346.

83. Mohler LR, Pedowitz RA, Lopez MA, et al. Effect of tourniquet compression of neuromuscular function. Clin Orthop 1999;359:213–220.

84. Hodgson AJ. A proposed etiology for tourniquet-induced neuropathies. J Biomech Eng 1994;116:224–227.

85. Palmer SH, Graham G. Tourniquet-induced rhabdomyolysis after total knee replacement. Ann R Coll Surg Engl 1994;76:416–417.

86. Kaufman RD, Walts LF. Tourniquet induced hypertension. Br J Anaesth 1982;54:333–336.

87. Bradford EMW. Haemodynamic changes associated with the application of lower limb tourniquets. Anaesthesia 1969;24:190–197.

88. Valli H, Rosenberg PH, Kytta J, et al. Arterial hypertension associated with the use of a tourniquet with either general or regional anaesthesia. Acta Anaesthesiol Scand 1987;31:279–283.

89. Gielen MJ, Stienstra R. Tourniquet hypertension and its prevention: a review. Reg Anesth 1991;16:191–194.

90. Townsend HS, Goodman SB, Schurman DJ, et al. Tourniquet release: systemic and metabolic effects. Acta Anaesthesiol Scand 1996;40:1234–1237.

91. Kadoi Y, Ide M, Saito S, et al. Hyperventilation after tourniquet deflation prevents an increase in cerebral flow velocity. Can J Anaesth 1999;46:259–264.

92. Lam AM, Slee T, Hirst R, et al. Cerebral blood flow velocity following tourniquet release in humans. Can J Anaesth 1990;37:S29.

93. Sparling RJ, Murray AW, Choksey M. Raised intracranial pressure associated with hypercarbia after tourniquet release. Br J Neurosurg 1993;7:75–78.

94. Kokki H, Vaatainen U, Pantila J. Metabolic effects of a low pressure tourniquet system compared with a high pressure tourniquet system in arthroscopic anterior crucial ligament reconstruction. Acta Anaesthesiol Scand 1998;42:418–424.

95. Berman AT, Parmet JL, Harding SP, et al. Emboli observed with use of transesophageal echocardiography immediately after tourniquet release during total knee arthroplasty with cement. J Bone Joint Surg Am 1998;80:389–396.

96. Parmet JL, Berman AT, Horrow JC, et al. Thromboembolism coincident with tourniquet deflation during total knee arthroplasty. Lancet 1993;341:1057–1058.

97. McGrath BJ, Hsia J, Boyd A, et al. Venous embolization after deflation of lower extremity tourniquets. Anesth Analg 1994;78:349–353.

98. Morawa LG, Manley MT, Edidin AA, et al. Transesophageal echocardiographic monitored events during total knee arthroplasty. Clin Orthop 1996;331:192–198.

99. Barnette RE, Eriksson LI, Cooney GF, et al. Sequestration of vecuronium bromide during extremity surgery involving use of a pneumatic tourniquet. Acta Anaesthesiol Scand 1997;41:49–54.

100. Shaw JA, Murray DG. The relationship between tourniquet pressure and underlying soft-tissue pressure in the thigh. J Bone Joint Surg Am 1982;64:1148–1152.

101. Van Roekel HE, Thurston AJ. Tourniquet pressure: the effect of limb circumference and systolic blood pressure. J Hand Surg (Br) 1985;10:142–144.

102. Fabian TC, Hoots AV, Stanford DS, et al. Fat embolism syndrome: prospective evaluation in 92 fracture patients. Crit Care Med 1990;18:42–46.

103. Kallenbach J, Lewis M, Zaltzman M, et al. "Low-dose" corticosteroid prophylaxis against fat embolism. J Trauma 1987;27:1173–1176.

104. Lindeque BGP, Schoeman HS, Dommisse GF, et al. Fat embolism and the fat embolism syndrome. A double-blind therapeutic study. J Bone Joint Surg Br 1987;69:128–131.

105. Schonfeld SA, Ploysongsang Y, DiLisio R, et al. Fat embolism prophylaxis with corticosteroids. A prospective study in high-risk patients. Ann Intern Med 1983;99:438–443.

106. Bulger EM, Smith DG, Maier RV, et al. Fat embolism syndrome. A 10-year review. Arch Surg 1997;132:435–439.

107. Robert JH, Hoffmeyer P, Broquet PE, et al. Fat embolism syndrome. Orthop Rev 1993;22:567–571.

108. Johnson MJ, Lucas GL. Fat embolism syndrome. Orthopedics 1996;19:41–50.

109. Byrick RJ. Fat embolism and postoperative coagulopathy [editorial]. Can J Anaesth 2001;48:618–621.

110. Jacobsen DM, Terrance CF, Reinmuth OM. The neurologic manifestations of fat embolism. Neurology 1986;36:847–851.

25
Transurethral Prostatectomy Syndrome and Other Complications of Urologic Procedures

Daniel M. Gainsburg

Elderly patients undergo numerous urologic procedures. This chapter presents some of the more common concerns and complications associated with these procedures.

The Transurethral Prostatectomy Syndrome

Transurethral prostatectomy (TURP) is considered the gold standard for the surgical treatment of benign prostatic hyperplasia (BPH).[1] During the past decade, the annual number of TURPs performed in the United States has declined from 400,000 to 100,000 because of advances in medical management, the introduction of minimally invasive thermal therapies (laser, radiofrequency, and microwave),[2] and the development of patient-care guidelines for patients with BPH.[3]

BPH is the most common nonmalignant tumor of the prostate, causing urinary symptoms in more than 50% of the aging male population.[4] TURP patients, who are often elderly, tend to have coexisting problems of which the most common are pulmonary (14.5%), gastrointestinal (13.2%), myocardial infarction (12.5%), arrhythmia (12.4%), and renal insufficiency (4.5%).[5] Therefore, these patients should be carefully evaluated preoperatively to determine the status of any coexisting diseases.

Complications of TURP include (1) absorption of irrigating solution; (2) circulatory overload, hyponatremia, and hypoosmolality; (3) glycine and ammonia toxicity; (4) bladder perforation; (5) transient bacteremia and septicemia; (6) hypothermia; (7) bleeding and coagulopathy; and 8) TURP syndrome.[6] The 30-day mortality rate of TURP is reported to be between 0.2% and 0.8%.[5] Common causes of death include myocardial infarction, pulmonary edema, and renal failure.[7] The postoperative morbidity rate was noted to be 18% and increased morbidity was found in patients with resection times exceeding 90 minutes, gland size greater than 45 g, acute urinary retention, and age older than 80 years.[5] TURP syndrome is a general term used to describe a collection of signs and symptoms caused primarily by excessive absorption of irrigating fluid through the opened venous sinuses of the prostate.

The Surgical Procedure

TURP is performed by inserting a resectoscope through the urethra and resecting prostatic tissue in an orderly manner with an electrically powered cutting-coagulating metal loop. Prostatic tissue is then resected without perforating the prostatic capsule. If the capsule is violated, large amounts of irrigation solution may be absorbed into the circulation, and the periprostatic and retroperitoneal spaces.[6,8] It is this rapid absorption of irrigation solution into the circulation that differentiates this complication from that of bladder perforation. (See also the section on Bladder Perforation.) Prostatic capsular perforation occurs in about 2% of patients and presents with symptoms of restlessness, nausea, vomiting, and abdominal pain—even under spinal anesthesia.[1] If perforation is suspected, the operation should be terminated as quickly as possible and hemostasis obtained.[1]

Bleeding often occurs during TURP, but is usually controllable. Arterial bleeding is controlled by electrocoagulation.[1] However, when large venous sinuses are opened, hemostasis becomes difficult. If this venous bleeding becomes uncontrollable, the procedure should be terminated as quickly as possible, and a Foley catheter should be inserted into the bladder and traction applied.[6,8] Attempts at estimating blood loss during TURP are usually extremely inaccurate, because the shed blood is mixed with ample amounts of irrigating solution. Intraoperative blood loss has been estimated to range from 2 to 4 mL/min of resection time and 20 to 50 mL/g of prostate tissue.[9] Bleeding requiring transfusion occurs in 2.5% of patients undergoing TURP.[5]

TABLE 25-1. Osmolality of various irrigation solutions used for transurethral prostatectomy.

Solution	Concentration (%)	Osmolality (mOsm/kg)
Glycine	1.2	175
Glycine	1.5	220
Cytal		178
Mannitol	5	275
Sorbitol	3.5	165
Glucose	2.5	139
Urea	1	167
Water		0

Irrigation Solutions

The ideal irrigating solution for use during TURP would be isotonic, nonhemolytic, electrically inert, transparent, nonmetabolized, nontoxic, rapidly excreted, and inexpensive.[10] Originally, distilled water was the fluid of choice because it was nonconductive and transparent. However, its absorption into the circulation caused massive hemolysis, dilutional hyponatremia, rare renal failure, and central nervous system (CNS) symptoms.[6,11]

These complications eventually led to abandonment of distilled water and to the use of isosmotic or nearly isosmotic solutions for TURP. Solutions such as normal saline and Ringer's lactate are isosmotic and would be well tolerated if absorbed intravascularly; however, they are highly ionized and cause dispersion of the high-frequency current from the resectoscope. Recently, in a small study, normal saline was used as the irrigating solution in which a bipolar electrocautery resectoscope replaced the customary monopolar resectoscope. None of the patients developed hyponatremia or TURP syndrome.[2]

The introduction of nonconductive and also nonhemolytic solutions, such as glycine, Cytal (a mixture of sorbitol 2.7% and mannitol 0.54%), sorbitol, mannitol, glucose, and urea, have replaced distilled water (Table 25-1).[6,8] Glycine and Cytal are currently the two most frequently used solutions.[6] Although all are nonconductive solutions that allow for electrocautery resection, they are purposely prepared moderately hypotonic to maintain transparency.[2,8]

Even though they cause no significant hemolysis, excessive absorption of modern irrigation solutions can be associated with numerous perioperative complications, including circulatory overload, hyponatremia, and hypoosmolality. Additionally, the solutes in the solutions may cause adverse effects: glycine may cause cardiac, neurologic, and retinal effects[8,12,13]; mannitol rapidly expands intravascular volume and might lead to pulmonary edema in cardiac patients[6]; sorbitol is converted to fructose and lactate, which may cause hyperglycemia and/or lactic acidosis[14]; and glucose may cause severe hyperglycemia in the diabetic patient.[15]

Signs and Symptoms

TURP syndrome may occur anytime intraoperatively or postoperatively. It has been observed as early as a few minutes after the start of surgery[16] and as late as several hours after completion of surgery.[17] Recent reports noted that TURP syndrome occurs in 2% of patients.[5,18]

Clinical manifestations of TURP syndrome include neurologic, cardiovascular, and respiratory effects (Table 25-2). The effects on the CNS include headache, dizziness, restlessness, agitation, confusion, seizures, and eventually coma. The clinical picture may be further compounded by the neurotoxic effects of glycine and ammonia.[6] TURP syndrome is usually described as being caused by hyponatremia and water intoxication. It is now thought that the classic CNS effects of TURP syndrome are not caused by hyponatremia, in itself, but are caused by the acute decrease in serum osmolality that results in the development of cerebral edema.[19,20]

Cardiovascular and respiratory effects occur from volume overload and hyponatremia. Acute hypervolemia will initially cause hypertension and bradycardia, which may progress to congestive heart failure, pulmonary edema, and cardiac arrest.[21] Rapidly decreasing serum sodium levels are associated with negative inotropic effects on the heart manifesting in hypotension, pulmonary edema, and congestive heart failure.[9,20] Electrocardiogram changes, such as widened QRS complexes and ventricular ectopy are often observed.[9,20]

TABLE 25-2. Signs and symptoms of transurethral prostatectomy syndrome.

Cardiovascular and respiratory	Central nervous system	Metabolic	Other
Hypertension	Restlessness	Hyponatremia	Hypoosmolality
Pulmonary edema	Agitation	Hyperglycinemia	Hemolysis
Congestive heart failure	Confusion	Hyperammonemia	
Hypotension	Seizures		
Arrhythmias	Coma		
Respiratory arrest	Blindness		
Cardiac arrest			

Absorption of Irrigating Solution

Excessive absorption of irrigating solution through opened venous sinuses of the prostate is the primary cause of TURP syndrome. The amount of absorption correlates with (1) the height of the irrigating fluid above the patient which determines hydrostatic pressure, (2) amount of distention of the bladder by the surgeon, (3) extent of opened venous sinuses, and (4) the length of time of resection.[22] The average rate of fluid absorption is 10–30 mL/min of resection time and as much as 8 L may be absorbed during a procedure.[6] A quick estimation of fluid volume absorbed, which compares serum sodium levels before and after the procedure, can be made by using the following equation:

Volume absorbed
= {(preoperative [Na$^+$]/postoperative [Na$^+$]) × ECF} − ECF

where extracellular fluid (ECF) volume comprises 20%–30% of body weight.[8,23]

Circulatory Overload, Hyponatremia, and Hypoosmolality

The replacement of distilled water with the present generation of irrigating solutions has eliminated hemolysis as a complication of TURP. At the same time, there has been a decrease in the incidence of severe CNS complications associated with hyponatremia.[20] However, excessive absorption of irrigating solution still occurs and leads to circulatory overload. Initially, hypertension and bradycardia are seen with acute volume overload, which may progress to congestive heart failure, pulmonary edema, and eventually cardiac arrest.[21]

The classic CNS signs of TURP syndrome are now thought to be caused by acute serum hypoosmolality, movement of water into the cells, and consequent cerebral edema.[19,20] With the use of solute-based nearly isosmotic solutions, the incidence of severe CNS symptoms has been reduced because acute serum hypoosmolality does not occur; however, CNS symptoms can still occur secondary to hyponatremia.[19,20]

Sodium is an electrolyte that is essential for the ability of excitable cells, particularly those of the heart and brain, to depolarize and produce an action potential.[6,8] With acute decreases in serum sodium levels to 120 mEq/L, CNS symptoms and cardiovascular effects are observed (Table 25-3).[8,14] Initially, confusion and restlessness are noted, and with decreasing serum sodium levels, may progress to loss of consciousness and seizures.[24] Rapidly decreasing serum sodium levels are associated with hypotension, pulmonary edema, congestive heart failure, and electrocardiogram changes. At levels near 100 mEq/L, respiratory and cardiac arrest may occur.[24,25] Acute changes in serum sodium levels are more harmful than chronic hyponatremia.[26] Also, it is often impossible to separate these symptoms of cardiovascular compromise secondary to hyponatremia from those caused by fluid overload.

Glycine and Ammonia Toxicity

Glycine is a nonessential amino acid. When absorbed in significant amounts, glycine may cause cardiac and neurologic effects.[8,12,13] It is metabolized in the liver into ammonia and glyoxylic acid.[12] The cardiac effect of glycine is myocardial depression; the mechanism is unknown.[27] Glycine has been implicated as the cause of transient blindness in TURP patients. It acts as an inhibitory neurotransmitter in the brain, spinal cord, and retina. Centrally acting mechanisms, such as cerebral edema, may cause visual impairment, but these patients have normal papillary light reflexes. In contrast, TURP patients with transient blindness have sluggish or nonreactive pupils, suggesting a retinal effect. Therefore, TURP blindness may be caused by increased glycine levels exerting an inhibitory effect on the retina.[28,29]

Signs of ammonia toxicity, nausea and vomiting, usually occur within 1 hour after surgery. With increasing ammonia levels, the patient lapses into a coma lasting about 10–12 hours, and then awakens as the ammonia levels decrease below 150 μmol/L.[8] A possible explanation for hyperammonemia in TURP patients is arginine deficiency. Ammonia is metabolized to urea in the liver, in a reaction that requires arginine. Patients who are

TABLE 25-3. Signs and symptoms associated with acute hyponatremia.

Serum Na$^+$ (mEq/L)	Central nervous system changes	Cardiovascular effects	Electrocardiogram changes
<120	Restlessness Confusion	Hypotension Pulmonary edema Congestive heart failure	
<115	Somnolence Nausea		Widened ORS complex Ventricular ectopy ST segment increase
<110	Seizures Coma		
<100		Respiratory arrest Cardiac arrest	

arginine deficient are unable to convert the excess ammonia created in the body when glycine solutions are absorbed, therefore leading to hyperammonemia.[30,31]

Bladder Perforation

Accidental perforation of the bladder is another common complication of TURP with an incidence of approximately 1% and most perforations occurring retroperitoneally. (See also the section on Transurethral Resection of Bladder Tumors.) It usually results from surgical instrumentation or overdistension of the bladder with irrigating fluid. An early sign of perforation, often unnoticed, is a decrease in return of irrigating solution from the bladder. Eventually, a significant volume of fluid will accumulate in the abdomen causing abdominal distention: patients under regional anesthesia may start to complain of abdominal pain and/or experience nausea and vomiting. Other clinical signs are hypotension followed by hypertension. Symptoms of intraperitoneal perforation are similar, develop sooner, and include severe shoulder pain secondary to diaphragmatic irritation. Diagnosis of bladder perforation is made by cystourethrography and treated with a suprapubic cystotomy.[8]

Transient Bacteremia and Septicemia

The prostate harbors a variety of bacteria, which can be the source of perioperative bacteremia through open prostatic venous sinuses. The presence of an indwelling urinary catheter will increase the risk. Therefore, the prophylactic administration of antibiotics is recommended in TURP patients. The bacteremia is usually transient and symptomless, and easily treated with frequently used antibiotic combinations. Nevertheless, 6%–7% of these patients will develop septicemia.[5] Common signs are fever, chills, hypotension, tachycardia, and/or bradycardia. In severe cases, cardiovascular collapse may occur, with mortality rates from 25% to 75%.[32]

Hypothermia

The use of room temperature irrigating solutions during TURP may cause shivering and hypothermia in many patients, especially in the elderly, who have a reduced thermoregulatory capacity.[14] Using warmed irrigating solutions will decrease heat loss and shivering.[33] The concern that warmed irrigating solutions may cause increased bleeding because of vasodilation has not been shown to be of clinical importance.[34]

Coagulopathy

Abnormal bleeding after TURP occurs in fewer than 1% of cases.[9] Possible causes include dilutional thrombocytopenia and systemic coagulopathy. The absorption of large volumes of irrigating solution might result in dilution of platelets and coagulation factors. Systemic coagulopathy in TURP patients is probably caused by either primary fibrinolysis or disseminated intravascular coagulopathy. In primary fibrinolysis, a plasminogen activator, which converts plasminogen into plasmin, is released from the prostate. Plasmin then causes fibrinolysis with the resultant increase in bleeding. Suggested treatment for primary fibrinolysis is epsilon aminocaproic acid.[9] Fibrinolysis that is secondary to disseminated intravascular coagulopathy is triggered by the systemic absorption of prostate tissue, which is rich in thromboplastin.[35] This will, in turn, cause a depletion of coagulation factors and platelets. Treatment is supportive with fluid and blood products administered as needed.[14]

Anesthetic Considerations for Transurethral Prostatectomy

Regional anesthesia, particularly spinal anesthesia, has long been considered the anesthetic technique of choice for TURP.[5] By allowing the patient to remain awake, this anesthetic technique allows early detection of mental status changes caused by TURP syndrome or the extravasation of irrigating solution. Restlessness and confusion are early signs of hyponatremia and/or serum hyperosmolality and should not be assumed to be signs of inadequate anesthesia. The administration of sedatives or the induction of general anesthesia in the presence of TURP syndrome can lead to severe complications and even death.[36] As discussed above, extravasation of irrigating solution secondary to either the perforation of the prostatic capsule or the bladder will cause the awake patient to complain of abdominal pain and/or experience nausea and vomiting.

There is controversy concerning whether anesthetic technique influences blood loss during TURP surgery. Some studies have reported less bleeding under regional anesthesia,[37–39] whereas others found no significant difference in blood loss between regional and general anesthesia.[40–43] In those studies that demonstrated decreased bleeding with regional anesthesia, the authors postulated that regional anesthesia reduces blood loss not only by decreasing systemic blood pressure, but also by decreasing central and peripheral venous pressures.[6,37–39]

Numerous comparative studies using neuropsychologic testing have been conducted to test whether the incidence of postoperative cognitive dysfunction would be less with regional anesthesia than general anesthesia. One small prospective study comparing spinal anesthesia with intravenous sedation versus general anesthesia on elderly TURP patients found a significant decrease in mental status in both groups at 6 hours after surgery, but there were no differences in perioperative mental function at any time between the groups during the first 30 days after surgery.[44] In a recent study of 438 elderly patients undergoing various types of surgical procedures, it was found that the incidence of postoperative cognitive dysfunction after 1 week was significantly greater after general than regional anesthesia, but no difference was found after 3 months.[45] Incidentally, this study found significantly greater mortality after general than regional anesthesia, noting that postoperative respiratory complications and need for prolonged intensive care occurred only after general anesthesia.[45]

If regional anesthesia is chosen for TURP, a T10 sensory level is needed to block the pain of bladder distention. Sensory levels above T9 are undesirable because the patient will not feel abdominal pain caused by perforation of the prostatic capsule.[6] Spinal anesthesia is often preferred over epidural anesthesia, because of the need to block sacral segments, which provide sensory innervations to the prostate, bladder neck, and penis.[14] Another advantage of regional anesthesia for TURP is improved postoperative pain control and decreased requirement for postoperative analgesics.[46]

Treatment of Transurethral Prostatectomy Syndrome

Prompt treatment is essential when the signs and symptoms of TURP syndrome are recognized. Initially, oxygenation, ventilation, and cardiovascular support should be provided based on the patient's symptomatology, while, at the same time, considering other treatable conditions such as diabetic coma, hypercarbia, or drug interactions.[10] The surgeon should be asked to terminate the procedure as rapidly as possible. Blood samples should be rapidly analyzed for electrolytes, creatinine, glucose, and arterial blood gases. A 12-lead electrocardiogram recording should be obtained.[8,14]

Treatment of hyponatremia and volume overload is dictated by the severity of the patient's symptoms. If the symptoms are mild and the serum sodium level is greater than 120 mEq/L, then fluid restriction and the administration of a loop diuretic, usually furosemide, are all that is necessary in returning serum sodium to normal levels. In severe cases, serum sodium less than 120 mEq/L, the recommended treatment is intravenous administration of hypertonic saline. A 3% sodium chloride solution should be infused at a rate no greater than 100 mL/h and the patient's hyponatremia should be corrected at a rate no greater than 0.5 mEq/L/h.[8,47] Rapid correction of hyponatremia with hypertonic saline has been associated with cerebral edema and central pontine myelinolysis.[20,48]

The Future of Transurethral Prostatectomy Syndrome

With advances in medical treatment and the introduction of new surgical techniques for the treatment of symptomatic BPH, TURP syndrome will become a rare complication of prostate surgery. In the near future, it seems that the new gold standard for the surgical treatment of BPH will be holmium laser enucleation of the prostate (HoLEP).[49] Advantages of HoLEP over TURP are its ability to be used on any size of prostate gland, decreased blood loss, can be performed as an ambulatory procedure, decreased absorption of irrigating solution, and the elimination of TURP syndrome.[49] Long-term complications of HoLEP are urethral stricture, bladder neck contracture, and reoperation rate higher than TURP. However, in a recent retrospective study of 552 patients, these complications were less than reported elsewhere for TURP and open prostatectomy.[5,18,49] Because of these advantages, HoLEP is becoming the preferred surgical procedure for BPH, especially in elderly patients with significant comorbidities.

Complications of Other Urologic Procedures

Transurethral Resection of Bladder Tumors

Bladder cancer is the second most common urologic malignancy and these tumors occur with a male to female ratio of approximately 3:1.[14] Most patients undergo an endoscopic procedure of transurethral resection of bladder tumor (TURBT). This procedure can be performed with either general or regional anesthesia. If a regional anesthesia is chosen, then a T10 sensory level is required to block the pain of bladder distention. As in TURP, bladder perforation can occur during TURBT with the same signs and symptoms that have been previously discussed. Bladder perforation can also occur if the bladder tumor lies near the obturator nerve. As the obturator nerve courses through the pelvis, it passes near the lateral bladder wall, bladder neck, and prostatic urethra. Inadvertent bladder perforation may occur if stimulation of the obturator nerve by electrocautery during the procedure causes the thigh muscles to contract forcefully. In this situation, general anesthesia with muscle relaxation would be the preferred technique.[50,51]

Extracorporeal Shock Wave Lithotripsy

In the United States, the annual incidence of urolithiasis is 16–24 cases per 10,000 persons and accounts for 7–10 of every 1000 hospital admissions.[52] Traditionally, renal stones were treated with open surgical procedures that required general anesthesia; however, in the late 1970s, a minimally invasive procedure, percutaneous nephrolithotomy, was introduced. Percutaneous nephrolithotomy also required general anesthesia, but had the advantage of shorter convalescence for patients. In 1980, a major noninvasive advance was made with the introduction of extracorporeal shock wave lithotripsy (ESWL), which has become the initial treatment modality for most patients with urinary tract stones.[53] Basically, the lithotripter generates repetitive high-energy shock waves that are focused on the stone and cause it to eventually fragment. The fragments are then excreted down the urinary tract over several weeks.[53]

First-generation lithotripters required immersion of the patient into a water bath and could cause physiologic effects in patients. Immersion causes compression of peripheral veins, resulting in an increase in cardiac preload, along with an increase in central venous, right atrial, and pulmonary pressures. As central venous pressure increases, arterial pressure and cardiac output will typically increase. This may lead to congestive heart failure and decreased systemic blood pressure in patients who have limited cardiac reserve.[54] Immersion of a patient to the level of their clavicles increases the work of breathing and respirations often become shallow and rapid.[55] The temperature of the water bath is of concern, especially in the elderly who have impaired thermoregulatory capacity. Cold water may induce vasoconstriction and shivering, whereas warm water may cause vasodilatation and hypotension.[54]

Cardiac arrhythmias have been observed in patients treated with first-generation lithotripters. It is thought that these arrhythmias are caused by the mechanical effects of the shock waves on the myocardium during the repolarization phase of the heart. By using electrocardiographic gating, the shock waves can be delivered milliseconds after the R wave during the refractory period of the heart. Newer generation lithotripters use a nonsynchronized mode in order to improve treatment times, but if induced arrhythmias are detected, a return to a gated mode will eliminate them.[53,56]

Because of the intense pain associated with first-generation lithotripters, general or regional anesthesia was required. Newer generations of lithotripters use a lower working voltage and have eliminated the water bath. Although they cause less pain, most patients still require intravenous sedation during treatments. Because the newer lithotripters use less power, the efficiency of stone fragmentation has decreased, causing the rate of re-treatment to increase.[53]

Absolute contraindications to ESWL are pregnancy, coagulopathy, and an active urinary tract infection. Relative contraindications include distal urethral stricture or obstruction, large stones, calcification or aneurysm of the renal artery or aorta, and/or renal insufficiency.[14,53] Surgical complications from ESWL include urinary obstruction from stone fragments; subcapsular, parenchymal, and perinephric hematomas of the kidney; transient renal failure; and damage to adjacent organs, such as the liver, pancreas, spleen, and lung.[14,53]

Laparoscopic Surgery in Urology

Just as other surgical specialists have adapted to laparoscopic techniques, so have urologists. Initially, pelvic lymph node dissection was the most common urologic laparoscopic procedure performed; however, in recent years, the complexity of surgeries performed laparoscopically has become greater to include radical or donor nephrectomies, adrenalectomy, and radical prostatectomy. The advantages of this minimally invasive technique, although often taking longer to perform, are decreased postoperative pain, decreased blood loss, shorter hospital stays, and quicker return to normal function compared with open surgery.[14,57]

In addition to all the conventional complications and concerns associated with laparoscopic surgery, urologic laparoscopic procedures have their own unique set of problems. Because many urogenital structures are retroperitoneal, urologists often prefer insufflating the retroperitoneal space during laparoscopic surgery. Several studies have shown that CO_2 absorption is greater with retroperitoneal than intraperitoneal insufflation.[58–60] Because the large retroperitoneal space and its connections with the thorax and subcutaneous tissue are exposed to insufflated CO_2, subcutaneous emphysema is a common complication. Subcutaneous emphysema is observed late in the procedure, is preceded by an increase in end-tidal CO_2, may extend all the way up to the head and neck, and is confirmed by palpation for crepitus.[57,61] In severe cases, the upper airway may be compromised secondary to pharyngeal swelling caused by submucous CO_2; therefore, extubation may have to be delayed and ventilation adjusted in these patients.[6,57]

General anesthesia with controlled ventilation is preferred because insufflation of CO_2 and use of the steep Trendelenburg position causes increased intraabdominal and intrathoracic pressures. Some urologic laparoscopic procedures tend to be lengthy, thereby allowing sufficient absorption of CO_2 to cause hypercapnia and acidosis.[6,61] Oliguria may occur intraoperatively during prolonged periods of gas insufflation and then be followed by diuresis in the postoperative period.[6] Two possible mechanisms for the cause of this oliguria have been postulated: the first being that insufflation causes decreased renal cortical blood flow and renal vein obstruction[62]; and the second is an increase in stress hormone levels, such as antidiuretic hormone.[63] Because intraoperative oliguria during prolonged laparoscopic procedures may not truly reflect intravascular volume depletion, treatment with fluid administration may lead to circulatory overload.[14]

Radical Prostatectomy

Prostate cancer is the most frequently diagnosed cancer in men.[64] Radical prostatectomy involves the removal of the entire prostate gland, the ejaculatory ducts, the seminal vesicles, and a portion of the bladder neck.[57] The procedure can be performed with either a retropubic or perineal approach; however, in the United States, most urologists use the retropubic approach.[57] Prostate cancer is a disease of older men with an incidence estimated at 75% for patients over 75 years old.[65] Preoperative evaluation should therefore focus on other coexisting conditions that are prevalent in elderly patients.[57] The perioperative mortality rate has been reported to be approximately 0.2%.[66]

The most common intraoperative complication is hemorrhage with reported blood loss ranging from less than 500 mL to greater than 1500 mL.[57] Because of the potential for rapid blood loss, the use of invasive arterial pressure monitoring as well as adequate venous access are recommended.[14,57] Patients undergoing radical prostatectomy are often placed in a hyperextended supine position along with Trendelenburg,[57] which places the pubis above the head.[6] Significant venous air embolism from the prostatic fossa may occur as a result of a gravitational gradient between the prostatic veins and head.[67] The Trendelenburg position can also produce edema of the upper airway.[14] Early postoperative complications, which occur in 0.5%–2% of cases, include deep vein thrombosis, pulmonary embolism, hematoma, seroma, and wound infection,[66] whereas late surgical complications are incontinence, impotence, and bladder neck contracture.[68]

General or regional anesthesia with sedation may be used for this procedure. If regional anesthesia is chosen, then a sensory level of T6 is recommended.[57] Because many patients may not tolerate lengthy surgery in the Trendelenburg position, one needs to be prepared for conversion to general anesthesia.[57] The choice of anesthetic technique does not seem to influence postoperative morbidity[69] or quality of life.[70]

Radical Cystectomy

The treatment of muscle-invasive bladder cancer is a radical cystectomy. The patient is usually male, a cigarette smoker, and/or had occupational chemical exposure who presents with painless, gross hematuria.[57] In men, it involves the removal of the bladder, prostate gland, seminal vesicles, and proximal urethra; in women, the bladder, uterus, fallopian tubes, ovaries, and the anterior vaginal wall are removed. After the bladder is removed, a urinary diversion is performed; an ileal conduit, bowel segments for continent reservoirs, or ureterostomies are frequently used.[57,71]

The intraoperative problems that may occur during radical retropubic prostatectomy may also arise in this procedure. However, radical cystectomy is an intraperitoneal procedure with increased fluid requirements. In addition to adequate venous access, the use of invasive arterial pressure monitoring and/or central venous monitoring to guide intravenous fluid therapy may be helpful because urinary output cannot be assessed.[57] Because of the length and extent of surgery, general or a combined general-epidural anesthetic technique is mandated.[14,57] A recent study of 50 patients undergoing radical cystectomy comparing combined epidural-general anesthesia (CEGA) to general anesthesia concluded that the CEGA group had significantly less blood loss than the general anesthesia group. There were no significant differences in intraoperative hemodynamics or postoperative complications, and the CEGA group had better postoperative pain control.[72]

Radical Nephrectomy

Renal cell carcinoma is the most common malignancy of the kidney. Because it is refractory to chemotherapy and radiation therapy, radical nephrectomy is the treatment of choice. Radical nephrectomy involves the excision of the kidney, surrounding fascia, the ipsilateral adrenal gland, and the upper ureter.[14,57] Partial nephrectomy is considered in those patients with small lesions or bilateral tumors or those at risk because of other diseases such as diabetes and hypertension.[73] This malignancy has a peak age of incidence of 60 years, and cigarette smoking has been identified as a risk factor.[57] Therefore, coronary artery disease as well as chronic obstructive pulmonary disease is common in these patients.[57]

Frequently used approaches for radical nephrectomy are the flank, subcostal, or thoracoabdominal. Potential complications of these approaches include significant pneumothorax with possible insertion of a chest tube; pulmonary contusion, caused by lung retraction, necessitating prolonged postoperative ventilation; and injuries to adjacent organs, in particular, splenic injury, which has a 10% incidence in association with a left nephrectomy.[57] These tumors tend to be very vascular and extensive blood loss may occur.[57] General anesthesia with invasive arterial pressure monitoring and adequate intravenous access is recommended.[57]

In 5%–10% of patients, the tumor extends into the renal vein and vena cava; therefore, the extent of the lesion must be defined preoperatively. Several potential problems can occur in these patients, ranging from circulatory failure as a result of total occlusion by tumor of the vena cava, to acute pulmonary embolization of tumor fragments.[6] Cardiopulmonary bypass is necessary when control of the vena cava above the tumor thrombus cannot be obtained.[57] If the tumor thrombus extends into the right atrium, then right heart catheterization is contraindicated.[57] The use of transesophageal echocardiography during resection of renal cell carcinoma with vena cava involvement has been shown to be helpful in the management of these complex cases.[74,75]

Summary

With the continuing decline in the annual number of TURPs being performed and the introduction of HoLEP, anesthesiologists will rarely, if at all, experience a patient with TURP syndrome. Because of its advantages over TURP, HoLEP will become the new gold standard for the surgical treatment of BPH in the elderly patient. As urologists become more proficient at laparoscopic techniques, the number of laparoscopic procedures performed on the elderly will increase. Because of their age and increased prevalence of comorbid disease, elderly patients are at higher risk for perioperative morbidity and mortality than their younger counterparts, especially during major surgery. Elderly patients may therefore benefit the most if current and future advances in urologic surgical techniques continue to improve outcomes.

References

1. Fitzpatrick JM, Mebust WK. Minimally invasive and endoscopic management of benign prostatic hyperplasia. In: Walsh PC, ed. Campbell's Urology. 8th ed. Philadelphia: WB Saunders; 2002:1379–1422.
2. Issa MM, Young MR, Bullock AR, et al. Dilutional hyponatremia of TURP syndrome: A historical event in the 21st century. Urology 2004; 64:298–301.
3. McConnell JD, Barry MD, Bruskewitz RC, et al. Benign prostatic hyperplasia: diagnosis and treatment. Clinical practice guideline. Rockville, MD: Agency for Health Care Policy and Research; 1994. Publication No. 94-0582.
4. Issa MM, Marshall FF. Contemporary diagnosis and management of diseases of the prostate. 2nd ed. Newton, PA: Handbook in Health Care Co.; 2004:13–14.
5. Mebust WK, Holtgrewe HL, Cockett ATK, et al. Transurethral prostatectomy: immediate and postoperative complications—cooperative study of 13 participating institutions evaluating 3885 patients. J Urol 1989;141:243–247.
6. Malhota V, Sudheendra V, Diwan S. Anesthesia and the renal and genitourinary systems. In: Miller RD, ed. Miller's Anesthesia. 6th ed. Philadelphia: Elsevier; 2005:2175–2207.
7. Melchior J, Valk WL, Foret JD, et al. Transurethral prostatectomy: computerized analysis of 2223 consecutive cases. J Urol 1974;112:634–642.
8. Azar I. Transurethral prostatectomy syndrome and other complications of urological procedures. In: McLeskey CH, ed. Geriatric Anesthesia. 1st ed. Baltimore: Williams & Wilkins; 1997:595–607.
9. Hatch PD. Surgical and anaesthetic considerations in transurethral resection of the prostate. Anaesth Intensive Care 1987;15:203–211.
10. Jensen V. The TURP syndrome. Can J Anaesth 1991;38: 90–96.
11. Marx GF, Orkin LR. Complications associated with transurethral surgery. Anesthesiology 1962;23:802–813.
12. Roesch RP, Stoelting RK, Lingeman JE, et al. Ammonia toxicity resulting from glycine absorption during a transurethral resection of the prostate. Anesthesiology 1983;58: 577–579.
13. Hoekstra PT, Kahnoski R, McMamish MA, et al. Transurethral prostatic resection syndrome—a new perspective: encephalopathy with associated hyperammonemia. J Urol 1983;130:704–707.
14. Monk TG, Weldon BC. The renal system and anesthesia for urologic surgery. In: Barash PG, Cullen BF, Stoeling RK, eds. Clinical Anesthesia. 4th ed. Philadelphia: Lippincott Williams & Wilkins; 2001:1005–1033.
15. Creevy CD. Reactions peculiar to transurethral resection of the prostate. Surg Clin North Am 1967;47:1471–1472.
16. Hurlbert BJ, Wingard DW. Water intoxication after 15 minutes of transurethral resection of the prostate. Anesthesiology 1979;50:355–356.
17. Still AJ, Modell JA. Acute water intoxication during transurethral resection of the prostate using glycine solution for irrigation. Anesthesiology 1973;38:98–99.
18. Borboroglu PG, Kane CJ, Ward JF, et al. Immediate and postoperative complications of transurethral prostatectomy in the 1990s. J Urol 1999;162:1307–1310.
19. Hahn RG. The transurethral resection syndrome—not yet a finished story [editorial]. Reg Anesth Pain Med 1998; 23:115.
20. Gravenstein D. Transurethral resection of prostate (TURP) syndrome: a review of pathophysiology and management. Anesth Analg 1997;84:438–446.
21. Hahn RG. The transurethral resection syndrome. Acta Anaesthesiol Scand 1991;35:557–567.
22. Rao PN. Fluid absorption during urological endoscopy. Br J Urol 1987;60:93–99.
23. Agin C. Anesthesia for transurethral prostate surgery. Int Anesthesiol Clin 1993;31:25–46.
24. Henderson DJ, Middleton RG. Coma from hyponatremia following transurethral resection of the prostate. Urology 1980;15:267–271.
25. Narins RG. Therapy of hyponatremia: does haste make waste? N Engl J Med 1986;314:1573–1575.
26. Osborn DE, Rao PN, Green MJ, et al. Fluid absorption during transurethral resection. Br Med J 1980;281:1549–1550.
27. Mebust WK, Brady TW, Valk WL. Observations on cardiac output, blood volume, central venous pressure, fluid and electrolyte changes in patients undergoing transurethral prostatectomy. J Urol 1970;103:632–636.
28. Rose FC. Transient blindness. Br Med J 1964;3:763–764.
29. Barletta JP, Fanous MM, Hamed LM. Temporary blindness in the TUR syndrome. J Neuroophthalmol 1994;14:6–8.
30. Fahey JL. Toxicity and blood ammonia rise resulting from intravenous amino acid administration in man: the protective effect of L-arginine. J Clin Invest 1957;36:1647–1655.

31. Nathans D, Fahey JL, Ship AG. Sites of origin and removal of blood ammonia formed during glycine infusion: effect of L-arginine. J Lab Clin Med 1958;51:124–133.

32. Murphy DM, Falkiner FR, Carr M, et al. Septicemia after transurethral prostatectomy. Urology 1983;22:133–135.

33. Allen TD. Body temperature changes during prostatic resection as related to the temperature of the irrigating solution. J Urol 1973;110:433–435.

34. Heathcote PS, Dyer PM. The effect of warm irrigation on blood loss during transurethral prostatectomy under spinal anesthesia. Br J Urol 1986;58:669–671.

35. Ladehoff AA, Rasmussen J. Fibrinolysis and thromboplastic activities in relation to hemorrhage in transvesical prostatectomy. Scand J Clin Lab Invest 1961;13:231–244.

36. Aasheim GM. Hyponatremia during transurethral surgery. Can Anaesth Soc J 1973;20:274–280.

37. Abrams PH, Shah PJR, Bryning K, et al. Blood loss during transurethral resection of the prostate. Anaesthesia 1982;37:71–73.

38. Mackenzie AR. Influence of anesthesia on blood loss in transurethral prostatectomy. Scott Med J 1990;35:14–16.

39. Madsen RE, Madsen PO. Influence of anesthesia form on blood loss in transurethral prostatectomy. Anesth Analg 1967;46:330–332.

40. McGowan SW, Smith GFN. Anaesthesia for transurethral prostatectomy. Anaesthesia 1980;35:847–853.

41. Nielsen KK, Andersen K, Asbjorn J, et al. Blood loss in transurethral prostatectomy: epidural versus general anesthesia. Int Urol Nephrol 1987;19:287–292.

42. Fraser I, Scott M, Campbell I, et al. Routine cross-matching is not necessary for a transurethral resection of the prostate. Br J Urol 1964;56:399–405.

43. Slade N, Andrews GL, Tovey GH, et al. Blood loss in prostatic surgery. Br J Urol 1964;36:399–405.

44. Chung FF, Chung A, Meier RH, et al. Comparison of perioperative mental function after general anaesthesia and spinal anaesthesia with intravenous sedation. Can J Anaesth 1989;36:382–387.

45. Rasmussen LS, Johnson T, Kuipers HM, et al. Does anaesthesia cause post-operative cognitive dysfunction? A randomized study of regional versus general anaesthesia in 438 elderly patients. Acta Anaesthesiol Scand 2003;47:260–266.

46. Bowman GW, Hoerth JW, McGlothlen JS, et al. Anesthesia for transurethral resection of the prostate: spinal or general? AANA J 1981;49:63–68.

47. Sterns RH, Riggs JE, Schochet SS Jr. Osmotic demyelinization syndrome following correction of hyponatremia. N Engl J Med 1986;314:1535–1542.

48. Malhotra V. Transurethral resection of the prostate. Anesthesiol Clin North Am 2000;18:883–897.

49. Elzayat EA, Habib EI, Elhilahi MM. Holmium laser enucleation of the prostate: a size-independent new "gold standard." Urology 2005;66(Suppl 5A):108–113.

50. Hobika JH, Clarke BG. Use of neuromuscular blocking drugs to counteract thigh-adductor spasm induced by electrical shocks of obturator nerve during transurethral resection of bladder tumors. J Urol 1961;85:295–296.

51. Prentiss RJ, Harvey GW, Bethard WF, et al. Massive adductor muscle contraction in transurethral surgery: cause and prevention; development of new electrical circuitry. J Urol 1965;93:263–271.

52. Pahira JJ, Razack AA. In: Hanno PM, Malkowitz SB, Wein AJ, eds. Nephrolithiasis: Clinical Manual of Urology. 3rd ed. New York: McGraw Hill; 2001:231–252.

53. Gravenstein D. Extracorporeal shock wave lithotripsy and percutaneous nephrolithotomy. Anesthesiol Clin North Am 2000;18:953–971.

54. Weber W, Madler C, Keil B, et al. Cardiovascular effects of extracorporeal shock wave lithotripsy. In: Gravenstein D, Peter K, eds. Extracorporeal Shock Wave Lithotripsy for Renal Stone Disease: Technical and Clinical Aspects. Stoneham, MA: Butterworth; 1986:101–112.

55. Bromage PR, Bonsu AK, el-Faqih S, et al. Influence of Dornier HM3 system on respiration during extracorporeal shock wave lithotripsy. Anesth Analg 1989;68:363–367.

56. Greenstein A, Kaver I, Lechtman V, et al. Cardiac arrhythmias during non-synchronized extracorporeal shock wave lithotripsy. J Urol 1995;154:1321–1322.

57. Whalley DG, Berrigan MJ. Anesthesia for radical prostatectomy, cystectomy, nephrectomy, pheochromocytoma, and laparoscopic procedures. Anesthesiol Clin North Am 2000;18:889–917.

58. Mullett CE, Viale JP, Sagnard PE, et al. Pulmonary CO_2 elimination during surgical procedures using intra- or extraperitoneal CO_2 insulation. Anesth Analg 1993;76:622–626.

59. Wolf JS Jr, Monk TG, McDougall EM, et al. The extraperitoneal approach and subcutaneous emphysema are associated with greater absorption of carbon dioxide during laparoscopic renal surgery. J Urol 1995;154:959–963.

60. Wolf JS Jr, Clayman RV, Monk TG, et al. Carbon dioxide absorption during laparoscopic pelvic operation. J Am Coll Surg 1995;180:555–560.

61. Weingram J, Sosa RE, Stein B, et al. Subcutaneous emphysema (SCE) during laparoscopic pelvic lymph node dissection (LPLND). Anesth Analg 1993;S460:76.

62. McDougall EM, Monk TG, Hicks M, et al. The effect of prolonged pneumo-peritoneum on renal function in an animal model. J Am Coll Surg 1996;182:317–328.

63. Ortega AE, Peters JH, Incarbone R, et al. A prospective randomized comparison of the metabolic and stress hormonal responses of laparoscopic and open cholecystectomy. J Am Coll Surg 1996;183:249–256.

64. Brawer MK. How to use prostate-specific antigen in the early detection or screening for prostatic carcinoma. Cancer J Clin 1995;45:148–164.

65. Morgan GE Jr, Mikhail MS, Murray MJ. Anesthesia for genitourinary surgery. In: Clinical Anesthesia. 4th ed. New York: Lange Medical Books; 2006:757–772.

66. Monk TG. Cancer of the prostate and radical prostatectomy. In: Malhotra V, ed. Anesthesia for Renal and Genitourinary Surgery. New York: McGraw Hill; 1996:177–195.

67. Albin MS, Ritter RR, Reinhart R, et al. Venous air embolism during radical retropubic prostatectomy. Anesth Analg 1992;74:151–153.

68. Catalona WJ. Surgical management of prostate cancer. Contemporary results with anatomic surgical prostatectomy. Cancer 1995;75:1903–1908.

69. Shir Y, Frank SM, Brendler CB, et al. Postoperative morbidity is similar in patients anesthetized with epidural and

general anesthesia for radical prostatectomy. Urology 1994; 44:232–236.

70. Haythornthwaite JA, Raja SN, Fisher B, et al. Pain and quality of life following radical retropubic prostatectomy. J Urol 1998;160:1761–1764.

71. Maffezzini M, Gerbi G, Campodonico F, et al. Peri-operative management of ablative and reconstructive surgery for invasive bladder cancer in the elderly. Surg Oncol 2004;13: 197–200.

72. Ozyuvaci E, Altran A, Karadeniz T, et al. General anesthesia verus epidural and general anesthesia in radical cystectomy. Urol Int 2005;74:62–67.

73. Shah N. Radical cystectomy, radical nephrectomy and retroperitoneal lymph node dissection. In: Malhotra V, ed. Anesthesia for Renal and Genitourinary Surgery. New York: McGraw Hill; 1996:197–226.

74. Hasnain JU, Watson RJN. Transesophageal echocardiography during resection of renal cell carcinoma involving the inferior vena cava. South Med J 1994;87: 273–275.

75. Mizoguchi T, Koide Y, Ohara M, et al. Multiplane transesophageal echocardiographic guidance during resection of renal cell carcinoma extending into the inferior vena cava. Anesth Analg 1995;81:1102–1105.

26
Thoracic Procedures

Steven M. Neustein and James B. Eisenkraft

From 1900 to 1990, the fraction of the population aged 65 years and older tripled to 13%.[1] Persons aged 80 years and older now constitute the fastest-growing elderly group in the United States.[2] Between 2000 and 2020, this segment of the United States population is expected to increase by approximately 35%.

Aging increases the susceptibility to pulmonary disease.[3] Lung cancer is the leading cause of cancer death in persons older than 70 years.[4] More than half of all lung cancers occur in people who are older than 65 years. From 1955 to 1992, worldwide mortality from lung cancer has increased by 180% and 580% in 65- to 82-year-old men and women, respectively.[5]

Most lung cancers become manifest in the geriatric population because they are associated with a long latency period after prolonged exposure to tobacco smoke or other predisposing factors. Surgical resection is currently the only available means for curing lung cancer. Those patients with unresectable tumors often receive chemotherapy and radiation treatment. Surgery is also the treatment of choice for localized non–small cell carcinomas, because often they can be excised completely.

Lung resection for tumor is a common procedure in the elderly. Resection is often preceded by bronchoscopy to evaluate tumor involvement of the airway and to determine the resectability. If there is mediastinal adenopathy on computed tomography scan of the chest, a mediastinoscopy is performed to determine if this enlargement is the result of malignant spread of the tumor, which, if present, would contraindicate surgical resection.

Although surgery is necessary to cure most lung cancers, the risk of operating on the elderly is increased.[6] Patients in this segment of the population are offered surgery less often than younger counterparts.[7] Elderly patients who are not treated survive an average 1–5 years.[8] Overall, the 5-year survival rate for patients with lung cancer is 18.5% for those younger than 65 and 13.8% for those 65 years or older.[9] This may be attributable to a lower rate of surgery in elderly patients with lung cancer.

Morbidity and Mortality of Thoracic Surgical Procedures in the Elderly

Among elderly patients undergoing pneumonectomy and lobectomy, the associated mortality has been twice that of patients younger than 65 years.[10] A series of 476 patients were studied by Kohman et al.[11] to identify predictors of mortality after thoracotomy for lung cancer. Hospital mortality for patients undergoing pulmonary resection was 5.6%. The only statistically significant risk factors for mortality were age 60 years or older, the presence of premature ventricular contractions on the admission electrocardiogram (EKG), and the need for pneumonectomy (versus lobectomy). Patients younger than 60 years had a mortality rate of 2.4%, as compared with 7.4% in patients aged 60 years or older. Hospital mortality after pneumonectomy and lobectomy was 11.7% and 3.7%, respectively. More recently, a 30-day mortality rate of 22% in patients older than 70 years has been reported after pneumonectomy.[12] In another report of patients more than 80 years undergoing thoracic surgery for lung cancer, there was a mortality rate of only 3%.[13] In a study of 296 patients who were 65–89 years of age, and underwent resection with video-assisted thoracoscopy (VAT) for stage 1 lung cancer, there was a 15% incidence of morbidity, and only a 1% mortality rate.[14]

Gerson et al.[15] studied 177 patients who were 65 years of age or older and scheduled for major elective abdominal or noncardiac thoracic surgery. The inability to exercise, defined as the inability to perform supine bicycle pedaling for 2 minutes or to increase the heart rate to at least 100 beats per minute, was the best predictor of postoperative cardiopulmonary complications. Patients capable of this exercise had a perioperative cardiac or pulmonary complication rate of 9.3%, as compared with 42% for those who could not perform the exercise. The comparative mortality rates were 0.9% and 7.2%, respectively. Perioperative pulmonary complications occurred in 24 patients (14%). Twenty-three of these patients had pneumonia, and one patient had a pulmonary embolism. Arterial blood gases were not predictive of the incidence of perioperative pulmonary complications in this study, but this may have been caused by the paucity of patients with increased carbon dioxide levels. A history of congestive heart failure or neurologic disease has been associated with an increased risk of postoperative pulmonary dysfunction in the elderly.[16]

Perioperative chest physical therapy in the elderly, when combined with postoperative chest physical therapy, can further decrease the incidence of atelectasis.[17] In this study of elderly patients who underwent cardiac and other thoracic surgical procedures, none of the 67 patients with chronic obstructive pulmonary disease (COPD) who received both preoperative and postoperative chest physical therapy developed pulmonary complications, as compared with all 34 patients with COPD who only received postoperative chest physical therapy ($p < 0.02$).[17] In a more recent study, patients with COPD who had a perioperative chest physical therapy program that was begun preoperatively also had a reduction in postoperative pulmonary complications.[18] Elderly patients have decreased pulmonary function because of aging and increased duration of exposure to cigarette smoke, and are less likely to tolerate removal of lung tissue.

In the study by Gerson et al.,[15] perioperative cardiac complications occurred in 25 of 177 patients (14%). Ninety-two percent of patients who had a perioperative pulmonary complication, and 88% of patients who had a perioperative cardiac complication, were unable to perform 2 minutes of exercise and increase their heart rates to at least 100 beats per minute. A previous study also demonstrated this test to be a predictor of perioperative cardiac complications in noncardiac thoracic geriatric surgery.[19]

Cardiorespiratory Physiology in the Elderly

A thorough preoperative assessment is essential for any patient scheduled to undergo thoracic surgery. It is particularly important for the geriatric patient, because with advancing age comes a decline in cardiopulmonary function. There is decreased elastic tissue in both peripheral and coronary arteries, leading to systolic hypertension, left ventricular hypertrophy, and decreased coronary reserve. There is also a decrease in the maximum achievable stroke volume and heart rate, and thus in maximum cardiac output.

A decrease in elastic tissue occurs in the lungs with age, leading to an increase in lung compliance. However, the thorax is more rigid because of calcification so that total thoracic compliance may be unchanged. The decrease in the amount of elastic tissue leads to airway closure, and there is an increase in both anatomic and alveolar dead space. The closing capacity, closing volume, and residual volume increase. In addition to a decreased ventilatory response to hypoxia and hypercarbia, elderly patients may have periodic breathing during sleep, putting them at increased risk of apnea in the postanesthesia care unit.[20] The vital capacity and PaO_2 decrease with increasing age.[21] A frequently used formula for estimating the PaO_2 according to age is, $PaO_2 = 100 -$ age (in years)/3. With aging, there is a decrease in both immune function, and ciliary function, which accounts for an increased rate of respiratory infections in the elderly.[22]

The patient with a preoperative forced vital capacity (FVC) of less than 20 mL/kg or postbronchodilator forced expiratory volume in 1 second (FEV_1)/FVC of less than 50% is at increased risk for pulmonary complications. Preoperative teaching of breathing exercises and planned bronchial therapy can decrease postoperative pulmonary complications.[23]

The elderly have decreased anesthetic requirements. There is an increase in sensitivity to anesthetic agents, which parallels the loss of cortical neurons and decrease in brain neurotransmitters that occur with aging. Premedication of the elderly patient for thoracic surgery should be light, because of the decreased pulmonary reserve and increased sensitivity to anesthetics. In many cases, premedication is best omitted. Anticholinergics to decrease secretions may be helpful, especially if bronchoscopy is planned.

Preoperative Evaluation

Postoperative pulmonary complications are a major source of morbidity and mortality after thoracic surgery.[24] The best evaluation of pulmonary function is a careful history. The information to be collected includes history of smoking, presence of respiratory systems, and functional status.

As described by Slinger and Johnston,[25] pulmonary function can be evaluated by assessing three aspects: mechanics, gas exchange, and cardiopulmonary function. The single most important test of respiratory mechanics is the FEV_1. Patients with an FEV_1 <70% predicted undergoing a pulmonary resection for lung cancer have been reported to have an increased 30-day mortality rate.[26,27] A predicted postoperative FEV_1 can be estimated. Patients with values >40% are at decreased risk, whereas those with values <30% are at increased risk.[28]

Gas exchange can be evaluated by the diffusing capacity for carbon monoxide (DLCO). Similar to the FEV_1, a predicted postoperative DLCO can be estimated based on how much functioning lung tissue will be removed.

A predicted postoperative DLCO <40% carries an increased risk.[29]

The third aspect is the overall cardiopulmonary function of the patient. This can be estimated from the history. The inability to climb two flights of stairs indicates an increased risk. More objectively, the maximal oxygen consumption can be determined. A maximal oxygen consumption >15 mL/kg/min is associated with reduced risk,[30] and <10 mL/kg/min has been reported to indicate very high risk.[31]

A careful preoperative evaluation and proper selection of surgical candidates may be partially responsible for the lower mortality rates that now accompany thoracic surgery in the elderly.[1]

Bronchoscopy

Rigid bronchoscopy may be performed by the thoracic surgeon for therapeutic reasons, such as for placement of an airway stent or debulking of a tracheal tumor. A rigid ventilating bronchoscope is essentially a hollow tube with a blunted beveled distal tip and an eyepiece at the proximal end. Side holes at the distal end permit ventilation of lung segments proximal to the tip of the bronchoscope. A side arm can be connected to an anesthesia circuit for ventilation and anesthesia administration. The increase in chest wall stiffness with aging may make ventilation more difficult. It may be necessary to use a smaller tidal volume and a greater ventilatory rate. During rigid bronchoscopy, monitoring should include an EKG, blood pressure cuff, precordial stethoscope, and pulse oximeter. If a thoracoscopy or thoracotomy is to follow, an arterial catheter should be placed, depending on the medical condition of the patient and the planned procedure.

Choice of Anesthesia

For rigid bronchoscopy, general anesthesia is preferred over local anesthesia. This is to prevent patient movement and possible airway trauma. Local anesthesia can be applied in addition to general anesthesia to minimize the hemodynamic response to bronchoscopy and decrease the amount of general anesthesia required. Ventilation may be decreased by a leak around the bronchoscope, and the use of a high inspired concentration of oxygen (FIO_2) and high fresh gas flows may be necessary. Paralysis of the patient for bronchoscopy using neuromuscular blocking agents reduces the likelihood of patient movement and therefore the risk of trauma from the rigid bronchoscope.

Ventilation and Oxygenation

A number of techniques have been described for ventilating, oxygenating, and anesthetizing the patient under-

going rigid bronchoscopy.[32] Apneic oxygenation with oxygen insufflation at 10–15 L per minute through a catheter whose tip is located above the carina has been reported to provide adequate oxygenation for 55 minutes.[33] However, during apnea, arterial carbon dioxide tension ($PaCO_2$) increases at the rate of approximately 3 mm Hg per minute and may limit the duration of apneic oxygenation that is possible. Hyperventilation of the patient before the apneic period in order to lower the starting $PaCO_2$ is a useful adjunct to this technique. The use of a pulse oximeter is especially critical if apneic oxygenation is used.

Another method for ventilation during rigid bronchoscopy is manual intermittent positive pressure ventilation (IPPV), which is accomplished by manually compressing the reservoir bag of the anesthesia circuit. With this technique, high fresh gas flows are often needed to compensate for the gas leak around the distal end of the bronchoscope. Ventricular arrhythmias are common, usually because of light anesthesia and/or hypercarbia, and they respond to hyperventilation and further increasing depth of anesthesia. Coordination with the surgeon is important, because squeezing the reservoir bag while the eyepiece of the bronchoscope is removed for suctioning or biopsy will direct any debris inside the bronchoscope at the surgeon. Packing of the pharynx by the surgeon can limit the leak.

The Sanders injection system can be used for jet ventilation of the patient during rigid bronchoscopy.[34] Manual depression of an in-line toggle switch allows a jet of oxygen that entrains air to be delivered from a high-pressure oxygen source. The jet of oxygen is delivered to the patient through a 16- or 18-gauge needle inside and as parallel as possible to the long axis of the bronchoscope. A pressure-reducing valve is also present in the system that adjustably decreases the driving pressure from the 50 pounds per square inch gauge pressure (PSIG) pipeline value to 30–35 PSIG. The pressure that results in the tracheal lumen is determined by the driving pressure from the reducing valve, the radius of the jet needle, and the cross-sectional area of the bronchoscope. If the bronchoscope fits tightly in the trachea, the oxygen driving pressure should be decreased because there may be increased risk of barotrauma.[32]

An advantage of the Sanders injection system is the ability to ventilate the patient without the eyepiece in place, thereby allowing continuous ventilation. Entrainment of air, however, produces a variable FIO_2 at the distal tip. Ventilation may be inadequate in the presence of low thoracic compliance. High-frequency positive pressure ventilation (HFPPV) may also be used to ventilate the patient's lungs during rigid bronchoscopy. Some bronchoscopes have a port that is designed for ventilation with HFPPV. This mode of ventilation uses a small jet of fresh gas from a high pressure source (50 PSIG) delivered at rates greater than 100 breaths per minute. A high-pressure air-oxygen supply is modulated by a solenoid valve, producing frequent jet pulses that result in forward motion of airway gas. HFPPV at rates of up to 150 breaths per minute has produced similar blood gas values to those obtained with the Sanders injector system.[35] The tracheobronchial wall is immobile during HFPPV, which may be an important advantage during laser surgery.[35] Complications of rigid bronchoscopy include damage to teeth, hemorrhage, bronchial or tracheal perforation, airway edema, and barotrauma. These risks are greater if the patient moves while the rigid bronchoscopy is in place. Flexible fiberoptic bronchoscopy is associated with fewer complications.

Flexible Fiberoptic Bronchoscopy

An examination of the airway with the flexible fiberoptic bronchoscope is typically performed before a lung resection. Preoperatively, an antisialagogue should be administered to decrease secretions that would otherwise interfere with visualization. Although scopolamine is the most potent drying agent, it may cause confusion in the elderly and should therefore be avoided. Glycopyrrolate is the drying agent of choice. It has a longer duration of action than atropine, and does not cross the blood–brain barrier.

Flexible fiberoptic bronchoscopy can be performed using either local or general anesthesia. Local anesthetic solution can be sprayed onto the base of the tongue, or the patient can gargle with viscous lidocaine (2%). Bilateral superior laryngeal nerve blocks can be performed either percutaneously or by using Krause forceps to hold local anesthetic-soaked pledgets in each piriform fossa. The trachea and vocal cords are anesthetized by direct injection of local anesthetic into the trachea through the cricothyroid membrane, by spraying of local anesthetic under direct vision, or by injection via the working channel of the fiberscope.

Instead of using the blocks described above, a nebulizer can be used to topically anesthetize the whole airway. A disposable ("acorn") nebulizer filled with lidocaine (4 mL of 4%) is attached to a closely fitting face mask. The flow of oxygen to the nebulizer creates a mist of lidocaine that is inhaled by the patient, who is instructed to hold the mist in the airway for as long as possible. The nasal mucosa should also be anesthetized if the fiberoptic bronchoscope is to be passed nasally. This can be accomplished with cocaine, or a mixture of lidocaine (3 mL of 4%) and phenylephrine (1 mL of 1%).

The technique of flexible fiberoptic bronchoscopy in an awake patient requires considerable cooperation from the patient. The elderly patient with lung disease may not tolerate much sedation; therefore, good topical anesthesia of the airway with local anesthetic is important.

Fiberoptic bronchoscopy can also be performed with the patient under general anesthesia. The trachea is first intubated, and then the fiberscope is inserted through an adapter that will create a gas-tight seal around the instrument such that the patient's lungs may be ventilated around the fiberscope. The passage of a fiberscope through an endotracheal tube during IPPV may cause a positive end-expiratory pressure (PEEP) effect. If PEEP is already being applied via the anesthesia circuit, it should be discontinued while the fiberscope is in place.[33] A smaller-diameter fiberscope should be used if the endotracheal tube being used is less than 8.0 mm in internal diameter. Problems associated with fiberoptic bronchoscopy include local anesthetic toxicity, bleeding, and airway obstruction because of passage of the fiberscope through a stenosed portion of the trachea, or bleeding into an already narrowed airway, hypoxemia, and bronchospasm.[32]

Mediastinoscopy

Mediastinoscopy was initially described by Carlens[36] as a method for assessing spread of bronchial carcinoma. The procedure enables examination of the superior mediastinal lymph nodes lying posterior to the aortic arch. The lymphatic drainage of the lungs is first to the subcarinal and paratracheal nodes and then to the supraclavicular nodes and thoracic duct. Through biopsy of these nodes, a diagnosis can be established, and suitability for thoracotomy and tumor resection can be determined. Proximal bronchial lesions often metastasize to the mediastinum, whereas peripheral lesions do not. Mediastinoscopy is less useful in patients with left lung tumors because these tumors usually spread to the subaortic lymph nodes that are not accessible via the mediastinoscope. These subaortic nodes are approached by an anterior thoracotomy through the second or third intercostal space (Chamberlain operation). Malignant spread of the tumor to the contralateral mediastinal nodes is an absolute contraindication to surgical resection of the tumor, whereas metastasis to the ipsilateral nodes does not rule out resection.

Traditional mediastinoscopy is performed via a transverse incision just above the suprasternal notch. Following anteriorly to the trachea, the tip of the mediastinoscope is passed behind the innominate (brachiocephalic) vessels and the aortic arch. Mediastinoscopy is usually not performed if the patient has had a previous mediastinoscopy. This is because of scarring and loss of usual tissue planes.

Mediastinoscopy can be performed under local anesthesia, but an awake patient breathing spontaneously would be at increased risk for venous air embolism because of negative intrathoracic inspiratory pressure and for mediastinal trauma if the patient moves. It has been claimed that performing mediastinoscopy under local anesthesia is safer in those patients with limited pulmonary reserve and cerebrovascular disease, both of which are more common in the elderly.[37] However, general anesthesia is usually preferred for mediastinoscopy and should include paralysis to prevent patient movement and coughing that could lead to intrathoracic venous congestion and possible intrathoracic trauma.

Mediastinoscopy is performed with the patient in the supine position and the neck hyperextended. The elderly patient may not be able to tolerate this position as well as the younger individual, and it is advisable to test the patient's range of neck motion before induction of general anesthesia.

The most common complication of mediastinoscopy is hemorrhage, which can be sudden and massive. Blood should therefore be available before starting the procedure. Emergency thoracotomy or sternotomy may be required to stop the bleeding, although surgical tamponade via the mediastinoscope may be done as a temporizing measure. Needle aspiration of any structure before its biopsy is done so that a major vessel will not be accidentally biopsied. If the bleeding is venous, a large-bore intravenous catheter should be placed in a vein in a lower extremity, because fluid and medications given into an upper extremity vein in this situation will drain into the mediastinum.[38] A torn mediastinal vein may also lead to an air embolus, especially if the patient is breathing spontaneously. The reverse Trendelenburg position can decrease venous pressure and therefore bleeding, but this also increases the potential for venous air embolism.

A pneumothorax may occur during mediastinoscopy, which may necessitate placement of a chest tube. The recurrent laryngeal nerve may be injured. The nerve may be damaged by the mediastinoscope or compressed by the tumor. Bilateral recurrent laryngeal nerve injury may lead to airway obstruction after tracheal extubation and spontaneous ventilation by the patient. An additional potential complication is arrhythmias that may occur because of stimulation of pressor receptors in the aortic arch.

The mediastinoscope may compress the innominate (brachiocephalic) artery, leading to a decrease in blood flow in the common carotid and right subclavian arteries. This has been misdiagnosed as a cardiac arrest.[39] Transient left hemiparesis has also been reported after mediastinoscopy.[40] The elderly patient is more likely to have a history of neurovascular insufficiency and be at risk for this complication. The blood pressure can be measured in the left arm, but the pulse in the right arm should be monitored continuously. The pulse is monitored most sensitively by an arterial catheter and pressure transducer system and less sensitively by a pulse oximeter.

A damped right radial pulse pressure is an indication for repositioning of the mediastinoscope, relieving compression of the innominate artery. Other complications of mediastinoscopy include tracheal collapse, tension pneumomediastinum, hemothorax, and chylothorax. A chest radiograph should be obtained in the immediate postoperative period if a pneumothorax is suspected, and is taken routinely in many centers.

Thoracotomy

Pulmonary resection (pneumonectomy or lobectomy) is the most frequently performed thoracic surgical procedure. Whenever possible, a lobectomy rather than a pneumonectomy is done for a primary tumor, because this procedure is associated with a lower morbidity and mortality but offers a similar prognosis to the more extensive procedure.[11]

The elderly have a higher mortality rate than younger patients undergoing thoracotomy.[1] In one series, the operative mortality in elderly patients undergoing pneumonectomy was 22%, compared with 3.2% in younger patients.[41]

Cardiovascular Complications

Arrhythmias are a common perioperative complication after pulmonary resection and may not be as well tolerated in the elderly. The older patient is more likely to have diastolic dysfunction and the less compliant ventricle is more dependent on the atrial contraction for proper filling. Atrial arrhythmias are more likely to cause hypotension in the geriatric patient. Arrhythmias are more common in patients older than 50 years undergoing pulmonary resection and are more frequently related to right pneumonectomy as compared with left pneumonectomy.

In a retrospective study of 236 patients, a 22% incidence of perioperative arrhythmias has been reported in the perioperative period of pneumonectomies.[42] Atrial fibrillation, which made up 64% of all arrhythmias, was the most common. In 55%, the arrhythmias persisted, and there was a 31% in-hospital mortality rate in this group. Prophylactic perioperative digitalization can reduce the incidence of arrhythmias[43,44] but has the potential for toxicity and contributing to arrhythmias. A prospective, controlled, randomized clinical study in 140 consecutive patients reevaluated the role of prophylactic digoxin in relation to thoracic surgical procedures.[45] Patients were randomly allocated to receive no digoxin or digoxin 0.5mg twice on the night before surgery, followed by 0.25mg with premedication. Postoperatively, patients received digoxin 0.25mg per day for 9 days. The dose of digoxin was adjusted according to serum level, and patients were monitored by EKG. The overall mortality was 5.7%. The investigators found no significant difference in the incidence of arrhythmias between the two groups and concluded that prophylactic digitalization in elective thoracic operations is not justified.

The use of perioperative metoprolol can reduce the incidence of atrial fibrillation after thoracotomy for lung resection.[46] In this prospective, randomized, double-blind study, the incidence of arrhythmias was 6.7% after metoprolol versus 40% in the control group.

Monitoring

Hypoxemia is likely during one-lung ventilation, and continuous monitoring using pulse oximetry is the standard of care. Patients undergoing pulmonary resection should have an indwelling arterial catheter for continuous blood pressure monitoring and arterial blood sampling. Central venous access allows for central delivery of drugs for treatment of arrhythmias, hypotension, measurement of pressure, and can guide the anesthesia provider in fluid therapy management.

Elderly patients are more likely to have cardiovascular disease, and their management may be facilitated by the use of a pulmonary artery catheter. Patients are at greater risk for pulmonary edema after pneumonectomy because of a decreased pulmonary vasculature cross-sectional area (increased pulmonary vascular resistance); thus, a pulmonary artery catheter may be of even more value in these cases. If a pulmonary artery catheter is placed for pneumonectomy, it is imperative that its tip not be in the pulmonary artery of the lung to be resected at the time of ligation. It may be necessary to withdraw the catheter at the time of pulmonary artery ligation and to then re-advance the catheter after the ligation.

Transesophageal echocardiography (TEE) may be useful during thoracic surgery. It may help to delineate the anatomy if a tumor is invading or compressing the heart.[47] It can provide real-time estimation of myocardial function and ventricular filling. The elderly patient is more likely to have a decrease in cardiac function and therefore is more likely to require central venous monitoring and/or TEE monitoring.

Airway Management

The placement of a double-lumen endobronchial tube allows collapse of the operated lung, making the surgical resection easier. It also facilitates suctioning and application of continuous positive airway pressure to the nonventilated lung. The most common approach to lung separation is the use of a left-sided double-lumen tube, except when the left mainstem bronchus is diseased. The left mainstem bronchus, being longer than the right mainstem bronchus, permits placement of a left-sided endobronchial tube with a smaller chance of upper lobe obstruction. In the case of a left pneumonectomy, the tube must be withdrawn into the trachea before ligation of the bronchus.

Another alternative is placement of an endobronchial tube into the nonoperative side, so as to avoid disruption of a potentially diseased bronchus and to avoid repositioning in the case of a pneumonectomy. A disadvantage of this method is that upper lobe obstruction is likely to cause hypoxemia during one-lung ventilation, because this is the lung to be ventilated during surgery of the contralateral lung.

A third method is placement of the endobronchial tube into the operated side. The advantage of this method is that upper lobe obstruction during one-lung ventilation is not more likely to lead to hypoxemia, because this lung will be collapsed during one-lung anesthesia. However, in the case of a right thoracotomy, the presence of the tube in this short bronchus may interfere with the surgeon's ligation of the bronchus.

Intubation is more likely to be difficult in the elderly if there is arthritis of the neck, with consequent limitation of mobility. Arthritis of the temporomandibular joint may cause limitation of mouth opening. However, if the patient is edentulous, which is also more likely in the elderly, the intubation may be easier. Thus, increased age may have the effect of making intubation easier or more difficult. Each patient must therefore be evaluated individually.

In the case of a difficult intubation, it may be preferable to begin by placing a single-lumen tube. A tube exchanger can then be used to replace the single-lumen tube with a double-lumen tube. Alternatively, one-lung ventilation could be facilitated with a bronchial blocker placed through the single-lumen tube into the bronchus of the lung to be deflated. Two blockers that are now available are the Arndt and the Cohen tip-deflecting blocker. The Arndt blocker (Cook Critical Care, Bloomington, IN) has a lumen with a wire extending through it, ending in a loop. A fiberscope is passed through the loop and is used to guide the blocker into place. More recently, the Cohen tip-deflecting blocker (Cook Critical Care) has been introduced. This blocker has an internal wire, which allows the tip to be angled and directed into either bronchus. There is a wheel at the proximal end that, when turned, bends (flexes) the tip of the blocker.

Intraoperative Anesthetic Management

Most pulmonary resections are performed with the patient in the lateral decubitus position and via a posterolateral incision. After transection of the chest wall muscles, the pleural space is entered either by rib resection or via an intercostal space. The lung should be collapsed before this entry to prevent injury. The lung resection is accomplished with ligation of the arterial and venous vessels, and the bronchus of the diseased lobe or lung.

Blood loss is usually not severe enough to require transfusion during lobectomy or pneumonectomy, but blood should be available. Blood loss is likely to be greater during pleuropneumonectomy, pleurectomy, or decortication, and the patient is more likely to require blood transfusion. Measurement of central venous pressure and hematocrit, and estimation of blood loss assist in guiding fluid administration. A fluid warmer is important because heat loss may occur during thoracotomy, and hypothermia will delay extubation and increase the likelihood of arrhythmias.

After lung resection, there is a reduction in the pulmonary vascular bed and an increased risk of pulmonary edema, especially after a pneumonectomy.[48] Fluids should therefore be given cautiously during and after pneumonectomy. Fluid overload in this situation may also cause right atrial distention and arrhythmias. The elderly have a decreased ability to tolerate these hemodynamic aberrations and, with a reduced cardiac function, would be more likely to develop pulmonary edema. Hypotension could lead to inadequate coronary artery perfusion, myocardial ischemia, and possibly infarction.

Maintenance of general anesthesia can be accomplished using a potent inhaled anesthetic agent and neuromuscular blocking drug to prevent movement of the diaphragm. The elderly patient with limited cardiac reserve may not tolerate a potent inhaled agent and may require a high-dose opioid technique in which case ventilation must be continued postoperatively.[49] However, in contrast to high-dose fentanyl, an infusion of remifentanil can decrease the requirement for a potent inhaled agent and still allow the patient to awaken promptly after the surgery. A high F_{IO_2} is needed during one-lung anesthesia, but, after this, the addition of nitrous oxide can also facilitate an earlier extubation by allowing use of lesser amounts of potent inhaled anesthetic agent.

After lung resection and before reinflation of remaining lung tissue, the endobronchial tube should be suctioned. The bronchial suture line is tested by applying 20–40 cm H_2O pressure using manual compression of the anesthesia circuit reservoir bag. Before closure of the chest, complete reexpansion of remaining lung tissue should be visually confirmed. Thoracostomy tubes are placed for drainage of air and fluid after a lobectomy. These tubes are not placed if a pneumonectomy has been performed, because there is no remaining lung tissue to reexpand. In this case, the use of nitrous oxide can lead to a tension pneumothorax once the chest is closed, because there is no tube to vent the space. After skin closure and return of the patient to the supine position, pressure in the postpneumonectomy thoracic cavity space is relieved by needle aspiration. The trachea may be extubated immediately after surgery, depending on the preoperative condition of the patient, temperature, hemodynamic stability, and extent of surgery and technique used (e.g., opioid versus potent inhaled agent). Early return to spontaneous ventilation is advantageous, because it can decrease an air leak from the lung and reduce stress on bronchial sutures. The double-lumen tube is generally replaced with a single-lumen endotracheal tube if the trachea is to remain intubated postoperatively. However, the airway may be edematous, and if intubation before the procedure was difficult, it may be prudent to change the tube over a guide or perhaps even not change the tube at all. The surgeon may request that the double-lumen tube be changed to a single-lumen tube after the resection in order to perform bronchoscopy.

Postoperative Complications

Several life-threatening complications may occur after thoracic surgery, and individual outcome is related to the underlying condition of the patient, which may be further impaired by aging. Outcome is also related to the extent of surgery.

Cardiopulmonary complications include arrhythmias, which are more frequent after pneumonectomy. Factors predisposing to arrhythmias include sympathetic stimulation from pain, intraoperative cardiac manipulation, and a reduced vascular bed from the pulmonary resection.[50] Arrhythmias that frequently occur after pneumonectomy include atrial tachycardia, atrial flutter, and atrial fibrillation. Multifocal atrial tachycardia is common in patients with obstructive pulmonary disease and right-sided heart strain. The elderly in particular are prone to circulatory compromise from these arrhythmias.[51] Right-sided heart failure may present in the postoperative period from a reduction in the pulmonary vascular bed.

Other postoperative pulmonary complications include atelectasis, which may be related to intraoperative lung retraction and manipulation, impaired clearance of secretions, splinting from pain, or incomplete reexpansion of the remaining lung tissue after one-lung anesthesia. Atelectasis may lead to pneumonia, which can be fatal in the setting of the reduced lung tissue postthoracotomy.[50] The elderly patient is more likely to have limited pulmonary reserve and be more affected by a pneumonia. The removal of lung tissue, especially a right-sided pneumonectomy, puts the patient at risk for pulmonary edema because of a reduced vascular bed and increased pulmonary arterial pressures. Fluid is therefore more likely to move into the lung interstitium according to the Starling forces. Pulmonary embolism may occur in the postoperative period, possibly originating from the remaining pulmonary artery stump or tumor tissue. An elderly patient with limited cardiopulmonary reserve may require a longer period of postoperative ventilatory support than a younger person undergoing a similar procedure.

Potential structural complications requiring rapid surgical treatment include cardiac herniation, tension pneumothorax, and hemorrhage. Cardiac herniation is a rare but catastrophic complication. It may occur after pneumonectomy, in which the heart herniates through a pericardial defect. To help avoid this complication, *the patient should not be turned lateral, with the operative side dependent.*

A tension pneumothorax can occur, even if chest tubes are placed, if they are not functioning properly or become occluded. A pneumothorax created by the placement of a central venous catheter into the nonoperative side of the chest is particularly hazardous both intraoperatively and postoperatively, because this is the only lung to be ventilated during one-lung anesthesia, and takes on an even greater role after resection of the other lung.

Hemorrhage may be caused by slipped sutures or ligatures, bleeding from raw lung surfaces, or damaged bronchial or intercostal arteries. Postoperative neurologic complications may be related to the surgery or to positioning. Surgical injuries can affect the phrenic nerve, recurrent laryngeal nerve, and spinal cord. The lateral decubitus position can lead to damage to the brachial plexus, radial nerve, ulnar nerve, sciatic nerve, and common peroneal nerve.

A bronchopleural fistula may develop after pulmonary resection, either immediately or even years later.[52] It carries a mortality rate of >20%. It may result from dehiscence of the bronchial stump after lung resection. Treatment includes reduction of the air leak and prevention of infection. Surgical intervention may be required. Placement of a double-lumen endobronchial tube into the contralateral mainstem bronchus can allow exclusive contralateral ventilation and isolation of the contralateral lung. An alternative is the use of high-frequency jet ventilation, which allows ventilation with lower airway pressures.[32]

Postthoracotomy Pain Management

Thoracic surgery is often followed by pain and pulmonary dysfunction because of the thoracic incision. There is a decreased functional residual capacity and vital capacity, which in association with pain produces atelectasis, hypoxia, and CO_2 retention.[53] Traditionally, opioids have been administered intravenously or intramuscularly to treat postthoracotomy pain. The disadvantage of these methods is that administering an amount of opioid adequate to relieve pain is likely to cause sedation and respiratory depression. The elderly patient is more likely to have pulmonary dysfunction and decreased central nervous system activity and is even more likely to have postoperative impairment of pulmonary function.

Patient-controlled analgesia (PCA) is preferred over the intermittent administration of pain medications. A basal continuous delivery of medication can be programmed in addition to boluses. Patients have been reported to have less pain and sedation with PCA as compared with intramuscular opioids.[54,55] Patients who receive PCA after thoracotomy have been reported to require less pain medication and have a lower incidence of pulmonary complications.[56] PCA also allows patients to feel less dependent and helpless, and it is generally well accepted. The elderly patient is also more sensitive to the respiratory depressant effects of systemically administered opioids. It may be preferable to not use a basal infusion rate, but rather to use only demand dosing in the interest of safety.

Ketorolac, a nonsteroidal antiinflammatory agent, does not cause respiratory depression and therefore may be a useful adjunct in the elderly. Ketorolac should not be used if there has been significant bleeding because it inhibits platelet function and can lead to further bleeding.

Cryoanalgesia can be accomplished by the direct application of a cryoprobe intraoperatively by the surgeon to the intercostal nerves, which reduces but does not eliminate postthoracotomy pain; it is usually used together with other analgesic treatments. Disadvantages include prolonged anesthesia, possible permanent nerve trauma, and the loss of intercostal muscle tone.[57]

Spinal opioids administered into either the epidural or subarachnoid space provide excellent analgesia for patients after thoracotomy. Spinal opioids work by binding to opioid receptors in the substantia gelatinosa of the spinal cord. Intrathecal (subarachnoid) opioids can bind directly to the spinal cord, whereas those administered into the epidural space travel to the spinal cord by either passing through the dura[58] or by being absorbed into blood vessels that supply the spinal cord.[59] The analgesia provided by spinal opioids is attributable to the effect on the spinal cord, as opposed to a systemic effect.

The subarachnoid injection of morphine can produce analgesia with a much smaller dose ($10–15\mu g/kg$) than produced by the intravenous, intramuscular, or oral routes.[60,61] Patients are more comfortable postoperatively, and less sedated when given subarachnoid opioids.[62,63] If given before the surgical incision, subarachnoid opioids have been reported to decrease the intraoperative general anesthetic requirement.[64] This technique would limit the amount of opioids required for analgesia. The use of intrathecal morphine carries with it the risk of delayed respiratory depression. The rostral spread of intrathecal morphine is greater than that of other opioids that are lipophilic and therefore bind to spinal opioid receptors rapidly and are reabsorbed into blood vessels.

The placement of an epidural catheter allows for repeated doses and therefore provides a longer duration of analgesia than the "one-shot" injection of subarachnoid morphine. Epidural fentanyl has been administered as a continuous infusion to provide postoperative analgesia. If given through a lumbar epidural catheter, the fentanyl should be diluted to a volume of at least 20 mL so that the fentanyl can reach the thoracic levels of the spinal cord.[65,66] Patient-controlled epidural analgesia may allow for improved pain treatment, compared with intravenous PCA.[67,68] In a large series of patients, epidural analgesia resulted in less intravenous morphine usage.[69] This would be an important consideration in the elderly.

The intravenous administration of ketorolac may be helpful, even in the presence of an epidural, to treat shoulder pain that may occur from being in the lateral position for an extended period of time. Epidurally administered local anesthetic is not effective in treating shoulder pain of this origin.

In a recent review of 165 studies, which included almost 20,000 patients, the results of three methods of postoperative analgesia after major surgery were reported.[70] The three different routes of treatment studied were intramuscular, PCA, and epidural. The highest degree of oxygen hemoglobin desaturation was associated with intramuscular analgesia (37%). The incidence of respiratory depression, as reflected by usage of naloxone, was highest with intramuscular PCA (1.9%). Hypotension was most often associated with the epidural route (5.6%).

The technique of interpleural analgesia was first described in 1986.[71] The injection of local anesthetic between the visceral and parietal layers of pleura may either block multiple intercostal nerves or the thoracic sympathetic chain. For patients undergoing thoracotomy, the catheter can be placed through an epidural needle under direct vision while the chest is open. This method of placement can avoid the risk of pneumothorax and aberrant placement of the catheter when performed percutaneously.

The results of interpleural block for postoperative pain relief after thoracotomy have been mixed, ranging from poor[72,73] to excellent analgesia.[74–76] Chest tubes should not be placed on suction for approximately 15 minutes after the injection of local anesthetic, because this would lead to removal of local anesthetic and a decrease in analgesic effect of the block.[72] Systemic toxicity is more likely in the presence of pleural abnormality.[73] This technique may be an option when neuraxial analgesia is contraindicated. The elderly patient is more likely to have kyphoscoliosis, which may make placement of an epidural more difficult.

Videothoracoscopy

VAT is now being used for a variety of thoracic procedures, including pleural biopsy, lung biopsy and resection, closure of bronchopleural fistulas, pericardial biopsy, pleurodesis, and laser ablation of emphysematous bullae.[77–80] Even lobectomy can be performed by VAT. VAT uses small incisions to accommodate the video camera for on-screen visualization, and working instruments. This technique does not involve spreading of the ribs, and there is no need for the large incision that is required for open thoracotomy. There generally is less postoperative pain and respiratory impairment than after a conventional thoracotomy. Postthoracotomy pain can otherwise cause splinting and limit deep breathing, coughing, and clearing of secretions. There is a lower incidence of morbidity after thoracoscopy compared with thoracotomy. Thoracoscopy is better tolerated than thoracotomy by high-risk patients, which would include the elderly who have reduced cardiac and pulmonary function. Arrhythmias may still occur after VAT.[81] The use of epidural analgesia may help to reduce the incidence of arrhythmias.[81,82] Ketorolac may be a useful adjunct, especially if an epidural has not been placed.

A procedure such as diagnostic VAT and pleural biopsy can be performed under general anesthesia, thoracic epidural anesthesia, or intercostal block. For procedures in which there is a high likelihood that thoracoscopy may not be adequate and a conventional thoracotomy may be required, unless it is expected that the patient can be easily tracheally intubated in the lateral position, general anesthesia is the best option. A double- or single-lumen tube with a bronchial blocker is required during general anesthesia to provide adequate surgical exposure. Insufflation of gas is usually not needed for visualization under these conditions.

Videoscopic surgery, which carries a lower risk of morbidity and mortality, may be preferable in the elderly patient, who is at increased risk.[1] Patients undergoing either wedge resection or lobectomy for stage I lung cancer, which are tumors that have not spread to lymph nodes, have been reported to have similar 5-year survival rates.[83,84] Patients undergoing video-assisted lobectomies have been reported to have a lower incidence of complications than patients undergoing lobectomy with thoracotomy.[85] Although long-term survival may be a less important consideration for the elderly than short-term results and complications, the long-term survival after video-assisted lobectomy seems to be similar to lobectomy via thoracotomy. A limited resection in the elderly may be preferable, because of a possible reduction in risk, and an increased incidence of diagnosis of stage I tumors.[1] Age is a risk factor for mortality after thoracotomy; therefore, the increased usage of VAT is particularly advantageous in the elderly.[86]

Conclusion

The anesthesia considerations for the elderly patient undergoing the most frequently performed thoracic surgical procedures have been briefly reviewed. Optimum anesthesia care of the elderly patient undergoing thoracic surgery requires an understanding of the principles of anesthesia for thoracic surgery coupled with an appreciation of the changes associated with aging. Most lung cancers occur in people older than 65 years of age, and surgical treatment should not be withheld based on age alone.[1]

References

1. Jaklitsch MJ, Mery CM, Audisio RA. The use of surgery to treat lung cancer in elderly patients. Lancet 2003;4: 463–471.
2. Etzioni DA, Liu JH, O'Connell JB, Maggard MA, Ko CY. Elderly patients in surgical workloads: a population-based analysis. Am Surg 2003;69:901–905.
3. Hurria A, Kris MG. Management of lung cancer in older adults. CA Cancer J Clin 2003;53:325–341.
4. Cangemi V, Volpino P, D'Andrea N, et al. Lung cancer surgery in elderly patients. Tumori 1996;82:237–241.
5. Levi F, La Vecchia C, Lucchini F, Negri E. Worldwide trends in cancer mortality in the elderly, 1955–1992. Eur J Cancer 1996;32:652–672.
6. Smetana GW. Preoperative pulmonary assessment of the older adult. Clin Geriatr Med 2003;19:35–55.
7. Mery CM, Pappas AN, Lukanich JM, et al. Long-term survival of patients with early stage non-small cell lung cancer as a function of age and treatment modality. Chest 2001;120:176.
8. Damhuis RA, Schutte PR. Resection rates and perioperative mortality in 7899 patients with lung cancer. Eur Respir J 1996;9:7–10.
9. National Cancer Institute. SEER Cancer Statistics Review 1973–1997. Bethesda, MD: National Cancer Institute; 2000.
10. Hall SW. Cancer: special considerations in older patients. Geriatrics 1984;39:74–78.
11. Kohman, LJ, Meyer JA, Ilkins PM, Oates RP. Random versus predictable risks of mortality after thoracotomy for lung cancer. Thorac Cardiovasc Surg 1986;91:551–554.
12. Mizushima Y, Noto H, Sugiyama S, et al. Survival and prognosis after pneumonectomy in the elderly. Ann Thorac Surg 1997;64:193–198.
13. Osaki T, Shirakura T, Kodte M, et al. Surgical treatment of lung cancer in the octogenarian. Ann Thorac Surg 1994; 57:188–193.
14. Jaklitsch MT, DeCamp MM Jr, Liptay MJ, et al. Video assisted thoracic surgery in the elderly: a review of 307 cases. Chest 1996;110:751–758.
15. Gerson MC, Hurst JM, Hertzberg VS, Baughman R, Rouan GS, Ellis K. Prediction of cardiac and pulmonary complications related to elective abdominal and non-cardiac thoracic surgery in geriatric patients. Am J Med 1990;88:101–107.
16. Liu LL, Leung JM. Predicting adverse postoperative outcomes in patients aged 80 years or older. J Am Geriatr Soc 2000;48:405–412.
17. Castillo R, Haas A. Chest physical therapy: comparative efficacy of preoperative and postoperative in the elderly. Arch Phys Med Rehabil 1985;66:376–379.
18. Warner DO. Preventing postoperative pulmonary complications. Anesthesiology 2000;92:1467–1471.
19. Gerson MC, Hurst JM, Hertzber VS, et al. Cardiac prognosis in non-cardiac geriatric surgery. Ann Intern Med 1985; 103:832–837.
20. Shore ET, Millman RD, Silage DA, et al. Ventilatory and arousal patterns during sleep in normal young and elderly subjects. J Appl Physiol 1985;59:1607.
21. Rossi A, Ganassini A, Tantucci C, Grassi V. Aging and the respiratory system. Aging (Milano) 1996;8:143–161.
22. Ganguly R, Craig CP, Waldman RH. Respiratory tract immunity in the aged. Z Erkr Atmungsorgane 1984;163: 112–120.
23. Van Dewater JM. Preoperative and postoperative techniques in the prevention of pulmonary complications. Surg Clin North Am 1980;60:1339–1348.
24. Naunheim KS, Kesler KA, D'Orazio SA, et al. Lung cancer surgery in the octogenarian. Eur J Cardiothorac Surg 1994; 8:453–456.
25. Slinger P, Johnston MR. Preoperative assessment for pulmonary function. J Cardiothorac Vasc Anesth 2000;14: 202–211.
26. Ploeg AJ, Kappefeim P, van Tangeren, et al. Factors associated with perioperative complications and long-term results after pulmonary resection for primary carcinoma of the lung. Eur J Cardiothorac Surg 2003;23:26–29.
27. Bernard L, Ferrand O, Benoit L. Identification of prognostic factors determining risk groups for lung resection. Ann Thorac Surg 2000;70:1161–1167.
28. Nakahara K, Ohno K, Hashimoto J, et al. Prediction of postoperative respiratory failure in patients undergoing lung resection for cancer. Ann Thorac Surg 1988;46:549–552.
29. Ferguson MK, Reeder LB, Mick R. Optimizing selection of patients for major lung resection. J Thorac Cardiovasc Surg 1995;109:275–283.
30. Walsh GL, Morice RC, Putnam JB, et al. Resection of lung cancer is justified in high risk patients selected by oxygen consumption. Ann Thorac Surg 1994;58:704.
31. Bollinger CT, Wyser C, Roser H, et al. Lung scanning and exercise testing for the prediction of postoperative performance in lung resection candidates at increased risk for complications. Chest 1995;108:341–348.
32. Eisenkraft JB, Neustein SM. Anesthesia for special problems in thoracic surgery. Probl Anesth 1990;4:326–354.
33. Frumin MJ, Epstein R, Cohen G. Apneic oxygenation in man. Anesthesiology 1959;20:789.
34. Sanders RD. Two ventilating attachments for bronchoscopes. Del Med J 1967;39:1270.
35. Vourc'h G, Fishler M, Michon F, et al. Manual jet ventilation vs. high frequency jet ventilation during laser resection of tracheobronchial stenosis. Br J Anaesth 1983;55:973.
36. Carlens E. Mediastinoscopy: a method for inspection and tissue biopsy stenosis. Br J Anaesth 1983;55:973.

37. Morton JR, Guinn GA. Mediastinoscopy using local anesthesia. Am J Surg 1971;122:696.
38. Roberts JT, Gissen AJ. Management of complications encountered during anesthesia for mediastinoscopy. Anesthesiol Rev 1979;6:31.
39. Lee J, Salvatore AJ. Innominate artery compression simulating cardiac arrest during mediastinoscopy. Anesth Analg 1976;55:748.
40. Ashbaugh DG. Mediastinoscopy. Arch Surg 1970;100:568.
41. Morandi U, Stefani A, Golinelli M, et al. Results of surgical resection in patients over the age of 70 years with non small-cell lung cancer. Eur J Cardiothorac Surg 1997;11:432–439.
42. Krowke MJ, Pairolero PC, Trustek F, Payne WS, Bernatz PE. Cardiac dysrhythmia following pneumonectomy: clinical correlates and prognostic significance. Chest 1987;91:490–495.
43. Burman SO. The prophylactic use of digitalis before thoracotomy. Ann Thorac Surg 1972;14:359–368.
44. Shields TW, Unik GT. Digitalization for prevention of arrhythmias following pulmonary surgery. Surg Gynecol Obstet 1968;126:743–746.
45. Ritchie AJ, Bowe P, Gibbons JRP. Prophylactic digitalization for thoracotomy: a reassessment. Ann Thorac Surg 1990;50:86–88.
46. Jakobsen CJ, Billie S, Ahlburg P. Perioperative metoprolol reduces the frequency of atrial fibrillation after thoracotomy for lung resection. J Cardiothorac Vasc Anesth 1997;11:746–751.
47. Neustein SM, Cohen E, Reich D, et al. Transesophageal echocardiography and the intraoperative diagnosis of left atrial invasion by carcinoid tumor. Can J Anaesth 1993;40:664–666.
48. Licker M, de Perrot M, Spiliopoulos A. Risk factor for acute lung injury after thoracic surgery for lung cancer. Anesth Analg 2003;97:1558–1565.
49. Eisenkraft JB. Effects of anaesthetics on the pulmonary circulation. Br J Anaesth 1990;65:63–78.
50. Gallagher C, Sladen RN, Lubarsky D. Thoracotomy. Postoperative complications. Probl Anesth 1990;4:393–415.
51. Breyer RH, Sippe C, Pharr WF, et al. Thoracotomy in patients over age seventy years: ten year experience. J Thorac Cardiovasc Surg 1981;81:187.
52. Hankins JR, Miller JE, Atlar S, et al. Bronchopleural fistula: thirteen-year experience with 77 cases. J Thorac Cardiovasc Surg 1978;76:755–762.
53. Craig DB. Postoperative recovery of pulmonary function. Anesth Analg 1981;60:46–52.
54. Bennett RL, Battenhorst RL, Graves D, et al. Patient-controlled analgesia—a new concept of postoperative relief. Ann Surg 1982;195:700–705.
55. Bennett RL, Baumann TJ, Graves DA, Griffen WD Jr. Patient controlled analgesia and analgesic outcome, nocturnal sleep, and spontaneous activity. Surg Forum 1987;35:57–59.
56. Lange MP, Dahn MS, Jacobs LA. Patient-controlled analgesia versus intermittent analgesia dosing. Heart Lung 1988;17:495–498.
57. Maiwand O, Makey AR, Rees A. Cryoanalgesia after thoracotomy. Improvement of technique and review of 600 cases. J Thorac Cardiovasc Surg 1986;92:291–295.
58. Nordberg G, Hedner T, Mellstrand T, et al. Pharmacokinetic aspect of epidural morphine analgesia. Anesthesiology 1983;58:545–551.
59. Cousins MJ, Mather LE. Intrathecal and epidural administration of opioids. Anesthesiology 1984;61:276–310.
60. Gray JR, Fromme GA, Nauss LA, Wang JK, Istrup DM. Intrathecal morphine for post-thoracotomy pain. Anesth Analg 1986;65:873–876.
61. Kotob HIM, Hand CV, Moore RA, et al. Intrathecal morphine and heroin in humans: six-hour drug levels in spinal fluid and plasma. Anesth Analg 1986;65:718–722.
62. Shulman M, Sandler AN, Bradley JW, Young PS, Brobrer J. Post-thoracotomy pain and pulmonary function following epidural and systemic morphine. Anesthesiology 1984;61:509–575.
63. Samii J, Chavim M, Viars P. Postoperative spinal analgesia with morphine. Br J Anaesth 1981;53:817–820.
64. Neustein SM, Cohen E. Intrathecal morphine during thoracotomy. Part II. Effect on postoperative meperidine requirements and pulmonary function tests. J Cardiothorac Vasc Anesth 1993;7:157–159.
65. Whiting WG, Sandler AN, Lau LC, Chovaz PM. Analgesic and respiratory effects of epidural sufentanil in post-thoracotomy patients. Anesthesiology 1988;609:36–42.
66. Melendez J, Cirella VN, Delphin ES. Lumbar epidural fentanyl analgesia after thoracic surgery. J Cardiothorac Anesth 1989;3:150–153.
67. Mann C, Pouzeratte J, Eledjam JJ. Postoperative patient-controlled analgesia in the elderly: risks and benefits of epidural versus intravenous administration. Drugs Aging 2003;20:337–345.
68. Alon E, Jaquenod M, Schaepp B. Post-operative epidural versus intravenous patient-controlled analgesia. Minerva Anestesiol 2003;69:473–476.
69. Flisberg P, Rudin A, Linne R, et al. Pain relief and safety after major surgery. A prospective study of epidural and intravenous analgesia in 2696 patients. Acta Anaesthesiol Scand 2003;47:457–465.
70. Cashman JN, Dolin SJ. Respiratory and hemodynamic effects of acute postoperative pain management: evidence from published data. Br J Anaesth 2004;93:212–223.
71. Reiestad F, Stromskag KE. Interpleural catheter in the management of postoperative pain: a preliminary report. Reg Anaesth 1986;11:89–91.
72. el-Baz N, Faber LP, Ivankovic AD, et al. Intrapleural infusion of local anesthetic: a word of caution. Anesthesiology 1988;68:809–810.
73. Rosenberg PH, Scheinin BWA, Lepantalo MJ, et al. Continuous intrapleural infusion of bupivacaine for analgesia after thoracotomy. Anesthesiology 1987;67:811–813.
74. Reddy Kanbam J, Hammon J, Parris WC, et al. Intrapleural analgesia for postthoracotomy pain and blood levels of bupivacaine following intrapleural injection. Can J Anaesth 1989;36:106–109.
75. Symreng T, Gomez MN, Rossi N. Intrapleural bupivacaine and saline after thoracotomy: effects on pain and lung function—a double blind study. J Cardiothorac Anaesth 1989;3:144–149.
76. Tetik O, Islamoglu F, Ayan E, et al. Intermittent infusion of 0.25% bupivacaine through an intrapleural catheter for

post-thoracotomy pain relief. Ann Thorac Surg 2004;77: 284–288.

77. Hasnin JU, Krasna MJ, Barker SJ, Weiman DS, Whitman GJR. Anesthetic consideration for thoracoscopic procedures. J Cardiothorac Vasc Anesth 1992;6:624–627.

78. Wakabayashi A. Thoracoscopic ablation of blebs in the treatment of recurrent or persistent spontaneous pneumothorax. Ann Thorac Surg 1989;48:651–653.

79. Torre M, Belloni P. Nd:YAG laser pleurodesis through thoracoscopy: new curative therapy in spontaneous pneumothorax. Ann Thorac Surg 1989;47:887–889.

80. Barker SJ, Clarke C, Hyatt J, Le N, Bhakta C. Thoracoscopic laser ablation of bullous emphysema: an anesthetic case study. Anesth Analg 1991;72:S11.

81. Neustein SM, Kahn P, Krellenstein D, et al. Incidence of arrhythmias after thoracic surgery: thoracotomy vs video-assist thoracoscopy. J Cardiothorac Vasc Anesth 1998;12:659–661.

82. Oka T, Ozawa Y, Ohkubo Y. Thoracic epidural bupivacaine attenuates supraventricular tachyarrhythmias after pulmonary resection. Anesth Analg 2001;93:253–259.

83. Faulkner SI. Is lobectomy the gold standard for stage I lung cancer in year 2000? Chest 2000;118:119S.

84. Swanson SJ, Bueno R, Jaklitsch MT, et al. Subcentimeter non-small cell lung cancer: a program for detection and resection is warranted. Proceedings of the 80th Annual Meeting of the American Association of Thoracic Surgery, Toronto, Canada; 2000:70.

85. Roberts JR, DeCamp MM, Mentzer SJ, Sugarbaker DJ. Prospective comparison of open and video assisted lobectomy. Chest 1996;110:45S.

86. Jaklitsch MT, Pappas-Estocin A, Bueno R. Thoracoscopic surgery in elderly lung patients. Crit Rev Oncol Hematol 2004;49:165–171.

27
Cardiac Procedures

James H. Abernathy III

Our population, both nationally and worldwide, is getting increasingly older. The proportion of people aged 65 and older in the United States is projected to increase from 35 million (12.4%) to 71 million (19.6%) by 2030 and 82 million by 2050.[1] Global trends are similar: people aged 65 and older are expected to make up 12% of the population by 2030 and 20% of the population by 2050. Considering that older patients have invasive procedures at almost four times the frequency of people younger than 65, this will significantly affect our health care system.[2] Because there are a greater number of older patients, surgery for cardiovascular disease is increasing. Compounding this, patients are increasingly presenting at an older age and later in their disease processes. For instance, in 1983, 12% of coronary artery bypass graft (CABG) patients were older than 65 years of age. Just 10 years later, half the patients undergoing CABG were older than 65 years of age.[3] Today, the average age of CABG surgery patients is 66 years of age.[4] For cardiac surgery, the 30-day mortality is estimated to increase by a factor of 1.55 per decade of age, compared with noncardiac surgery at 1.35 per decade of age.[5] However, despite the increasing age of our patients and the increased risk of morbidity and mortality as the patient population has aged, operative mortality from cardiac surgery has not substantially increased. The reasons for this are multifactorial including improved surgical techniques, dedicated cardiac anesthesiologists, better cardiopulmonary bypass (CPB) machines, improved pharmacologic interventions, and better anesthesia techniques and technology such as transesophageal echocardiography and epiaortic ultrasound.

This chapter concentrates on the surgical interventions for elderly patients with heart disease. Surgical frequency, morbidity, and mortality between the aged population and younger patients are explored. In addition, strategies for preventing adverse outcomes in this unique patient cohort are presented.

The Society of Thoracic Surgeons (STS) Cardiac Surgery Database was initiated in 1986 with the goal of providing risk-adjusted outcomes compared with the national experience. The data set contains detailed clinical information on more than 1.5 million registered patients undergoing cardiac surgical procedures from 541 academic, private, military, and Veterans Affairs hospitals from 48 of the United States and Canada. It is the single best place to investigate risk factors and outcomes of cardiac operations. Most of what has been published regarding age and cardiac surgery revolves around multiple series from single institutions.[6-12] We focus mostly on those few studies that have utilized large databases such as the STS database.

Coronary Artery Disease

Coronary artery disease (CAD) continues to be a major contributor to mortality in the elderly. An even larger proportion of the elderly population experiences morbidity from their CAD. Approximately 40% of Americans will reach the age of 80 and, of these, 40% will have symptomatic heart disease.[13] Eighty-three percent of all cardiovascular deaths occur in patients older than 65 years of age.[14] As the population ages, it is not surprising, therefore, that the median age of coronary artery bypass grafting has steadily increased to 66 years of age. Despite this increase in age at operation, there has been a significant decline in overall operative mortality and risk-adjusted mortality for CABG patients[15] (Figure 27-1).

Anesthesiologists and surgeons are faced with caring for older and sicker patients to palliate CAD. As previously discussed in this book, elderly patients present with multiple organ system disease resulting in less physiologic reserve than their younger counterparts. They are more likely to have hypertension, diabetes mellitus, cerebral

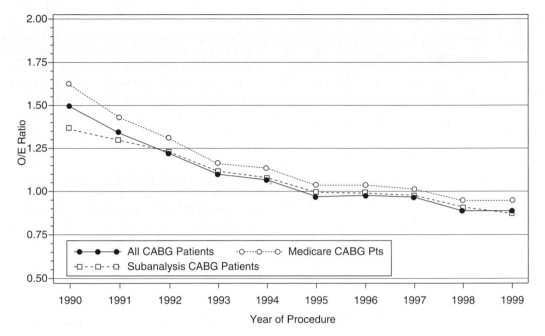

FIGURE 27-1. Observed mortality to expected mortality ratio (O/E), 1990–1999. CABG = coronary artery bypass graft. (Reprinted with permission from Ferguson et al.[15] Copyright © 2002. With permission of The Society of Thoracic Surgeons.)

and peripheral vascular disease. Elderly patients presenting for coronary revascularization are more likely to be women, in New York Heart Association (NYHA) heart failure class IV, and have left main CAD.[16] Interestingly, in reviewing the STS database of more than 1 million patients, Ferguson et al.[15] found that, when compared with younger patients, fewer elderly patients are undergoing reoperative CABG, likely reflecting patient selection.

Examining the extremes of the elderly population, Bridges et al.[17] investigated 575,389 nonagenarians and centenarians undergoing CABG. Patients older than 90 years of age were more likely to be women, undergo urgent or emergent operations, have left main disease, unstable angina, and preoperative renal failure, and be in NYHA class IV. The overall operative mortality for these patients was 11% compared with 2.8% for those younger than 80 years of age. The multivariate analysis for operative mortality showed an increased risk for emergent or salvage operation [odds ratio (OR) 2.26], preoperative intraaortic balloon pump (IABP) (OR 2.79), perioperative renal failure (OR 2.08), defined as creatinine >2.0 and also more than twice the baseline value or a new requirement for dialysis, peripheral or cerebral vascular disease (OR 1.39), and mitral insufficiency (OR 1.50). This trend was evident in morbidity measures as well as with patients older than 90 having an increased risk of perioperative stroke (2.9%), renal failure (9.2%), prolonged ventilation (12.2%), and postoperative length of stay (median 7 days).[17] In this population, if the patient did not have the

preoperative risk factors of emergent operation, IABP, renal failure, peripheral vascular disease, or cerebral vascular disease, their operative mortality was only 7.2%. Surprisingly, this subpopulation accounted for 57% of the nonagenarians and centenarians undergoing CABG.

Valvular Heart Disease

As we age, the fibromuscular skeleton of the heart changes, including myxomatous degeneration and collagen infiltration, termed sclerosis. Aortic valve sclerosis is estimated to occur in 30% of elderly persons. Other age-related changes include calcium deposition on the leaflets of the aortic valve, base of the semilunar cusps, and the mitral annulus. Fibrosis with valve calcification is the most common etiology of valvular stenosis in the elderly. Valvular regurgitation often occurs as a result of ischemia or hypertensive disease, especially at the mitral valve.[18] The age of the patient presenting for a valve operation is ever increasing (Figure 27-2).

Aortic Valve

Aortic stenosis in patients older than 65 years of age is estimated to be 2% for severe stenosis, 5% for moderate stenosis, and 9% for mild stenosis.[18,19] Consequences of aortic stenosis, left ventricular hypertrophy, decreased left ventricular compliance, and decreased stroke volume are independent of etiology. The same process that causes

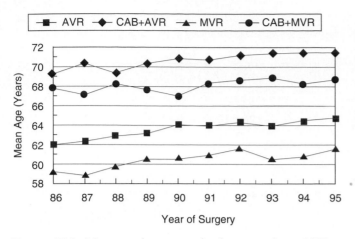

FIGURE 27-2. Mean age by year and valve procedure. AVR = aortic valve replacement, CAB = coronary artery bypass, MVR = mitral valve replacement. (Reprinted with permission from Jamieson et al.[21] Copyright © 1999. With permission of The Society of Thoracic Surgeons.)

sclerosis of the aortic valve seems to also affect the coronaries and helps to explain the association between aortic valve disease and CAD.

Aortic regurgitation also occurs with increasing frequency in the elderly. In one study, 13% of those older than 80 had mild aortic regurgitation, and 16% had either moderate or severe regurgitation. Patients with heart failure and pulmonary congestion from acute aortic regurgitation have a 50%–80% mortality.[20]

Morbidity and mortality data for elderly patients undergoing aortic valve replacement (AVR) has mostly come from small, single institution case series. The mortality rates have been quoted from 5% to 10%, depending on comorbidities. Using the STS database, Jamieson et al.[21] better quantified the operative mortality risk for patients undergoing valve replacements with or without CABG. Table 27-1 delineates the increased risk of mortality with increasing age. The operative risk for AVR almost doubles with every decade over 60 years of age. Independent predictors of mortality have been consistently shown to include age, emergent procedures, advanced NYHA class, and renal failure. However, in the STS analysis by Jamieson et al.,[21] age was not an independent risk factor. Those of statistical significance included salvage status (OR 7.12), perioperative renal failure (OR 4.32), emergent case (OR 3.46), reoperation (OR 2.27), cardiogenic shock (OR 1.67), NYHA class IV (OR 1.56), prior cerebrovascular accident (OR 1.44), previous myocardial infarction (OR 1.36), female gender (OR 1.25), and diabetes mellitus (OR 1.23).

Chiappini et al.[22] retrospectively studied 115 patients with a mean age of 82 years who underwent AVR alone or in combination with CABG. The most common presenting symptoms were dyspnea in 99%, congestive heart failure in 15%, and angina in 77%. As expected in an extreme elderly population presenting for heart surgery, 20% had an ejection fraction lower than 50%, 44% had significant CAD, and 78% presented in NYHA class III

TABLE 27-1. Operative mortality rate by age group and valve position and population size (1986–1995, The Society of Thoracic Surgeons database).

Procedure	Age (years)				
	50–59	60–69	70–79	80–89	90–99
AVR					
Mortality rate (%)	2.9	3.2	5.3	8.5	14.5
Population	3,686	7,001	8,468	2,756	69
AVR + CABG					
Mortality rate (%)	4.7	5.1	8.6	12.5	18.8
Population	1,709	6,120	10,617	3,717	64
MVR					
Mortality rate (%)	4.1	6.1	9.8	13.4	25
Population	2,815	4,062	3,576	621	4
MVR + CABG					
Mortality rate (%)	8.6	12.3	18.4	25.1	42.9
Population	1,050	2,889	3,782	730	7
Multiple valves					
Mortality rate (%)	5.5	9.9	15.7	23.7	0
Population	803	998	854	177	2
Multiple + CABG					
Mortality rate (%)	10.3	16.5	21.4	26.6	100
Population	155	430	612	154	2

Source: Adapted with permission from Jamieson et al.[21] Copyright © 1999, with permission from The Society of Thoracic Surgeons.
AVR = aortic valve replacement, CABG = coronary artery bypass graft, MVR = mitral valve replacement.

or greater. The 30-day mortality rate was 8.5% with an actuarial survival rate of 86.4% at 1 year and 69% at 5 years. There was no statistically significant difference in the death rate, either in hospital or out of hospital, between AVR or AVR-CABG groups. Logistical regression analysis revealed that reduced preoperative ejection fraction, perioperative heart failure, and type of implanted device were predictors of late death. Those patients who received a bioprosthetic valve did much better than those who received a mechanical or stentless valve. Having a patient survive an operation is not the only endpoint worth discussing. The elderly have to do better in life post-repair than before. In this patient population, 98% of survivors were satisfied with their choice. There was a statistically significant improvement in NYHA class, 2.9 ± 0.6 versus 1.6 ± 0.6, p < 0.01.[22]

Mitral Valve

The aging process has a similar effect on the mitral valve as it does on the aortic valve. These same factors also predispose patients to worse outcomes after mitral valve surgery. Left ventricular diastolic function, decreased systemic vascular compliance, increased left ventricular mass index, and altered neurohormonal and autonomic influ-ences have been attributed to adverse outcomes in those undergoing mitral valve repair.

Mehta et al.[23] analyzed data on all patients undergoing mitral valve replacements, either alone or in combination with CABG or tricuspid valve operation between January 1997 to December 2000 who were enrolled in the STS database. Of the 262,718 patients in the database, 31,688 met the criteria. Mitral valve replacement represents the only cardiac operation done more frequently in those patients who are older than 70 years of age than in any other age group. The elderly patients (>60 years of age) were more likely to undergo an urgent operation, have a concomitant CABG, and need the assistance of an IABP. Pump times and cross-clamp times were similar across all age groups.

All in-hospital adverse events increased with advancing age including stroke, prolonged ventilation, reoperation for bleeding, renal failure, atrial fibrillation, and mortality. Multivariate models show that the risk of operative mortality increases with age, even after adjusting for other variables (Figure 27-3). Sadly, this indicates that a vigorous 80 year old has increased risk of mortality independent of other comorbidities. Using their multiple regression model, Mehta et al. proposed a classification tree for those older than 75 years of age contemplating mitral valve replacement (shown in Figure 27-4).

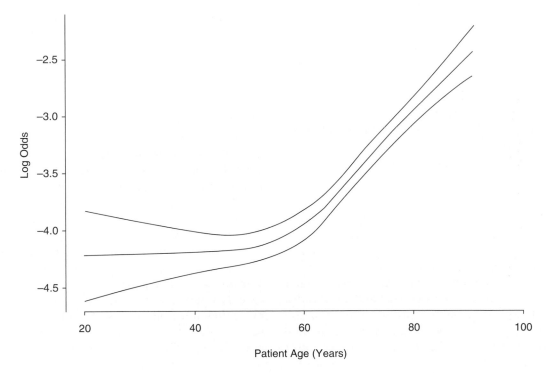

FIGURE 27-3. Plot of log odds of operative mortality for mitral valve replacement versus age, after adjusting for other risk factors. (Reprinted with permission from Mehta et al.[23] Copyright © 2002. With permission from The Society of Thoracic Surgeons.)

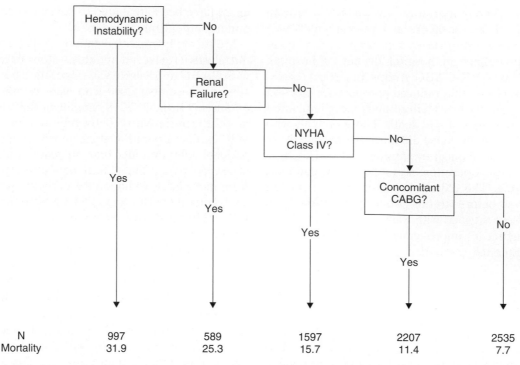

FIGURE 27-4. Risk classification tree for elderly patients (>75 years) undergoing mitral valve replacement. NYHA = New York Heart Association, CABG = coronary artery bypass graft.

(Reprinted with permission from Mehta et al.[23] Copyright © 2002. With permission of The Society of Thoracic Surgeons.)

Preventing Adverse Outcomes

Despite the existence of an increase in both morbidity and mortality for elderly patients undergoing cardiac surgery, relatively little is known about how to prevent it. Improvements in anesthesia techniques, medications, surgical techniques, and perfusion practices have improved cardiac surgical outcomes despite a population of advancing age. What little is known is covered in the following section.

Cardiovascular

Atrial fibrillation is a morbid event occurring in up to 30% of elderly patients after cardiac surgery. Because of the elderly's lower physiologic reserve, it is imperative to avoid beta-blocker and statin withdrawal, two offenders in postoperative atrial fibrillation. Additionally, their peripheral vascular system is more calcified and less distendable than younger patients. This increases their risk of aortic dissection and embolization with cannulation and initiation of CPB. Severe aortic disease or lower extremity vascular disease may increase the risk associated with IABP. Furthermore, poor coronary vasculature may predispose patients to incomplete revascularization and further ischemia after CPB. Ferguson et al.[24] demon-

strated that the internal mammary artery was underutilized in elderly patients (77% for elderly versus 93% for younger). Those elderly patients who received an internal mammary artery bypass had a lower operative and postoperative mortality, even after controlling for other causative factors.

Central Nervous System/Neurologic

Neurologic injury remains one of the largest sources of morbidity and mortality after cardiac surgery. Its risk clearly increases with age, with quoted stroke risks ranging from 1% to 30% depending on age and operation. Figure 27-5 demonstrates the increased risk of neurologic insult with increasing age. Roach et al.[25] studied adverse cerebral outcomes after CABG surgery in 2108 patients. Type I injuries were defined as death attributable to stroke or hypoxic encephalopathy, nonfatal stroke, transient ischemic attack, or stupor or coma at the time of discharge. Type II injuries were defined as new deterioration in intellectual function, confusion, agitation, disorientation, memory deficit, or seizure without evidence of focal injury. The predominant predictor of both type I and II injury was age: 6.1% of patients who were older than 70 experienced a type I injury, and 5.8% experienced a type II compared with 1.9% and 1.8%, respectively, for those patients younger than 70 years of age.[25]

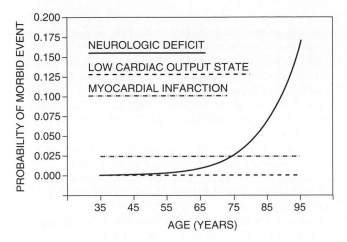

FIGURE 27-5. Probability of incurring a morbid event during the perioperative cardiac surgical period and its association with age. Neurologic deficits increase dramatically beginning at age 65, whereas low cardiac output state and myocardial infarction remain relatively stable. (Reprinted with permission from Tuman KJ, McCarthy RJ, Najafi H, Ivankovich AD. Differential effects of advanced age on neurologic and cardiac risks of coronary artery operations. J Thorac Cardiovasc Surg 1992;104(6):1510–1517. Copyright © 1992. With permission of the American Association for Thoracic Surgery.)

Suggested mechanisms of cerebral injury include global hypoperfusion, focal occlusion of the cerebral vasculature, or thermal injury on rewarming. It seems that, despite reductions in cerebral blood flow during CPB in the elderly, there is a concomitant reduction in cerebral metabolic rate of oxygen consumption keeping the difference in arterial-venous oxygen content normal.[26] Embolic phenomena have been blamed as the most likely culprit in central nervous system damage in the elderly. It is for this reason that combined carotid endarterectomy and CABG in the elderly remains a debated topic. Detecting ascending aortic atheroma either by surgical palpation or epiaortic ultrasound has been shown to reduce embolic events and improve post-bypass cerebral outcomes.[27,28] pH management by either alpha-stat or pH-stat and the association with cerebral outcomes has been vigorously studied. pH stat, through increased CO_2, is associated with increased cerebral blood flow, but alpha-stat preserves cerebral autoregulation[29] (also J.P. Mathew et al., in press, Anesthesiology). Because most neurologic injuries are secondary to embolic phenomena, more cerebral blood flow may be detrimental. One prospective, randomized trial failed to show a difference between alpha-stat and pH-stat management in adult patients.[30] Based on preserving autoregulation, alpha-stat blood gas management would be recommended in the elderly. No intervention, however, has been studied in a population exclusive to those aged more than 65.

Renal

The prevalence of renal failure after cardiac operation varies from 2% to 15%, depending on the procedure and degree of preoperative renal dysfunction.[23] If it occurs, the mortality rate may be as high as 80%. Because the elderly have lower baseline glomerular filtration rate, are likely to have hypertension and an altered renal autoregulatory curve, and are more likely to have diabetes mellitus, they are at a higher risk of renal failure than their younger counterparts. The use of preoperative diuretics for those with depressed ejection fraction and radiopaque dyes often worsens preoperative renal function. Unfortunately, there has been no large investigation regarding the prevention of renal dysfunction in the elderly patient undergoing CPB. Mannitol as a scavenger of oxygen free-radicals and Lasix are often used but have not been specifically studied in the elderly population. The most important principle might be that recovery of renal function after bypass is directly related to the recovery of cardiac function.

Cardiopulmonary Bypass Management

CPB provides many alterations to the normal physiologic milieu. The optimal mean arterial pressure, perfusion flow, mode of perfusion (pulsatile versus nonpulsatile), pH and CO_2 management, temperature, and hematocrit have not been established for the elderly patient undergoing CPB. As previously mentioned, aortic cannula sites should be carefully chosen with the assistance of epiaortic ultrasound scanning to minimize embolized atheromatous debris. Perfusion flows range from 1.2 to 2.4 L/min/m², with perfusion pressures varying from 30 to 80 mm Hg. No difference in outcomes has been demonstrated for flows within this range or for pulsatile versus nonpulsatile flows. The appropriate temperature management (normothermia versus hypothermia) for the elderly patient has not been studied.

The optimum hematocrit while on CPB and immediately after for the elderly patient has not been determined. The absolute safe level will depend on many variables, including adequacy of myocardial revascularization, myocardial function, and, possibly, the age of the patient. The adequacy of tissue oxygenation and perfusion as determined by the mixed venous oxygen saturation determines transfusion in most centers. Blood-sparing strategies such as cell salvage techniques and retrograde autologous prime should routinely be used to conserve hematocrit and decrease the need for transfusion. The elderly might be a group for whom a higher hematocrit is beneficial; however, transfusion delivers new risks, most of which are related to the inflammatory response. Increased sternal wound infection, longer intensive care unit stays, and increased renal failure associated with blood transfusion should be weighed against evidence of poor tissue oxygen delivery.

With admittedly little scientific evidence to support their assertions, some authors empirically recommend the following: (1) alpha-stat blood gas management, (2) higher perfusion pressures throughout the perioperative period, (3) higher mean arterial pressures while on CPB, (4) higher hematocrit before termination of CPB (>24%), (5) mild hypothermia (32°C) during CPB, and (6) careful selection of the aortic cannulation site with the assistance of epiaortic ultrasound scanning.[31]

Conclusion

We have demonstrated over the past several decades that, with continued focus on improving outcomes in cardiac surgery, we can be successful. Cardiac surgical patients are older, but their overall outcomes have improved. As our population ages, so too will our patients, and we will continue to push the envelope. Despite our successes, however, there are many unanswered questions. With continued vigilance, one day our recommendations will be more than empiric: they will be well-proven scientific assertions.

References

1. Centers for Disease Control and Prevention. Trends in aging—United States and worldwide. MMWR Morb Mortal Wkly Rep 2003;52(6):101.
2. Lichtor J. Sponsored research reveals postoperative mortality stats. Anesth Patient Safety Found Newslett 1988;3:9–11.
3. Gersh BJ, Kronmal RA, Schaff HV, et al. Long-term (5 year) results of coronary bypass surgery in patients 65 years old or older: a report from the Coronary Artery Surgery Study. Circulation 1983;68(3 Pt 2):II190–199.
4. Acinapura AJ, Jacobowitz IJ, Kramer MD, Adkins MS, Zisbrod Z, Cunningham JN Jr. Demographic changes in coronary artery bypass surgery and its effect on mortality and morbidity. Eur J Cardiothorac Surg 1990;4(4):175–181.
5. Khuri SF, Daley J, Henderson W, et al. Risk adjustment of the postoperative mortality rate for the comparative assessment of the quality of surgical care: results of the National Veterans Affairs Surgical Risk Study. J Am Coll Surg 1997;185(4):315–327.
6. Utley JR, Leyland SA. Coronary artery bypass grafting in the octogenarian. J Thorac Cardiovasc Surg 1991;101(5):866–870.
7. Edmunds LH Jr, Stephenson LW, Edie RN, Ratcliffe MB. Open-heart surgery in octogenarians. N Engl J Med 1988;319(3):131–136.
8. Samuels LE, Sharma S, Morris RJ, et al. Cardiac surgery in nonagenarians. J Card Surg 1996;11(2):121–127.
9. Akins CW, Daggett WM, Vlahakes GJ, et al. Cardiac operations in patients 80 years old and older. Ann Thorac Surg 1997;64(3):606–614; discussion 614–615.
10. Avery GJ 2nd, Ley SJ, Hill JD, Hershon JJ, Dick SE. Cardiac surgery in the octogenarian: evaluation of risk, cost, and outcome. Ann Thorac Surg 2001;71(2):591–596.
11. Sundt TM, Bailey MS, Moon MR, et al. Quality of life after aortic valve replacement at the age of >80 years. Circulation 2000;102(19 Suppl 3):III70–74.
12. Fiore AC, Naunheim KS, Barner HB, et al. Valve replacement in the octogenarian. Ann Thorac Surg 1989;48(1):104–108.
13. National health interview survey 1983–1985. Hyattsville, MD: National Center for Health Statistics; 1986.
14. National Center for Health Statistics: Advance report of final mortality statistics, 1988. Monthly Vital Stat Rep 1990;39(7 Suppl):1–48.
15. Ferguson TB Jr, Hammill BG, Peterson ED, DeLong ER, Grover FL. A decade of change—risk profiles and outcomes for isolated coronary artery bypass grafting procedures, 1990–1999: a report from the STS National Database Committee and the Duke Clinical Research Institute. Society of Thoracic Surgeons. Ann Thorac Surg 2002;73(2):480–489; discussion 489–490.
16. Khan SS, Kupfer JM, Matloff JM, Tsai TP, Nessim S. Interaction of age and preoperative risk factors in predicting operative mortality for coronary bypass surgery. Circulation 1992;86(5 Suppl):II186–190.
17. Bridges CR, Edwards FH, Peterson ED, Coombs LP, Ferguson TB. Cardiac surgery in nonagenarians and centenarians. J Am Coll Surg 2003;197(3):347–356; discussion 356–357.
18. Otto CM, Lind BK, Kitzman DW, Gersh BJ, Siscovick DS. Association of aortic-valve sclerosis with cardiovascular mortality and morbidity in the elderly. N Engl J Med 1999;341(3):142–147.
19. Zipes D, Libby P, Bonow R, Braunwald E. Braunwald's Heart Disease: A Textbook of Cardiovascular Medicine. 7th ed. Philadelphia: Saunders; 2005.
20. Aronow WS, Ahn C, Kronzon I. Comparison of echocardiographic abnormalities in African-American, Hispanic, and white men and women aged >60 years. Am J Cardiol 2001;87(9):1131–1133, A10.
21. Jamieson WR, Edwards FH, Schwartz M, Bero JW, Clark RE, Grover FL. Risk stratification for cardiac valve replacement. National Cardiac Surgery Database. Database Committee of The Society of Thoracic Surgeons. Ann Thorac Surg 1999;67(4):943–951.
22. Chiappini B, Camurri N, Loforte A, Di Marco L, Di Bartolomeo R, Marinelli G. Outcome after aortic valve replacement in octogenarians. Ann Thorac Surg 2004;78(1):85–89.
23. Mehta RH, Eagle KA, Coombs LP, et al. Influence of age on outcomes in patients undergoing mitral valve replacement. Ann Thorac Surg 2002;74(5):1459–1467.
24. Ferguson TB Jr, Coombs LP, Peterson ED. Internal thoracic artery grafting in the elderly patient undergoing coronary artery bypass grafting: room for process improvement? J Thorac Cardiovasc Surg 2002;123(5):869–880.
25. Roach GW, Kanchuger M, Mangano CM, et al. Adverse cerebral outcomes after coronary bypass surgery. Multicenter Study of Perioperative Ischemia Research Group and the Ischemia Research and Education Foundation Investigators. N Engl J Med 1996;335(25):1857–1863.

26. Newman MF, Croughwell ND, Blumenthal JA, et al. Effect of aging on cerebral autoregulation during cardiopulmonary bypass. Association with postoperative cognitive dysfunction. Circulation 1994;90(5 Pt 2):II243–249.

27. Gold JP, Torres KE, Maldarelli W, Zhuravlev I, Condit D, Wasnick J. Improving outcomes in coronary surgery: the impact of echo-directed aortic cannulation and perioperative hemodynamic management in 500 patients. Ann Thorac Surg 2004;78(5):1579–1585.

28. Marshall WG Jr, Barzilai B, Kouchoukos NT, Saffitz J. Intraoperative ultrasonic imaging of the ascending aorta. Ann Thorac Surg 1989;48(3):339–344.

29. Murkin JM, Farrar JK, Tweed WA, McKenzie FN, Guiraudon G. Cerebral autoregulation and flow/metabolism coupling during cardiopulmonary bypass: the influence of $PaCO_2$. Anesth Analg 1987;66(9):825–832.

30. Bashein G, Townes BD, Nessly ML, et al. A randomized study of carbon dioxide management during hypothermic cardiopulmonary bypass. Anesthesiology 1990; 72(1):7–15.

31. Schell RM, Newman M, Reves J. Interventional therapy to palliate coronary artery disease in the elderly. In: McLeskey CH, ed. Geriatric Anesthesiology. Baltimore: Williams & Wilkins; 1997:609–635.

28
Vascular Procedures

Leanne Groban* and Sylvia Y. Dolinski

Anesthesia for vascular surgery is predominantly geriatric anesthesia. Atherosclerosis, the underlying disease process in the patient with peripheral vascular disease, has an insidious onset but typically presents about 10 years after the diagnosis of coronary artery disease. Given that persons aged 65 years and older comprise the fastest-growing segment of the United States population, the prevalence of vascular interventions, including minimally invasive angioplasty, endovascular stents, and open reconstructive procedures, will undoubtedly increase. This chapter focuses on anesthetic management for the geriatric patient undergoing aortic and peripheral vascular surgery. Preoperative preparation is a key feature, because various comorbidities associated with advanced age, such as ischemic heart disease, renal insufficiency, and diabetes are robust predictors of cardiac complications in the vascular patient.[1] A brief discussion of postoperative care follows the discussion of surgical procedures.

Preoperative Evaluation and Preparation

Fundamental to perioperative management is an understanding of the specific anesthetic and overall goals for care of the elderly vascular patient (Table 28-1). A critical step to achieving these perioperative goals and obtaining the best possible outcome from the surgical procedure is a careful preoperative evaluation. Knowledge of the age-related structural and functional changes that may have an impact on anesthesia for the geriatric patient is also important (Table 28-2). The aims of the preoperative assessment for the older vascular patient are to: (1) estimate risk; (2) optimize cardiovascular, respiratory, renal, and endocrinologic status; (3) undertake further investigation when necessary; (4) plan the anesthetic manage-

ment; and (5) arrange appropriate postoperative care. Given that the elderly patient is at an increased risk for postoperative complications, because of increased comorbid illnesses and diminished organ functional reserve,[2] a detailed evaluation of both cardiac and respiratory systems reserve is warranted.

Cardiac Risk Assessment and Intervention

Regardless of age, cardiovascular complications (e.g., myocardial infarction, pulmonary edema, arrhythmias) are among the most serious postoperative problems in patients undergoing noncardiac surgery.[3] Assessment of the perioperative cardiac risk and its impact on long-term health should be accomplished during preoperative evaluations to ascertain potential interventions that may modify the cardiac risk. However, one must also take particular caution when applying generalizations about the elderly population to specific elderly persons, because the aging process is very heterogeneous. That is, even major vascular procedures are accompanied by low risk when cardiac functional status is good, coronary artery disease is absent, and the multifactorial risk index is low.[4]

The Revised Cardiac Risk Index (RCRI) is often used to predict the risk of major cardiac complications among patients undergoing major, nonemergent, noncardiac surgery.[1] The index was derived from 2893 patients and validated in 1422 patients, all aged 50 or older. The six independent predictors of cardiac risk identified from the study that are currently used include high-risk surgery (Table 28-3), history of ischemic heart disease, history of congestive heart failure, history of cerebrovascular disease, insulin therapy, and serum creatinine more than 2.0 mg/dL. The presence of zero, one, two, and three or more predictors has been associated with cardiac complication rates of nearly 0.5%, 1%, 7%, and 12%, respectively.[1,5] Thus, the higher the score based on the presence of risk indices, the greater the risk for cardiac morbidity.

*Partially funded by the Dennis Jahnigen Career Development Award and Paul Beeson Scholars Award (K08-AG026764-01) to Dr. Groban.

TABLE 28-1. Perioperative goals.

For vascular surgery
- Maintain cardiovascular stability
- Maintain circulating blood volume
- Decrease stress response
- Preserve renal function

For the geriatric surgical patient
- Optimize medical and physical status
- Minimize perioperative starvation and inactivity
- Minimize the stresses of hypothermia, hypoxemia, and pain
- Promote rapid recovery and avoid declines in functional status
- Meticulous perioperative care to avoid complications from:
  - Fluid and electrolyte perturbations
  - Impaired cardiorespiratory function
  - Inappropriate pharmacotherapy

TABLE 28-3. Surgery-specific cardiac risk stratification for noncardiac surgical procedures.

High (reported cardiac risk often >5%)
  Emergent major operations, particularly in the elderly
  Aortic and other major vascular surgery (suprainguinal, abdominal, or thoracic)
  Peripheral vascular surgery
  Anticipated prolonged surgical procedures associated with large fluid shift and/or blood loss

Intermediate (reported cardiac risk generally <5%)
  Carotid endarterectomy
  Head and neck surgery
  Intraperitoneal and intrathoracic surgery
  Orthopedic surgery
  Prostate surgery

Low (reported cardiac risk generally <1%)
  Endoscopic procedures
  Superficial procedure
  Cataract surgery
  Breast surgery

Source: Reprinted with permission from Eagle et al.[6] Copyright © 2002 with permission from The American College of Cardiology Foundation.

Interestingly, the RCRI does not include advanced age as an independent predictor of cardiovascular outcome presumably because ischemic heart disease, insulin-dependent diabetes, and renal insufficiency are already highly associated with age.

The American College of Cardiology/American Heart Association guidelines for perioperative cardiovascular evaluation for noncardiac surgery[6] advocate identification of functional status in the assessment algorithm. This can be done by estimating energy demands of daily activities using the unit of metabolic equivalents (METs). The MET is a ratio comparing the energy consumption of an activity to energy consumption at rest. Usually, healthy elders can achieve 4.0 METs (e.g., showering while standing, toweling off, fishing, sweeping floors, playing with children) without dyspnea or fatigue.[7] Poor functional status, described as patients' inability to perform activities of <4.0 METs (e.g., cooking, sweeping floors, making the bed, food shopping with cart, or walking on level

ground at 3mph) without dyspnea or fatigue, is associated with nearly a 2 times greater cardiac risk than those who can perform this level of activity symptom-free. Interestingly, patients with intermediate- to high-risk profiles who can achieve >4.0 METs (e.g., washing windows, mopping floors, doing home calisthenics, walking upstairs with light load) or those who can achieve >75%–85% of their maximum age-predicted heart rate with a nonischemic electrocardiogram (ECG) response, are at low risk for postoperative cardiac events.[8]

Except in the case of emergent vascular surgery (when additional testing is obviated and the patient

TABLE 28–2. Age-related physiologic changes and anesthetic implications.

Structural and functional changes	Physiologic consequences	Clinical consequences
Myocyte		Greater reliance on ventricular filling and increases in stroke volume (rather than ejection fraction) to achieve increases in cardiac output. Intolerance to hypovolemia
Impaired calcium homeostasis	Impaired LV relaxation	
Reduced number (apoptosis) and increased size	Increased myocardial stiffness	
Reduced beta receptor responsiveness	Impaired Ca_2^+ homeostasis, reduced LV relaxation, increased circulating catecholamines	
Extracellular matrix	Increased LV stiffness	
Increased interstitial fibrosis		
Amyloid deposition		
Conduction system	Conduction block, atrial fibrillation, decreased contribution of atrial contraction to diastolic volume	Intolerance to tachycardia. dysrhythmias, including atrial fibrillation
Apoptosis of pacemaker and His-bundle cells		
Valvular apparatus	Aortic stenosis leads to LVH, reduced compliance, impaired relaxation	Prone to large swings in blood pressure with clamping and unclamping
Fibrosis and calcification		
Vasculature	Increased arterial stiffness, increased vascular impedance, early reflected waves, increase pulse wave velocity—decreasing LV compliance	
Increased diameter of large arteries		
Increased medial and intimal thickness		
Decreased endothelial nitric oxide production		

LV = left ventricular, LVH = left ventricular hypertrophy.

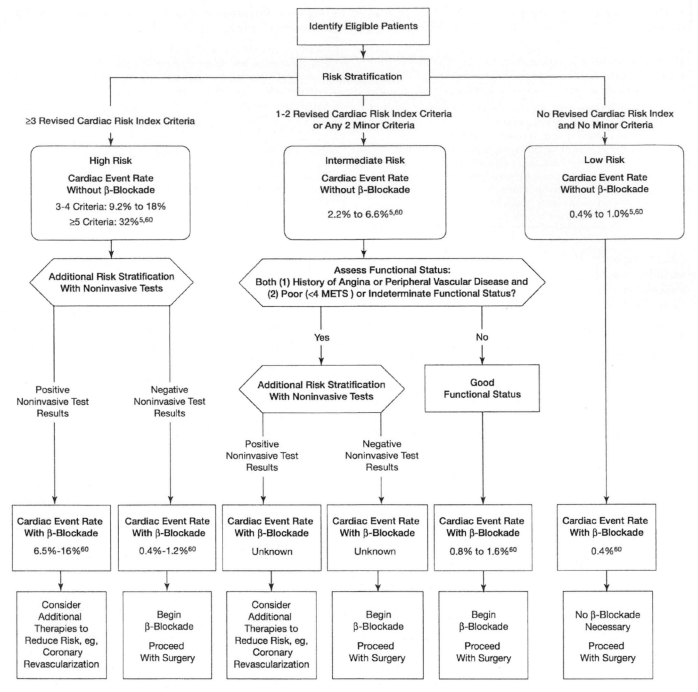

FIGURE 28-1. Perioperative beta-blockers: patient selection and preoperative risk stratification. The six independent predictors of complications in the Revised Cardiac Risk Index include: high-risk surgery, history of ischemic heart disease, congestive heart failure or cerebral vascular accident, preoperative insulin therapy, or serum creatinine >2.0 mg/dL. METS = metabolic equivalents. (Reprinted with permission from Auerbach and Goldman.[9] Copyright © 2002 American Medical Association. All rights reserved.)

proceeds directly to the operating room), the decision to perform noninvasive testing is based on the presence of clinical risk factors, the patient's functional status, and the type of surgery scheduled. Although little evidence exists showing that noninvasive imaging tests lead to therapeutic strategies that reduce cardiac risk, they remain a useful stratification tool for those elderly patients with age-related musculoskeletal changes that limit their functional status. For nonemergent vascular surgery, noninvasive testing (e.g., dobutamine stress echocardiography) may be indicated for (1) patients with stable angina, (2) patients scheduled for major aortic surgery who have either poor functional status or one clinical predictor, and (3) patients undergoing intermediate surgery (e.g., carotid endarterectomy), who have poor functional status and/or two or more clinical predictors. Given that perioperative beta-blockade lowers cardiac risk,[9] it should be initiated in all patients undergoing major aortic surgery who carry, at minimum, one cardiac risk factor. If beta-blockade is contraindicated, alpha-adrenergic agonists can be substituted.[10] One clinical algorithm for preoperative risk stratification and perioperative beta-blockade is shown in Figure 28-1.[9]

Optimization Strategies

Beta-Blocker Therapy

Perioperative administration of beta-adrenergic receptor blockers reduces the incidence of postoperative cardiac complications and death in high-risk patients undergoing noncardiac, major vascular procedures,[9,11–15] with beneficial effects lasting up to 2 years.[11,14,16] Perioperative myocardial infarctions are not necessarily all caused by unstable plaque rupture and subsequent thrombosis that occludes coronary arteries. Many occur in the absence of plaque rupture and in areas not supplied by known severely stenosed arteries.[17] Postoperative changes in sympathetic activity and stress response lead to changes in heart rate and blood pressure predisposing to myocardial ischemia perhaps from imbalances in supply and demand of coronary perfusion. This is where beta-blocker therapy enters the perioperative therapeutic picture, to help reduce these changes in heart rate and blood pressure. The strongest evidence to date that beta-blockade decreases the incidence of postoperative myocardial infarction and death is from Poldermans et al.[12] These investigators showed that high-risk patients with positive dobutamine stress echocardiograms administered bisoprolol (7 days preoperatively to 30 days postoperatively) had a tenfold decrease in morbidity and mortality compared with untreated patients. Despite overwhelming evidence in support of perioperative beta-blockade, these agents remain underutilized[18–20] because of classic concerns from described contraindications of diabetes, chronic obstructive lung disease, and heart failure. However, beta-blockers are often well tolerated in these individuals, especially when carefully titrated.[21,22] The reluctance of some physicians may be attributable to the lack of published data regarding their beneficial effects in the geriatric patient. A given trial in the elderly may have insufficient power to promote evidenced-based therapy, because the elderly are often excluded from studies, and thus the results, in fact, may not be generalizable. However, in a subgroup analysis of those >80 years, the mortality after myocardial infarction is reduced by 30%.[18–20]

In a small prospective study of 63 elderly patients (>65 years) undergoing noncardiac surgery, Zaugg et al.[23] showed no difference in in-hospital myocardial infarction rates between patients who received perioperative atenolol and those who did not receive prophylactic treatment. However, the perioperative use of beta-blockade in this study was associated with reduced analgesic requirements, faster recovery times from anesthesia, and improved hemodynamic stability, suggesting that perioperative beta-blockade may be not only safe, but provide additional beneficial effects in the elderly. Similarly, in the nonsurgical Metoprolol CR/XL Randomized Intervention Trial,[24,25] a subgroup of elderly patients ≥65 years (n = 1920) with chronic systolic heart failure treated with metoprolol exhibited risk reductions in total mortality (37%), sudden death (43%), death from worsening heart failure (36%), and hospitalizations from worsening heart failure (36%). These results were as favorable as the benefits observed in younger (<65 years) beta-blockade–treated patients. Given these data and the finding that metoprolol is also well tolerated, safe, and efficacious in heart failure patients >75 years of age,[26] beta-blockers should not be withheld from any surgical, high-risk patient with evidence of or known risk factors for coronary artery disease. One must keep in mind that older patients have decreased beta receptor responsiveness and, thus, may not exhibit the expected negative chronotropic response. Also, because of the rapid changes in blood volume that occur during aortic cross-clamping and unclamping and the age-related reductions in baroreceptor responsiveness,[27] the authors choose to use an esmolol infusion during the intraoperative period.

Alpha Agonists

Alpha-2 agonists provide an alternative therapy for prevention of cardiac morbidity and mortality in patients with or at risk for coronary artery disease who undergo vascular surgery.[10,28] In a recent study by Wallace et al.,[28] perioperative administration of oral (0.2 mg) or transdermal clonidine (0.2 mg/day) for 4 days reduced the incidence of perioperative myocardial ischemia (clonidine group, 14% versus placebo group, 31%) and also reduced the incidence of postoperative mortality in patients >60 years of age undergoing noncardiac surgery for up to 2 years. Mivazerol, an alpha-2 agonist administered by continuous infusion, significantly reduced the incidence of myocardial infarction in major vascular surgery patients who had cardiac disease.[29] However, with the potential for hypotension[30–32] and reductions in coronary perfusion pressure, the authors prefer using beta-blockers rather than alpha-2 agonists in the elderly in light of an increased prevalence of aortic stenosis with advancing age. Clearly, direct-comparison studies are needed to determine which class of sympatholytic agents provides the greatest cardiovascular benefit with the fewest side effects in this expanding surgical cohort.

Statins

Statins may also have cardiac protective effects in major vascular surgery. The mechanisms through which statins confer their beneficial effect include antithrombotic and antiinflammatory effects,[33] normalization of sympathetic outflow,[34] improved vasodilation,[35] and attenuation of cardiac remodeling.[36] In two case-control studies, statins were associated with lower perioperative[37] and long-term[38] mortality after major noncardiac vascular surgery. In two retrospective studies, preoperative use of statins significantly decreased cardiovascular complications (statin: 9.9% versus nonstatin: 16.5%)[39] and in-hospital mortality (statin users had a 38% reduction in the odds of in-hospital mortality).[40] Only the former, an observational study,[39] was specific to older patients (median age 71; range 63–78). Thus, even though the latter study[40] included 780,591 patients, it is not clear how well the results apply to older patients. Whether statins should be given to octogenarians for the prevention of cardiac disease and perioperative complications remains controversial.[41,42] Interestingly, Alter et al.[43] projected that if a combined therapy of statins and beta-blockers in acute coronary syndromes would have a 25% efficacy rate, one would need to treat 15 elderly patients compared with 175 in the youngest age group to show a benefit (Table 28-4). Findings from the Prospective Study of Pravastatin in the Elderly at Risk primary prevention trial[44] show that even though statins reduce death from heart disease, non-fatal myocardial infarction, and fatal or nonfatal stroke in the elderly, they may increase risks of myositis, rhab-domyolysis, and cancer.[42] Thus, until more trials are conducted in the older high-risk patient, the decision to prescribe a statin for prophylaxis against perioperative cardiac complications awaits additional study. Also, the effect of abrupt discontinuation of statin therapy in the elderly, high-risk patient remains unclear.[45]

Preoperative Assessment

A detailed cardiovascular history and examination with standard laboratory studies including a hematocrit, platelets, electrolytes, creatinine, and clotting profile are suffi-cient. A relatively recent 12-lead ECG is also indicated. Cardiovascular symptoms should be carefully determined, because preoperative ECG abnormalities do not predict postoperative cardiac complications in the elderly.[46] Chronic stable angina represents a low risk, whereas unstable angina has been associated with a high risk of perioperative ventricular dysfunction, ischemia, myocardial infarction, and arrhythmias. The high-risk patient should be referred to a cardiologist for additional testing and coronary therapies, if deemed necessary, before vascular surgery. Because many elderly patients have limited exercise capacity (because of arthritis, osteoporosis, and claudication) and atypical features of coronary artery disease, the authors recommend dobuta-mine stress echocardiography or dipyramidole-thallium scanning. Patients ultimately having either coronary stenting or angioplasty should then wait 2–4 weeks before their vascular procedure. Failure to wait for recovery after coronary intervention places these patients at high risk for lethal intraoperative bleeding or myocardial infarction.[47,48]

Patients with congestive heart failure are also at increased risk for postoperative cardiac complications. B-type natriuretic peptide (BNP) plasma level is useful in determining the etiology of pulmonary congestion.[49,50] With BNP levels of ≤100 pg/mL, heart failure is highly unlikely. However, BNP levels are increased in healthy elderly[51] and should not be used in isolation from clinical context. BNP trends in the chronic heart failure patient may help determine whether medical optimization is required before surgery. In the elderly hypertensive patient with concentric left ventricular hypertrophy and normal systolic function, diastolic dysfunction can lead to congestive heart failure. These patients are exquisitely sensitive to factors that alter diastolic filling such as tachycardia, atrial fibrillation, and hypovolemia. Thus, identifying these patients preoperatively, with Doppler echocardiographic indices of diastolic performance,[52] could help to establish the perioperative goals of fluid and blood pressure management.[53]

Because there is a paucity of data on patients >75 years of age, with normal systolic function and impaired diastolic function or diastolic heart failure, management of

TABLE 28-4. The relation between baseline risk (1-year mortality) and number needed to treat by various relative efficacies of treatment.

Age group (years)	1-Year mortality	Number needed to treat assuming a relative efficacy of 10%	Number needed to treat assuming a relative efficacy of 25%	Number needed to treat assuming a relative efficacy of 50%
<50	2.3	437	175	87
50–64	4.8	209	84	42
65–74	11.1	90	36	18
≥75	27.0	37	15	7

Source: Reprinted with permission from Alter et al.[43] Copyright © 2004 with permission from Excerpta Medica Inc.

these patients remains largely empiric and should be weighed on a case-by-case basis. Intraoperative and postoperative management emphasis should be placed on control of arterial hypertension (no higher than 130–140/80–90 mm Hg), maintenance of normal sinus rhythm and a low, normal heart rate (60–70 bpm), avoidance of ischemia, and the prevention of volume overload as well as an insufficient LV preload. In general, control of hypertension is easily done by anesthesia (to a desirable systolic blood pressure of 120 mm Hg). The authors also use a combination of low-dose infusions of nitroglycerin and phenylephrine titrated to maintain systolic blood pressure within 10% of baseline and to prevent increases in pulse pressure (e.g., pulse pressure > diastolic blood pressure $\cong$ increased impedance) and low diastolic blood pressures (e.g., <40 mm Hg), which, if ignored, could lead to myocardial ischemia.[54–56] Indeed, these agents administered alone might be detrimental to some elderly patients with diastolic dysfunction. That is, a nitroglycerin-induced reduction in vascular tone could lead to an insufficient LV preload and a reduction in cardiac output. Similarly, phenylephrine alone could increase vascular impedance such that the workload of the noncompliant heart increases. Thus, our goal of maximizing stroke volume with minimal cardiac work can be achieved using nitroglycerin and phenylephrine; this preserves distensibility of the vascular system while avoiding reductions in vascular tone. Maintenance of a low, normal heart rate (60–70 bpm) is achieved with low-dose beta-blockade after appropriate anesthesia and analgesia are assured. Albeit there are no convincing data that beta-blockers are of benefit to patients with diastolic heart failure. In the operating room setting, a titratable esmolol infusion can easily be used to maximize diastolic filling time. Certainly, too low a heart rate in the elderly (e.g., <50 bpm) could be detrimental. Specifically, with very low heart rates (<50 bpm), a longer time interval becomes available for reflected waves to merge with incident waves (forward stroke volume) in the aorta, ultimately increasing the workload of the heart.[57] Finally, volume status and preload adequacy are continuously assessed (and subsequently treated) using information from the arterial pressure waveform contour, central venous or pulmonary artery diastolic pressures, urine output, and the transesophageal short-axis ultrasound view of the left ventricle, if the transesophageal echocardiograph monitor and probe are available. Particularly, in the case of major aortic surgery, we have found that patients with diastolic dysfunction may actually require mild volume loading just before the placement of an infraceliac aortic cross-clamp. That is, if the splanchnic venous tone is low, an infraceliac clamp may shift blood volume into the splanchnic circulation, resulting in a decrease in venous return and preload.[58]

The prevalence of hypertension, specifically systolic hypertension, increases with aging.[59] Systolic hypertension in the absence of major risk factors and target organ damage is defined as systolic blood pressure $\geq$140 mm Hg. In the presence of normal diastolic blood pressure (<90 mm Hg), systolic hypertension is referred to as isolated hypertension. Given that systolic pressure increases with age and diastolic pressures plateau or even decrease, isolated diastolic hypertension is rare in the elderly. In fact, systolic blood pressure and pulse pressure are more important predictors of cardiovascular risk than diastolic blood pressure.[60–62] However, the optimal period of therapy before surgery is unclear, and in the elderly, acute treatment may cause more harm than the underlying disorder. The authors advocate that in general, patients continue to receive all their medications in the perioperative period (especially beta-blockers) to avoid reflex hypertension and tachycardia from drug withdrawal.[63] Hypertensive patients treated with either angiotensin-converting enzyme inhibitors or angiotensin receptor blockers are more prone to prolonged hypotension during induction and early maintenance of anesthesia, so these medications should be discontinued.[64–67] However, in the patient with hypertension and heart failure there is strong evidence to continue these medications. This evidence is lacking for the heart failure patient in the absence of hypertension.[68–70]

The elderly often encounter pulmonary complications after vascular surgery. In one study, the risk of postoperative pneumonia was found to be 5 times greater in patients aged 80 years or older than in those younger than 50 years.[71] In another study, the combination of age 60 years or older and an American Society of Anesthesiologists (ASA) status $\geq$2 identified almost 90% of patients who had respiratory complications after abdominal surgery.[72] Because of this, and the high prevalence of chronic obstructive pulmonary disease and active pulmonary infections related to smoking in the elderly, patients should be encouraged to stop smoking 6–8 weeks before surgery. Incentive spirometry breathing exercises should commence 2–3 days before surgery, and airflow obstruction should be treated with bronchodilators and inhaled glucocorticoids. Active respiratory infections should be resolved, even if it means delaying surgery.

Renal

Progressive decline in renal function in the aged and the compromise to renal blood flow associated with aortic cross-clamping puts the elderly vascular patient at high risk of developing postoperative renal failure. Accordingly, renal function (e.g., creatinine clearance) should be investigated preoperatively, and intraoperative renal preservation strategies used. The Cockcroft-Gault equation [(in mL/min): $(140 - \text{age}) \times \text{wt (kg)}/\text{serum creatinine (mg/dL)} \times 72$ ($\times 0.85$ in female subjects)] can help estimate creatinine clearance to make renal dose adjustments of medications. At present, there are no published guidelines of measures to prevent perioperative renal failure, although the use of acetylcysteine pre- and post-IV contrast has appeared in the literature.[73] Indeed, the use of magnetic resonance angiography as the sole imaging modality is an acceptable alternative for the preoperative evaluation of vascular architecture in high-risk patients, and it does not have harmful renal effects.[73] Nonetheless, the authors strive to maintain circulating blood volume and cardiac output in an attempt to maintain renal blood flow and perfusion pressure. The two "renal protective" strategies often used during aortic surgery include low-dose dopamine ($1-3\,\mu g/kg/min$) for its antialdosterone effect and mannitol ($12.5-25\,mg/70\,kg$), given before aortic cross-clamp application, for its potential free-radical scavenging and osmotic diuretic effects. Although dopamine has not been shown to have direct renal protective effects, it can be used to augment cardiac output, thus improving renal blood flow.[74] Mannitol increases tubular flow through its osmotic effects and by reducing renal tubular cellular swelling. Its renal protective effects were demonstrated in the renal transplant literature.[75] There are no large randomized controlled studies of its conclusive benefit in the vascular patient; however, one small study revealed reduced tubular injury by measured urinary albumin and N-acetyl glucosaminidase levels.[76]

Some anesthesiologists also advocate the use of loop diuretics in an attempt to "poison" the energy requiring Na^+/K^+-adenosine triphosphatase pump, thereby reducing renal metabolic O_2 demand.[58,77] However, with the high prevalence of diastolic dysfunction in geriatric patients,[78] the authors do not advise the routine use of loop diuretics for fear of compromising stroke volume and cardiac output. It has been suggested that low-dose fenoldopam ($0.03\,\mu g/kg/min$), a selective dopaminergic-1 receptor agonist, may have renal protective effects.[73,79,80] At this dose, it is unlikely to contribute to the hypotension one often sees postoperatively in these patients.

Cognitive Function/Delirium

Postoperative delirium is common in elderly patients and is a predictor of prolonged hospital stay and functional decline.[81] Risk factors for postoperative delirium include preexisting dementia, visual impairment, alcohol use, duration of anesthesia, use of benzodiazepines and narcotics, and postoperative infection. In an effort to identify patients at risk, the Mini-Mental State Examination is a reliable screening tool that is easy to use. (See Chapter 9 for more discussion on delirium.) In those patients considered to be at risk for postoperative delirium, the authors recommend a regional technique, if possible with no sedation. Although there is no evidence that regional anesthesia decreases the incidence of postoperative delir-

ium, the authors think this is attributable to the common use of various sedatives (e.g., midazolam, fentanyl, propofol, and ketamine) during surgical procedures performed under regional anesthesia.

Intraoperative Management

General Anesthesia for the Vascular Patient

After arrival in the warm operating room, standard noninvasive monitors are applied. Supplemental oxygen by nasal cannula is initiated at the time of low-dose premedication with either midazolam ($0.5-1.0\,mg$) or fentanyl ($25-50\,\mu g$). All patients should be attached to an ECG system capable of monitoring V5 and all limb and augmented leads. Normally, leads II and V5 are monitored simultaneously with ST segment trending. The only patients for whom the authors do not routinely place an arterial line are those presenting for a lower extremity bypass or amputation procedure. One has access to the wrists during these surgeries and often they can be managed without direct arterial pressure monitoring, unless the procedure is prolonged, the noninvasive blood pressure monitor cannot detect a regular pulse (e.g., chronic atrial fibrillation), or multiple activated clotting times are requested by the surgeon. Unless peripheral intravenous access is poor, a 16-gauge peripheral intravenous is started for induction. Central venous or pulmonary artery pressure monitoring is performed after induction in only those patients who are undergoing open aortic aneurysm/aortobifemoral bypass, because these surgeries predispose to large volume shifts. Central venous access allows assessment of right-sided filling pressure, the administration of vasoactive drugs, if necessary, and the facilitation of rapid blood transfusion. The elderly maintain their cardiac output by increasing stroke volume and preload. This preload dependency results in significant hypotension when hypovolemia is encountered. Therefore, acute blood loss during surgery is not well tolerated.[53] The noncompliant, older heart is exquisitely sensitive to volume overload. Thus, the delicate balance between hypotension and congestive heart failure warrants the use of central monitoring both intraoperatively and postoperatively in the geriatric patient undergoing major aortic surgery under general anesthesia. Transesophageal echocardiography is frequently used by one author (L.G.), because it provides real-time information about filling status, myocardial function, and ischemia. Monitoring of central and peripheral temperature is desirable. The aim is to maintain normothermia during surgical procedures using active measures including forced air, fluid warming devices, and warm ambient temperatures. The geriatric patient has less-efficient mechanisms of heat conservation, production, and dissipation.

Maintaining intraoperative normothermia reduces wound infections, cardiac events, and length of stay.[82,83]

Before preoxygenation, esmolol boluses or an esmolol infusion is titrated to achieve a heart rate 10%–20% below the patient's baseline. The advantages of esmolol include its high specificity for the beta$_1$ receptor, and its short duration of action. It can be used in severe chronic obstructive pulmonary disease patients, because it does not affect forced expiratory volume in 1 second, even at high infusion rates.[84] Preoxygenation in the geriatric patient is very important because an increased closing volume and a delayed onset of neuromuscular blockade predisposes them to rapid and profound desaturation and hypoxemia-induced cardiac events.[85] If rushed for time, 8 breaths at 100% oxygen over 1 minute at a 10 L/min flow rate is recommended.[86]

No matter if the approach to anesthesia is opioid-based supplemented with a volatile agent or a combined general and regional technique, the goals are the same (Table 28-1). Induction is undertaken with short-acting opioids, any intravenous induction agent (etomidate 0.2 mg/kg; propofol 0.5–0.7 mg/kg; thiopental 3 mg/kg), and cisatracurium. General anesthesia and sedative/hypnotics have a direct negative effect on sympathetic output, cardiac contractility, vascular tone, and cardiac filling pressures predisposing the older patient to a greater risk of hypotension. After the patient either stops breathing or becomes obtunded, the inhalational agent is slowly added to maintain normotension while neuromuscular blockade takes effect. Long-acting neuromuscular agents such as pancuronium should be avoided, because even when reversed these agents are associated with postoperative pulmonary complications.[87] The authors prefer cisatracurium for its forgiving pharmacodynamic profile. All neuromuscular blockers, including cisatracurium, have an increased onset time by about 1 minute in the geriatric patient. Recovery times for pancuronium, vecuronium, and rocuronium are also longer, whereas recovery times with cisatracurium are not altered by advanced age.[88] Heart rate responses to laryngoscopy are prevented by the use of the esmolol infusion (vide supra beta-blocker therapy). Anesthesia is maintained with any of the volatile agents, additional fentanyl, and a cisatracurium infusion at 1–3 μg/kg/min. Because minimal alveolar concentration (MAC) requirements are reduced in the elderly, bispectral index (BIS) monitoring may be useful. Longer-acting opioids (e.g., morphine) may be given toward the end of surgery to provide postoperative pain control if an epidural is not in place. However, one must keep in mind that the volume of distribution of morphine is smaller in the elderly, plasma and tissue drug levels are greater for a fixed dose, and the drug disappears more slowly from cerebral spinal fluid. Taken together, these effects can account for the more marked respiratory depression seen in the morphine-treated 80-year-old versus the morphine-treated 50-year-old. Moreover, plasma morphine concentration and morphine clearance also depend on renal function.

Patients are extubated provided they are warm and have an arterial pH of >7.35. The elderly are less able to mount a respiratory compensation for a metabolic acidosis, especially in the face of pain or narcotic loads. They have less muscle strength, and their hypoxic drive to breathe is also easily blunted with residual 0.1 MAC inhalational agent on board. Patients with postoperative epidural analgesia may be more readily extubated. Patients not extubated at the end of surgery receive infusions of either low-dose propofol (15 μg/kg/min) or dexmedetomidine (0.2–0.7 μg/kg/h). Dexmedetomidine has no respiratory depressant effects and minimal blood pressure–lowering effects in euvolemic patients.[89,90] Heart rates are lower with dexmedetomidine than with placebo during emergence and up to 48 hours after major vascular surgery, suggesting a cardioprotective benefit as well.[91]

Epidural Anesthesia/Regional Techniques

Neuraxial/regional anesthesia alone, or in combination with general anesthesia, has several potential benefits including attenuation of the stress response and the production of a sympathectomy (Table 28-5). These effects may reduce the tendency to form clots and enhance graft patency through improved blood flow.[92,93] Numerous studies, however, have failed to show that regional anesthesia is superior to general anesthesia for vascular surgeries for other outcomes such as death.[94] With the emphasis on administration of beta-blockers and maintenance of normothermia, morbidity and mortality in patients undergoing general anesthesia may be reduced, negating any difference one might see between regional and general anesthesia groups.[95] In addition, an inadequate or failed regional technique resulting in untreated tachycardia and hypertension, which leads to an increased need for supplementation of narcotics and anxiolytics, may produce hypercarbia or hypotension that likely will have a more adverse effect on outcome than a well-executed general.

Elderly patients at risk for postoperative delirium may benefit from epidural pain control as opposed to systemic

TABLE 28-5. Potential benefit of epidural anesthesia for vascular surgery.

Reduce stress response to surgery
Improve myocardial oxygen supply/demand balance
Improve endocardial blood flow
Reduce minimal alveolar concentration
Improve graft patency
Preserve pulmonary function
Reduce postoperative narcotic requirements

opiates in addition to the possibility of minimal sedation during the surgery.[95,96] T2 epidural anesthesia reduces MAC and MAC_{awake} by 50%.[97,98] The concentration of inhalational agent required during combined general/epidural technique is markedly reduced. In fact, BIS levels are reduced with the combination technique.[99] Intraoperative anticoagulation is not a contraindication for a neuraxial technique as long as the heparin is dosed 1 hour after the epidural insertion.[100] Lower extremity surgeries require a T-12 level. Presently, there seems to be little evidence in the literature that regional anesthesia provides a benefit in length of hospital stay, mortality, and cardiac morbidity over general anesthesia.[94] This may be because in randomized controlled trials both the study and control groups are closely watched, and it is close perioperative watching that makes a difference in outcome.

However, on subgroup analysis of aortic surgery, Park et al.[96] found that patients who had epidurals had fewer postoperative complications including less cardiovascular and respiratory failure. A meta-analysis of randomized controlled trials addressing the postoperative effects of epidurals on pulmonary function revealed that there is a decreased incidence of respiratory infections and overall pulmonary complications, compared with systemic opioid administration.[98] Another recent meta-analysis also showed reductions in the pulmonary complications of pulmonary embolism, pneumonia, and respiratory depression.[101]

When the authors place epidurals for abdominal aortic surgeries at T6–8, the patients undergo test dosing with 2% lidocaine. Before incision, morphine (2–3 mg) is administered epidurally. It is not until after the cross-clamp has been removed and the patient is hemodynamically stable, that the epidural is redosed with 2% lidocaine, and a continuous 0.25% bupivacaine infusion through the epidural catheter is begun at a rate of 3 mL/h. As the blood pressure increases, the patient is given a 1- to 2-mL 2% lidocaine bolus, and the bupivacaine infusion is increased by 1 mL/h. This is repeated until the patient is on an infusion of 4–6 mL/h at the end of the case. In the postanesthesia care unit, the 0.25% bupivacaine infusion is stopped once the postoperative infusion of 0.125% bupivacaine with 0.005% morphine sulfate is available, thereby continually controlling postoperative pain.

In the postoperative period, if the patient is anticoagulated with prophylactic low-molecular-weight heparin (LMWH), the epidural should be removed at least 10–12 hours after the last LMWH dose, and 2 hours before the next dose,[100] to reduce the risk of epidural or spinal hematoma associated with anticoagulation. The epidural is continued if the patient receives prophylactic unfractionated heparin for a few days postoperatively. The authors discourage their surgical colleagues from using fractionated heparin in the elderly despite creatinine

values in the normal range. There is some evidence that the elderly are at increased risk of bleeding when given fractionated heparin.[102]

Infraaortic Vascular Procedures

These procedures are amenable to either neuraxial techniques alone or combined with general anesthesia depending on the length of surgery and/or type of surgery. An ileofemoral bypass requires abdominal muscle relaxation better afforded by neuromuscular blockade (and hence, general anesthesia) than by only a neuraxial technique. However, patients undergoing such procedures are frequently already receiving anticoagulants such as intravenous heparin or have been recently dosed with platelet inhibitors such as clopidogrel, which preclude any neuraxial technique. Other regional techniques such as lumbar plexus/sciatic blocks have been associated with increased bleeding risks.[103] Below the knee amputations have successfully been performed by popliteal blocks, and distal foot amputations are amenable to ankle blocks.

Aortic Surgeries

The risk of rupture for aneurysms <4 cm in diameter is minimal. For those >6 cm, the annual rupture risk is >25%. The best predictor of rupture risk is an aneurysm that increases in size more than 1.0 cm/year. Current standard of care dictates that aneurysms >5.0 cm in size should be repaired. Advanced age is a risk factor for increased death and complication rates. Postoperative mortality in octogenarians for open aortic repair has been reported to be between 1.4%–9.6% (Table 28-6). Dardik et al.[104] showed that mortality was 2.9% in those in their sixth decade of life compared with 7.9% in octogenarians (Table 28-6, Figure 28-2). Increased postoperative complications have also been reported with advanced age (Figure 28-3). Octogenarians undergoing endovascular abdominal aneurysm repair (EVAR), however, had a mortality rate of 1.9% versus 5.3% for open surgeries.[105]

Before aortic cross-clamp placement, heparin (100 U/kg) is administered and an activated clotting time is con-

TABLE 28-6. Perioperative mortality rates after elective open surgical repair of abdominal aortic aneurysm in octogenarians.

Source	Patients (no.)	Mortality rate (%)
Treiman (1982)	35	8.6
Paty (1993)	116	3.0
Akkersdijk (1994)	75	8.3
Ohara (1995)	94	9.6
Van Damme (1998)	52	45.7
Kazmers (1998)	206	8.3
Dardik (1999)	246	7.9
Mailapur (2001)	62	1.4

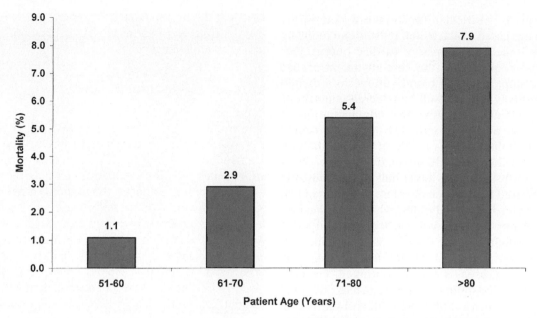

FIGURE 28-2. Rate of in-hospital mortality after repair of intact abdominal aortic aneurysm compared across age groups (p < 0.001). (Reprinted with permission from Vemuri C, Wainess RM, Dimick JB, et al. Effect of increasing patient age on complication rates following intact abdominal aortic aneurysm repair in the United States. J Surg Res 2004;118:26–31. Copyright © 2004. With permission from Elsevier.)

firmed to be longer than 250 seconds. Depth of anesthesia is increased and a nitroglycerin drip is also started before clamp placement. Venodilatation aids in volume loading of the patient during aortic cross-clamping. The physiologic response to aortic cross-clamping is dependent on the preoperative myocardial function, site of clamp application, aortic pathology (e.g., occlusive versus aneurysmal), and the volume status. A diaphragmatic-level aortic clamp is associated with increases in central venous, pulmonary artery end diastolic, and pulmonary artery mean pressures along with increases in mean arterial pressure. The cardiac output also increases in patients with normal myocardial function because of a shift in blood volume proximal to the clamp. In patients with ischemic heart

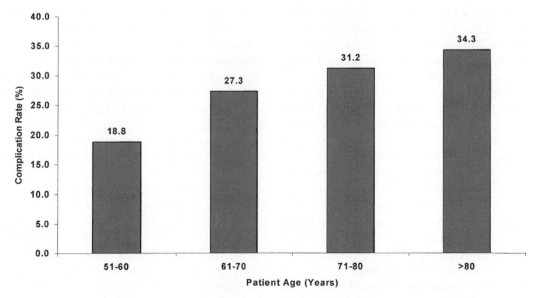

FIGURE 28-3. Percentage of patients with one or more complications after surgery for repair of intact abdominal aortic aneurysm according to age group (p < 0.001). (Reprinted with permission from Vemuri C, Wainess RM, Dimick JB, et al. Effect of increasing patient age on complication rates following intact abdominal aortic aneurysm repair in the United States. J Surg Res 2004;118:26–31. Copyright © 2004. With permission from Elsevier.)

disease, however, ventricular function can deteriorate secondary to increased wall tension. If afterload reducing agents and volume do not restore cardiac output, inotropes may be required. In the case of an infraceliac aortic cross-clamp, a shift in blood volume to a dilated splanchnic bed may in fact result in a decrease in venous return and preload, prompting the administration of fluids at the time of cross-clamp.[58] Distal to the clamp, anaerobic metabolism ensues as blood flow to the gut, kidney, and legs decrease. Upon removal of the cross-clamp and reperfusion of the lower half of the body, the patient is subjected to a sudden decrease in afterload and washout of anaerobic metabolites which can lead to hypotension if not properly volume loaded. Cell saver blood and autologous blood units as well as saline are infused to optimize preload before unclamping. The nitroglycerin drip, if used, is now discontinued. The concentration of the inhalational agent is reduced, fractional inspired oxygen concentration increased, and ventilation increased to counteract the released acid load. Phenylephrine is readily available, and the surgeon releases the cross-clamp slowly while volume is rapidly infused to counteract the vasodilation and hypotension.

Endovascular Abdominal Aortic Aneurysm Repair

Since 1991, the number of endovascular graft surgeries has surged. Three studies looking at EVAR in the elderly have shown >82%–95% success rate in placement with a <3.3% 30-day mortality.[106–108] EVAR advantages include decreased operating room time, decreased blood loss, avoidance of general anesthesia and aortic cross-clamping with its inherent hemodynamic perturbations and organ dysfunction. The intensive care unit (ICU) and hospital stays are reduced. There is less cardiac and respiratory dysfunction associated with EVAR than major abdominal surgery.[108] A large endovascular stent delivery device is advanced under fluoroscopic guidance through the femoral artery to the diseased aortic target site. Here it is deployed to exclude the diseased segment from aortic blood flow. There are several types of endovascular stents: the aortic tube stent, the aorto-bi-iliac, and the aorto-uni-iliac graft (Figure 28-4). The tube graft is less popular for infrarenal aortic aneurysm repair, because it requires a fairly long aortic segment to be present below the renal arteries to ensure its secure attachment before the aorta bifurcates. The aorto-bi-iliac stent results in less subsequent leakage or stenosis, but requires more exact measurement of graft dimensions before deployment. The aorto-uni-iliac graft is deployed in the aorta and one iliac vessel. The contralateral iliac artery is permanently occluded. A femoral–femoral bypass is then performed to provide circulation to the contralateral extremity.

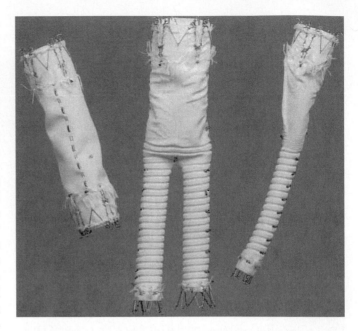

FIGURE 28-4. Ancure (Guidant, Menlo Park, CA) aortic tube endograft (left), single-piece bifurcated (center), and aorto-uni-iliac aortic (right) endograft. (Reprinted with permission from Makaroun MS. The Ancure endografting system: an update. J Vasc Surg 2001;33:S129–134. Copyright © 2001. With permission from The Society for Vascular Surgery.)

Finally, there is a bifurcated modular device. Here the proximal component is attached to the infrarenal aorta and extends into one iliac artery. A second (module) is anchored to the first component and extends into the contralateral iliac artery. This device has the greatest risk of leakage and stenosis, because it has twice as many attachments as the single piece graft.

Complications of this technique include endoleaks, which may be subtle and heal over or become apparent with sudden hypotension in the operating room or postanesthesia care unit. One should never dismiss hypotension as a complication of a neuraxial technique. Other complications include continued aneurysmal growth, and device dislodgement or failure. Because of the use of renal contrast, worsening postoperative renal function is also a concern. Postoperative renal morbidity in octogenarians after EVAR was reported to be between 0%–14%. However, even in the higher group, there was no increased hemodialysis requirement, length of stay, or mortality.[109,110]

Which treatment option is best (endovascular versus open repair) depends on the patient and the aneurysm. Forty to sixty percent of patients are candidates for endovascular repair, if their aneurysm has a proximal neck of at least 15 mm and they have one straight iliac artery for insertion. Other anatomic criteria have been published.[111,112] Patient factors that make open abdominal aortic aneurysm repair more risky include older age, pul-

TABLE 28-7. Descriptive analyses of in-hospital mortality rates according either to age and significant risk factors or to ASA scoring.

	TEAM		Open surgery		
	%	N	%	N	p Value
Patients <72 years of age					
Without pulmonary or renal risk	0	0 of 54	0.9	1 of 115	0.492
With pulmonary or renal risk	3	1 of 33	6.7	2 of 30	0.498
Patients ≥72 years of age					
Without pulmonary or renal risk	1.6	1 of 62	4	3 of 75	0.409
With pulmonary or renal risk	5.3	3 of 57	21.4	6 of 28	0.023
ASA score					
1 and 2	0.0	0 of 10	1.1	1 of 88	0.735
3	0.9	1 of 111	4.5	6 of 134	0.094
4	4.7	4 of 85	19.2	5 of 26	0.018

Source: Reprinted with permission from Teufelsbauer et al.[113]
ASA = American Society of Anesthesiologists.

monary dysfunction, creatinine >1.8 mg/dL, and congestive heart failure. Life expectancy after abdominal aortic aneurysm repair for individuals aged 70, 75, 80, and 85 years is 10, 8, 6, and 5 years, respectively.[108] The 4-year survival rate was 43% compared with 17% in those octogenarians deemed too high a risk for surgery in the past, half of whom died from aneurysm rupture.[107] One study of ASA 4 patients showed an in-hospital mortality rate of 4.7% in EVAR patients compared with the open repair rate of 19.2% (p < 0.02). Patients older than 72 with pulmonary or renal risk factors had a 21.4% mortality in the open group compared with the EVAR group of 5.3%. In the same age group, those without pulmonary or renal risks had a 4% mortality in the open group compared with the EVAR of 1.6%[113] (Table 28-7).

Two large-bore IVs and an arterial line are placed. The authors do not routinely place central venous catheters for EVAR. A phenylephrine drip is prepared. Blood is kept in the room in case of intraoperative aortic rupture. The authors prefer to place a combined spinal-epidural catheter as the primary anesthetic for the procedure. The spinal injection of 12.5 mg plain isobaric 0.5% bupivacaine typically provides anesthesia/analgesia for the duration of the procedure. During placement of the neuraxial catheter, the patient receives minimal amounts of midazolam. Intraoperatively, the patient is sedated via a continuous infusion of dexmedetomidine (0.2–0.7 μg/kg/h) or a propofol/ketamine (190:10 mg) mixture.

Carotid Endarterectomy

Two landmark randomized prospective trials showed that endarterectomy performed in patients who are symptomatic and have >70% internal carotid stenosis reduces the risk of ipsilateral stroke from 26% to 9% over the course of 2 years.[114,115] During surgery, the patient is at risk for an intraoperative stroke, and it is thought that placing a shunt across the clamped artery may improve on the ischemia. Some surgeons routinely place a shunt in patients undergoing a general anesthetic, because the ischemia that leads to a stroke cannot be recognized until after the operation. Some place a shunt only in patients at high risk for perioperative stroke, whereas others try not to place a shunt at all because the majority of patients do tolerate cross-clamping of the carotid. Shunting has its inherent risks of dissection or shedding of atheroemboli. High-risk patients are considered those with a 100% contralateral carotid occlusion.

This procedure can be performed under regional or general anesthetic techniques. Sensory blockade in the C2–C4 dermatome can be achieved with a superficial cervical or deep cervical plexus block with minimal or no sedation. Local infiltration of lidocaine by the surgeons is an alternative option. This allows monitoring for optimal cerebral blood flow perfusion during the carotid cross-clamping by conversing with the patient. There is little need for more invasive or complex cerebral monitoring and often less need for shunting. However, with high carotid bifurcations, the regional technique usually fails to control all the intraoperative mandibular retraction pain and local anesthetic supplementation by the surgeon is required.

A recent Cochrane review of nonrandomized trials suggests that surgery performed under local anesthesia is associated with a reduction in the odds of death, stroke, myocardial infarction, and pulmonary complications within 30 days of the operation. In the seven randomized controlled trials, there were no differences in the aforementioned outcomes. The ongoing General Anesthetic versus Local Anesthetic for Carotid Surgery trial is a randomized controlled trial designed to determine if regional anesthesia leads to a reduction in postoperative strokes.[116]

Regional anesthesia may be associated with occasional intense pain and anxiety that can lead to myocardial stress. Not all patients are candidates for regional anesthesia, particularly those who are claustrophobic, very anxious, or experience a lot of pain from lying on a hard surface.

Two intravenous lines are placed. Both phenylephrine and nitroglycerin drips are attached to a T-port connector on one of the lines close to the intravenous catheter insertion site, thereby ensuring little dead space. The authors typically perform a superficial cervical block with 0.25% ropivacaine because the cardiac safety profile seems to be better than the other long-acting local anesthetics, especially if the drug is inadvertently bolused into a large vessel in the neck.[117] After the block is placed, an arterial line is inserted in the arm opposite of the surgical site if both arms are not tucked. Intravenous fluids are kept to a minimum, blood pressure is kept at or above baseline, and the patient is monitored by engaging the patient in conversation. If necessary, the surgeon can supplement with 1% lidocaine if pain arises from the carotid sheath. During removal of the plaque, it is useful to warn the patient that this will feel like a dull toothache. Before cross-clamping, a 100 mg/kg bolus of heparin is given, and after the cross-clamping of the carotid, the patient is monitored for 1–2 minutes by squeezing the patient's untucked hand and listening to the patient's speech. If any change in the patient's behavior is noted, the surgeon is alerted, the cross-clamp removed, the blood pressure increased by 20% above base line, and the clamp replaced. If the patient again exhibits signs of decreased cerebral perfusion, the surgeon places a shunt.

If a general anesthetic is required because of surgeon or patient preference and cooperation, then induction proceeds as previously described under General Anesthesia for the Vascular Patient. Typically, only 1–2 µg/kg of fentanyl (or a maximum of 150 µg) is given to maximize the chances for a rapid emergence. Alternatively, remifentanil can be used and titrated off as the patient is allowed to spontaneously breathe; fentanyl is then titrated to a respiratory rate of 8–12. The authors typically hold pressure over the surgical site dressing until the patient is extubated. The goal is a smooth emergence with minimal coughing.

Intraoperatively, there are numerous techniques for the monitoring of cerebral ischemia, and the authors have typically used cerebral oximetry or spectral edge frequency. Other techniques include full 16-lead electroencephalography, jugular venous saturation, stump pressures, evoked potentials, and transcranial Doppler monitoring.[118] None is as good as an awake, cooperative, communicative patient. In fact, when awake patients were simultaneously monitored by electroencephalography, there was a 6.7% false-positive and a 4.5% false-negative rate in detection of neurologic deficits.[119]

Carotid Stents

Of the endovascular techniques used for treating carotid stenosis, stenting is the preferred technique because it reduces the restenosis and dissection rates compared with angioplasty.[120] The first randomized controlled trial comparing carotid stent placement with open surgery in high-risk patients was conducted in 2002.[121] The 30-day mortality, stroke, or myocardial infarction rate was 5.8% for the stent group and 12.6% for the carotid endarterectomy group (p < 0.05). At 1-year follow-up, the differences were still remarkable for the same endpoints: 11.9% in the stent group compared with 19.9% in the carotid endarterectomy group.[122] However, the Cochrane review of the five trials comparing endovascular with open carotid endarterectomy showed that there was no significant difference in the risk of perioperative stroke, myocardial infarction, or death. It did show a reduction in cranial neuropathy.[123] This technique allows very high-risk patients and high, surgically inaccessible cervical carotid lesions to be treated. However, unlike stents placed in a coronary vessel or aorta, carotid surgery is relatively safe, inexpensive, and associated with a short hospital stay. Atheromatous emboli are devastating, and neuroprotective devices such as balloon catheter or microfilter systems are used by surgeons.[120] Local anesthesia and standard noninvasive monitors are used.

Postoperative Care

Most elderly patients have comorbidities that warrant their admission to the ICU. These include cardiac, respiratory, and renal insufficiency. The elderly are more prone to delirium. Bohner et al.[124] documented the incidence to be 38.9% with longer ICU treatment needed. Early restoration to preoperative physiologic and cognitive functioning is most important. Longer-term postoperative cognitive dysfunction is also not uncommon in the elderly. A large study revealed that 9.9% of patients had some postoperative cognitive deficits compared with their cohort who did not have any anesthesia.[125] Of those >75 years of age, 14% had a persistent cognitive deficit. Deeper anesthesia has also been suggested to affect mortality in the elderly.[126] Patients 60 years and older who were subjected to deeper BIS values (<40) had a 16% increased incidence of mortality at 1 year (Figure 28-5).[127] This intriguing finding has not been validated as a direct cause and effect relationship and awaits further study.

One might surmise that there would be less mortality with regional anesthesia. This has not yet been found to be true.[128] However, this may be related to the fact that all patients received some form of sedation. No studies have been conducted that looked at regional without sedation, regional with sedation, and general anesthesia.

The recent Transfusion Requirement in Critical Care trial compared a "restrictive" versus a "liberal" transfusion strategy for ICU patients. The restrictive group received transfusions at a hemoglobin level of 7 mg/dL

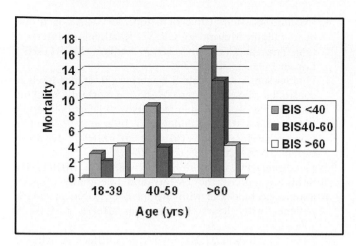

FIGURE 28-5. Mortality tends to be higher if the bispectral index (BIS) levels are <40 in patients 40 years and older. (Data from Weldon et al.[127])

and maintained between a range of 7–9 mg/dL. The liberal group received a transfusion at a hemoglobin level of 10 mg/dL and was maintained in a range of 10–12 mg/dL.[129] There was no difference in mortality between the groups. In a subgroup analysis of those same patients who had cardiovascular disease, there also was no difference between the liberal and restrictive cohorts in 30-day mortality. Additionally, they had a 50% reduction in the number of transfusions. However, this was based on a small number of patients. In a study limited to vascular surgery patients, myocardial infarction occurred in 14% of patients whose hematocrit was >28%, whereas it occurred in 77% of those whose hematocrit was <28%.[130] In patients aged 65 and older who had a myocardial infarction, those who were transfused for a hematocrit <33% had a reduced 30-day mortality.[131] There are three reasons why the authors still adhere to keeping their elderly vascular patient's hemoglobin at >9.0 mg/dL. First, the elderly who have left-ventricular hypertrophy may be more prone to subendocardial ischemia in the face of anemia. Second, the authors are advocating beta-blocker therapy that reduces the compensatory mechanism of increasing heart rate. Third, a study in vascular surgery patients comparing a transfusion trigger of 9.0 versus 10 mg/dL showed no difference in mortality.[132]

All of the ICU patients receive deep venous thrombosis and ulcer prophylaxis. The blood glucose is kept <200 mg/dL with an insulin infusion. This is based on the study by van den Berghe et al.,[133] which showed a reduction in mortality, acute failure, and number of transfused red blood cell units to a postsurgical ICU population. Although the blood glucose levels were kept at 110 mg/dL and the majority of the patients were post–cardiac surgery, there is little reason to believe that maintaining euglycemia is harmful.

Finally, as pointed out in the beta-blocker therapy section, it is not enough to write for postoperative beta-blockers, but one must titrate to a heart rate effect. Prolonged increased heart rate (>95 bpm for >12 hours) is associated with increased myocardial infarctions and cardiac death.[134]

Increased heart rate, especially in the elderly, is associated with the development of atrial fibrillation. Both myocardial infarction and atrial fibrillation result in prolonged ICU stays.

Conclusions

The geriatric vascular patient faces not only complications related to predictable structural and functional changes in the heart and vasculature, but also because of the existence of a number of comorbid diseases. Without clear-cut contraindications, beta-blockers should be used in the elderly vascular patient. Future studies should examine comprehensive care strategies targeted toward the geriatric patient to improve cognitive and functional outcomes.

References

1. Lee TH, Marcantonio ER, Mangione CM, et al. Derivation and prospective validation of a simple index for prediction of cardiac risk of major noncardiac surgery. Circulation 1999;100:1043–1049.
2. Rothschild JM, Bates DW, Leape LL. Preventable medical injuries in older patients. Arch Intern Med 2000;160:2717–2728.
3. Fleisher LA. Preoperative cardiac evaluation. Anesthesiol Clin North Am 2004;22:59–75.
4. Golden MA, Whittemore AD, Donaldson MC, et al. Selective evaluation and management of coronary artery disease in patients undergoing repair of abdominal aortic aneurysms. A 16-year experience. Ann Surg 1990;212:415–420; discussion 420–423.
5. Grayburn PA, Hillis LD. Cardiac events in patients undergoing noncardiac surgery: shifting the paradigm from non-invasive risk stratification to therapy. Ann Intern Med 2003;138:506–511.
6. Eagle KA, Berger PB, Calkins H, et al. American College of Cardiology; American Heart Association. ACC/AHA guideline update for perioperative cardiovascular evaluation for noncardiac surgery—executive summary: a report of the American College of Cardiology/American Heart Association Task Force on Practice Guidelines Committee to Update the 1996 Guidelines on Perioperative Cardiovascular Evaluation for Noncardiac Surgery. J Am Coll Cardiol 2002;39:542–553.
7. Studenski S. Exercise. In: Landefeld CS, Palmer RM, Johnson MAG, et al., eds. Current Geriatric Diagnosis and Treatment. New York: McGraw Hill; 2004:441.
8. Lette J, Waters D, Lassonde J, et al. Multivariate clinical models and quantitative dipyridamole-thallium imaging to

predict cardiac morbidity and death after vascular recon-struction. J Vasc Surg 1991;14:160–169.

9. Auerbach AD, Goldman L. β-Blockers and reduction of cardiac events in noncardiac surgery: scientific review. JAMA 2002;287:1435–1444.

10. Wijeysundera DN, Naik JS, Beattie WS. Alpha-2 adrenergic agonists to prevent perioperative cardiovascular complications: a meta-analysis. Am J Med 2003;114:742–752.

11. Mangano DT, Layug EL, Wallace A, et al. Effect of atenolol on mortality and cardiovascular morbidity after noncardiac surgery. Multicenter Study of Perioperative Ischemia Research Group. N Engl J Med 1996;335:1713–1720.

12. Poldermans D, Boersma E, Bax JJ, et al. The effect of bisoprolol on perioperative mortality and myocardial infarction in high-risk patients undergoing vascular surgery. Dutch Echocardiographic Cardiac Risk Evaluation Applying Stress Echocardiography Study Group. N Engl J Med 1999;341:1789–1794.

13. Raby KE, Brull SJ, Timimi F, et al. The effect of heart rate control on myocardial ischemia among high-risk patients after vascular surgery. Anesth Analg 1999;88:477–482.

14. Wallace A, Layug B, Tateo I, et al. Prophylactic atenolol reduces postoperative myocardial ischemia. McSPI Research Group. Anesthesiology 1998;88:7–17.

15. Boersma E, Poldermans D, Bax JJ, et al. DECREASE Study Group (Dutch Echocardiographic Cardiac Risk Evaluation Applying Stress Echocardiography). Predictors of cardiac events after major vascular surgery: role of clinical characteristics, dobutamine echocardiography, and beta-blocker therapy. JAMA 2001;285:1865–1873.

16. Poldermans D, Boersma E, Bax JJ, et al. Dutch Echocardiographic Cardiac Risk Evaluation Applying Stress Echocardiography Study Group. Bisoprolol reduces cardiac death and myocardial infarction in high-risk patients as long as 2 years after successful major vascular surgery. Eur Heart J 2001;22:1353–1358.

17. Landesberg G. The pathophysiology of perioperative myocardial infarction: facts and perspectives. J Cardiothorac Vasc Anesth 2003;17:90–100.

18. Warltier DC. Beta-adrenergic-blocking drugs: incredibly useful, incredibly underutilized. Anesthesiology 1998;88:2–5.

19. Mendelson G, Aronow WS. Underutilization of beta-blockers in older patients with prior myocardial infarction or coronary artery disease in an academic, hospital-based geriatrics practice. J Am Geriatr Soc 1997;45:1360–1361.

20. Soumerai SB, McLaughlin TJ, Spiegelman D, et al. Adverse outcomes of underuse of beta-blockers in elderly survivors of acute myocardial infarction. JAMA 1997;277:115–121.

21. Sirak TE, Jelic S, Le Jemtel TH. Therapeutic update: nonselective beta- and alpha-adrenergic blockade in patients with coexistent chronic obstructive pulmonary disease and chronic heart failure. J Am Coll Cardiol 2004;44:497–502.

22. Di Bari M, Marchionni N, Pahor M. Beta-blockers after acute myocardial infarction in elderly patients with diabetes mellitus: time to reassess. Drugs Aging 2003;20:13–22.

23. Zaugg M, Tagliente T, Lucchinetti E, et al. Beneficial effects from beta-adrenergic blockade in elderly patients undergoing noncardiac surgery. Anesthesiology 1999;91:1674–1686.

24. [No authors listed.] Effect of metoprolol CR/XL in chronic heart failure: Metoprolol CR/XL Randomised Intervention Trial in Congestive Heart Failure (MERIT-HF). Lancet 1999;353:2001–2007.

25. Hjalmarson A, Goldstein S, Fagerberg B, et al. Effects of controlled-release metoprolol on total mortality, hospitalizations, and well-being in patients with heart failure: the Metoprolol CR/XL Randomized Intervention Trial in Congestive Heart Failure (MERIT-HF). MERIT-HF Study Group. JAMA 2000;283:1295–1302.

26. Deedwania PC, Gottlieb S, Ghali JK, et al. MERIT-HF Study Group. Efficacy, safety and tolerability of beta-adrenergic blockade with metoprolol CR/XL in elderly patients with heart failure. Eur Heart J 2004;25:1300–1309.

27. Ebert TJ, Morgan BJ, Barney JA, et al. Effects of aging on baroreflex regulation of sympathetic activity in humans. Am J Physiol 1992;263:H798–803.

28. Wallace AW, Galindez D, Salahieh A, et al. Effect of clonidine on cardiovascular morbidity and mortality after noncardiac surgery. Anesthesiology 2004;101:284–293.

29. Oliver MF, Goldman L, Julian DG, et al. Effect of mivazerol on perioperative cardiac complications during noncardiac surgery in patients with coronary heart disease: the European Mivazerol Trial (EMIT). Anesthesiology 1999;91:951–961.

30. Jalonen J, Hynynen M, Kuitunen A, et al. Dexmedetomidine as an anesthetic adjunct in coronary artery bypass grafting. Anesthesiology 1997;86:331–345.

31. Boldt J, Rothe G, Schindler E, et al. Can clonidine, enoximone, and enalaprilat help to protect the myocardium against ischaemia in cardiac surgery? Heart 1996;76:207–213.

32. Myles PS, Hunt JO, Holdgaard HO, et al. Clonidine and cardiac surgery: haemodynamic and metabolic effects, myocardial ischaemia and recovery. Anaesth Intensive Care 1999;27:137–147.

33. Undas A, Brozek J, Musial J. Anti-inflammatory and anti-thrombotic effects of statins in the management of coronary artery disease. Clin Lab 2002;48:287–296.

34. Hayashidani S, Tsutsui H, Shiomi T, et al. Fluvastatin, a 3-hydroxy-3-methylglutaryl coenzyme a reductase inhibitor, attenuates left ventricular remodeling and failure after experimental myocardial infarction. Circulation 2002;105:868–873.

35. Laufs U, La Fata V, Plutzky J, et al. Upregulation of endothelial nitric oxide synthase by HMG CoA reductase inhibitors. Circulation 1998;97:1129–1135.

36. Hasegawa H, Yamamoto R, Takano H, et al. 3-Hydroxy-3-methylglutaryl coenzyme A reductase inhibitors prevent the development of cardiac hypertrophy and heart failure in rats. J Mol Cell Cardiol 2003;35:953–960.

37. Poldermans D, Bax JJ, Kertai MD, et al. Statins are associated with a reduced incidence of perioperative mortality in patients undergoing major noncardiac vascular surgery. Circulation 2003;107:1848–1851.

38. Kertai MD, Boersma E, Westerhout CM, et al. Association between long-term statin use and mortality after successful abdominal aortic aneurysm surgery. Am J Med 2004;116:96–103.

39. O'Neil-Callahan K, Katsimaglis G, Tepper MR, et al. Statins decrease perioperative cardiac complications in patients undergoing noncardiac vascular surgery: the Statins for Risk Reduction in Surgery (StaRRS) study. J Am Coll Cardiol 2005;45:336–342.

40. Lindenauer PK, Pekow P, Wang K, et al. Lipid-lowering therapy and in-hospital mortality following major noncardiac surgery. JAMA 2004;291:2092–2099.

41. Stone NJ. Are statins indicated for the primary prevention of coronary heart disease in octogenarians? Protagonist viewpoint. Am J Geriatr Cardiol 2003;12:351–356.

42. Foody JM, Krumholz HM. Are statins indicated for the primary prevention of CAD in octogenarians? Antagonist viewpoint. Am J Geriatr Cardiol 2003;12:357–360.

43. Alter DA, Manuel DG, Gunraj N, et al. Age, risk-benefit trade-offs, and the projected effects of evidence-based therapies. Am J Med 2004;116:540–545.

44. Shepherd J, Blauw GJ, Murphy MB, et al. PROSPER Study Group. PROspective Study of Pravastatin in the Elderly at Risk. Pravastatin in elderly individuals at risk of vascular disease (PROSPER): a randomised controlled trial. Lancet 2002;360:1623–1630.

45. McGowan MP. Treating to New Target (TNT) Study Group. There is no evidence for an increase in acute coronary syndromes after short-term abrupt discontinuation of statins in stable cardiac patients. Circulation 2004;110: 2333–2335.

46. Liu LL, Dzankic S, Leung JM. Preoperative electrocardiogram abnormalities do not predict postoperative cardiac complications in geriatric surgical patients. J Am Geriatr Soc 2002;50:1186–1191.

47. Kaluza GL, Joseph J, Lee JR, et al. Catastrophic outcomes of noncardiac surgery soon after coronary stenting. J Am Coll Cardiol 2000;35:1288–1294.

48. Posner KL, Van Norman GA, Chan V. Adverse cardiac outcomes after noncardiac surgery in patients with prior percutaneous transluminal coronary angioplasty. Anesth Analg 1999;89:553–560.

49. Maisel AS. The diagnosis of acute congestive heart failure: role of BNP measurements. Heart Fail Rev 2003;8: 327–334.

50. Cowie MR, Jourdain P, Maisel A, et al. Clinical applications of B-type natriuretic peptide (BNP) testing. Eur Heart J 2003;24:1710–1718.

51. Wallen T, Landahl S, Hedner T, et al. Brain natriuretic peptide in an elderly population. J Intern Med 1997;242: 307–311.

52. Zile MR, Brutsaert DL. New concepts in diastolic dysfunction and diastolic heart failure. Part I. Diagnosis, prognosis, and measurements of diastolic function. Circulation 2002; 105:1387–1393.

53. Groban L. Diastolic dysfunction in the older heart: a review. J Cardiothorac Vasc Anesth 2005;19:228–236.

54. Somes GW, Pahor M, Shorr RI, et al. The role of diastolic blood pressure when treating isolated systolic hypertension. Arch Intern Med 1999;159:2004–2009.

55. Mitchell GF, Parise H, Benjamin EJ, et al. Changes in arterial stiffness and wave reflection with advancing age in healthy men and women: the Framingham Heart Study. Hypertension 2004;43:1239–1245.

56. Pauca AL, Kon ND, O'Rourke MF. The second peak of the radial artery pressure wave represents aortic systolic pressure in hypertensive and elderly patients. Br J Anaesth 2004;92:651–657.

57. London GM. Large artery function and alterations in hypertension. J Hypertens Suppl 1995;13:S35–38.

58. Gelman S. The pathophysiology of aortic cross-clamping and unclamping. Anesthesiology 1995;82:1026–1060.

59. Franklin SS, Jacobs MJ, Wong ND, et al. Predominance of isolated systolic hypertension among middle-aged and elderly US hypertensives: analysis based on National Health and Nutrition Examination Survey (NHANES) III. Hypertension 2001;37:869–874.

60. Kannel WB. Elevated systolic blood pressure as a cardiovascular risk factor. Am J Cardiol 2000;85:251–255.

61. Staessen JA, Gasowski J, Wang JG, et al. Risks of untreated and treated isolated systolic hypertension in the elderly: meta-analysis of outcome trials. Lancet 2000;355:865–872.

62. Vaccarino V, Berger AK, Abramson J, et al. Pulse pressure and risk of cardiovascular events in the systolic hypertension in the elderly program. Am J Cardiol 2001;88: 980–986.

63. Shammash JB, Trost JC, Gold J, et al. Perioperative beta-blocker withdrawal and mortality in vascular surgical patients. Am Heart J 2001;141:148–153.

64. Comfere T, Sprung J, Kumar MM, et al. Angiotensin system inhibitors in a general surgical population. Anesth Analg 2005;100:636–644.

65. Ryckwaert F, Colson P. Hemodynamic effects of anesthesia in patients with ischemic heart failure chronically treated with angiotensin-converting enzyme inhibitors. Anesth Analg 1997;84:945–949.

66. Coriat P, Richer C, Douraki T, et al. Influence of chronic angiotensin-converting enzyme inhibition on anesthetic induction. Anesthesiology 1994;81:299–307.

67. Bertrand M, Godet G, Meersschaert K, et al. Should the angiotensin II antagonists be discontinued before surgery? Anesth Analg 2001;92:26–30.

68. Prys-Roberts C. Hypertension and anesthesia—fifty years on. Anesthesiology 1979;50:281–284.

69. Goldman L, Caldera DL. Risks of general anesthesia and elective operation in the hypertensive patient. Anesthesiology 1979;50:285–292.

70. Howell SJ, Hemming AE, Allman KG, et al. Predictors of postoperative myocardial ischaemia. The role of intercurrent arterial hypertension and other cardiovascular risk factors. Anaesthesia 1997;52:107–111.

71. Arozullah AM, Khuri SF, Henderson WG, et al. Development and validation of a multifactorial risk index for predicting postoperative pneumonia after major noncardiac surgery. Ann Intern Med 2001;135:847–857.

72. Hall JC, Tarala RA, Hall JL, et al. A multivariate analysis of the risk of pulmonary complications after laparotomy. Chest 1991;99:923–927.

73. Swaminathan M, Stafford-Smith M. Renal dysfunction after vascular surgery. Curr Opin Anaesthesiol 2003;16:45–51.

74. Sadovnikoff N, Gelman S. Perioperative renal protection. Curr Opin Anaesthesiol 1999;12:337–341.

75. Tiggeler RG, Berden JH, Hoitsma AJ, et al. Prevention of acute tubular necrosis in cadaveric kidney transplantation

by the combined use of mannitol and moderate hydration. Ann Surg 1985;201:246–251.

76. Nicholson ML, Baker DM, Hopkinson BR, et al. Randomized controlled trial of the effect of mannitol on renal reperfusion injury during aortic aneurysm surgery. Br J Surg 1996;83:1230–1233.

77. Gelman S. Renal protection during surgical stress. Acta Anaesthesiol Scand Suppl 1997;110:43–45.

78. Phillip B, Pastor D, Bellows W, et al. The prevalence of preoperative diastolic filling abnormalities in geriatric surgical patients. Anesth Analg 2003;97:1214–1221.

79. Gilbert TB, Hasnain JU, Flinn WR, et al. Fenoldopam infusion associated with preserving renal function after aortic cross-clamping for aneurysm repair. J Cardiovasc Pharmacol Ther 2001;6:31–36.

80. Halpenny M, Rushe C, Breen P, et al. The effects of fenoldopam on renal function in patients undergoing elective aortic surgery. Eur J Anaesthesiol 2002;19:32–39.

81. Moller JT, Cluitmans P, Rasmussen LS, et al. Long-term postoperative cognitive dysfunction in the elderly ISPOCD1 study. ISPOCD investigators. International Study of Post-Operative Cognitive Dysfunction. Lancet 1998;351:857–861.

82. Frank SM, Fleisher LA, Breslow MJ, et al. Perioperative maintenance of normothermia reduces the incidence of morbid cardiac events. A randomized clinical trial. JAMA 1997;277:1127–1134.

83. Kurz A, Sessler DI, Lenhardt R. Perioperative normothermia to reduce the incidence of surgical-wound infection and shorten hospitalization. Study of Wound Infection and Temperature Group. N Engl J Med 1996;334:1209–1215.

84. Gold MR, Dec GW, Cocca-Spofford D, et al. Esmolol and ventilatory function in cardiac patients with COPD. Chest 1991;100:1215–1218.

85. Roy RC. What's New in Geriatric Anesthesia? 55th Annual Refresher Course Lectures and Basic Science Reviews. Park Ridge, IL: American Society of Anesthesiologists; 2004:109.

86. Benumof JL. Preoxygenation: best method for both efficacy and efficiency. Anesthesiology 1999;91:603–605.

87. Berg H, Roed J, Viby-Mogensen J, et al. Residual neuromuscular block is a risk factor for postoperative pulmonary complications. A prospective, randomised, and blinded study of postoperative pulmonary complications after atracurium, vecuronium and pancuronium. Acta Anaesthesiol Scand 1997;41:1095–1103.

88. Moore EW, Hunter JM. The new neuromuscular blocking agents: do they offer any advantages? Br J Anaesth 2001; 87:912–925.

89. Arain SR, Ruehlow RM, Uhrich TD, et al. The efficacy of dexmedetomidine versus morphine for postoperative analgesia after major inpatient surgery. Anesth Analg 2004;98:153–158.

90. Herr DL, Sum-Ping ST, England M. ICU sedation after coronary artery bypass graft surgery: dexmedetomidine-based versus propofol-based sedation regimens. J Cardiothorac Vasc Anesth 2003;17:576–584.

91. Talke P, Chen R, Thomas B, et al. The hemodynamic and adrenergic effects of perioperative dexmedetomidine infusion after vascular surgery. Anesth Analg 2000;90:834–839.

92. Cook DJ, Rooke GA. Priorities in perioperative geriatrics. Anesth Analg 2003;96:1823–1836.

93. Rosenfeld BA, Beattie C, Christopherson R, et al. The effects of different anesthetic regimens on fibrinolysis and the development of postoperative arterial thrombosis. Perioperative Ischemia Randomized Anesthesia Trial Study Group. Anesthesiology 1993;79:435–443.

94. Norris EJ, Beattie C, Perler BA, et al. Double-masked randomized trial comparing alternate combinations of intraoperative anesthesia and postoperative analgesia in abdominal aortic surgery. Anesthesiology 2001;95:1054–1067.

95. Roy RC. Choosing general versus regional anesthesia for the elderly. Anesthesiol Clin North Am 2000;18: 91–104.

96. Park WY, Thompson JS, Lee KK. Effect of epidural anesthesia and analgesia on perioperative outcome: a randomized, controlled Veterans Affairs cooperative study. Ann Surg 2001;234:560–569; discussion 569–571.

97. Hodgson PS, Liu SS, Gras TW. Does epidural anesthesia have general anesthetic effects? A prospective, randomized, double-blind, placebo-controlled trial. Anesthesiology 1999;91:1687–1692.

98. Inagaki Y, Mashimo T, Kuzukawa A, et al. Epidural lidocaine delays arousal from isoflurane anesthesia. Anesth Analg 1994;79:368–372.

99. Ishiyama T, Kashimoto S, Oguchi T, et al. Epidural ropivacaine anesthesia decreases the bispectral index during the awake phase and sevoflurane general anesthesia. Anesth Analg 2005;100:728–732.

100. Horlocker TT, Wedel DJ, Benzon H, et al. Regional anesthesia in the anticoagulated patient: defining the risks (the second ASRA Consensus Conference on Neuraxial Anesthesia and Anticoagulation). Reg Anesth Pain Med 2003;28:172–197.

101. Rodgers A, Walker N, Schug S, et al. Reduction of postoperative mortality and morbidity with epidural or spinal anaesthesia: results from overview of randomised trials. BMJ 2000;321:1493.

102. Siguret V, Pautas E, Gouin I. Low molecular weight heparin treatment in elderly subjects with or without renal insufficiency: new insights between June 2002 and March 2004. Curr Opin Pulm Med 2004;10:366–370.

103. Weller RS, Gerancher JC, Crews JC, et al. Extensive retroperitoneal hematoma without neurologic deficit in two patients who underwent lumbar plexus block and were later anticoagulated. Anesthesiology 2003;98:581–585.

104. Dardik A, Lin JW, Gordon TA, et al. Results of elective abdominal aortic aneurysm repair in the 1990s: a population-based analysis of 2335 cases. J Vasc Surg 1999;30: 985–995.

105. Sicard GA, Rubin BG, Sanchez LA, et al. Endoluminal graft repair for abdominal aortic aneurysms in high-risk patients and octogenarians: is it better than open repair? Ann Surg 2001;234:427–435; discussion 435–437.

106. Lobato AC, Rodriguez-Lopez J, Malik A, et al. Impact of endovascular repair for abdominal aortic aneurysms in octogenarians. Ann Vasc Surg 2001;15:525–532.

107. Minor ME, Ellozy S, Carroccio A, et al. Endovascular aortic aneurysm repair in the octogenarian: is it worthwhile? Arch Surg 2004;139:308–314.

108. Al-Omran M, Verma S, Lindsay TF, et al. Clinical decision making for endovascular repair of abdominal aortic aneurysm. Circulation 2004;110:e517–523.

109. Brinkman WT, Terramani TT, Najibi S, et al. Endovascular abdominal aortic aneurysm repair in the octogenarian. Ann Vasc Surg 2004;18:401–407.

110. Biebl M, Lau LL, Hakaim AG, et al. Midterm outcome of endovascular abdominal aortic aneurysm repair in octogenarians: a single institution's experience. J Vasc Surg 2004;40:435–442.

111. Chaikof EL, Blankensteijn JD, Harris PL, et al. Ad Hoc Committee for Standardized Reporting Practices in Vascular Surgery of The Society for Vascular Surgery/American Association for Vascular Surgery. Reporting standards for endovascular aortic aneurysm repair. J Vasc Surg 2002;35:1048–1060.

112. Kahn RA, Moskowitz DM, Marin M, et al. Anesthetic considerations for endovascular aortic repair. Mt Sinai J Med 2002;69:57–67.

113. Teufelsbauer H, Prusa AM, Wolff K, et al. Endovascular stent grafting versus open surgical operation in patients with infrarenal aortic aneurysms: a propensity score-adjusted analysis. Circulation 2002;106:782–787.

114. European Carotid Surgery Trialists' Collaborative Group. MRC European Carotid Surgery Trial: interim results for symptomatic patients with severe (70–99%) or with mild (0–29%) carotid stenosis. Lancet 1991;337:1235–1243.

115. North American Symptomatic Carotid Endarterectomy Trial Collaborators. Beneficial effect of carotid endarterectomy in symptomatic patients with high-grade carotid stenosis. N Engl J Med 1991;325:445–453.

116. Rerkasem K, Bond R, Rothwell PM. Local versus general anaesthesia for carotid endarterectomy. Cochrane Database Syst Rev 2004;(2):CD000126.

117. Groban L, Deal DD, Vernon JC, et al. Cardiac resuscitation after incremental overdosage with lidocaine, bupivacaine, levobupivacaine, and ropivacaine in anesthetized dogs. Anesth Analg 2001;92:37–43.

118. Ackerstaff RG, van de Vlasakker CJ. Monitoring of brain function during carotid endarterectomy: an analysis of contemporary methods. J Cardiothorac Vasc Anesth 1998; 12:341–347.

119. Stoughton J, Nath RL, Abbott WM. Comparison of simultaneous electroencephalographic and mental status monitoring during carotid endarterectomy with regional anesthesia. J Vasc Surg 1998;28:1014–1021; discussion 1021–1023.

120. Wholey MH, Wholey M. Current status in cervical carotid artery stent placement. J Cardiovasc Surg (Torino) 2003;44: 331–339.

121. Mozes G, Sullivan TM, Torres-Russotto DR, et al. Carotid endarterectomy in SAPPHIRE-eligible high-risk patients: implications for selecting patients for carotid angioplasty and stenting. J Vasc Surg 2004;39:958–966.

122. Bettmann MA, Dake MD, Hopkins LN, et al. American Heart Association. Atherosclerotic Vascular Disease Conference: Writing Group VI: revascularization. Circulation 2004;109:2643–2650.

123. Coward LJ, Featherstone RL, Brown MM. Percutaneous transluminal angioplasty and stenting for carotid artery stenosis. Cochrane Database Syst Rev 2004;(2): CD000515.

124. Bohner H, Friedrichs R, Habel U, et al. Delirium increases morbidity and length of stay after vascular surgery operations. Results of a prospective study [German]. Chirurg 2003;74:931–936.

125. Moller JT, Cluitmans P, Rasmussen LS, et al. Long-term postoperative cognitive dysfunction in the elderly ISPOCD1 study. ISPOCD Investigators. International Study of Post-Operative Cognitive Dysfunction. Lancet 1998;351:857–861.

126. Monk TG, Saini V, Weldon BC, et al. Anesthetic management and one-year mortality after noncardiac surgery. Anesth Analg 2005;100:4–10.

127. Weldon BC, Mahla ME, van der Aa MT, et al. Advancing age and deeper intraoperative anesthetic levels are associated with higher first year death rates. Anesthesiology 2002;97(Suppl):A1097.

128. Rasmussen LS, Johnson T, Kuipers HM, et al. ISPOCD2 (International Study of Postoperative Cognitive Dysfunction) Investigators. Does anaesthesia cause postoperative cognitive dysfunction? A randomised study of regional versus general anaesthesia in 438 elderly patients. Acta Anaesthesiol Scand 2003;47:260–266.

129. Hebert PC, Wells G, Blajchman MA, et al. A multicenter, randomized, controlled clinical trial of transfusion requirements in critical care. Transfusion Requirements in Critical Care Investigators, Canadian Critical Care Trials Group. N Engl J Med 1999;340:409–417.

130. Nelson AH, Fleisher LA, Rosenbaum SH. Relationship between postoperative anemia and cardiac morbidity in high-risk vascular patients in the intensive care unit. Crit Care Med 1993;21:860–866.

131. Wu WC, Rathore SS, Wang Y, et al. Blood transfusion in elderly patients with acute myocardial infarction. N Engl J Med 2001;345:1230–1236.

132. Bush RL, Pevec WC, Holcroft JW. A prospective, randomized trial limiting perioperative red blood cell transfusions in vascular patients. Am J Surg 1997;174:143–148.

133. van den Berghe G, Wouters P, Weekers F, et al. Intensive insulin therapy in the critically ill patients. N Engl J Med 2001;345:1359–1367.

134. Sander O, Welters ID, Foex P, et al. Impact of prolonged elevated heart rate on incidence of major cardiac events in critically ill patients with a high risk of cardiac complications. Crit Care Med 2005;33:81–88; discussion 241–242.

29
Abdominal Procedures

Jeffrey H. Silverstein

Operations on the abdominal viscera are common among the elderly. Few of the operations are truly elective, with the majority being either scheduled reasonably shortly after a diagnostic procedure or truly emergent procedures necessitated by the presence of an intraabdominal catastrophe. The impact of abdominal surgery on the elderly is significant and the potential for complications is high. This chapter synthesizes current thought to provide an approach to the elderly abdominal surgical patient including both emergent and elective surgeries. It should be stated that there are relatively few prospective trials regarding the perioperative management of abdominal surgery in the elderly. There is a good amount of retrospectively acquired information that provides direction to both current care paradigms as well as ongoing research. Major vascular surgery may involve an abdominal approach; however, vascular surgery, particularly in the elderly, is becoming the province of endovascular surgery and is not covered in this chapter.

General Principles

Presentation

The presentation of abdominal symptoms in the elderly is frequently diminished, muted, or less specific than in younger patients. Significant numbers of patients over the age of 65 do not manifest classic symptoms of cholecystitis.[1] Sixty percent did not have typical upper quadrant pain and 5% had no pain at all. Less than half were febrile. Approximately 30% of patients with peptic ulcer disease do not complain of pain and frequently the first sign of ulcer disease is perforation.[2] However, pain out of proportion to all physical findings remains the most common and prominent symptom of acute mesenteric ischemia, a frequently fatal disease in older patients. Lyon and Clark[3] have recently reviewed the general approach to the diagnosis of abdominal pain in the elderly. Anes-

thesiologists do not generally participate in the diagnosis of abdominal disease; however, they should be aware that, because symptoms are frequently nonspecific, by the time the patient arrives in the operating room (OR) they are potentially sicker than would be the case for younger patients. It is not uncommon for a patient to be relatively stable at the beginning of the operation only to become very unstable as the pathology evolves either in the OR or not long thereafter.

Outcomes from Abdominal Surgery

As explained in the first chapter, many patients approach the outcomes from their proposed surgery not in terms of whether their wound will heal, but on how it will affect their function and independence. The return to preoperative levels of independent activities of daily living can take up to 6 months after abdominal surgery. The landmark study by Lawrence et al.[4] indicated that function returns in a progressive manner with activities of daily living returning before the independent activities which, in turn, recover quicker than some measures of physical strength. It should be noted that the data of Lawrence et al. were collected before widespread use of laparoscopic surgical techniques. There have been a number of reports of a combined multimodal approach to primarily colonic surgery patients.[5] Included in the program is early ambulation and discharge home within 2 days of surgery. These programs have reported some success and seem to indicate a capacity to recover more rapidly from abdominal surgery than the cases reported by Lawrence.

The risk of surgery in patients older than 90 years was evaluated by Denney and Denson.[6] Their report on 272 patients undergoing 301 operations at the University of Southern California Medical Center found that the risk was more than justified in at least 70% of the nonagenarians. However, they did find that serious bowel obstruction was associated with a prohibitive perioperative mortality rate (63%), even though there is rarely an alternative to surgery. Reviewing their experience many years ago, Djokovic and Hedley-Whyte[7] reported that mortality in 500 patients older than 80 years was predicted by the American Society of Anesthesiologists (ASA) physical status classification. Fewer than 1% of ASA 2 patients died whereas 25% of ASA 4 patients died. At the time (1979), myocardial infarction was the leading cause of postoperative death. In a cohort of 2291 patients evaluated between 1982 and 1991, pulmonary complications were found to be more frequent and associated with longer hospital stays than cardiac complications.[8] The data support the idea that risk is not a function of chronologic age but rather of coexisting disease and physical status. The ASA physical score does not specifically include age as a factor, although many clinicians probably factor their assessment of the impact of age on their assessment of functional status.

Both the relative risks and potential benefits associated with anesthesia and major abdominal surgery need to be individually assessed for each elderly patient. The elderly patient, as described in many of the preceding chapters, may have relatively intact function of all systems with limited alterations that limit the ability to respond to stress, or they may have function that is suboptimal and limiting even at rest. The heterogeneity between patients and even within a patient is important to keep in mind as any given patient is assessed. The goals of the planned therapy should be clear to the anesthesia and surgical teams. Maximization of longevity by means of a definitive or curative major surgical procedure may be a very appropriate option for elderly patients, but some patients may prefer a functional result short of cure. Patients may have alternative needs based on their perception of risk, concerns regarding independence and immediate responsibilities for spouses among myriad issues. Although the anesthesiologist must carefully assess all systems to understand the physiologic status of any given patient, the decision to pursue a surgical procedure has typically been made by the patient and their surgeon. Emergency surgery has repeatedly been shown to be an independent predictor of adverse postoperative outcomes in older surgical patients undergoing noncardiac surgery.[9,10] It has long been speculated that poorer preoperative physiology and preparation have a large influence on these results. The challenge is to prepare the patient expeditiously and minimize risks where intervention has the potential to make a difference.

Consent and Health Proxy

The care team should have a clear idea of how decisions will be made should the patient not be able to decide for themselves for some period of time after surgery. Regulations regarding health care proxies, next of kin and surrogate decision making, and the role of physicians in emergency decision making vary state by state. Particularly for emergent surgeries on patients with impaired capacity to consent, how the decision to proceed with surgery is made should be clear to the anesthesia team. Some jurisdictions allow physicians to make decisions regarding the need for emergency treatment, others do not and, surprisingly, some states do not have clear regulation for surrogate decision making in the absence of a formal health proxy. Assessment of the capacity to consent to a procedure is not clearly standardized. A reasonable expectation is that an individual consenting to surgery should be able to reiterate what procedure is being done and why. Asking a patient to reiterate the risks of a procedure may indicate understanding, but can also increase anxiety and is rarely required. Some jurisdictions require a separate anesthesia consent. It is best if there is a standard procedure to follow if there is a disagreement among the perioperative staff as to the patient's capacity to consent. The appropriate local approach to "do not resuscitate" orders in place for patients brought to the OR should be clear to the anesthesia team. This area remains controversial.[11] If policy and time permit, the anesthesiologist should have a clear discussion with the patient and appropriate family members regarding the appropriate approach to different circumstances that occur in the immediate perioperative period. Even if the do not resuscitate order remains in effect, once intubated for general anesthesia it is not possible to remove an endotracheal tube in the absence of a reasonable assessment that the patient will breathe spontaneously. Patients and families who have indicated that they do want to "end up intubated on a ventilator" need to understand how endotracheal intubation will be managed in a given patient.

Preoperative Care

Preanesthetic Evaluation

For emergency surgery, a comprehensive geriatric assessment may be difficult. Given the opportunity, the perioperative team should have a complete understanding of the physical, psychosocial, and environmental factors that can affect the health of the patient, with the goal of optimizing functional outcomes.[12] (See also Chapter 1.) Although the anesthesiologist might not be the obvious person to collect this information, there is no existential reason opposing it. Regardless of how the preparation of elderly surgical patients is organized, there must be mechanisms to capture this information, which will be important to properly design postoperative care plans.

Frailty is a term used to characterize the weakest and most vulnerable subset of older adults. Frailty does not

TABLE 29-1. Changes in cardiovascular parameters in elderly patients at rest and with exercise.

Cardiovascular parameter	Aging effect at rest	Aging effect with exercise
Heart rate	No change or slight decrease	Less increase
Systolic blood pressure	Increased	Greater increase
Diastolic blood pressure	No change	Slightly greater increase
Cardiac output	No change	Slightly less increase
Ejection fraction	No change	Less increase
Stroke volume	No change or slight increase	Greater increase

fit neatly into a system-based assessment for preanesthetic evaluation and is almost never the chief complaint or presenting symptom for a surgical patient. The current clinical model for frailty focuses on muscle loss (sarcopenia) and diminished strength,[13] although many of those interested in the field tend to refer to the broader concept of homeostenosis or decreased ability to respond to a broad array of stressors.[14] The majority of work on this concept has been applied retrospectively to cohorts of medical patients and has demonstrated that frailty is related to increased vulnerability and poor health outcomes.[13] Specific research into the utility of frailty as a means of assessment and risk stratification or as a target of perioperative intervention is just beginning. Although it seems reasonable to be concerned about the frail elderly, it is not currently possible to make any specific or general evidence-based recommendations.

Age-related changes in cardiac function have been described as emanating primarily from alterations in the stiffness of the aorta, ultimately resulting in systolic hypertension, concentric left ventricular hypertrophy, and delayed relaxation of the left ventricle. Nonetheless, the resting cardiac function of an elderly patient, in the absence of specific cardiovascular disease, should be fairly normal (Table 29-1) and the ability to respond to stress (or exercise) is somewhat, but not seriously, limiting. If noticeable cardiac functional decline is present, this should not be attributed to old age, but rather requires a coherent pathophysiologic explanation.

Diastolic function is currently conceived as an important aspect of aging and age-related cardiovascular disease. Phillip et al.[15] reported on 251 patients whose mean age was 72 ± 7 years to determine the prevalence of diastolic abnormalities. They found that only 36.5% of the patients had normal diastolic filling. Mild dysfunction was most common (48.3%), but 9.6% had mild to moderate abnormalities, 3.9% had pseudonormal filling properties, and 1.7% of patients were considered to have severe abnormalities suggestive of a restrictive pattern. Of the patients with ejection fractions >50%, 61.5% had diastolic filling abnormalities.

Pulmonary function gradually declines in the elderly, even in those who exercise in order to maintain aerobic capacity. Aging is associated with structural changes such as decreases in lung static elastic recoil and chest wall compliance, and functional changes such as impaired respiratory muscle strength and alterations in responses to hypoxia. In the absence of pathology, the aging process does not limit a patient's respiratory capacity, although the capacity to markedly increase respiration in response to a challenge is markedly limited. How these factors interact with the stress associated with surgery and anesthesia is of primary importance because postoperative respiratory complications account for approximately 40% of the perioperative deaths in patients over 65 years of age.[16] In evaluating a patient, the practitioner should keep in mind that the breathing pattern of elderly patients typically involves smaller tidal volumes and an increased respiratory rate. This can be further exacerbated by intraabdominal pathology. Between the ages of 40 and 75, the PaO_2 (mm Hg) decreases, with significant relationship to changes in both $Paco_2$ and the body mass index (BMI). The following equation provides a reasonable estimate: PaO_2 (mm Hg) = 143.6 − (0.39 × age) − (0.56 × BMI) − (0.57 × $Paco_2$). After 75 years of age, arterial oxygen tension remains unaffected by BMI and PaO_2, and remains relatively stable at around 83 mm Hg.[17] A deterioration of protective mechanisms of cough and swallowing in the elderly may lead to ineffective clearance of secretions and increased susceptibility to aspiration. Loss of protective upper-airway reflexes has been postulated to be related to an age-related peripheral deafferentation together with a decreased central nervous system reflex activity.[18]

Renal Assessment

Multiple alterations in normal renal function and fluid and electrolyte balance are seen in the aging (Table 29-2). Assessment of fluid status is problematic in the older patient. Skin turgor is difficult to interpret because the loss of elasticity and thinning of the dermis makes skin appear dehydrated. The decrease in thirst sensation makes a lack of thirst not useful. Even urine output is suspect because of the possibility of inappropriately dilute urine being excreted. Estimating the patients glomerular filtration rate allows the practitioner to develop an expectation of how quickly administered fluid and medications may be excreted. Estimating equations provide some guidance but are often not accurate for

TABLE 29-2. Alteration in fluid balance in the elderly.

Decrease in total body water	Young body is 65% water, 80-year-old body 50%
Kidney	
Decrease in renal cortical mass	20% loss, primarily cortex by age 85
Decline in renal blood flow	10% decline/decade
Decrease in glomerular filtration rate	Down 10 mL/decade, 50% by age 80
Decrease in urinary concentrating ability	Less sensitivity to antidiuretic hormone
Increase in antidiuretic hormone	Increase relative to osmolality, decreased in Alzheimer's disease
Increase in atrial natriuretic peptide	Fivefold over basal levels
Decrease in aldosterone	
Decrease in thirst mechanism	
Decrease in free water clearance	

a given patient. Therefore, an actual measurement of glomerular filtration rate is preferable.[19] When medications that require careful control of plasma levels are used, drug levels should be measured. The combination of senescence in fluid management and the current understanding of cardiovascular aging suggest that the therapeutic window for intravenous fluid is markedly narrowed.

Patients presenting for emergent surgery, particularly those with bowel obstruction, present an important dilemma regarding preoperative fluid preparation. Patients who have been vomiting and or undergoing upper gastrointestinal decompression with a nasogastric tube may be significantly intravascularly dehydrated. Ideally, rehydration of these patients should begin immediately upon their admission to the hospital and continue through any diagnostic procedures that are undertaken. If the patient's rehydration is not accomplished before surgery, the anesthesiologist is faced with the decision to delay operation in order to resuscitate the patient and hopefully ameliorate cardiovascular instability during induction and maintenance of anesthesia. Most studies of hemodynamic optimization have involved the use of a pulmonary artery catheter and have produced extremely controversial results. A meta-analysis and review in 1996 concluded that achieving supranormal hemodynamic goals did not reduce mortality in critically ill patients.[20] In subsequent years, the distinction between patients who had signs of organ failure at the time of resuscitation compared with those whose organ function was intact when therapy was instituted suggested that such therapy applied sufficiently early in the clinical course could be effective. In a recent review of nearly 2000 patients in 17 randomized controlled trials designed to increase tissue perfusion in the perioperative period, Boyd[21] concluded

that there was a significant reduction in mortality in the treatment group [odds ratios 0.45 (95% confidence interval 0.33–0.60)]. A similar review from Kern and Shoemaker[22] essentially agreed, indicating that patients who achieved an increase in oxygen delivery before the onset of organ dysfunction had decreased perioperative mortality. Essentially, all of the published trials of optimization of oxygen delivery for elderly patients undergoing either elective or emergent abdominal surgery have been conducted preoperatively in intensive care units, rather than in the OR. However, the ability to undertake preoperative optimization is frequently limited by facilities and staff. Therefore, it seems prudent to advise that patients who are assessed to have a high risk of organ failure (signs of severe dehydration and particularly those showing early signs of shock physiology) should undergo an attempt to improve oxygen delivery, initially using fluids but potentially including autonomic stimulation as well, before the induction of anesthesia. If feasible, this tune-up is probably best done over a number of hours in an intensive care environment. Preoperative optimization of elderly patients presenting for most elective surgeries is generally not necessary. Indeed, as discussed below, there is a strong argument to be made for the administration of significantly less intravenous fluid than is frequently prescribed.

Bowel Preparation

Many patients presenting for bowel surgery have undergone some type of preparation to clean out their bowel. These preparations have the potential for altering the fluid and electrolyte balance of the patient. Although not the general province of the anesthesiologist, a short overview of what is used and the associated side effects is useful. The literature for bowel preparation has been developed primarily by endoscopists and is the subject of a recent consensus statement and addendum prepared by a task force from the American Society of Colon and Rectal Surgeons, the American Society for Gastrointestinal Endoscopy, and the Society of American Gastrointestinal and Endoscopic Surgeons.[23] Tolerance and effectiveness of preparations for bowel surgery vary. Most preparations use either polyethylene glycol, an osmotically balanced electrolyte lavage solution or other osmotic laxatives such as sodium phosphate (NaP) or magnesium citrate. The polyethylene glycol preparations are effective, but 4 L of fluid can be difficult to tolerate. NaP preparations may be safe in selected healthy elderly patients. Elderly patients were found to be at an increased risk for phosphate intoxication. Administration of NaP causes a significant increase in serum phosphate, even in patients with normal creatinine clearance. Hypokalemia is more prevalent in frail patients.[24] Other adverse effects on the elderly using oral preparations range from confusion, dehydration with tongue dryness, and upper-body muscle weakness to electrolyte disturbances.

There is considerably less agreement on the need for orthograde bowel preparation for colorectal surgery. Although this is clearly the standard of care in many facilities, a recent meta-analysis of 10 randomized trials comparing cleansing with no bowel preparation showed a significant increase in anastomotic dehiscences and a trend toward increased surgical infections and reoperation even though mortality was unchanged by orthograde bowel cleansing.[25] The anesthesiologist caring for colorectal surgery patients should inquire as to whether they underwent some type of bowel preparation.

Interaction with Geriatricians

Excellent results have been reported for programs specifically designed to address issues that are uniquely or primarily geriatric that could be easily integrated into perioperative care regimens.[26,27] The Hospital Elder Life Program (Table 29-3) is designed to prevent delirium. Although the results of this and other programs have been promising in early trials, the ability to implement such plans varies among institutions[28,29] and much remains to be learned about the general utility as well as applicability of these programs to the perioperative period.[30] Much of the care offered by these geriatric-focused programs are not specifically reimbursable under current insurance programs, such that funding for these programs can be difficult to obtain. However, these are the types of programs you would want in place if your grandmother needed surgery.

TABLE 29-3. Contents of the Hospital Elder Life Program.

- Daily Visitor Program: cognitive orientation, communication, and social support
- Therapeutic Activities Program: cognitive stimulation and socialization
- Early Mobilization Program: daily exercise and walking assistance
- Non-Pharmacologic Sleep Protocol: promotes relaxation and sufficient sleep
- Hearing and Vision Protocol: hearing and vision adaptations and equipment
- Oral Volume Repletion and Feeding Assistance Program: assistance and companionship during meals
- Geriatric Interdisciplinary Care: nursing, medicine, rehabilitation therapies, pharmacy, nutrition and chaplaincy care, and support for patients and their families
- Provider Education Program: geriatric education for professional staff
- Links with Community Services: assist with the transition from hospital to home

Data from Inouye et al.,[26] and from McDowell JA, Mion LC, Lydon TJ, Inouye SK. A nonpharmacologic sleep protocol for hospitalized older patients. J Am Geriatr Soc 1998;46(6):700–705.

Intraoperative Care

Intravenous Access and Choice of Monitoring

There are no studies that have specifically addressed intravenous access in the elderly. The following suggestions are based on the author's personal experience. The skin of the elderly is thin with relatively diminished elasticity. A catheter size that will easily fit in the vein selected for cannulation should be chosen. A tight fit will easily disrupt the vein, causing a potentially large widespread hematoma. The skin surrounding the vein must be stretched and fixed with the nondominant hand to facilitate entrance of the intravenous catheter into the vein. This maneuver also straightens and fixes tortuous veins. The vein is usually not as "deep" as younger patients. Once in the vein, the catheter itself should be advanced without releasing the tension on the surrounding skin. This generally requires advancing the catheter with the index finger of the dominant hand. Cannulation of a vein, as well as general comfort for the elderly, can be facilitated by the institution of a forced-air warming system immediately upon entrance to the OR. The patient does not shiver and the veins dilate slightly in response to the warmth. At least two intravenous cannulas should be considered for major surgical cases. When the arms are not visually accessible to the anesthesiologists, great concern for vein rupture should always be considered when an infusion set ceases to flow easily. The arms should be visualized before any pressure is applied to the infusion system.

Particularly fragile skin on the upper arm or an upper arm with excess skin relative to muscle mass may predispose to bruising from the blood pressure cuff. This can be prevented to a certain extent by a layer or two of cotton wadding (Webril and others) typically available from the OR nurses. Oscillometric blood pressure measurement can be difficult in the presence of substantial arrhythmias. A decision to place an intraarterial cannula for invasive blood pressure measurement and frequent blood sampling is based on the same considerations applied to younger patients. Age per se is not an indication for intraarterial blood pressure measurement; however, age-related alterations and coexisting disease may easily persuade the experienced practitioner to institute such monitoring. Whether such monitoring is instituted before or after induction of anesthesia is based on experience and local practice, because no clear evidence exists to specifically recommend either practice.

The evidence regarding measurement of central venous versus pulmonary artery pressure has not been specifically addressed regarding elderly patients. To the extent that central venous pressures or pulmonary artery pressures reflect intravascular volume, they can be useful. Multiple recent randomized studies of the pulmonary artery catheter have failed to demonstrate an advantage over central venous pressure monitoring and have been associated with increased complication rates.[31,32] Transesophageal echocardiography has been proposed as a particularly effective tool for evaluating the geriatric heart.[15] Echocardiography is the only means currently available for detecting diastolic dysfunction, which is present in a significant number of the elderly. Echocardiography requires expensive equipment and extensive training, particularly to distinguish findings such as diastolic dysfunction. In the absence of direct outcome data, it is not possible to recommend routine echocardiographic monitoring of elderly abdominal surgery patients. Noninvasive monitoring of physiologic variables (primarily cardiac output), which has been successfully used in elderly trauma patients, should also be helpful in surgical cardiovascular management.[33]

Renna and Venturi[34] found that although age-related electroencephalogram differences exist in the normal population, the bispectral index (BIS, Aspect Systems) still correlates with the depth of sedation independently of age. Senile dementia may be associated with significantly lower BIS values.

Urinary catheters provide important information during longer surgeries but their use may promote urinary incontinence and urinary tract infections in the elderly. Studies of elderly patients undergoing orthopedic surgery tend to favor avoidance of a catheter if the indication is weak, and removal of the catheter within 24 hours with the use of intermittent straight catheterization. These approaches tend to diminish urinary retention, but not infection rates.[35,36] A more intensive infection prevention program has recently demonstrated a decrease in the incidence of urinary tract infection from 10.4 to 3.9 episodes per 100 patients.[37]

The physiology of thermal stability and the importance of maintaining normothermia in elderly patients are described in detail in Chapter 8. Every effort should be engaged to maintain normal temperatures in abdominal surgery patients.

Patient positioning can be important.[38] At times, the patient's ability to move extremities into certain positions should be explored with the patient awake in order to avoid damaging an extremity under anesthesia. Look for pressure spots, particularly around the sacrum and heels and provide padding. Patients with severe spine deformities can represent a challenge to pad appropriately; however, this should be done with the goal of not only preventing nerve damage, but also avoiding skin breakdown and undue stretch on contracted tendons and ligaments.

Choosing an Epidural Catheter

There is a longstanding debate regarding whether neuraxial techniques such as epidural analgesia reduces the frequency of postoperative complications. Pulmonary and central nervous system complications (delirium and postoperative cognitive dysfunction) have been the principal focus. Although there is no doubt that these techniques provide excellent analgesia and patient satisfaction, their benefit regarding various outcomes is much less clear.[39] Epidural anesthesia/analgesia is an integral part of the multiple modal approach to abdominal surgery developed by Kehlet and colleagues in Denmark.[40] This approach to anesthesia for abdominal surgery is described below. Some meta-analyses have concluded that there is benefit to epidural analgesia; however, many of the studies used in these analyses are plagued with several problems.

Jayr et al.[41] studied 153 patients undergoing abdominal cancer surgery randomized to receive either continuous epidural bupivacaine and morphine, or subcutaneous morphine infusion. This carefully designed study found no difference in pulmonary complications even in patients with preexisting pulmonary dysfunction. The authors did note that the epidural provided superior postoperative analgesia. Norris et al.[42] randomized 168 patients undergoing abdominal aortic aneurysm and found essentially the same result.

Variations on Anesthetic Plans for the Elderly

Most abdominal surgery is accomplished using general anesthesia. Lower abdominal procedures can be done using a primarily regional technique with the addition of sedation. Adjustments to regional technique for elderly patients are described in Chapter 19. Despite numerous attempts to show superiority of regional versus general anesthesia, substantive reviews of the subject[39,43,44] have failed to show a substantial difference in outcomes. Because many, if not most, procedures are currently undertaken using laparoscopic techniques, the need to create a pneumoperitoneum and to frequently adjust the position of the patient makes the use of general endotracheal anesthesia the preferred technique. Patients presenting for emergency surgery are typically administered general anesthesia, although there may be cases that can appropriately be accomplished with regional techniques.

Laparoscopic surgery has been promoted as being less stressful, particularly for elderly patients. The actual advantage has yet to be clearly delimited; however, there is little reason to specifically select an open surgical technique if a laparoscopic technique is technically feasible.[45,46]

Elderly patients being prepared for general anesthesia require additional time to successfully achieve proper denitrogenation (preoxygenation). Patients with severe abdominal pain or distension can have limited respiratory effort. Supplemental oxygen should be considered early in the treatment plan for such patients and continued 4–5 days into the postoperative period.[47,48] It has been suggested that a full 3-minute period for preoxygenation be used in elderly patients to effectively prevent hypoxemia during the induction and intubation process.[49] Elderly patients are prone to decreased muscular pharyngeal support and decreased upper airway reflexes thought to be secondary to age-related neural deafferentation.[50] The general approach to patients with a propensity for aspiration is to use a rapid sequence induction of general anesthesia, which incorporates cricothyroid pressure to occlude the upper esophagus. Occlusion of the esophagus is purported to prevent passive regurgitation. There have been no studies that support this beneficial result from cricoid pressure although there are substantial numbers of reports indicating that it is ineffective and at times hampers intubation.[51,52] This procedure is so ingrained in United States anesthesia practice that it is hard to suggest that it not be used. Practitioners should at least be willing to release cricoid pressure should it appear to be impeding intubation.

There is little to suggest a specific drug choice for either induction or maintenance of anesthesia based on aging physiology. Most comparisons of specific agents are based on recovery times. Regimens are usually found to be safe and effective without clinically significant advantages.[53–55] It is clear that the doses of most common agents, with the primary exception of neuromuscular blocking agents, are decreased in aged patients (Table 29-4). Particular care should be taken with those patients whose hemodynamic stability is in question at the beginning of an anesthetic.

A multimodal approach to perioperative care that seeks to reduce the stress response and organ dysfunction leading to earlier recovery has been extensively studied and promoted by Kehlet.[56] One of the principal endpoints of this approach, which is also referred to as fast-track surgery, is to accelerate the recovery process and get the patient out of the hospital quickly. This approach to elective surgery has been used primarily in colon surgery. The approach begins with extensive preoperative counseling with the patient. The patients do not undergo bowel preparation (except enemas), receive no sedative premedication, and are not fasted but rather receive carbohydrate-loaded liquids until 2 hours before surgery. The anesthetic combines a thoracic epidural catheter plus short-acting inhalational anesthetic agents. Patients are mobilized and fed early on the first postoperative day (Table 29-5). Results from fast-track colonic surgery suggest that postoperative pulmonary, cardiovascular, and muscle function are improved and body composition preserved as well as providing the potential to achieve a normal oral intake of energy and protein. In a recent controlled study of 160 patients, hospital stay was reduced from 7.5 days to 3.4 days.[5] In this group, functional recovery, as measured by activities of daily living, was not improved. Despite a higher risk for readmissions, overall costs and morbidity seem to be reduced. This approach has been shown clearly to be safe for elderly patients. For those who recover more rapidly, the program seems to be beneficial; however, one cannot expect all elderly patients to recover more rapidly. The utility of this approach has yet to be explored extensively in the United States. Because the program includes not only specific medical interventions (e.g., thoracic epidural analgesia) but also behavioral components that require a different approach by both the patient as well as doctors and nurses, it is necessary to reserve judgment as to whether this approach will effectively save resources in the United States system. Hopefully, this information will be available in the near future.

These considerations should not discourage the use of these valuable techniques in the elderly, but the evidence does not support their use to minimize pulmonary complications. The use of a full range of adjunctive analgesia techniques, such as infiltration with local anesthetics, peripheral nerve blocks, nonsteroidal antiinflammatory agents, and others as part of a "multimodal" approach is appropriate.

The one study that has evaluated atelectasis formation in the elderly included 45 patients between the ages of 23 and 69. Although 87% of subjects developed some atelectasis, the degree of atelectasis was not associated with age.[57] Nonetheless, in the presence of limited reserve capacity, the impact of atelectasis can be severe and is best prevented. The application of positive end-expiratory pressure does not predictably reverse atelectasis or increase arterial oxygenation unless preceded by a prolonged vital capacity breath with high inflation pressures, referred to as a "recruitment maneuver."[58–60] A peak opening inspiratory pressure of at least 40 cm H_2O is needed to fully reverse anesthesia-induced collapse of healthy lungs. Blood pressure should be monitored during a recruitment maneuver because of its potential to induce hypotension.

Fluid Management in the Elderly

There is a continuing debate about the type and quantity of fluid that should be administered during elective major surgery, particularly in the elderly. There is a substantial collection of publications that describe the adverse effects of excess fluid. Persistent positive fluid balance in older surgical patients is associated with prolonged mechanical ventilation.[61] Itobi et al.[62] found that elderly patients were more likely to develop edema and that the presence of edema was associated with a delay in tolerating solid food, opening bowels, a prolonged hospital stay [median 17 (range 8–59) versus 9 (range 4–27) days], and more postoperative complications (13 of 20 versus 4 of 18 patients; p = 0.011). Fluid replacement for abdominal

TABLE 29-4. Age-related pharmacologic changes of anesthetics and drugs in anesthesia practice.

Anesthetic/drug	Pharmacodynamics	Pharmacokinetics	Anesthetic management
Inhalational anesthetics	Sensitivity of the brain↑ (cerebral metabolic rate)↓	Ventilation/perfusion mismatch with slow increase of alveolar/inspired ratio of inhaled gases; maximal cardiac output;↓ volume of distribution↑	Minimal alveolar concentration down 30%; slower induction and emergence; delayed but more profound onset of anesthesia
Hypnotics			
Thiopental	No changes	Central volume of distribution;↓ intercompartmental clearance↑	Induction dose reduced by 15% (20-year-old patient: 2.5–5.0 mg/kg IV; 80-year-old patient: 2.1 mg/kg IV). Maintenance dose: same requirements 60 minutes after starting a continuation infusion. Emergence: slightly faster
Propofol	No changes	Central volume of distribution;↓ intercompartmental clearance↑	Induction dose reduced by 20% (slower induction requires lower doses) (20-year-old: 2.0–3.0 mg/kg IV; 80-year-old: 1.7 mg/kg IV). Maintenance dose: same requirements 120 minutes after starting a continuous infusion. Emergence: slightly faster (?)
Midazolam	Sensitivity of the brain↑	Clearance↓	Sedation/induction dose reduced by 50% (20-year-old: 0.07–0.15 mg/kg IV; 80-year-old: 0.02–0.03 mg/kg IV). Maintenance dose reduced by 25%. Recovery: delayed (hours)
Etomidate	No changes	Central clearance;↓ volume of distribution↑	Induction dose reduced by 20% (20-year-old: 0.3 mg/kg IV; 80-year-old: 0.2 mg/kg IV). Emergence: slightly faster (?)
Ketamine	?	?	Use with caution: hallucinations, seizures, mental disturbance, release of catecholamines; avoid in combination with levodopa (tachycardia, arterial hypertension)
Opioids			
Fentanyl, alfentanil, sufentanil	Sensitivity of the brain↑	No changes	Induction dose reduced by 50%. Maintenance doses reduced by 30%–50%. Emergence: may be delayed
Remifentanil	Sensitivity of the brain↑	Central volume of distribution;↓ intercompartmental clearance↓	Induction dose reduced by 50%. Maintenance dose reduced by 70%. Emergence: may be delayed
Muscle relaxants			
Mivacurium, succinylcholine	No changes	Plasma cholinesterase;↓ muscle blood flow;↓ cardiac output;↓ intercompartmental clearance↓	Onset time.↑ Maintenance dose requirements.↓ Duration of action↑ clinically indistinguishable from mivacurium. Differences: no changes in initial dose, prolonged block with metoclopramide
Pancuronium, doxacuronium, pipecuronium, vecuronium, rocuronium	No changes	Muscle blood↓ flow; cardiac output;↓ intercompartmental clearance;↓ clearance; (volume of distribution)↓	Onset time.↑ Maintenance dose requirements.↓ Duration of action.↑ Recommended dose reduced by 20%
Atracurium	No changes	No changes	No changes
Reversal agents			
Neostigmine, pyridostigmine	No changes	Clearance↓	Duration of action;↑↑ because muscle relaxants have a markedly prolonged duration of action, larger doses of reversal agents are needed in elderly patients
Edrophonium	No changes	No changes	No change
Local anesthetics	Sensitivity of the nervous tissue (?)↑	Hepatic microsomal metabolism of amide local anesthetics [lidocaine (lignocaine), bupivacaine];↓ plasma protein binding;↓ cephalad spread↑	Epidural (and spinal) dose requirements.↓ Duration of spinal and epidural anesthesia seems clinically independent of age, toxicity↑ (percent free drug)↑

↑, increase; ↓, decrease.

Source: Modified with permission from Silverstein JH, Zaugg M. Geriatrics. In: Hemmings HC, Hopkins PM, eds. Foundations of Anesthesia: Basic and Clinical Science. 2nd ed. London: Elsevier Mosby; 2006.

TABLE 29-5. Care program in patients undergoing colonic resection with fast-track care.

Preoperatively
Information of surgical procedure, expected length of stay, and
daily milestones for recovery

Day of surgery
Mobilized 2 hours
Drink 1 L
2 protein-enriched drinks
Solid food

Postoperative day 1
Mobilized >8 hours
Drink >2 L
4 protein-enriched drinks
Solid food
Remove bladder catheter
Plan discharge

Postoperative day 2
Normal activity
Remove epidural catheter
Discharge after lunch

Source: Reprinted with permission from Jakobsen et al.[5]

surgery is based on the idea that there is a large amount of insensible or unmeasurable loss through evaporation and that a substantial amount of fluid is transudated into an area often referred to as the third space. In a recent review, Brandstrup[63] concluded that:

- current standard fluid therapy is not at all evidence-based;
- the evaporative loss from the abdominal cavity is highly overestimated;
- the nonanatomic third space loss is based on flawed methodology and probably does not exist;
- the fluid volume accumulated in traumatized tissue is very small; and
- volume preloading of neuroaxial blockade is not effective and may cause postoperative fluid overload.

Many of the trials reviewed by Brandstrup refer to "restricted" intravenous fluid therapy. In a randomized controlled study, Brandstrup et al.[64] used two different fluid regimens in patients undergoing colon surgery. The principal difference was the absence of a preload and lack of replacement for third space loss (Table 29-6). The administered intravenous fluid volume on the day of operation was significantly less in the restricted group [median 2740 mL (range 1100–8050) versus 5388 mL (range 2700–11083); $p < 0.0005$]. The patients receiving less fluid had significantly lower complication rates [28 (33%) versus 44 (51%) in the standard group ($p = 0.013$)]. In another study, patients receiving on average 5.9 L for colon surgery had a longer duration of ileus, more complications after surgery, and longer hospital stays than patients who received about 3.6 L.[65] However, in the largest study (n = 253), there was no difference in wound healing or hospital stay between patients randomized who received approximately 5.7 versus 3.1 L of crystalloid perioperatively.[66] As compared with major abdominal surgery, patients undergoing ambulatory surgery seem to benefit from administration of >1–1.5 L of fluid, compared with patients who receive <1000 mL.[67] In a superb review of the literature to date, Holte and Kehlet[67] concluded that until more outcome studies are performed, care should be taken to avoid fluid overload during major surgery procedures and 1–1.5 L of fluid should be routinely administered to ambulatory surgical patients.

One of the seldom discussed consequences of limited fluid resuscitation is more liberal use of vasopressors. In general, direct-acting agents, such as phenylephrine, are preferred over indirect-acting agents in the elderly based on the idea that adrenergic tone is increased at baseline so that there are smaller vasoactive stores in the nerve endings. There is much variation found in clinical practice, so an initial trial of ephedrine is warranted. Continuous support with infusion therapy is performed in an

TABLE 29-6. Intraoperative fluid therapy.

	Restricted regimen	Standard regimen
Preloading of epidural analgesia	No preloading	500 mL HAES 6%*
Third space loss	No replacement	Normal saline 0.9%; 7 mL/kg/h first hour; 5 mL/kg/h second and third hour; 3 mL/kg/h following hours
Loss during fast (maintenance)	500 mL of glucose 5% in water, less oral fluid intake during fast	500 mL of normal saline 0.9% independent of oral intake
Blood loss	Volume-to-volume with HAES 6% with allowance for maximun 500 mL extra.	Loss up to 500 mL: 1000–1500 mL of normal saline; loss >500 mL, additional HAES 6%
	Blood-component therapy started at approximate loss >1500 mL dependent on hematocrit	Blood-component therapy started at approximate loss >1500 mL dependent on hematocrit

*Hydroxyethyl starch 6% in normal saline.
Reprinted with permission from Brandstrup B, Tonnesen H, Beier-Holgersen R, Hjortso E, Ording H, Lindorff-Larsen K, Rasmussen MS, Lanng C, Wallin L, Iversen LH, Gramkow CS, Okholm M, Blemmer T, Svendsen PE, Rottensten HH, Thage B, Riis J, Jeppesen IS, Teilum D, Christensen AM, Graungaard B, Pott F. Effects of intravenous fluid restriction on postoperative complications: comparison of two perioperative fluid regimens: a randomized assessor-blinded multicenter trial. Ann Surg. 2003 November; 238(5): 641–648.

identical manner to younger patients with the dosage titrated to an effect rather than a specific dose.

Emergence and Extubation of the Elderly

The elderly may be particularly prone to the effects of inadequate reversal of muscle relaxation.[68] In elderly patients who are overly narcotized, hypoventilation may lead to respiratory acidosis that potentiates the effects of residual neuromuscular blockade in the recovery room, further increasing the rate of postoperative pulmonary complications.[69] There is little published guidance on making decisions regarding extubation of elderly patients after anesthesia. From clinical experience, emergence can sometimes be prolonged without obvious reason, and return of active upper airway reflexes can also be delayed. There are no data to suggest that standard extubation criteria should not be required in the elderly.

Postoperative Care

The postoperative care of the elderly abdominal surgery patient has been best described by Kehlet and colleagues. (See discussion of multimodal approach above and Table 29-5.) Apart from those efforts and geriatric programs that incorporate specific geriatric assessments, postoperative care for the elderly follows the same plans used for younger patients. Pain management can be more demanding in the elderly because the therapeutic ratio of the narcotic analgesics seems narrowed. Nonetheless, pain control is no less important for the elderly. (See Chapter 21.)

Postoperative Complications

Elderly patients have higher levels of complications than younger patients.[70] The impact of illness on the elderly is greater, such that the number of complications associated with disease is considerably higher in elderly patients with underlying disease. There are also a number of complications that are both more common in the elderly and associated with poor outcomes. These are highlighted here so that they are clearly in mind as the practitioner develops a perioperative care plan for a patient. Delirium and postoperative cognitive dysfunction are mentioned but are explored in greater detail elsewhere in this book. (See Chapter 9.) Postoperative ileus is treated somewhat more in depth. Finally, a predilection for pneumonia represents the most common complication of elderly surgical patients.

Postoperative Ileus

Ileus is the temporary absence of propulsive bowel function. Two forms of postoperative ileus can be distinguished: (1) an uncomplicated form that occurs after most abdominal surgery, particularly open abdominal surgery, and spontaneously resolves in 2 or 3 days, and (2) a paralytic form that lasts more than 3 days and generally prolongs hospital stay.

The list of potential etiologies for postoperative ileus is large. Contributory mechanisms may include alterations of autonomic nervous function, gastrointestinal hormones, inflammatory mediators, and the direct action of anesthetic agents. Although many factors have been implicated, no single mechanism or final common pathway has been identified.[71]

Traditional treatment for ileus has been based on nasogastric decompression and bowel rest. Unfortunately, these regimens have not been found to hasten the return of bowel function and seem to increase hospital stays and prolong recovery.[71] Interesting novel approaches to preventing or decreasing the duration of ileus include the use of nonsteroidal antiinflammatory agents, such as ketorolac.[72] The most promising therapeutic approach on the horizon is alvimopan, a selective, competitive mu-opioid receptor antagonist with limited oral bioavailability that may be used to reduce length of postoperative ileus. A recent meta-analysis of five trials including 2195 patients concluded that alvimopan was effective in restoring gastrointestinal function and reduced time to discharge after major abdominal surgery, with acceptable side effects.[73] The use of a midthoracic (T6–T8) epidural catheter with local anesthetic for pain relief is effective; however, lower thoracic and lumbar catheters are not effective in altering the duration of ileus.[71,74] In recent years, patients are being fed earlier, and the traditional marker of waiting for first flatus is no longer considered a reasonable endpoint.[71] Early small feedings are most appropriate.

Pneumonia

Concomitant pneumonia and influenza constitute the leading infectious cause of death in the elderly and the fourth most common cause of death overall. The presence of concomitant illness and delays in diagnosis contribute to significant mortality from this disease in the elderly. Senescence of the immune system seems less important in predisposition to pneumonia than the presence of concomitant illness. Mortality is generally higher in older than in younger patients, although outcome in pneumonia depends primarily on the presence of underlying illness and the causative organism.[75] Delay in diagnosis is frequently secondary to the atypical presentations of pneumonia in the elderly. The typical symptoms of sputum production, fever, chills, and rigors may be absent in the elderly; confusion may be the only presenting symptom. Tachypnea is frequent; however, this vital sign is poorly recorded in many facilities and is not sufficiently sensitive in making a diagnosis. Leukocytosis is common, but by no means specific. Chest roentgenograms frequently show incomplete consolidation, and the findings are difficult to distinguish from other diseases of the elderly, such as congestive heart failure, atelectasis, pulmonary embolism, and malignancy. Therefore, clinical diagnosis requires a high index of suspicion despite atypical clinical manifestations. In a recent review for the American College of Physicians, Lawrence et al.[76] concluded that few interventions have been shown to clearly or even possibly reduce postoperative pneumonia, noting that the quality of the evidence regarding the prevention of pneumonia in general was only fair. Thus, prevention of pneumonia in elderly patients remains a key, yet elusive goal in improving perioperative care.

Conclusion

The elderly patient presenting for abdominal surgery represents a challenge to the anesthesia practitioner. Patients may be sicker than one would presume from their clinical presentation. Given the likelihood of diminished reserve capacity in one or more organ systems, aggressive management to prevent organ dysfunction is in order. Fluid resuscitation remains a controversial issue, and determining appropriate endpoints for fluid administration is clinically challenging. In the absence of major preexisting disease, elderly patients should tolerate surgery and anesthesia and recover well if complications can be avoided. Certain postoperative complications, particularly central nervous system, gastrointestinal, and pulmonary complications, are most common in the elderly, are particularly troublesome, and their likelihood is possibly reducible by techniques that can be used in the perioperative period. Clinicians can hope to see additional data published in the next few years that should help to further fine-tune the perioperative approach to the elderly abdominal surgical patient.

References

1. Parker LJ, Vukov LF, Wollan PC. Emergency department evaluation of geriatric patients with acute cholecystitis. Acad Emerg Med 1997;4:51–55.
2. Hilton D, Iman N, Burke GJ, et al. Absence of abdominal pain in older persons with endoscopic ulcers: a prospective study. Am J Gastroenterol 2001;96:380–384.
3. Lyon C, Clark DC. Diagnosis of acute abdominal pain in older patients. Am Fam Physician 2006;74:1537–1544.
4. Lawrence VA, Hazuda HP, Cornell JE, et al. Functional independence after major abdominal surgery in the elderly. J Am Coll Surg 2004;199:762–772.
5. Jakobsen DH, Sonne E, Andreasen J, Kehlet H. Convalescence after colonic surgery with fast-track vs conventional care. Colorectal Dis 2006;8:683–687.
6. Denney JL, Denson JS. Risk of surgery in patients over 90. Geriatrics 1972;27:115–118.
7. Djokovic JL, Hedley-Whyte J. Prediction of outcome of surgery and anesthesia in patients over 80. JAMA 1979;242: 2301–2306.
8. Lawrence VA, Hilsenbeck SG, Mulrow CD, Dhanda R, Sapp J, Page CP. Incidence and hospital stay for cardiac and pulmonary complications after abdominal surgery. J Gen Intern Med 1995;10:671–678.
9. Hosking MP, Warner MA, Lobdell CM, Offord KP, Melton LJ III. Outcomes of surgery in patients 90 years of age and older. JAMA 1989;261:1909–1915.
10. Leung JM, Dzankic S. Relative importance of preoperative health status versus intraoperative factors in predicting postoperative adverse outcomes in geriatric surgical patients. J Am Geriatr Soc 2001;49:1080–1085.
11. Ewanchuk M, Brindley PG. Perioperative do-not-resuscitate orders—doing 'nothing' when 'something' can be done. Crit Care 2006;10:219.
12. Palmer RM. Geriatric assessment. Med Clin North Am 1999;83:1503–1523, vii–viii.
13. Fried LP, Tangen CM, Walston J, et al. Frailty in older adults: evidence for a phenotype. J Gerontol A Biol Sci Med Sci 2001;56:M146–M156.
14. Fried LP, Hadley EC, Walston JD, et al. From bedside to bench: research agenda for frailty. Sci Aging Knowledge Environ 2005;2005:e24.
15. Phillip B, Pastor D, Bellows W, Leung JM. The prevalence of preoperative diastolic filling abnormalities in geriatric surgical patients. Anesth Analg 2003;97:1214–1221.
16. Zaugg M, Lucchinetti E. Respiratory function in the elderly. Anesthesiol Clin North Am 2000;18:47–58, vi.
17. Cerveri I, Zoia MC, Fanfulla F, Spagnolatti L, Berrayah L, Grassi M, Tinelli C. Reference values of arterial oxygen tension in the middle-aged and elderly. Am J Respir Crit Care Med 1995;152:934–941.
18. Marik PE, Kaplan D. Aspiration pneumonia and dysphagia in the elderly. Chest 2003;124:328–336.
19. Malmrose LC, Gray SL, Pieper CF, et al. Measured versus estimated creatinine clearance in a high-functioning elderly sample: MacArthur Foundation Study of Successful Aging. J Am Geriatr Soc 1993;41:715–721.
20. Heyland DK, Cook DJ, King D, Kernerman P, Brun-Buisson C. Maximizing oxygen delivery in critically ill patients: a methodologic appraisal of the evidence. Crit Care Med 1996;24:517–524.
21. Boyd O. Optimisation of oxygenation and tissue perfusion in surgical patients. Intensive Crit Care Nurs 2003;19: 171–181.
22. Kern JW, Shoemaker WC. Meta-analysis of hemodynamic optimization in high-risk patients. Crit Care Med 2002;30: 1686–1692.
23. Wexner SD, Beck DE, Baron TH, et al. A consensus document on bowel preparation before colonoscopy: prepared by a Task Force from the American Society of Colon and Rectal Surgeons (ASCRS), the American Society for Gastrointestinal Endoscopy (ASGE), and the Society of American Gastrointestinal and Endoscopic Surgeons (SAGES). Surg Endosc 2006;20:1161.
24. Seinela L, Pehkonen E, Laasanen T, Ahvenainen J. Bowel preparation for colonoscopy in very old patients: a randomized prospective trial comparing oral sodium phosphate and

polyethylene glycol electrolyte lavage solution. Scand J Gastroenterol 2003;38:216–220.

25. Muller-Stich BP, Choudhry A, Vetter G, et al. Preoperative bowel preparation: surgical standard or past? Dig Surg 2006;23:375–380.

26. Inouye SK, Bogardus ST Jr, Baker DI, Leo-Summers L, Cooney LM Jr. The Hospital Elder Life Program: a model of care to prevent cognitive and functional decline in older hospitalized patients. Hospital Elder Life Program. J Am Geriatr Soc 2000;48:1697–1706.

27. Marcantonio ER, Flacker JM, Wright RJ, Resnick NM. Reducing delirium after hip fracture: a randomized trial. J Am Geriatr Soc 2001;49:516–522.

28. Bradley EH, Webster TR, Schlesinger M, Baker D, Inouye SK. Patterns of diffusion of evidence-based clinical programmes: a case study of the Hospital Elder Life Program. Qual Saf Health Care 2006;15:334–338.

29. Inouye SK, Baker DI, Fugal P, Bradley EH. Dissemination of the Hospital Elder Life Program: implementation, adaptation, and successes. J Am Geriatr Soc 2006;54: 1492–1499.

30. Landefeld CS. Improving health care for older persons. Ann Intern Med 2003;139:421–424.

31. Sandham JD, Hull RD, Brant RF, et al. A randomized, controlled trial of the use of pulmonary-artery catheters in high-risk surgical patients. N Engl J Med 2003;348:5–14.

32. Wheeler AP, Bernard GR, Thompson BT, et al. Pulmonary-artery versus central venous catheter to guide treatment of acute lung injury. N Engl J Med 2006;354:2213–2224.

33. Brown CV, Shoemaker WC, Wo CC, Chan L, Demetriades D. Is noninvasive hemodynamic monitoring appropriate for the elderly critically injured patient? J Trauma 2005;58: 102–107.

34. Renna M, Venturi R. Bispectral index and anaesthesia in the elderly. Minerva Anestesiol 2000;66:398–402.

35. Michelson JD, Lotke PA, Steinberg ME. Urinary-bladder management after total joint-replacement surgery. N Engl J Med 1988;319:321–326.

36. Skelly JM, Guyatt GH, Kalbfleisch R, Singer J, Winter L. Management of urinary retention after surgical repair of hip fracture. CMAJ 1992;146:1185–1189.

37. Stephan F, Sax H, Wachsmuth M, Hoffmeyer P, Clergue F, Pittet D. Reduction of urinary tract infection and antibiotic use after surgery: a controlled, prospective, before-after intervention study. Clin Infect Dis 2006;42:1544–1551.

38. Martin JT. Positioning aged patients. Anesthesiol Clin North Am 2000;18:105–121.

39. Roy RC. Choosing general versus regional anesthesia for the elderly. Anesthesiol Clin North Am 2000;18:91–104.

40. Kehlet H. Future perspectives and research initiatives in fast-track surgery. Langenbecks Arch Surg 2006;391:495–498.

41. Jayr C, Thomas H, Rey A, Farhat F, Lasser P, Bourgain JL. Postoperative pulmonary complications. Epidural analgesia using bupivacaine and opioids versus parenteral opioids. Anesthesiology 1993;78:666–676.

42. Norris EJ, Beattie C, Perler BA, et al. Double-masked randomized trial comparing alternate combinations of intraoperative anesthesia and postoperative analgesia in abdominal aortic surgery. Anesthesiology 2001;95:1054–1067.

43. Wu CL, Hsu W, Richman JM, Raja SN. Postoperative cognitive function as an outcome of regional anesthesia and analgesia. Reg Anesth Pain Med 2004;29:257–268.

44. Bryson GL, Wyand A. Evidence-based clinical update: general anesthesia and the risk of delirium and postoperative cognitive dysfunction. Can J Anaesth 2006;53:669–677.

45. Basse L, Jakobsen DH, Bardram L, et al. Functional recovery after open versus laparoscopic colonic resection: a randomized, blinded study. Ann Surg 2005;241:416–423.

46. Kehlet H, Kennedy RH. Laparoscopic colonic surgery—mission accomplished or work in progress? Colorectal Dis 2006;8:514–517.

47. Reeder MK, Goldman MD, Loh L, et al. Postoperative hypoxaemia after major abdominal vascular surgery. Br J Anaesth 1992;68:23–26.

48. Arunasalam K, Davenport HT, Painter S, Jones JG. Ventilatory response to morphine in young and old subjects. Anaesthesia 1983;38:529–533.

49. Valentine SJ, Marjot R, Monk CR. Preoxygenation in the elderly: a comparison of the four-maximal-breath and three-minute techniques. Anesth Analg 1990;71:516–519.

50. Pontoppidan H, Beecher HK. Progressive loss of protective reflexes in the airway with the advance of age. JAMA 2006; 174:2209–2213.

51. Brimacombe JR, Berry AM. Cricoid pressure. Can J Anaesth 1997;44:414–425.

52. Butler J, Sen A. Best evidence topic report. Cricoid pressure in emergency rapid sequence induction. Emerg Med J 2005; 22:815–816.

53. Iannuzzi E, Iannuzzi M, Viola G, Cerulli A, Cirillo V, Chiefari M. Desflurane and sevoflurane in elderly patients during general anesthesia: a double blind comparison. Minerva Anestesiol 2005;71:147–155.

54. Iannuzzi E, Iannuzzi M, Cirillo V, Viola G, Parisi R, Chiefari M. Small doses of remifentanil and alfentanil in continuous total intravenous anesthesia in major abdominal surgery. A double blind comparison. Minerva Anestesiol 2003;69: 127–136.

55. Heavner JE, Kaye AD, Lin BK, King T. Recovery of elderly patients from two or more hours of desflurane or sevoflurane anaesthesia. Br J Anaesth 2003;91:502–506.

56. Kehlet H. Fast-track colonic surgery: status and perspectives. Recent Results Cancer Res 2005;165:8–13.

57. Gunnarsson L, Tokics L, Brismar B, Hedenstierna G. Influence of age on circulation and arterial blood gases in man. Acta Anaesthesiol Scand 1996;40:237–243.

58. Hedenstierna G, Rothen HU. Atelectasis formation during anesthesia: causes and measures to prevent it. J Clin Monit Comput 2000;16:329–335.

59. Rothen HU, Sporre B, Engberg G, Wegenius G, Hedenstierna G. Reexpansion of atelectasis during general anaesthesia may have a prolonged effect. Acta Anaesthesiol Scand 1995;39:118–125.

60. Lachmann B. Open up the lung and keep the lung open. Intensive Care Med 1992;18:319–321.

61. Epstein CD, Peerless JR. Weaning readiness and fluid balance in older critically ill surgical patients. Am J Crit Care 2006;15:54–64.

62. Itobi E, Stroud M, Elia M. Impact of oedema on recovery after major abdominal surgery and potential value of

multifrequency bioimpedance measurements. Br J Surg 2006;93:354–361.

63. Brandstrup B. Fluid therapy for the surgical patient. Best Pract Res Clin Anaesthesiol 2006;20:265–283.

64. Brandstrup B, Tonnesen H, Beier-Holgersen R, et al. Effects of intravenous fluid restriction on postoperative complications: comparison of two perioperative fluid regimens: a randomized assessor-blinded multicenter trial. Ann Surg 2003;238:641–648.

65. Nisanevich V, Felsenstein I, Almogy G, Weissman C, Einav S, Matot I. Effect of intraoperative fluid management on outcome after intraabdominal surgery. Anesthesiology 2005; 103:25–32.

66. Kabon B, Akca O, Taguchi A, et al. Supplemental intravenous crystalloid administration does not reduce the risk of surgical wound infection. Anesth Analg 2005;101: 1546–1553.

67. Holte K, Kehlet H. Fluid therapy and surgical outcomes in elective surgery: a need for reassessment in fast-track surgery. J Am Coll Surg 2006;202:971–989.

68. Berg H, Roed J, Viby-Mogensen J, et al. Residual neuromuscular block is a risk factor for postoperative pulmonary complications. A prospective, randomised, and blinded study of postoperative pulmonary complications after atracurium, vecuronium and pancuronium. Acta Anaesthesiol Scand 1997;41:1095–1103.

69. Debaene B, Plaud B, Dilly MP, Donati F. Residual paralysis in the PACU after a single intubating dose of nondepolarizing muscle relaxant with an intermediate duration of action. Anesthesiology 2003;98:1042–1048.

70. Tiret L, Desmonts JM, Hatton F, Vourch G. Complications associated with anaesthesia—a prospective survey in France. Can Anaesth Soc J 1986;33:336–344.

71. Mattei P, Rombeau JL. Review of the pathophysiology and management of postoperative ileus. World J Surg 2006;30: 1382–1391.

72. Kelley MC, Hocking MP, Marchand SD, Sninsky CA. Ketorolac prevents postoperative small intestinal ileus in rats. Am J Surg 1993;165:107–111.

73. Tan EK, Cornish J, Darzi AW, Tekkis PP. Meta-analysis: alvimopan vs. placebo in the treatment of post-operative ileus. Aliment Pharmacol Ther 2007;25(1):47–57.

74. Delaney CP. Clinical perspective on postoperative ileus and the effect of opiates. Neurogastroenterol Motil 2004;16 (Suppl 2):61–66.

75. Fein AM. Pneumonia in the elderly: special diagnostic and therapeutic considerations. Med Clin North Am 1994;78: 1015–1034.

76. Lawrence VA, Cornell JE, Smetana GW. Strategies to reduce postoperative pulmonary complications after noncardiothoracic surgery: systematic review for the American College of Physicians. Ann Intern Med 2006;144:596–608.

Index

Printed in the United States of America.